AF478456

SARCOIDOSIS AND OTHER GRANULOMATOUS DISEASES OF THE LUNG

LUNG BIOLOGY IN HEALTH AND DISEASE

Executive Editor: **Claude Lenfant**

Director, National Heart, Lung, and Blood Institute
National Institutes of Health
Bethesda, Maryland

Volume 14   PULMONARY VASCULAR DISEASES,
edited by Kenneth M. Moser

Volume 15   PHYSIOLOGY AND PHARMACOLOGY OF THE AIRWAYS,
edited by Jay A. Nadel

Volume 16   DIAGNOSTIC TECHNIQUES IN PULMONARY DISEASE (in two parts),
edited by Marvin A. Sackner

Volume 17   REGULATION OF BREATHING (in two parts),
edited by Thomas F. Hornbein

Volume 18   OCCUPATIONAL LUNG DISEASES:
RESEARCH APPROACHES AND METHODS,
edited by Hans Weill and Margaret Turner-Warwick

Volume 19   IMMUNOPHARMACOLOGY OF THE LUNG,
edited by Harold H. Newball

Volume 20   SARCOIDOSIS AND OTHER GRANULOMATOUS
DISEASES OF THE LUNG,
edited by Barry L. Fanburg

Other volumes in preparation

SARCOIDOSIS AND OTHER GRANULOMATOUS DISEASES OF THE LUNG

Edited by

Barry L. Fanburg

New England Medical Center Hospital
Tufts University School of Medicine
Boston, Massachusetts

MARCEL DEKKER, INC.   New York • Basel

Library of Congress Cataloging in Publication Data
Main entry under title:

Sarcoidosis and other granulomatous diseases of the lung.

   (Lung biology in health and disease; v. 20)
   Includes bibliographies and indexes.
   1. Sarcoidosis. 2. Granuloma. 3. Lungs–Diseases.
I. Fanburg, Barry L. [DNLM: 1. Lung diseases.
2. Granulomatous disease, Chronic. 3. Sarcoidosis.
W1 LU62 v.20 / WF 600 S2435]
RC756.L83 vol. 20 616.2'4s [616.2'4] 82-23584
[RC182.S14]
ISBN 0-8247-1866-6

Marcel Dekker, Inc.
270 Madison Avenue, New York, New York 10016

Current printing (last digit):
10 9 8 7 6 5 4 3 2 1

Printed in the United States of America

CONTRIBUTORS

Dov L. Boros, Ph.D. Professor, Department of Immunology and Microbiology, Wayne State University School of Medicine, Detroit, Michigan

Solon R. Cole, M.D. Associate Pathologist and Director of Electron Microscopy, Department of Pathology, Hartford Hospital, and Assistant Professor of Pathology, University of Connecticut Health Center, Hartford, Connecticut

Ronald G. Crystal, M.D. Chief, Pulmonary Branch, Department of Health and Human Services, National Heart, Lung, and Blood Institute, National Institutes of Health, Bethesda, Maryland

Ronald P. Daniele, M.D. Associate Professor, Departments of Medicine and Pathology, University of Pennsylvania School of Medicine, Philadelphia, Pennsylvania

James H. Dauber, M.D.* Assistant Professor, Department of Medicine, University of Pennsylvania School of Medicine, Philadelphia, Pennsylvania

Barry L. Fanburg, M.D. Chief, Pulmonary Division, and Professor, Department of Medicine, New England Medical Center Hospital, Tufts University School of Medicine, Boston, Massachusetts

Jonathan E. Gottlieb, M.D. Fellow, Division of Clinical Decision Making, Department of Medicine, New England Medical Center Hospital, Tufts University School of Medicine, Boston, Massachusetts

---

Present Affiliation

*Associate Professor, Department of Medicine, University of Pittsburgh, and Chief of Pulmonary Service, VA Medical Center, Pittsburgh, Pennsylvania

Gary W. Hunninghake, M.D.* Senior Investigator, Pulmonary Branch, National Heart, Lung, and Blood Institute, National Institutes of Health, Bethesda, Maryland

Harold L. Israel, A.B., M.D., M.P.H. Professor Emeritus, Department of Medicine, Jefferson Medical College, Thomas Jefferson University, Philadelphia, Pennsylvania

D. Geraint James, M.D., M.A.M.D. (Cantab), F.R.C.P. (Lond.), LL.D. (Hon) Dean and Senior Physician, Royal Northern Hospital, and Physician, Ophthalmic Department, St. Thomas' Hospital, London, England; Adjunct Professor of Medicine and Epidemiology, University of Miami School of Medicine, Miami, Florida

Kent J. Johnson, M.D. Assistant Professor, Department of Pathology, The University of Michigan, Ann Arbor, Michigan

Sol Katz, M.D. Professor of Medicine (Pulmonary), Georgetown University School of Medicine; Professorial Lecturer in Medicine, George Washington University School of Medicine, Washington, D.C.

Homayoun Kazemi, M.D. Professor of Medicine, Harvard Medical School; Chief, Pulmonary Unit, and Physician, Massachusetts General Hospital, Boston, Massachusetts

Brendan A. Keogh, M.D. Senior Investigator, Department of Health and Human Services, National Heart, Lung, and Blood Institute, National Institutes of Health, Bethesda, Maryland

Marvin Lesser, M.D. Chief, Pulmonary Department, Bronx Veterans Administration Hospital, Bronx, New York, and Assistant Professor, Department of Medicine, Mount Sinai School of Medicine, New York, New York

Bruce R. Line, M.D.† Attending Physician, Department of Nuclear Medicine, Clinical Center, National Institutes of Health, Bethesda, Maryland

Donald N. Mitchell, M.D., M.R.C.P. Member, Clinical Scientific Staff, MRC Tuberculosis and Chest Diseases Unit; Honorary Consultant Physician, Brompton Hospital and Central Middlesex Hospital; Honorary Senior Lecturer, Cardiothoracic Institute, London, England

---

Present Affiliation

*Director, Pulmonary Disease Division, Department of Internal Medicine, University of Iowa Hospitals and Clinics, Iowa City, Iowa

†Professor of Radiology, Director of Nuclear Medicine, Department of Radiology, Albany Medical Center Hospital, Albany, New York

Stephen G. Pauker, M.D. Chief, Division of Clinical Decision Making, and Associate Professor, Department of Medicine, New England Medical Center Hospital, Tufts University School of Medicine, Boston, Massachusetts

Charles E. Putman, M.D. Professor and Chairman, Department of Radiology, Duke University Medical Center, Durham, North Carolina

R. J. W. Rees, C.M.G., M.R.C.S., L.R.C.P., M.B., F.R.C. Path.* Medical Research Council, Laboratory for Leprosy and Mycobacterial Research, National Institute for Medical Research, The Ridgeway, Mill Hill, London, England

Ross E. Rocklin, M.D. Chief, Allergy Division, Department of Medicine, New England Medical Center, Tufts University School of Medicine, Boston, Massachusetts

Bruce A. Rodan, M.D.† Associate, Department of Radiology, Duke University Medical Center, Durham, North Carolina

Edward C. Rosenow, III, M.D. Professor, Department of Internal Medicine, Division of Thoracic Diseases, Mayo Graduate School of Medicine, Mayo Clinic, Rochester, Minnesota

Milton D. Rossman, M.D. Assistant Professor, Department of Medicine, University of Pennsylvania School of Medicine, Philadelphia, Pennsylvania

Nancy L. Sprince, M.D., M.P.H. Co-Director, Occupational Medicine Clinic, Pulmonary Unit, Massachusetts General Hospital, Boston, Massachusetts

Alvin S. Teirstein, M.D. Professor, Department of Medicine, and Director, Pulmonary Division, The Mount Sinai Medical Center, New York, New York

K. Krishnan Unni, M.B. Associate Professor, Department of Surgical Pathology, Mayo Graduate School of Medicine, Mayo Clinic, Rochester, Minnesota

Peter A. Ward, M.D. Professor and Chairman, Department of Pathology, The University of Michigan, Ann Arbor, Michigan

M. Henry Williams, Jr., M.D. Professor of Medicine and Director, Pulmonary Division, Albert Einstein College of Medicine, Bronx, New York

---

Present Affiliation

*Visiting Worker, Division of Communicable Diseases, Clinical Research Centre, Harrow, Middlesex, England

†Staff Radiologist, Department of Radiology, Palm Beach–Martin County Medical Center, Jupiter, Florida

FOREWORD

Most of us who are asked to name how the great advances in modern
medicine and surgery have come about, would probably respond by listing
some Nobel laureates and the discoveries closely linked with their names:
for example, Roentgen and X-rays; Koch and the tubercle bacillus; Fleming
and penicillin; Enders and culture of polio virus; Banting and insulin. Yet,
once in awhile, an event that is ineligible for a Nobel Prize has had just as
important an impact on medical advance as one that was eligible and won
an award. One such event was Abraham Flexner's 1910 report "Medical
Education in the United States and Canada" that resulted in a considerable
decrease in the number of American medical schools and a considerable
increase in their quality and in the scientific content of their curricula.
Another was the opening of the Johns Hopkins Medical School in 1893,
staffed by four professors, each outstanding as a scientist in his specialty
and each believing in joining scientific research, medical education, and
patient care.

Sometimes a book or a series of books has had a strong influence on
the advance of medical science. One such book was the first edition of
Osler's *Medicine* (1892) because Osler's emphasis on how little physicians
knew for sure led John Rockefeller's adviser on philanthropy to recommend the building of the great Institute for Medical Research, which
opened in 1904 and for decades was the foremost institution for research
in basic medical sciences in the United States. Another was the first
(1941) edition of Goodman and Gilman's *Pharmacological Basis for
Medical Practice* that revolutionized teaching and research on the action
and use of drugs; as one professor of pharmacology stated in 1941, no
professional pharmacologist could from then on teach at a lower level
than that of the superb text used by his students!

In the field of respiration and the lungs, there are some classic
monographs and a comprehensive *Handbook of Physiology* that have

heightened the interest of scientists, students, and physicians in this subject and stimulated them to enter pulmonary research. One can safely predict that this new series of monographs, "Lung Biology in Health and Disease," will have an even greater impact on young (and older) researchers because it is the first truly comprehensive, monumental work in this field. It does not deal just with cellular processes or just with clinical problems but with the entire spectrum of basic sciences and of lung function, metabolic functions, and respiratory defense mechanisms. The series will also include volumes that apply modern biological knowledge to elucidate mechanisms of pulmonary and respiratory disorders (immunologic, infectious, and genetic disorders, physiology and pharmacology of airways, genesis and resolution of pulmonary edema, and abnormalities of respiratory regulation). Other volumes will deal with the biology of specific pulmonary diseases (e.g., cancer, chronic obstructive pulmonary disease, disorders of the pulmonary circulation, and abnormalities associated with occupational and environmental factors) and with early detection and specific diagnosis.

This series shows the lung as a challenging organ, with many problems calling for innovative research. If it attracts some imaginative, creative, and perceptive young scientists to attack these difficult problems, the tremendous effort in writing, editing, and publishing these volumes will be well worth-while. The volumes cannot win the Nobel Prize, but someone may who was challenged by them.

Julius H. Comroe, Jr.
San Francisco, California

PREFACE

The spectrum of granulomatous diseases of the lung is large and varies from those produced by identifiable causes, which include infectious agents (e.g., tuberculosis, schistosomiasis, fungi) and foreign materials (e.g., talc, lipid aspirates, beryllium, organic substances), to those where no etiological agent is currently known (e.g., sarcoidosis, Wegener's and "allergic" granulomatoses). Infections and the granulomatoses have been discussed previously in other volumes of this series and will be addressed only briefly here. Some attention will be given to the diseases associated with pulmonary granulomas produced by foreign materials such as noted in Chapter 19 (Beryllium Disease) and Chapter 20 (Drug-Induced Pulmonary Granulomas). However, the primary granulomatous disease discussed in this book is sarcoidosis, a fascinating, albeit enigmatic entity that, over the years, has produced a voluminous number of studies and publications, but no explanation of its etiology, and uncertainties regarding its diagnosis and therapy remain.

Early approaches to sarcoidosis were descriptive, and although not always identified or easily distinguished from other diseases, its usual modes of clinical presentation are generally recognized and agreed on. Dr. Sol Katz relates his many years of experience with the clinical presentation and natural history of sarcoidosis in Chapter 1. Similarly, although varied, radiological and physiological accompaniments of sarcoidosis have been generally identified, as noted in Chapters 2 and 3. Epidemiological and genetic factors of sarcoidosis have been studied extensively, but there are limitations associated with these sorts of studies. These limitations and available data are discussed in Chapters 4 and 5.

Although considerable comfort may be taken at times in the diagnosis of sarcoidosis by its clinical presentation, many physicians demand a more rigorous identification of this disease with the exclusion of other diseases with which it may be confused. Biopsy material is often useful in this respect and various approaches to and specificity of biopsy are discussed in Chapters 13 and 14. There has been a never-ending search for other methods of diagnosis, less invasive than biopsy. These methods include the Kveim reaction, available for many years and quite dramatic in its response, but limited by the lack of standardization of the test substance. The test is controversial and not available in all centers. It will be discussed in Chapter 11.

More recently other tests, such as the measurement of serum angiotensin 1-converting enzyme, examination of bronchoalveolar lavage material, and gallium lung scans have been used for both diagnosing and following the course of sarcoidosis. These tests are discussed in Chapters 9, 10, and 12. Since diagnosis and therapy are imperfect in this disease, the physician is often confronted with the need to make a decision about the management of these patients. Decision analysis provides a formalized and systematic approach for doing so, and the basic tenets of this approach plus their applications in the diagnosis and therapy of sarcoidosis will be discussed in Chapter 15.

It is currently recognized that there is an immunologic disorder associated with sarcoidosis. Whether this disorder is primary or secondary is not known. Nevertheless, a wide assortment of immunologic techniques are being applied to better define the disorder and its possible relationship to the eventual development of fibrosis. Our knowledge of the cellular and immunologic abnormalities of sarcoidosis, along with some background of basic immunology, is discussed in Chapters 7 and 8. The cellular immunologic alterations in the lung, as reflected in bronchial lavage, are discussed in Chapters 9 and 12. The chapter on pathology of sarcoidosis and other granulomas (Chapter 6) compares histological changes of sarcoidosis with those of other pulmonary granulomas and relates them to immunologic alterations.

There is currently no known spontaneous animal model of sarcoidosis. To bridge this deficiency in our knowledge, we must use information from other experimental granulomatous models developed in animals. Dr. Boros addresses these considerations in Chapter 18.

Finally, despite many investigations now in progress, it is clearly recognized that no etiological agent has yet been defined for sarcoidosis. If one were known, diagnosis and management of patients with this disease might change considerably. Such an agent, if discovered, may differ from currently known infectious organisms. Dr. Mitchell and Dr. Rees discuss our current meager knowledge of possible transmissible agents in sarcoidosis in Chapter 17. A better understanding of the pathogenesis of sarcoidosis is badly needed and awaits future innovative investigation. Perhaps a reader of this book will provide it.

Barry L. Fanburg

INTRODUCTION

Ever since sarcoidosis was described by Boeck in 1899, numerous investigators and clinicians have attempted to uncover the elusive cause(s) and pathogenesis of the disease. Unlike many other pathological entities, this one has attracted the attention and interest of experts in many internal medicine subspecialties and in several scientific disciplines. Yet, as of today, sarcoidosis remains as mysterious as it was at the turn of the century.

However, the extraordinary advances that we have witnessed during the last ten to fifteen years in morphology, ultrastructure, cell biology, and immunology, as well as in other disciplines, have truly paved the way to new and promising avenues of research. That sarcoidosis may one day be "eradicated" is of course at present unforeseeable, but that the disease will be understood and treatable has become a reasonable expectation.

Clinicians and scientists interested in sarcoidosis and other granulomatous lung diseases are working diligently and producing much new information. Throughout the world these individuals are many and they meet regularly to discuss their progress. The proceedings of their meetings are usually a reflection of past advances rather than a look into the future.

This volume, edited by Barry L. Fanburg, offers a prospective that has been lacking. When the series of monographs "Lung Biology in Health and Disease" was planned, it was anticipated that it would include eighteen volumes; the last of these was published in early 1981. Thus, in addition to being a springboard into the future, this volume is also the first of a second generation of monographs.

It is a personal pleasure to acknowledge Dr. Fanburg's efforts in planning this volume and in assembling such a distinguished list of authors. Undoubtedly this contribution will epitomize the new approaches to sarcoidosis and other granulomatosis lung diseases.

Claude Lenfant, M.D.
Bethesda, Maryland

CONTENTS

SARCOIDOSIS AND OTHER GRANULOMATOUS DISEASES OF THE LUNG

Part One

CLINICAL, RADIOLOGICAL, AND PHYSIOLOGICAL ASPECTS OF SARCOIDOSIS

1

Clinical Presentation and Natural History
of Sarcoidosis

SOL KATZ

Georgetown University School of Medicine
Washington, D.C.

I. General

Since diseases in which the etiology is unknown, such as a sarcoidosis,
cannot be simply defined, they must be described. A Subcommittee on
Classification and Definition of the Seventh International Conference on
Sarcoidosis (1976) adopted the following description:

> Sarcoidosis is a multisystem granulomatous disorder of unknown
> etiology, most commonly affecting young adults and presenting
> most frequently with bilateral hilar lymphadenopathy, pulmonary
> infiltration, and skin or eye lesions. The diagnosis is established
> most securely when clinicoradiographic findings are supported by
> histological evidence of widespread noncaseating epitheloid-cell
> granulomas in more than one organ or a positive Kveim-Siltzbach
> skin test. Immunological features are depression of delayed-type
> hypersensitivity suggesting impaired cell-mediated immunity and
> raised or abnormal immunoglobulins. There may also be hyper-
> calciuria, with or without hypercalcemia. The course and
> prognosis may correlate with the mode of onset: An acute onset
> with erythema nodosum heralds a self-limiting course and

"

spontaneous resolution, whereas an insidious onset may be
followed by relentless, progressive fibrosis. Corticosteroids
relieve symptoms and suppress inflammation and granuloma
formation.

A clinical diagnosis of sarcoidosis implies that widespread characteristic
granulomas are known or thought to be present in several organs. When
patients present with clinical manifestations related to only one organ, the
presence of additional clinical, radiological, or laboratory evidence supported
by immunological features allows the inference of the existence of a
generalized granulomatous disorder. Although establishment of multiple
organ involvement requires proof by biopsy, this is rarely required or
justified. However, it is necessary to exclude diseases which may mimic
sarcoidosis clinically, radiographically, and histologically. This exclusion
must be based on thorough testing and examinations to limit the possibility
of diagnostic error.

Although the clinical manifestations of sarcoidosis may be absent or
confined to a single organ, it is a generalized disease that may involve
almost any organ in the body in various combinations, thereby giving rise
to many clinical syndromes. The diverse presentations of sarcoidosis
embrace all branches of medicine. Therefore, this fascinating and exciting
disease should be of interest to all physicians.

Individuals with sarcoidosis may be asymptomatic or may present
with constitutional manifestations and pulmonary or extrapulmonary
complaints. The frequency of the modes of presentation and organ
involvement varies with the speciality interest of the physician. It is
apparent that dermatologic abnormalities occur in all patients observed by
dermatologists, and ocular aberrations are noted in most patients referred
to ophthalmologists. Variability in mode of onset is also influenced by
the country of origin as well as by the routine use of chest roentgenography. Further confusion with regard to the distribution of organ
involvement in sarcoidosis results from the failure to distinguish among
histological changes, clinical findings, and alterations in function. For
example, splenic and hepatic involvement as determined by enlargement
of these organs is low, whereas needle biopsy reveals a strikingly high
frequency of pathology (Klatskin 1976, Selroos 1976).

The onset of sarcoidosis, as can be best judged, is most commonly
between 20 and 40 years of age. However, it has been noted in children,
particularly between 9 and 15, and in some studies a significant number of
patients were over 40 years of age at presentation (James et al. 1969,
James et al. 1976, Selroos, 1969). There is no sex predominance although
in a few studies slightly more women are affected. In the United States
the majority of patients are black, with a black to white incidence of

10–20 to 1. Approximately 20–40% of patients are symptom-free and their disease is discovered by routine chest radiography. Males are more often asymptomatic than females.

Involvement of an organ may be great without clinical manifestations. Anatomical presence of disease without clinical dysfunction is one of the most important hallmarks of sarcoidosis. Symptoms are caused by mechanical interference with function so that if there is sufficient involvement or strategic location of the granulomas, there may be a clinical expression of the disease. Therefore, specific symptoms are related to the extent of organ involvement. Constitutional symptoms such as fever, fatigue, malaise, anorexia, and weight loss are usually absent or mild. However, in some patients with certain sarcoidal syndromes, constitutional symptoms may be striking. Perhaps 20–30% of patients with sarcoidosis have symptoms of a systemic nature. In some series these are more often noted in black patients.

The time of onset of sarcoidosis is difficult to assess unless an acute event such as erythema nodosum or acute iridocyclitis reflects the beginning of the process. Respiratory symptoms such as cough, dyspnea, chest pain, and nasal complaints may also announce the clinical onset. These symptoms are noted at the onset in 30–50% of most studies. Although the first awareness of sarcoidosis may be an abnormal routine chest roentgenogram, this finding does not necessarily reflect the time of onset unless it can be determined from serial radiographs. In less than 10% of patients other extrathoracic features such as skin lesions, peripheral lymphadenopathy, parotid enlargement, central nervous system symptoms, cardiac syndromes, liver involvement, splenic enlargement, and endocrine syndromes of arthralgia may reflect the onset of this protean disease.

II. Intrathoracic Sarcoidosis

Although the precise pathogenesis of sarcoidosis is not known, clinical evidence suggests that the lung is the first site of involvement. The process extends through the lymphatics to the hilar and mediastinal nodes. It is further speculated that, as in miliary tuberculosis, lymphohematogenous dissemination may then occur throughout the lung as well as other favored organs. Radiographically apparent mediastinal and hilar lymph node involvement occurs in about 90% of patients with sarcoidosis. By international agreement sarcoidosis is divided into several stages.

In stage 0 the chest roentgenogram is normal and only extrapulmonary disease is apparent. It is likely that, at least in some patients, mediastinoscopy and lung biopsy would reveal evidence of involvement. About 5–10% of patients with sarcoidosis have a normal chest roentgenogram at the time of initial presentation (James et al. 1976). This stage may reflect a late phase of sarcoidosis in which the intrathoracic manifestations originally present have cleared, leaving only the extrathoracic lesions. Others have suggested that isolated extrapulmonary sarcoidosis has a different pathogenesis. Thus, a normal chest roentgenogram may accompany sarcoidosis causing chronic ocular involvement, hepatosplenomegaly, nephrocalcinosis or hypercalcemia.

Stage I sarcoidosis is characterized by bilateral symmetrical hilar lymph node enlargement with or without paratracheal lymphadenopathy. This is the earliest clinically detectable form of sarcoidosis and the most common mode of presentation, being noted in about 40–60% of patients. Although the lung fields are roentgenographically clear, there is anatomical involvement of the lung parenchyma by granuloma formation in over half of these individuals as detected by transbronchial biopsy of the lung and pulmonary function testing. The right paratracheal nodes, especially the inferior group, or azygos nodes are enlarged along with the hilar nodes in about half of those with stage I disease.

Typically, but not invariably, in sarcoidosis the right hilar nodes are separated from the right heart border. However, in neoplastic hilar lymphadenopathy the nodal density frequently blends with the density of the right heart border. At times the hilar or paratracheal lymphadenopathy is predominately unilateral. In this event it is more often right-sided. Rarely, the mediastinum is compactly and irregularly stuffed with lymph nodes with little or no hilar lymph node enlargement. This last pattern resembles lymphoma. True anterior mediastinal retrosternal nodes are very infrequently encountered.

Patients with stage I sarcoidosis have minimal symptoms or are asymptomatic unless there is associated erythema nodosum. They may have a cough, which at times is distressing, or mild unimpressive substernal discomfort. About 10% of those with stage I disease have clinically apparent extrathoracic manifestations such as involvement of the eyes, lacrimal glands, salivary glands, skin, or central nervous system. They commonly (about 75%) have noncaseating granulomas on liver or scalene node biopsy. As a matter of fact, when a patient presents with such extrathoracic manifestations in the presence of bilateral symmetrical hilar lymphadenopathy, the diagnostic possibility of sarcoidosis should be immediately suspected. Not infrequently in stage I sarcoidosis with extrathoracic manifestations the hilar adenopathy has been present for years, thereby indicating the chronicity of both the thoracic and extrathoracic processes.

In 60–80% of those with stage I sarcoidosis the disease clears spontaneously in 1–2 years (Sharma 1975). In the presence of erythema nodosum the prognosis is especially good. About 10–20% will continue to have enlarged lymph nodes beyond 2 years and some of these patients will develop extrathoracic disease. The remainder, representing about 10–15% will remain unchanged or slowly develop pulmonary opacities usually within 2 years but occasionally as long as 5 years later.

Stage II sarcoidosis, pulmonary opacities associated with hilar lymphadenopathy, is noted at presentation in 25–35% of patients. The pulmonary infiltrations have a variable appearance on chest x-ray. They may be localized and unilateral, but more often they are diffuse and symmetrical. Fine or, less frequently, coarse reticular radiations appear to extend into the lung fields from the enlarged hilar nodes. The middle lung zones and perihilar areas show the most marked changes. Quite frequently as the parenchymal changes develop, there is regression of the lymph node enlargement. Diffuse disseminated miliary or isolated miliary lesions are seen. As these miliary patterns develop, the hilar lymph nodes may not regress in contrast to lymph node behavior in the presence of the linear-reticular parenchymal foci. The nodulations may be coarse and sharply circumscribed, or fluffy, ill-defined cotton-wool patches called alveolar sarcoidosis may develop. Combinations of patterns are also noted.

Patients with stage II sarcoidosis, especially those with miliary nodulations, are often asymptomatic or mildly symptomatic. They may have low-grade fever, cough, malaise, modest weight loss, or tachypnea. When pulmonary involvement is extensive, significant dyspnea may be present. However, stage II sarcoidosis often displays a striking disparity between the paucity of signs and symptoms and the extensive roentgenographic changes. In about one-half to two-thirds of patients with stage II sarcoidosis, roentgenographic resolution occurs. Irreversible pulmonary fibrosis occurs in about 15–20%, while the rest will show persistent infiltrates without fibrosis, symptoms, or signs.

Healed hilar and mediastinal nodes may undergo calcification in less than 5% of patients. Occasionally, there may be egg shell calcification. The lung parenchymal lesions practically never calcify.

Roentgenographic clearing of intrathoracic lymph nodes with persistence or progression of the pulmonary infiltrates characterizes stage III sarcoidosis. It must be appreciated that staging is arbitrary and based on radiological evaluation using routine posterior-anterior and lateral views. Even in disease classified as stage III, lymphadenopathy may be detected using computed tomography, gallium scanning, and mediastinoscopy. This stage is observed at presentation in approximately 5–15% of patients. The character of the pulmonary lesions is variable, but there is a distinct tendency toward fibrosis as the process ages. The changes are usually bilateral and less marked in the apices and bases. There are generalized or localized linear or nodular opacifications. The foci may progressively enlarge and become confluent. Frequently the nodulations are quite symmetrical.

Dense fibrosis with upward retraction of the hilar areas occurs as well as honeycombing and bulla formation, pulmonary hypertension, and right ventricular failure. Aspergillomas due to colonization by aspergilli in the emphysematous cavities may develop (Winterbauer and Kraemer 1976). Spontaneous pneumothorax is another complication in this group of patients (Sharma 1977). For those with diffuse progressive fibrosis, some physicians have used the designations stage IV, stage IIIb, or late stage III.

Cough and dyspnea are common complaints in the late stage of disease. The cough is usually dry, but there may be sputum production and rarely there may be hemoptysis. In the presence of the latter complaint aspergillomas should be sought. Extrathoracic sarcoidosis, which may include chronic skin and ocular lesions and occasionally bone cysts, accompanies stage III more often than stages I and II sarcoidosis. In fact, chronic skin lesions, chronic ocular manifestations, or bone cysts are indicators of pulmonary chronicity suggesting that the lung lesions are unlikely to resolve.

Transition from stage I to stage II to stage III is the usual course in progressive sarcoidosis. However, the reverse from stage III to stage II to stage I is not encountered. When mediastinal lymphadenopathy appears after stage III sarcoidosis another etiology for the lymph node enlargement should be considered.

III. Upper Respiratory Tract

Sarcoidosis of the upper respiratory tract may be present and asymptomatic so that the frequency of involvement can be assessed only by careful examination in all patients with systematic sarcoidosis. This has been done in several studies yielding a frequency of 5–20% (DiBenedetto and Lefrak 1970, Neville et al. 1976). Nasal mucosal lesions are the most frequent site of upper airways involvement. The mucosa may appear erythematous and granular. White-yellow papules with adhesions may be noted. A granulomatous polypoid mass involving the septum and turbinates can occur. Epistaxis, nasal stuffiness, crusting, and nasal discharge are seen. Ulcerations, septal perforation, as well as sarcoidosis of the nasal sinuses and osteolytic lesions of the nasal bones and cartilage with saddle nose deformity have been described (Allen 1978).

The incidence of laryngeal lesions is less than 1% of patients with sarcoidosis (Vico and Larsen 1979). Hoarseness is almost universally present. With laryngeal airway obstruction there is dyspnea, wheezing, and stridor. At laryngoscopy there may be thickening of the epiglottis, a granulomatous mass, and infiltrative and nodular lesions extending into the aryepiglottic folds, epiglottis, and false cords. True vocal cord lesions are rarely seen. Nasal sarcoidosis not infrequently accompanies laryngeal sarcoidosis.

Upper respiratory sarcoidosis is associated with lupus pernio about 50% of the time and these patients often have fibrotic pulmonary disease and other chronic extrathoracic findings of sarcoidosis.

IV. Endobronchial Sarcoidosis

With the increased use of fiberoptic bronchoscopy for transbronchial biopsy in sarcoidosis and simultaneously obtaining tissue by random bronchial biopsy, it is apparent that endobronchial sarcoidosis is present not infrequently even in asymptomatic individuals (Mitchell et al. 1980). The bronchial mucosa may appear normal or may show plaques or stenosis. Main stem, lobar, segmental, or subsegmental bronchi may be involved. Single or multiple sites may reveal pathology. The chest roentgenogram may be normal or show stage I, II, or III sarcoidosis with or without atelectasis and obstructive pneumonitis. Multiple segmental bronchial obstruction may result in the erroneous diagnosis of asthma. A bronchial tumor with atelectasis can be simulated. The frequency of bronchial sarcoidosis has been variously reported from 30 to 100% of patients with the greatest number of cases noted in stage III sarcoidosis.

Airways obstruction in sarcoidosis may occasionally be caused by extrabronchial compression from lymph nodes or loss of peribronchial support around small airways from pulmonary sarcoidosis.

V. Pleura

In the past pleural involvement due to sarcoidosis has been considered either not to occur or to be very rare. It would be more accurate to state that pleural effusion and clinical manifestations due to pleural involvement are unusual, but that histological changes due to sarcoidosis are encountered in 1–5% of patients (Beekman et al. 1976).

Pleural sarcoidosis cannot be established by roentgenographic findings. The diagnosis must be made by the demonstration of noncaseating granulomas of the pleura in a patient with sarcoidosis. Although pleural sarcoidosis has been reported in 73 cases in the world's literature since 1947, only 37 have been confirmed by histological involvement of the pleura and 20 of these had pleural effusion. In the presence of pleural involvement in a patient with sarcoidosis, concomitant diseases such as tuberculosis, fungal diseases, cancer, and congestive heart failure must be excluded.

In the 16 patients with established pleural effusion due to sarcoidosis in whom the pleural fluid was studied, the fluid was usually exudative with a lymphocyte predominance (Beekman et al. 1976). Bloody fluid has also been noted (Chusid and Siltzbach 1974, DeVuyst et al. 1979). Stage II and stage III sarcoidosis accompany the pleural process and extrathoracic findings are common. Because of the rarity of pleural sarcoidosis the diagnosis should not be assumed merely because of the presence of sarcoidosis elsewhere. Rather, the diagnosis should be pursued by pleural biopsy if examination of the fluid does not yield another diagnosis. If despite this evaluation there is no histological confirmation, it should be considered that the patient has sarcoidosis and an unexplained cause of pleural effusion.

The granulomas are present on either the visceral or parietal pleura or both. They form beneath the mesothelial surface and bulge into the pleural cavity.

VI. Extrathoracic Sarcoidosis

If stage I sarcoidosis is considered to announce the onset of sarcoidosis, then all areas of involvement, both intrapulmonary and extrapulmonary, usually appear within 2 years of the beginning of the disease. Approximately 10% of patients develop new manifestations after the first 2 years. It must be emphasized, however, that although new sites of involvement are unusual, the chronic (more than 2 years) granulomatous stage of sarcoidosis often persists for many years during which time the clinical manifestations may be severe and the pathological findings of fibrosis relentlessly progressive, compromising function of the associated organs.

Widespread involvement of many organs with few or mild constitutional features characterizes sarcoidosis. The clinical expressions are diverse. Some patients have extrathoracic manifestations as the major findings with or without abnormal chest roentgenograms.

VII. Skin

Skin involvement in sarcoidosis (Figs. 1–9) may be transient or chronic. Erythema nodosum is the most common dermatologic form of sarcoidosis. It occurs more frequently in Europe than in North America (Lofgren and Stanvenow 1961, Sones and Israel 1960). In the United States most studies give an incidence of less than 5% (Israel and Sones 1953). Scandinavian series, especially from Sweden, have noted erythema nodosum in as many as 67% of females compared to about 25% in other parts of Europe (Lofgren 1953). Irish female immigrants in London and Puerto Rican females in New York also have a high incidence of erythema nodosum

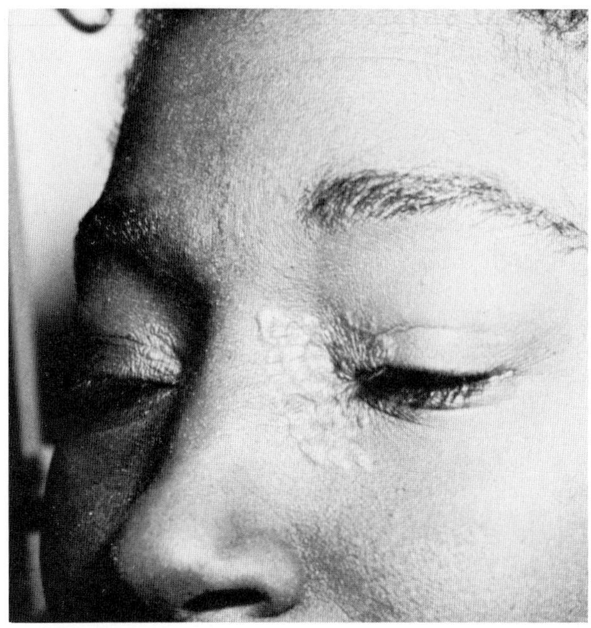

Figure 1 Silvery scaly papular lesions around the eyes were associated with chronic fibrosing sarcoidosis.

(Siltzbach 1967). The condition is encountered in women more often than in men at a ratio of 4:1 or greater. The ratio of erythema nodosum in females is highest in the age group 20–29. Caucasians show erythema nodosum much more often than blacks.

In all series of erythema nodosum over 90% of patients have stage I sarcoidosis and the remainder have stage II disease. In about 70% of patients polyarthralgia occurs within 2 weeks before or after the onset of the skin lesions. There may be accompanying fever, malaise, and fatigue. The constitutional, joint, and skin manifestations subside in 1–20 weeks with an average of 3 weeks. The prognosis for resolution of the intrathoracic manifestations is excellent with spontaneous resolution within 1–2 years.

It is a striking clinical phenomenon that stage I sarcoidosis is usually quite asymptomatic despite the presence of granulomas in intrathoracic lymph nodes and often in lung, liver, muscle, bone marrow, and other sites. Yet, with erythema nodosum there is a dramatic onset of stage I disease with systemic manifestations, as though the susceptible subject has

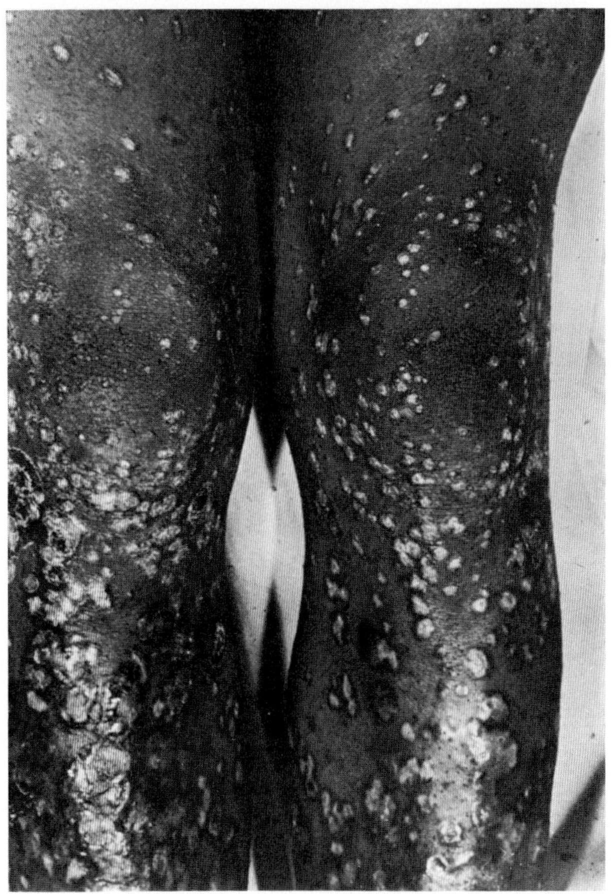

Figure 2 Extensive flat scaly lesions of sarcoidosis on the lower extremities.

been attacked by a sensitizing agent, albeit unidentified, which has pro-voked a generalized epithelioid granulomatous reaction.

Excluding erythema nodosum, granulomatous skin lesions have been reported in varying frequencies depending on the source of the patients. They are noted in 10–30% of patients and are observed especially fre-quently in American blacks (Scadding 1967). Skin lesions in general are much more frequent in women. Maculopapular lesions can be found in subacute sarcoidosis. They are found especially on the face near the eyelids and around the eyes and nares but may be found on the trunk and extremities. They are associated with stage I or stage II sarcoidosis.

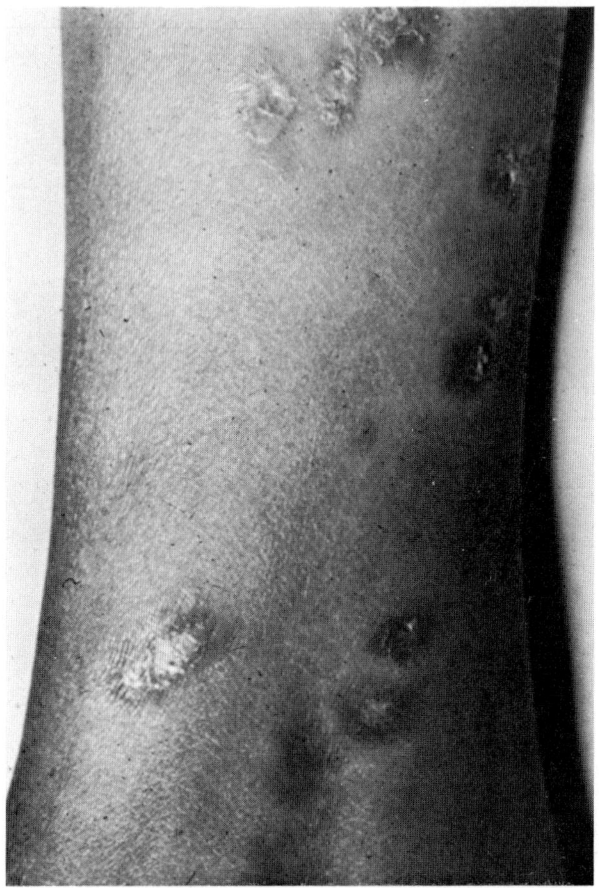

Figure 3 Chronic papular skin lesions in various phases of healing are characterized by scaling and pigmentation.

Lupus pernio is the most characteristic of all the cutaneous granulomas in sarcoidosis. Bluish-purple thickened elevations occur on the nose, cheeks, ear lobes, digits, lips, and knees. The changes are persistent and often disfiguring. The affected areas are swollen with a shining surface. Venectasia is seen especially over the red bulbous nasal tip and over the fingers. There may be scaly desquamation and even very small superficial erosions. The bulbous fingers and toes reflect phalangeal bone changes with multiple lacy rarefactions. Lupus pernio of the nose is usually associated with nasal mucosal changes and at times with nasal bone destruction.

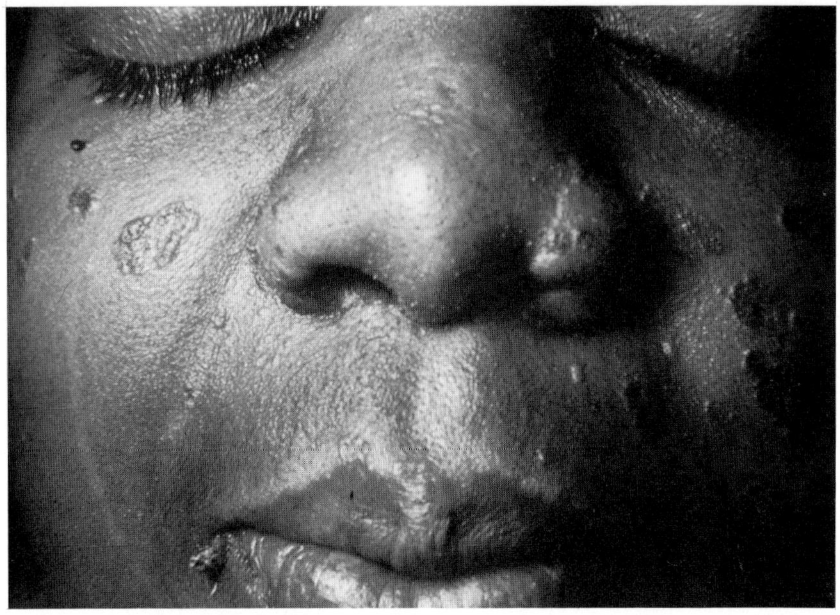

Figure 4 Some of the papular and nodular lesions on the face have pitted centers. On the right cheek there is coalescence into annular formation with central atrophy.

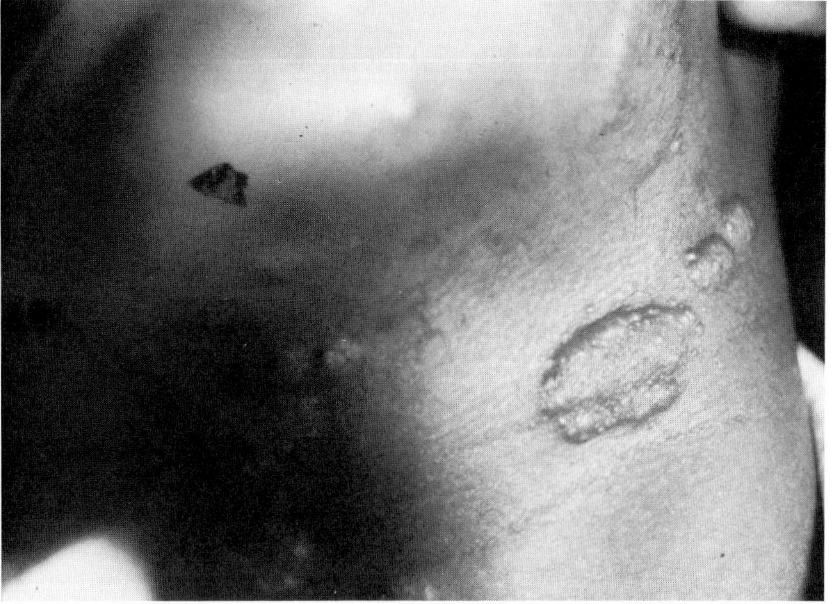

Figure 5 Indurated elevated reddish-purple plaques of lupus pernio on the neck.

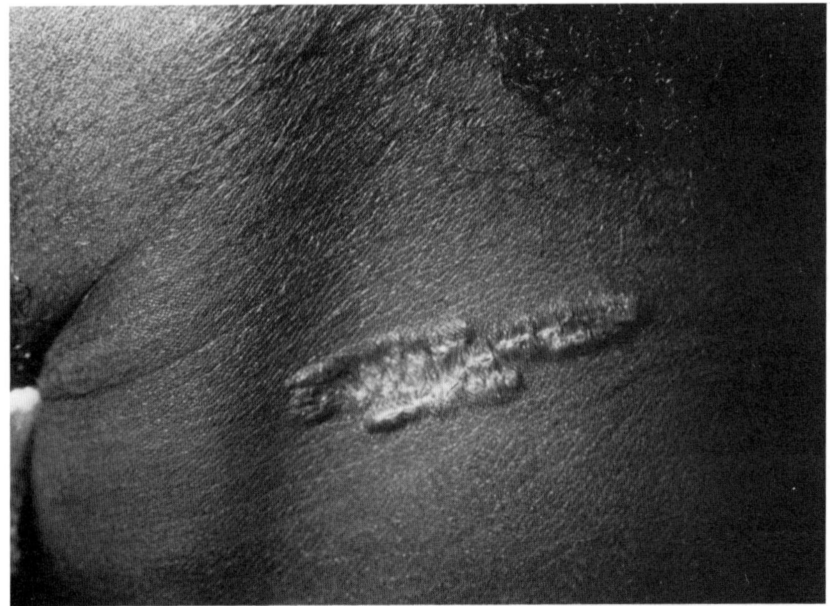

Figure 6 Raised lobulated indurated nodules at the hairline.

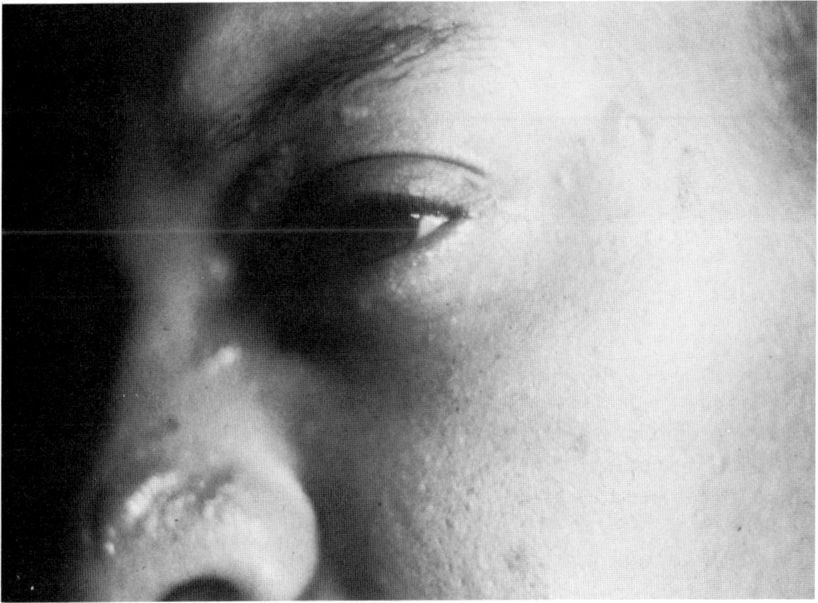

Figure 7 Nodules about the eyes and nose. The red bulbous nasal lesion progressed to distort the nostrils. Nasal mucosal lesions of sarcoidosis were also present.

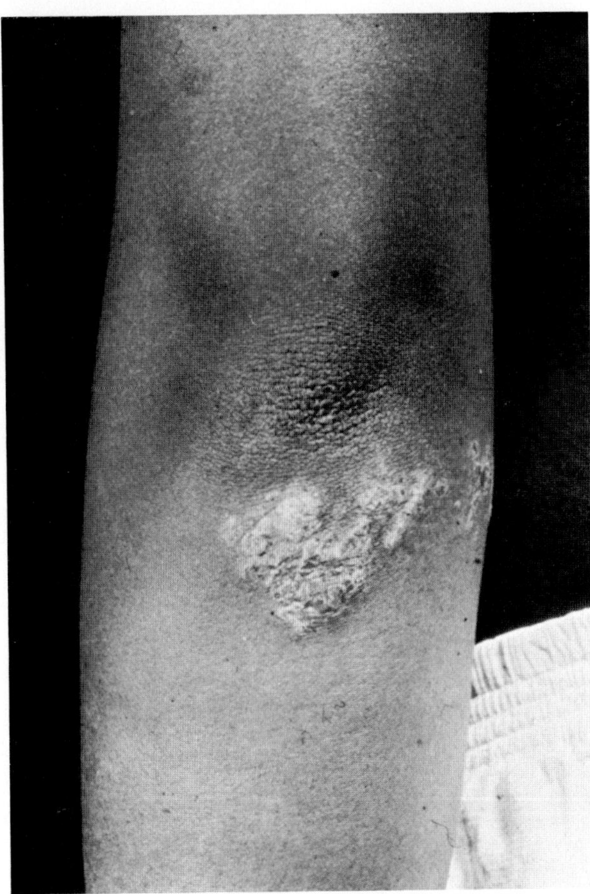

Figure 8 Psoriasiform cutaneous plaques on the elbow.

The nails are dystrophic, thick, and distorted when the terminal phalanges
are involved. Lupus pernio is also associated with other features of
chronic sarcoidosis such as progressive fibrosis of the lungs, chronic
uveitis, and nephrocalcinosis.

Skin plaques are indolent, violaceous, persistent, and slightly raised
especially at the edges. The plaque is annular and flat except for a
slightly elevated rim which is a little darker and scaly. The center is
paler and atrophic. The face and extremities are the usual sites of involvement. Often lesions on the limbs are symmetrical. When the scalp is
involved along with the forehead there are atrophic changes and scarring

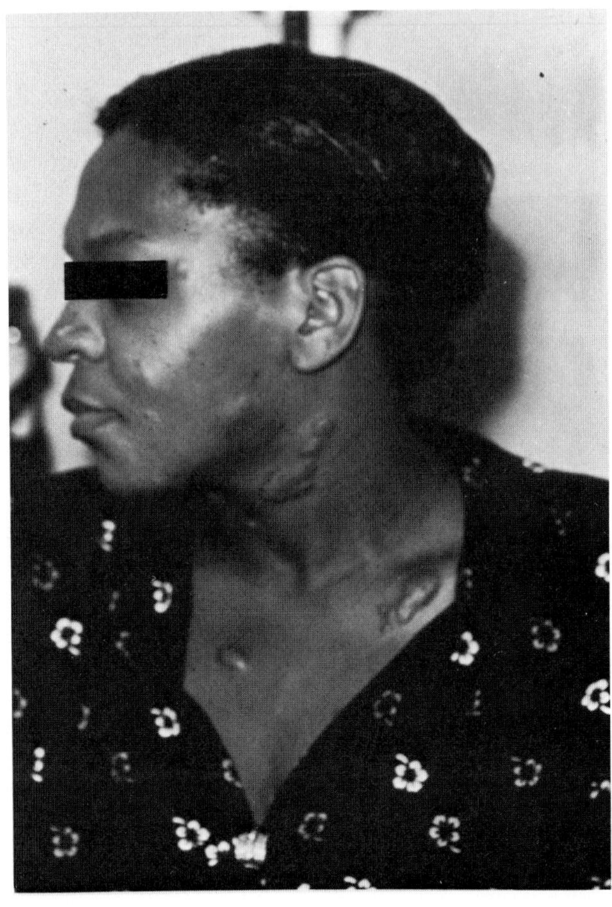

Figure 9 Old acneform keloids have been reactivated due to sarcoidosis.

alopecia. As in lupus pernio, the chronicity of the skin changes is reflected in the persistence and progression of pulmonary and extrapulmonary lesions, including, in particular, lymphadenopathy and splenomegaly.

Nodular lesions greater than 1 cm are elevated above the surrounding skin and are somewhat indurated; they seem to extend to the subcutaneous tissue. The infiltrations are round or oval and pink or reddish early, and as healing ensues they become purplish, then brown with superficial scaling. The skin lesions may appear at different phases of development and resolution and occur most frequently on the face, limbs, and trunk. As with lupus pernio and plaques, the larger nodular lesions tend to persist and are associated with pulmonary fibrosis. The smaller nodular lesions (less than 1 cm) develop earlier in the development of lung changes and tend to resolve, as do the lung changes.

Transformation of old or new cutaneous scars into active granulomas may occur as an interesting cutaneous phenomenon in sarcoidosis. Healed and inactive for years, scars may become edematous and purplish at the time of onset of the disease process and may become normal flat scars as the lung lesions resolve. Surgical, vaccination, and traumatic scars, acne scars and keloids are all subject to these changes. This form of cutaneous sarcoidosis is found equally in men and women.

Subcutaneous nodules arise deep in the dermis and subcutaneous tissue especially on the trunk and extremities. There may be associated erythema nodosum and stage I sarcoidosis, and the subcutaneous nodules in these cases will clear. In other patients the subcutaneous nodules are chronic and indolent. They are palpable only at the onset and later become larger and visible. Ultimately, they infiltrate the skin and appear as nodular sarcoidosis of the skin. These chronic subcutaneous nodules and skin nodules are known as Darier-Roussy sarcoidosis (Maloney and Combes 1936).

Psoriasiform cutaneous sarcoidosis is a violaceous or brownish plaque cutaneous lesion found only in blacks. The lichenified, heavy scaly lesion is found on the trunk and extremities. When nodules or plaques of sarcoidosis of the skin are covered with dilated superficial capillaries, the term angiolupoid sarcoidosis has been used. Generalized erythroderma due to extensive infiltration of the skin by sarcoidosis has been called erythro-dermic sarcoidosis. Although the skin appears deeply infiltrated, there is erythema without visual or tactile evidence of deep infiltration. These patients usually also have other more classical varieties of cutaneous sarcoidosis.

VIII. Bone

The incidence of bone involvement in sarcoidosis varies from 1 to 13% depending on the population being studied and the radiological criteria used (James et al. 1976, Mayock et al. 1963). Although figures up to 30% are quoted, most large series accept about 3–5% if stricter criteria are used. Bone changes are more common in chronic cases and are especially common in blacks with chronic skin involvement whose sarcoidosis is more florid and progressive. Thus, one may see sarcoidosis of the skin of the lupus pernio or plaque type without bone changes, but in the presence of sarcoidosis of the bone chronic skin lesions are frequently present.

Osteoporosis, cortical thinning, well-defined cysts, and rarefactions of variable size, giving an irregular fine or coarse latticelike reticulated appearance, are described (Neville et al. 1977). There is no periosteal reaction, no sclerosis except during healing, no sinus formation, and the joints are usually not involved except when bone adjacent to a joint is destroyed. Osteoporosis and cortical thinning are due to trophic disturbances secondary to interference with blood supply due to perivascular infiltration of the Haversian systems by sarcoid deposits. Cystic changes are caused by coalescence of contiguous lesions. As destruction continues, there is enlargement of bone lacunae resulting in mottled rarefaction and a lace-work appearance of bone. This lacy, honeycomb, and coarse reticulated pattern is more specific for sarcoidosis.

Bone changes are usually restricted to the phalanges, metacarpals, and metatarsals. The pathology is uneven and the distal ends of the proximal and middle phalanges and the proximal ends of the distal phalanges show radiological findings best. In some cases, particularly those with isolated cysts, the fingers and toes are not distorted and bone changes are found on routine radiography. In the presence of reticulated bone changes the

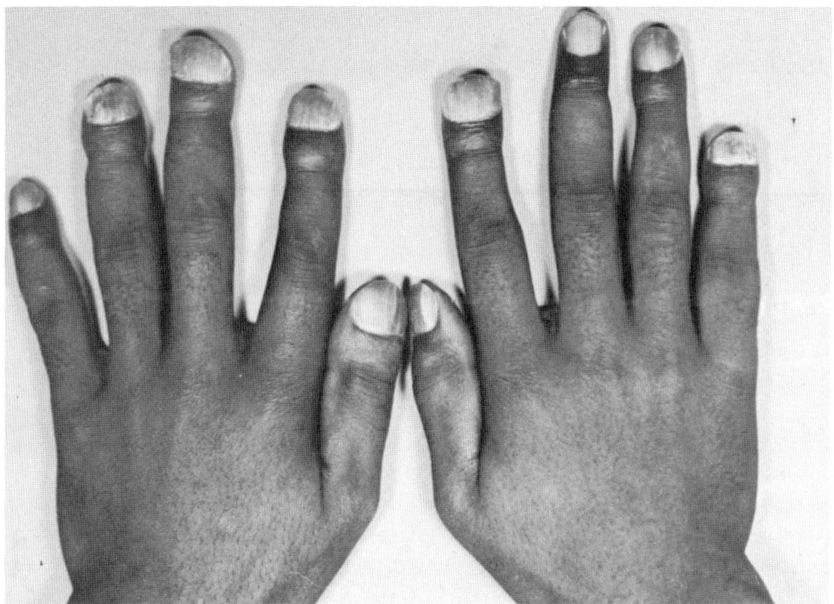

Figure 10 Distorted, deformed, and swollen digits in a patient with extensive bone sarcoidosis. The terminal phalanges are markedly affected as shown by the dystrophic nails which are ridged, thickened, and reveal an abnormal growth pattern.

affected digits are swollen and deformed (Fig. 10). The skin may be shiny and livid, ultimately reaching the complete picture of lupus pernio.

Medullary bone may be infiltrated without roentgenographic change. The carpal and tarsal bones, as well as the distal ends of long bones skull, pelvis, and vertebrae, may rarely be affected. However, the nasal bones are sometimes abnormal in lupus pernio of the nose. Since skeletal sarcoidosis is a feature of chronic sarcoidosis, associated irreversible pulmonary and ocular changes are fairly common. The bony involvement is usually asymptomatic, but there may be pain and tenderness.

IX. Joints

Joint involvement in sarcoidosis takes many forms (Grigor and Hughes 1976, Spilberg et al. 1969). The most common presentation is the arthralgia or arthritis accompanying erythema nodosum. There may be arthralgia associated with hilar adenopathy but without erythema nodosum. The latter occurs more often in men while the arthralgia associated with erythema nodosum is seen more frequently in women. The larger joints such as the ankles, knees, wrists, and elbows are affected. The arthralgia subsides within a few weeks or a few months. Roentgenograms are negative and there are no residual deformities. There are usually no recurrences.

Migratory polyarthralgia or polyarthritis resembling acute rheumatic fever is seen and may be the initial manifestation of sarcoidosis, preceding other features of the disease by months and even years. In the latter circumstance it is difficult to be certain of the relationship to sarcoidosis.

In bone sarcoidosis the articular surfaces contiguous to the involved bone may be invaded. Occasionally, even in the absence of bone involvement, a monoarticular or polyarticular arthritis occurs. Relapses can occur or the joint disease can be chronic and persistent with resulting deformity. Synovial granulomas are often present in the persistent or recurrent forms, and multiple organ involvement by sarcoidosis is present.

In the presence of monoarticular arthritis gout may be erroneously suspected because of the concomitant rise in uric acid seen in some patients with sarcoidosis. However, clinical gout may be seen as an unrelated finding. The combination of sarcoidosis with gout and psoriasis has been noted.

X. Muscle

Sarcoidosis of muscle is rarely apparent clinically. However, random muscle biopsy in early sarcoidosis frequently reveals noncaseating granulomas. Few systematic studies of muscle biopsy in sarcoidosis in the absence of clinical evidence of muscular disease have been performed. However, when this has been done the incidence of granulomas in skeletal muscle in systemic sarcoidosis varies from 50 to 80% with the highest percentage found in those with erythema nodosum and those patients with more organs affected in subacute sarcoidosis (Sharma 1975). Like sarcoidosis of the liver, which is also present frequently and is unaccompanied by symptoms in subacute sarcoidosis, asymptomatic sarcoidosis of muscle resolves completely. In the diagnosis of asymptomatic sarcoidosis of muscle many serial sections of a generous specimen are advised because the granulomas are thinly scattered and may be difficult to find. Although the finding of non-caseating granuloma is not specific for sarcoidosis, its presence in muscle beneath normal skin helps to exclude other conditions associated with granuloma such as tuberculosis, fungal infection, and carcinoma.

Palpable muscle nodules with or without muscle pain and tenderness occur rarely. These are often mistaken for erythema nodosum or sub-cutaneous sarcoidosis. Pathologically, the palpable muscle nodules often reveal both muscle granuloma and subcutaneous granulomas. Another form of symptomatic muscular sarcoidosis is acute myositis which is seen more often in women. There is fever, myalgia, and muscle tenderness especially in the proximal shoulder and pelvic girdle muscles. The myositis may be the first clinical manifestation of sarcoidosis, and electromyographic findings are compatible with nongranulomatous polymyositis.

Chronic myopathy with weakness and muscle wasting, although rare, may be associated with evidence of chronic sarcoidosis elsewhere. The onset is gradual, extending over months or years, with the average age about 50 and a preponderance in postmenopausal women. The muscle enzymes are elevated and electromyography shows myopathic potentials. Some patients appear to have isolated sarcoid myopathy without clinical evidence of sarcoidosis in other systems. These cases really do not represent isolated muscular involvement, for careful evaluation by diagnostic biopsy and other studies often reveals undetected sarcoidosis in the lungs, spleen, lymph nodes, and eyes. Furthermore, at autopsy other evidence of sarcoidosis is disclosed.

XI. Eyes

Ocular changes (Figs. 11–13) occur in about 25% of patients, with the highest incidence recorded among blacks and in those series in which thorough eye examinations, including slit lamp studies performed by an ophthalmologist, have been done (Katz 1976). Although sarcoidosis may affect any portion of the eye, the uveal tract is most often involved. Yet,

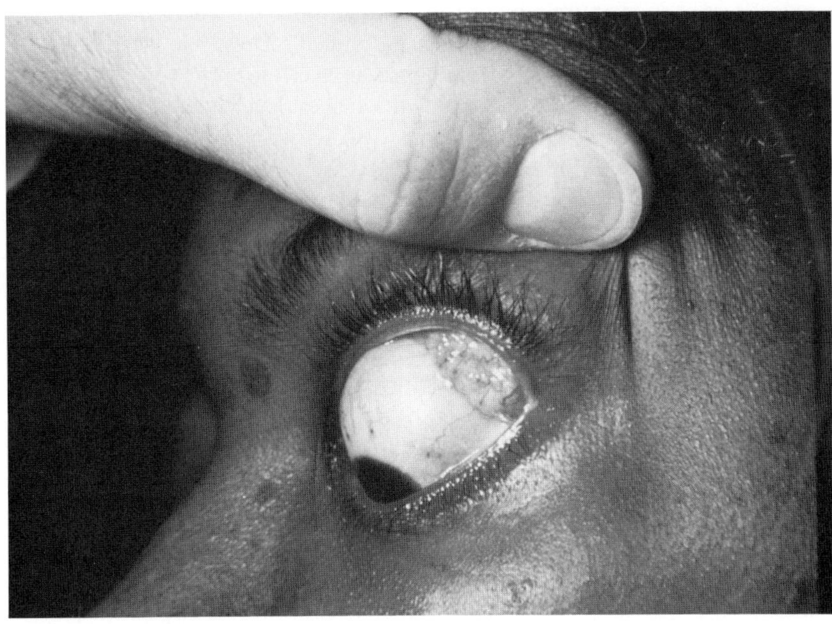

Figure 11 Enlarged lacrimal gland due to sarcoidosis. There are also flat pigmented skin plaques.

among all cases of uveitis in which a diagnosis is established, sarcoidosis comprises only 2–4%. Eye symptoms may be the first manifestation of the disease and appear usually as bilateral subacute or chronic inflammation of the anterior uveal tract with iridocyclitis. Conjunctival involvement is the second most common ocular finding.

Subacute iridocyclitis occurs quite suddenly with little or no pain, mild photophobia, misty vision, and tearing. The eyes are red with circumcorneal ciliary congestion, turbidity of the aqueous humor, pupil irregularity, and fine keratitic precipitates floating in the anterior chamber. Other early manifestations of sarcoidosis occur, including erythema nodosum and other transient skin lesions, bilateral hilar adenopathy, mottled lung densities, and lymphadenopathy. Some patients have transient cranial nerve palsies, subacute meningitis, and salivary gland enlargement. The complete or incomplete syndrome of uveoparotid fever (Heerfordt's syndrome) may be seen with uveitis, parotid enlargement, cranial nerve palsies (especially of the seventh cranial nerve), fever, lassitude, drowsiness, night sweats, arthralgia, anorexia, gastrointestinal symptoms, and pleocytosis of the cerebrospinal fluid. This syndrome is often incomplete, showing only

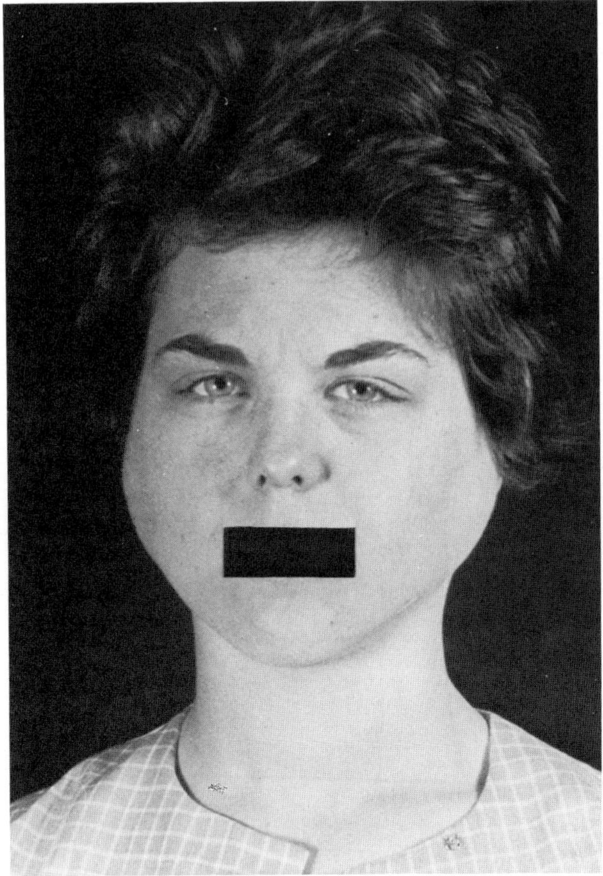

Figure 12 Uveoparotitis and bilateral lacrimal gland enlargement. Blurred vision and dryness of the eyes and mouth were present.

anterior uveitis and parotid enlargement without facial palsy. Subacute iridocylitis not only has a sudden onset but often clears within 6–12 months.

By contrast chronic iridocyclitis develops insidiously and may be persistent because of progressive fibrosis. There is no ciliary congestion, but pain and blurred vision are present. Gray fatty precipitates, picturesquely described as "mutton fat" keratitic precipitates, are present in the anterior chamber and posterior corneal surface. Troublesome chronic complications include posterior synechiae between the iris and lens, iris nodules, cataracts,

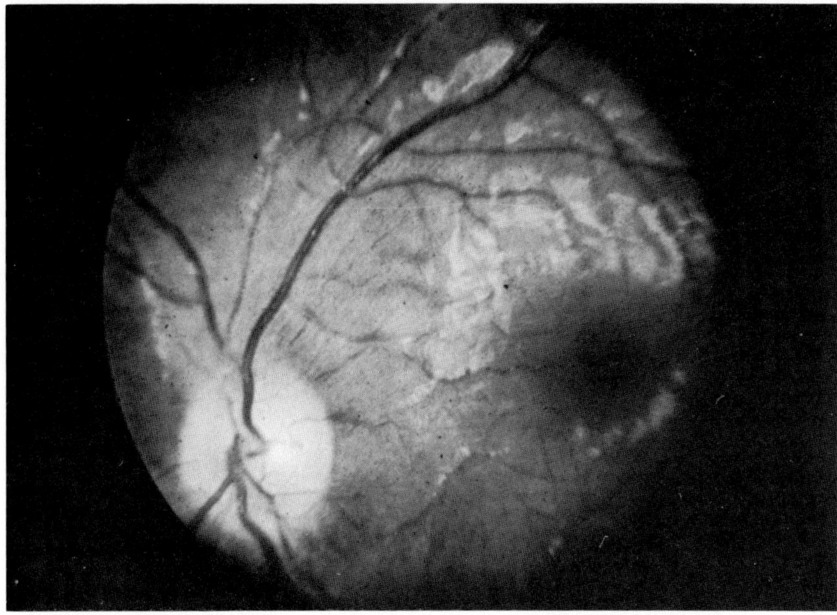

Figure 13 Severe choroidoretinitis associated with visual impairment.

corneal degeneration, and secondary glaucoma. Contrasting with the
transient accompanying clinical findings seen with subacute iridocyclitis,
patients with chronic iridocyclitis have chronic manifestations of sarcoidosis
such as skin plaques, lupus pernio, bone lesions, persistent lymphadenopathy,
splenomegaly, and fibrotic lung changes.

Posterior uveitis (choroidoretinitis) may occur more frequently than is
usually thought because it may be difficult to detect in the presence of
anterior uveitis. Choroiditis, choroidal tubercles, retinal edema, and retinal
degeneration have been noted. Choroidoretinitis causes blurring of vision
with moveable black spots in the field of vision. At times there may be
no symptoms with either subacute or chronic iridocyclitis, and the diagnosis
is established only by thorough ocular examination.

Phlyctenular conjunctivitis, small follicles, or large nodules, may be
seen in the palpebral conjunctiva, bulbar conjunctiva or cul-de-sac. Conjunctival lesions are associated with annoying symptoms of irritation which
cause the patient to seek medical attention.

Other manifestations of sarcoidosis are keratoconjunctivitis and peri-
phlebitis retinae with retinal hemorrhages and retinitis proliferans. The
lacrimal glands may be enlarged and painless but there may be keratocon-

junctivitis sicca with or without gland enlargement, causing dryness of the eyes and mouth resembling Sjögren's disease. Even in the absence of dry eyes a decrease in lacrimal secretion can be demonstrated indicating frequent lacrimal gland involvement in sarcoidosis. Enlarged lacrimal glands with associated enlargement of the parotid glands suggests Mikulicz's syndrome. In patients with sarcoidosis with long-standing hypercalcemia there may be deposits of calcium salts in the conjunctiva and cornea (band keratopathy). Exophthalmos due to infiltration of the orbital tissue by granulomas has been described (Melmon and Goldberg 1962).

Multiple sites of involvement of the eyes may be present concurrently. The eye changes in sarcoidosis cannot be identified with certainty by their appearance. However, during the evaluation of the eye lesions, associated findings of sarcoidosis may be uncovered not only in the eyes but elsewhere, and thus the diagnosis of the cause of the ocular disease can be inferred.

XII. Nervous System

The nervous system is affected in 1–5% of patients with sarcoidosis (Delaney 1977). Neurologic findings reflect involvement of any part of the nervous system, both central and peripheral. Central nervous system manifestations are diverse and include encephalopathy, meningitis, space-occupying lesions, seizures, and lesions of the hypothalamus, pituitary, brain stem, cerebellum, spinal cord, and cranial nerves. Both sensory and motor peripheral neuropathy is encountered. Neurologic dysfunction can be the presenting or only clinical manifestation of sarcoidosis.

Peripheral and cranial neuropathies are often associated with overt features of sarcoidosis, especially uveoparotid syndrome with its associated pulmonary findings. Patients with the other types of central nervous system sarcoidosis usually do not have the uveoparotid syndrome. Although any or several cranial nerves may be involved, the facial nerve is most often affected. The optic nerve is the second most frequently involved nerve. Papilledema, due to raised intracranial pressure, and optic nerve invasion, due to sarcoidosis, occur. The ninth and tenth cranial nerves comprise the third most frequently seen cranial nerve abnormality resulting in dysphagia, absent gag reflex, immobile soft palate, and vocal cord paralysis. The eighth nerve constitutes the fourth most frequently encountered cranial nerve abnormality; associated findings include deafness, vertigo, and tinnitus. The extraocular muscles are rarely abnormal. Although the trigeminal nerve may occasionally be affected, it is the sensory portion that shows the abnormality. Deficits of the spinal accessory nerve with paresis of the sternomastoid and trapezius muscles have occurred, as well as hypoglossal neuropathy resulting in dysarthria and atrophy of the tongue. Although olfactory dysfunction is thought to be rare, careful questioning and testing reveal anosmia, hyposmia, and dysosmia to occur more frequently than is usually appreciated. Those symptoms may be due to olfactory or trigeminal nerve pathology or to nasal mucosal sarcoidosis.

Mono- or polyneuropathy of the peripheral nerves with or without cranial neuropathy has been noted. Pain, weakness, muscle wasting, paresthesia, and sensory loss are experienced.

Meningeal infiltrations, especially at the base of the brain, can cause pressure or extension to the cranial nerves or obstruction of cerebrospinal fluid flow. Spinal meningeal sarcoidosis may involve the spinal cord or spinal nerves. The cerebrospinal fluid usually shows pleocytosis, elevated protein levels, and hypoglycorrhachia (low cerebrospinal fluid sugar). The spinal fluid pressure can be elevated. The meningitis is usually chronic and the preference of the meningitis for the basal portion of the brain explains the pituitary or hypothalamic disturbances.

Sarcoidosis of the brain can present as a space-occupying mass with headaches, seizures, lethargy, and focal signs. The sarcoid masses have been found in the ventricles, optic chiasm, basal ganglia, hypothalamus, cerebellum, brain stem, and spinal cord (Delaney 1977). Psychiatric, mental and personality changes have been observed (Katz 1976). Multiple sites of involvement of the nervous system can produce bizarre syndromes mimicking multiple sclerosis, cerebral degeneration, and malingering (Katz 1976).

XIII. Heart

Although sarcoidosis of the heart can be found at autopsy in about 20% of cases, clinical detection is noted in less than 5% (Silverman et al. 1978). Dysfunction of the heart in sarcoidosis may be due to cor pulmonale caused by extensive pulmonary fibrosis or to compression and invasion of the pulmonary vasculature (Battesti 1978). Primary sarcoid granuloma of the heart may be found as a part of generalized sarcoidosis, or the process may be confined to the heart. The granulomas occur most often in the free wall of the left ventricle, followed in frequency by the ventricular septum, right ventricle, papillary muscle, and atria (Roberts et al. 1977). Sarcoid granulomas have also been found very rarely in the aorta, pulmonary arteries, superior vena cava, and pulmonary veins. Unquestioned proof of sarcoidosis of the heart valves by the demonstration of granulomatous valvulitis, as well as clinical sarcoidosis and sarcoid lesions in other organs, is a unique phenomenon.

The patients with cardiac dysfunction are often older than the general population of patients with sarcoidosis and there are proportionately more males and whites than in the overall population of patients with sarcoidosis in the United States. The types of cardiac findings include arrhythmias (especially ventricular), high degrees of atrioventricular block and complete bundle branch block, sudden death, congestive heart failure, angina pectoris, simulated acute myocardial infarction, papillary muscle dysfunction, ventricular aneurysm, recurring pericardial effusion, and cardiac enlargement without clinical congestive heart failure.

Disturbance of rhythm is the most frequent clinical presentation of myocardial sarcoidosis, with premature ventricular beats and ventricular tachycardia the most commonly noted arrhythmias. However, if abnormal electrocardiographic changes are included in patients without cardiac complaints, such findings become the first indicator of cardiac disease. Conduction disturbances, arrhythmias, and ST- and T-wave changes are encountered. Since these changes may also be due to other causes, it is often difficult to prove their relationship to sarcoidosis.

Conduction disturbances are found in the form of first-degree heart block, varying types of intraventricular conduction defects, and complete heart block. Since the cephalad portion of the muscular ventricular septum is the major site of involvement in the intraventricular septum by granulomas or scars in sarcoidosis, the occurrence of complete heart block and complete bundle branch block may be readily understood.

Sudden death occurs frequently in patients with myocardial sarcoidosis and is the most common clinically significant cardiac manifestation of cardiac sarcoidosis. It has been reported in as many as two-thirds of these patients. In fact, sudden death may be the first manifestation of sarcoidosis in patients without clinical suspicion of myocardial involvement. Complete heart block, ventricular arrhythmias, and ventricular premature beats are present before sudden death in some of the patients. Atrial arrhythmias and bundle branch block may also precede sudden death.

Congestive heart failure resulting from extensive myocardial granulomas may be the mode of death. The heart may not be enlarged, although usually it is. Often there are accompanying cardiac arrhythmias.

Chest pain resembling angina pectoris or myocardial infarction may occur with electrocardiographic changes simulating myocardial ischemia or infarction. Papillary muscle dysfunction causing an apical systolic murmur due to mitral regurgitation can cause confusion in etiologic diagnosis (Raftery et al. 1966). The papillary muscle dysfunction may be due to sarcoid granulomas in the left ventricular papillary muscles and in the free myocardial walls beneath them, or to dilatation of the left ventricle.

Ventricular aneurysm in the absence of significant coronary artery disease is strongly suggestive of sarcoidosis (Roberts et al. 1977). The wall of the aneurysm contains mostly fibrous tissue, but residual sarcoid granulomas may also be present. Recurring pericardial effusion is infrequent, although the use of echocardiography will disclose pericardial effusion

more frequently. Pericardial effusion may be due to pericardial involvement by sarcoidosis or may be secondary to congestive heart failure or
coincidental pericardial disease. Granulomas confined to the epicardium
represent myocardial sarcoidosis with incidental extension into the epicardium.
Pericarditis caused by parietal pericardial sarcoidosis represents true pericardial sarcoidosis. In most cases the pericarditis is indolent and the fluid
is straw-colored and transudative, although it may be slightly hemorrhagic.
Retrosternal chest pain may be present. Although thallium 201 myocardial
imaging may prove useful in detecting subclinical myocardial sarcoidosis, its
precise role and practicality remain to be defined.

XIV. Liver

The liver is often affected in sarcoidosis although clinical expressions of
liver disease are uncommon. The frequency of sarcoidosis of the liver as
determined by liver biopsy and the exclusion of other diseases that can
cause similar granulomas varies from 60 to 90% (Scadding 1967). It is
striking that liver granulomas are noted most often in subacute sarcoidosis
especially when there is only hilar and mediastinal lymph node enlargement; 80–90% of liver biopsies are positive under these conditions. In
stage II sarcoidosis two-thirds to three-quarters of liver biopsies are positive, whereas in stage III sarcoidosis 60% or less are positive. In chronic
sarcoidosis the frequency of involvement is decidedly less.

The most prevalent hepatic involvement in sarcoidosis is asymptomatic
granulomatous infiltration. The liver may be slightly enlarged in less than
20% of patients and biochemical evidence of abnormality is often absent,
but there may be increased serum levels of alkaline phosphatase.

The lesions are scattered and healing is usual with little or no
fibrosis. However, the clinical spectrum of sarcoidosis of the liver includes
portal fibrosis and obliteration of the hepatic venous bed, either of which
can result in portal hypertension. Chronic intrahepatic cholestasis with or
without resulting biliary cirrhosis may occasionally occur in sarcoidosis with
jaundice, pruritus, hepatomegaly, and splenomegaly. Jaundice, with or
without portal hypertension or biliary cirrhosis, has been noted in late
chronic sarcoidosis; however, the role of hepatitis, alcohol, and malnutrition
in the genesis of jaundice must be considered.

Liver involvement may be extensive without apparent clinical, radiographic or laboratory evidence of multisystem sarcoidosis. Mediastinoscopy,
abdominal exploration, splenic aspiration, and conjunctival, bone marrow, or
other blind extrahepatic biopsies may show granulomas, thus separating

these patients from those with cryptogenic hepatic granulomatosis. Kveim test and serum angiotensin converting enzyme determination are usually not helpful in this form of clinically isolated hepatic sarcoidosis. It is likely that many cases of cryptogenic hepatic granulomatosis would be correctly diagnosed as sarcoidosis if a thorough search for extrahepatic granulomas were made.

XV. Peripheral Lymphadenopathy

Peripheral lymphadenopathy is one of the most common physical findings in subacute sarcoidosis. Since even small unimpressive lymph nodes may show sarcoid granulomas, the true prevalence of peripheral lymph node sarcoidosis is probably higher than usually given, approaching 75%. The lymph nodes may be barely palpable or massively enlarged to the extent that the patient may be aware of the adenopathy. All major lymph node groups or single sites or several groups may be enlarged. Cervical, axillary, epitrochlear, and inguinal lymphadenopathy occur in that order of frequency.

The cervical nodes are most often enlarged on the right side and, in particular, are present in the posterior triangle just above the clavicles and near the sternomastoid muscles. They are palpable in about 75% of patients with lymphadenopathy. Anterior triangle cervical nodes may be involved alone but usually are associated with palpable posterior triangle cervical lymph nodes. Preauricular, postauricular, submaxillary, and submental nodes are often felt, but occipital nodes are rarely involved. If they are carefully sought, epitrochlear nodes are palpable in about 25% of patients while axillary nodes are enlarged in about one-half of those with lymphadenopathy. It is difficult to assess the frequency of inguinal node lymphadenopathy because palpable nodes in this area are often present in normal individuals. Mesenteric and retroperitoneal lymph nodes can also enlarge and may even be palpable.

Sarcoid lymph nodes are usually only moderately enlarged. They are firm, rubbery, discrete, moveable, and not adherent. They are painless and cause no changes in the overlying skin, nor do they soften and ulcerate to form draining sinuses. They are often bilateral. At times lymphatic nodules are felt along the course of major lymphatic vessels in limbs, similarly to those of sporotrichosis or tularemia.

As is the case with microscopic muscle granuloma, liver involvement, and parotitis in subacute sarcoidosis, the lymph node enlargement clears so that persistent lymphadenopathy in chronic sarcoidosis is not common.

XVI. Spleen

Involvement of the spleen as determined by palpation has been reported
in 6–42% of patients, with most observers indicating palpability in 5–20%
of patients (Sharma 1975). Enlargement as determined by radioisotope
scanning is noted in about 50%. Fine-needle percutaneous aspiration
discloses nests of epithelioid cells also in about 50% of patients, with the
highest yield in those with extrathoracic dissemination of sarcoidosis
(Selroos 1976). Pathological involvement at autopsy ranges from 50 to 75%.
Although isolated splenic sarcoidosis occurs, in most cases the liver is also
affected. Very enlarged spleens are associated with chronic fibrosing
sarcoidosis. Slight splenic enlargement such as occurs in subacute sarcoidosis
is usually asymptomatic. However, more significant enlargement as seen in
chronic sarcoidosis can be associated with local discomfort, spontaneous
rupture, and hypersplenism. Along with the latter there may be throm-
bocytopenia with or without purpura, hemolytic anemia, and pancytopenia.

XVII. Endocrine Glands

The pituitary gland and hypothalamus are invaded by sarcoid granulomas
more often than any other endocrine gland. Dysfunction of the hypo-
thalamus-pituitary axis resulting in diabetes insipidus is the most frequently
encountered endocrinopathy. Most of these patients have other manifestations of sarcoidosis such as basal meningitis, uveoparotitis, or other systemic
features of the disease concurrently or in the past. However, when diabetes
insipidus represents the only obvious feature of the multisystem disease, the
diagnosis of sarcoidosis is difficult. Helpful is other evidence suggesting a
hypothalamic or pituitary disturbance such as somnolence, lethargy,
obesity, hypothermia, impotence, amenorrhea, sleep disturbances, hypo-
gonadism, and alveolar hypoventilation. Another clue to the diagnosis of
hypothalamic-pituitary sarcoidosis can be supplied by evidence of involvement of adjacent parts of the base of the brain resulting in visual disturbances, deafness, vertigo, anosmia, and other cranial nerve abnormalities.

Hypopituitarism of the anterior pituitary due to sarcoidosis is revealed
by deficiences of gonadotropin, thyroid-stimulating hormone, and adreno-
corticotropic hormone (Winnacker 1968). Although anterior hypopituitarism may occur as the only evidence of pituitary sarcoidosis, in most
cases hypopituitarism and diabetes insipidus occur simultaneously.

Anatomical involvement without unquestioned functional disturbance
due to sarcoidosis has been noted rarely in the pancreas, thyroid, and
parathyroid glands (Winnacker 1968).

XVIII. Genitourinary System

Granulomas in the kidney are found uncommonly at autopsy in cases of sarcoidosis. When present, they are few in number and do not interfere with renal function. Although renal failure has been described in patients with extensive sarcoid lesions of the kidney, there are usually additional findings such as nephrocalcinosis and pyelonephritis responsible for the impaired renal function. In some patients with sarcoidosis, thickening and hyalinization of the capsular membrane and hyalinization of glomeruli and arteriolar walls have been found (Vanhille et al. 1977, Waldek et al. 1978). Nephrotic syndrome has also been described along with proliferative glomerulonephritis. Interstitial nephritis has occasionally been observed.

The most common cause of renal impairment in sarcoidosis is nephrocalcinosis due to prolonged hypercalcemia and hypercalciuria. Renal calculi may also occur as a consequence of hypercalcemia. Although hypercalcemia and hypercalciuria have been reported in the past as being frequent, the older projections of 10–40% are currently considered to be excessive. Significant alterations in calcium metabolism are rarely present. Careful prospective studies with a controlled intake of calcium indicate that both total and diffusible calcium levels are elevated in only 2% of patients with sarcoidosis (Goldstein et al. 1971). Hypercalciuria without hypercalcemia is also infrequently observed. Hypercalcemia and hypercalciuria are associated with a decrease in fecal calcium suggesting that these individuals appear to absorb calcium excessively. Due to the rarity of hypercalcemia in sarcoidosis its presence should prompt an evaluation for hyperparathyroidism.

Sarcoidosis may very uncommonly affect any portion of the male and female reproductive system. Fertility is rarely affected.

XIX. Gastrointestinal Tract

Scattered case reports of gastrointestinal sarcoidosis exist; however, the digestive system appears to be rather resistant to the development of sarcoidosis. Sarcoidlike granulomas in the mucosa of the stomach arise as a local sarcoid tissue reaction rather than as a part of systemic sarcoidosis. True gastric sarcoidosis can result in infiltration of the stomach wall and submucosa resulting in antral or pyloric narrowing and a linitis plastica type deformity (Konda et al. 1980). Genuine sarcoidosis of the small intestine has not been positively proved. It is likely that the reported cases are examples of regional enteritis or Crohn's disease (Katz 1976). The pathologic similarity plus the reported high incidence of positive

Kveim tests in Crohn's disease in some series add to the mistaken identification of Crohn's disease as sarcoidosis.

XX. Course and Prognosis

From the viewpoints of course, prognosis, and response to therapy, it is helpful to categorize patients with sarcoidosis into two major subdivisions—those with subacute disease estimated to be of less than 2 years' duration and those with chronic lesions of more than 2 years' duration. Since these varieties are not always sharply defined, syndromes related to them will overlap.

Subacute sarcoidosis often develops in patients under the age of 30. The patients are often asymptomatic and the disease is discovered by routine chest roentgenography showing hilar adenopathy. The onset may also be announced by erythema nodosum, acute uveitis, peripheral lymphadenopathy or parotitis. The Kveim test is positive, and noncaseating granulomas are found on scalene node (thoracic duct node), mediastinal node, liver or muscle biopsy, or in an old cutaneous scar that has become violaceous or red. The prognosis is good because the lesions are likely to undergo spontaneous remission within 2 years. If there is later development of ocular lesions, salivary and lacrimal gland enlargement, peripheral lymphadenopathy or pulmonary lesions, they occur within 2 years of the onset of the disease.

Chronic sarcoidosis has an insidious onset with manifestations occurring later in the disease and persisting beyond 2 years. The patients are often over 30. Pulmonary or extrapulmonary findings may indicate the presence of disease. The chest roentgenograms show pulmonary mottling often with receding of absent hilar lymphadenopathy proceeding into the phase of fibrosis, bullae, and functional disability. Peripheral lymphadenopathy may persist as a residual finding from the subacute phase. In contrast to the subacute stage, skin plaques, lupus pernio, and chronic ocular findings (chronic uveitis, keratoconjunctivitis sicca, glaucoma, cataracts, or phthisis bulbi) may be seen. Nephrocalcinosis, central nervous system lesions (other than neuropathies), bone cysts, chronic myopathy, and chronic hepatosplenomegaly are less frequently encountered. The Kveim reaction is often negative except when mediastinal lymphadenopathy persists. Spontaneous remission is unlikely and the prognosis is unfavorable because unremitting fibrosis causes striking functional derangement in the affected organs.

To identify the stage of the disease requires knowledge of the element of time. Patients encountered during the chronic phase may have passed through the subacute phase which went unrecognized because symptoms

Table 1 Modes of Presentation of Sarcoidosis

Respiratory	*Cardiac features*
Wheezing	Unexplained dyspnea
Dyspnea	Heart failure
Cough	Cardiomyopathy
Abnormal chest roentgenogram	Arrhythmias
Cor pulmonale	Heart block
	Cor pulmonale
Abnormal roentgenograms	Abnormal ECG
Chest	Ventricular aneurysm
Bone	Sudden death
Cardiac enlargement	
	Rheumatologic symptoms
Ocular	Polyarthralgia
Iridocyclitis	Arthritis
Conjunctivitis	Myopathy
Choroidoretinitis	Bone cysts
Keratoconjunctivitis	Dactylitis
Cataract	
Glaucoma	*Endocrine manifestations*
Sjögren's syndrome	Diabetes insipidus
Enlarged lacrimal glands	Hypercalcemia
	Hypercalciuria
Dermatologic manifestations	
Erythema nodosum	*Gastroenterologic manifestations*
Lupus pernio	Hepatic granuloma
Nodules	Abnormal liver function tests
Plaques	Splenomegaly
Papules	Similarity to Crohn's disease
Scars	
Keloids	*General manifestations*
Transient maculopapular rash	Fever, weakness, malaise
Subcutaneous nodules	Weight loss
	Lymphadenopathy
Neurologic manifestations	Parotid enlargement
Cranial nerve palsy	Renal calculi
Peripheral neuropathy	Nasal stuffiness
Meningitis	Hoarseness
Myopathy	Hematologic abnormalities
Papilledema	"Sorting out" all modes of presentation
Space-occupying lesions	
Spinal cord manifestations	
Pituitary involvement	

Source: James (1970).

were absent. When old chest x-ray films made years earlier are resurrected, they may show hilar lymphadenopathy that was unrecognized.

Practically no organ is exempt from sarcoidosis. Clinical manifestations may include any branch of medicine. All physicians regardless of their specialty will encounter this disease (Table 1).

References

Allen, B. R. (1978). Sarcoid of nose with collapse of nasal cartilage. *Br. J. Dermatol.,* **99** (Suppl. 16):54–56.

Battesti, J. P., Georges, R., Basset, F., and Saumon, G. (1978). Chronic cor pulmonale in pulmonary sarcoidosis. *Thorax,* **33**:76–84.

Beekman, J. F., Zimmet, S. M., Chun, B. K., Miranda, A., and Katz, S. (1976). Spectrum of pleural involvement in sarcoidosis. *Arch. Intern. Med.,* **136**:323–330.

Chusid, E. L., and Siltzbach, L. E. (1974). Sarcoidosis of the pleura. *Ann. Intern. Med.,* **81**:190–194.

Delaney, P. (1977). Neurologic manifestations in sarcoidosis. *Ann. Intern. Med.,* **87**:336–345.

DeVuyst, P., DeTroyer, A., and Yernault, J. C. (1979). Bloody pleural effusion in a patient with sarcoidosis. *Chest,* **76**:607–609.

DiBenedetto, R., and Lefrak, S. (1970). Systemic sarcoidosis with severe involvement of the upper respiratory tract. *Am. Rev. Respir. Dis.,* **102**:801–807.

Goldstein, R. A., Israel, H. L., Becker, K. L., and Moore, C. F. (1971). The infrequency of hypercalcemia in sarcoidosis. *Am. J. Med.,* **51**: 21–30.

Grigor, R. R., and Hughes, G. R. (1976). Chronic sarcoid arthritis. *Br. Med. J.,* **2**:1044.

Israel, H. L., and Sones, M. (1953). Sarcoidosis: Clinical observation on 160 cases. *Arch. Intern. Med.,* **102**:766–776.

James, D. G. (1970). Sarcoidosis. *DM Disease-A-Month* Feb. 2–41.

James, D. G., Siltzbach, L. E., Sharma, O. P., and Carstairs, L. S. (1969). A tale of two cities: Comparison of sarcoidosis, London and New York. *Arch. Intern. Med.,* **123**:187–191.

James, D. G., Neville, E., Siltzbach, L. E., Turiaf, J., Battesti, J. P., Sharma, O. P., Hosoda, Y., Mikami, R., Odaka, M., Villar, T. G., Djuric, B., Douglas, A. C., Middleton, W., Karlish, A., Blasi, A., Olivieri, D., and Press, P. (1976). A worldwide review of sarcoidosis. *Ann. N.Y. Acad. Sci.,* **278**:321–333.

Katz, S. (1976). Slide presentation. Sarcoidosis: Medcom Famous Teachings in Modern Medicine

Klatskin, G. (1976). Hepatic granulomata. *Ann. N.Y. Acad. Sci.*, **278**: 427–432.

Konda, J., Ruth, M., Sassaris, M., and Hunter, F. M. (1980). Sarcoidosis of the stomach and rectum. *Am. J. Gastroenterol.* **73**:516–518.

Lofgren, S. (1953). Primary pulmonary sarcoidosis. I. Early signs and symptoms. *Acta Med. Scand.* **145**:424–431.

Lofgren, S., and Stanvenow, S. (1961). Course and prognosis of sarcoidosis. *Am. Rev. Respir. Dis.*, **84** (Suppl.):71–75.

Maloney, E. R., and Combes, F. C. (1936). Darier-Roussy's sarcoid. *Arch. Dermatol. Syph.*, **33**:709–724.

Mayock, R. L., Bertrand, P., Morrison, C. E., and Scott, J. H. (1963). Manifestations of sarcoidosis. Analysis of 145 patients with a review of nine series selected from the literature. *Am. J. Med.*, **35**:67–89.

Melmon, K. L., and Goldberg, J. S. (1962). Sarcoidosis with bilateral exophthalmos as the presenting symptom. *Am. J. Med.*, **33**:158–160.

Mitchell, D. M., Mitchell, D. N., Collins, J. V., and Emerson, C. J. (1980). Transbronchial lung biopsy through fibreoptic bronchoscope in diagnosis of sarcoidosis. *Br. Med. J.*, **280**:679–681.

Neville, E., Mills, R. G., and Jash, D. K. (1976). Sarcoidosis of the upper respiratory tract and its association with lupus pernio. *Thorax*, **31**:660–664.

Neville, E., Carstairs, L. S., and James, D. G. (1977). Sarcoidosis of bone. *Q. J. Med.*, **46**:215–227.

Raftery, E. B., Oakley, C., and Goodwin, J. F. (1966). Acute subvalvular mitral incompetence. *Lancet*, **2**:360–365.

Roberts, W. C., McAllister, H. A., and Ferrans, V. J. (1977). Sarcoidosis of the heart. *Am. J. Med.*, **63**:86–108.

Scadding, J. G. (1967). *Sarcoidosis.* London, Eyre and Spottiswoode.

Sharma, O. P. (1975). *Sarcoidosis: A Clinical Approach.* Springfield, Ill., Charles C. Thomas.

Sharma, O. P. (1977). Sarcoidosis: Unusual pulmonary manifestations. *Postgrad. Med.*, **61**:67–73.

Selroos, O. (1969). The frequency, clinical picture and prognosis of pulmonary sarcoidosis in Finland. Academic Dissertation: Faculty of Medicine of the University of Helsinki.

Selroos, O. (1976). Sarcoidosis of spleen. *Acta Med. Scand.*, **200**:337–340.

Siltzbach, L. E. (1967). Sarcoidosis: Clinical features and management. *Med. Clin. North Am.*, **51**:483–502.

Silverman, K. J., Hutchins, G. M., and Bulkley, B. H. (1978). Cardiac sarcoid: A clinicopathologic study of 84 unselected patients with systemic sarcoidosis. *Circulation*, **58**:1204–1211.

Sones, M., and Israel, H. L. (1960). Course and prognosis of sarcoidosis. *Am. J. Med.*, **29**:84–93.

Spilberg, I., Siltzbach, L. E., and McEwen, C. (1969). The arthritis of
    sarcoidosis. *Arthritis Rheum.,* **12**:126–137.
Vanhille, P., Dequiedt, P., Ruviart, B., Lelievre, G., and Tacquet, A. (1977).
    Renal insufficiency caused by granulomatous nephritis during
    sarcoidosis. *Lille Med.,* **22**:778–782.
Vico, J. J., and Larsen, C. R. (1979). Sarcoidosis of the larynx. *Radiology,*
    131:636.
Waldek, S., Agius-Ferrante, A. M., and Lawler, W. (1978). Renal failure
    due to glomerulonephritis in sarcoidosis. *Br. Med. J.,* **1**:1110–1111.
Winnacker, J. L., Becker, K. L., and Katz, S. (1968). Endocrine aspects of
    sarcoidosis. *N. Engl. J. Med.,* **278**:427–434, 483–492.
Winterbauer, R. H., and Kraemer, K. G. (1976). The infectious complica-
    tions of sarcoidosis: A current perspective. *Arch. Intern. Med.,* **136**:
    1356–1362.

2

Radiological Alterations in Sarcoidosis

BRUCE A. RODAN* and CHARLES E. PUTMAN

Duke University Medical Center
Durham, North Carolina

I. Introduction

Most patients with sarcoidosis exhibit abnormalities on their chest radiographs during the course of their disease and often it is these findings that first suggest the diagnosis in asymptomatic patients.

The differential diagnosis in some of these patients may be extensive and is based on the particular radiographic abnormality noted (Table 1). No single radiographic finding or combination of findings is diagnostic of sarcoidosis, although certain patterns are highly suggestive of this disease. However, when the chest radiograph is atypical, it may be difficult to make the diagnosis. An important aspect in the follow-up of patients with sarcoidosis is the evaluation of serial chest radiographs. These examinations should be performed with a standardized technique utilizing high KvP (130 KvP). Variation in technique is often responsible for misinterpreting changes in the disease process.

Present Affiliation
    *Palm Beach–Martin County Medical Center, Jupiter, Florida.

Table 1 Differential Diagnosis of Pulmonary Sarcoidosis

Radiographic abnormality	Differential diagnosis
Stage 1	
Lymphadenopathy alone	Lymphoma
	Bronchogenic carcinoma
	Lymph node metastases
	Tuberculosis
	Fungal diseases
	Histoplasmosis
	Coccidioidomycosis
	Brucellosis
Stage 2A	
Lymphadenopathy with parenchymal opacities	Lymphoma
	Lymphangitic carcinomatosis
	Tuberculosis
	Fungal diseases
	Silicosis
	Berylliosis
Stage 2B	
Parenchymal opacities alone	Tuberculosis
	Fungal diseases
	Collagen vascular diseases
	Rheumatoid arthritis
	Lupus erythematosus
	Scleroderma
	Hypersensitivity pneumonitis
	Eosinophilic granuloma
	Pneumoconiosis
	Alveolar proteinosis
Stage 3	
Advanced fibrosis	Fibrosing alveolitis
	Bullous emphysema
	Chronic tuberculosis
	Chronic fungal diseases
	Bronchiectasis
	Pneumoconiosis

Source: Data from Sharma (1975).

II. Radiographic Staging

Radiographic evidence of sarcoidosis is seen in over 90% of cases (Kirks et al. 1973, Smellie and Hoyle 1960). To aid classification of these findings, the International Congress on Sarcoidosis has established the following categories: (0) no abnormal radiographic findings, (1) lymph node enlargement without pulmonary abnormalities, (2A) a combination of diffuse pulmonary disease and lymph node enlargement, (2B) diffuse pulmonary disease without lymph node enlargement, and (3) pulmonary fibrosis. Almost 90% of patients fall into stage 1 or 2 (A or B) (Dunbar 1978).

A. Stage 0

At the time of their initial presentation, 5–10% of patients have a normal chest radiograph (Dunbar 1978). Although the radiograph may be normal, there may be other evidence of lung disease such as abnormalities on pulmonary function testing and biopsy evidence of granulomas. These findings will be discussed in other chapters. Many observers believe that stage 0 represents the earliest phase of the disease process.

B. Stage 1

Intrathoracic lymphadenopathy occurs in 75–90% of patients with sarcoidosis (Dunbar 1978). On initial chest radiograph, parenchymal disease is present in about half of these patients. Of 150 patients studied by Kirks et al. (1973), lymph node enlargement was the sole abnormality in 65 (43%), while in 61 (41%) nodal enlargement was associated with pulmonary disease. About one-half the patients with lymphadenopathy alone were asymptomatic. Lymph node enlargement is localized primarily to the bronchopulmonary, tracheobronchial, and paratracheal groups. These nodes are lobulated masses usually extending symmetrically throughout the hila, and when particularly large, have been referred to as "potato" nodes. Characteristically, there is a relatively translucent space between the mass of nodes and the cardiovascular margin (Fraser and Pare' 1978). This space is more apparent on the right side where the hilum is normally better seen than on the left.

Bilaterality is the hallmark of nodes involved in sarcoidosis. A characteristic radiograph is shown in Figure 1a and b. The distribution of thoracic adenopathy is shown in Figure 1c. Bilateral hilar adenopathy occurs in about 90% of patients with nodal enlargement (Kirks and Greenspan 1973). It may be associated with either right paratracheal or bilateral paratracheal adenopathy. The right paratracheal zone is more clearly seen than the left zone on posteroanterior (PA) chest radiographs.

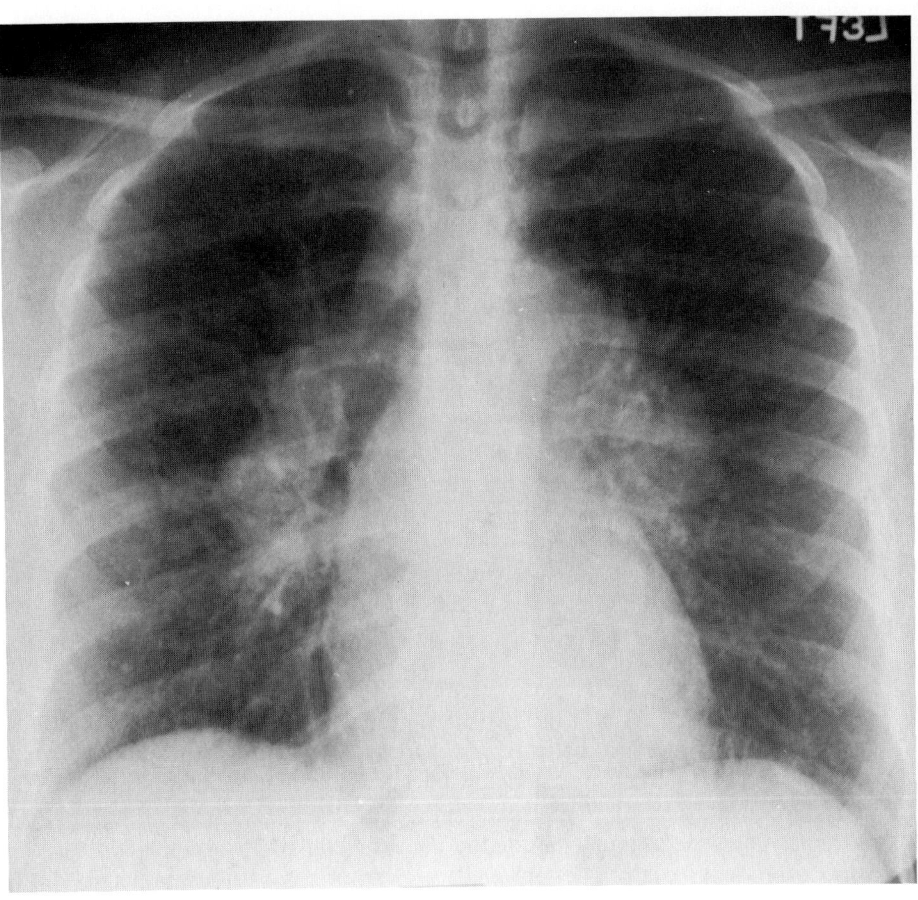

1a

Figure 1 PA (a) and lateral (b) chest radiographs (Stage 1 sarcoidosis) with classical distribution of lymph nodes. Bilateral symmetrical hilar and paratracheal adenopathy. (c) Distribution and frequency of lymphadenopathy in sarcoidosis. (Modified from Bein et al. [1978] © 1978, American Roentgen Ray Society.)

Left paratracheal adenopathy is at times difficult to detect because of partial superimposition of adjacent structures such as the aortic arch, bracheocephalic vessels, and manubrium. Loss of the normally straight or concave appearance of the aorticopulmonary window on the PA chest radiograph is considered a positive finding of lymphadenopathy. Involvement may be due to enlarged ductus nodes, which are the lowest of the

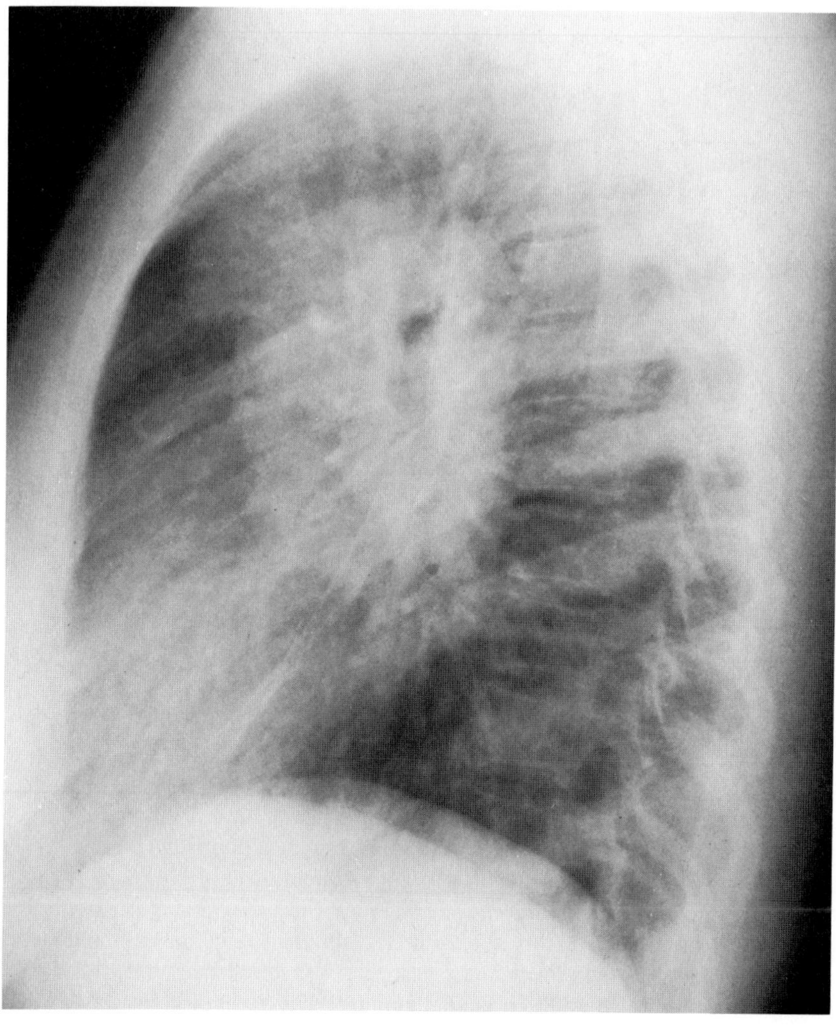

1b

left anterior mediastinal chain, or to enlarged inferior nodes in the left tracheobronchial chain (Bein et al. 1978). Bilateral hilar adenopathy with bilateral paratracheal adenopathy is found more often than bilateral hilar and right paratracheal adenopathy. However, the paratracheal nodes are frequently asymmetric.

Most lymph node groups may be affected, and unilateral hilar adenopathy (1–5%) (Kirks and Greenspan 1973, Rabinowitz et al. 1974)

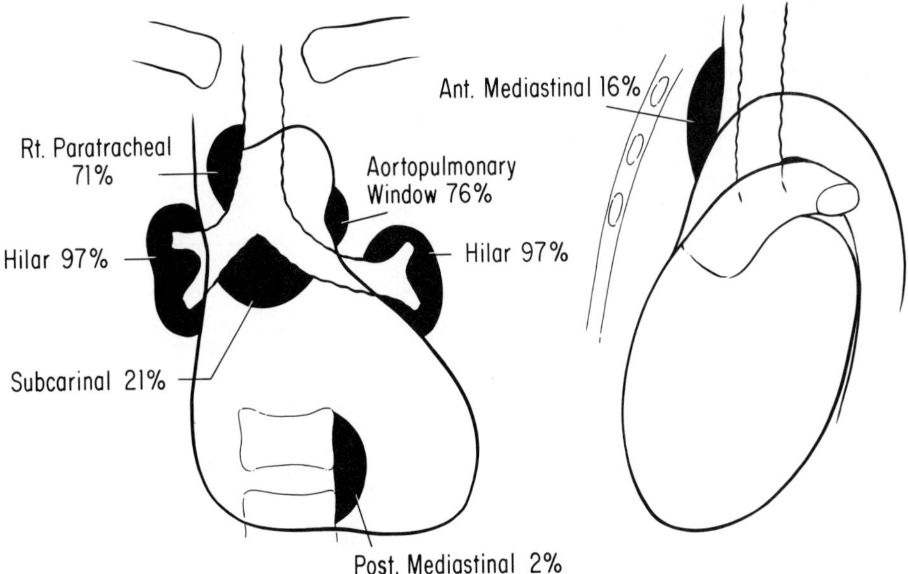

1c

and solitary paratracheal adenopathy (1–3%) (Dunbar 1978; Kirks and
Greenspan 1973) (Fig. 2a) are uncommon findings in sarcoidosis. Computed
tomography (CT) may be helpful in recording other nodes (Fig. 2b).
Recent studies show that subcarinal (Fig. 3) aorticopulmonary, anterior
mediastinal, and/or posterior mediastinal nodes may accompany the
characteristic lymphadenopathy of sarcoidosis (Bein et al. 1978, Schabel et
al. 1978). These new findings are contrary to the belief that adenopathy
in these groups is so rare that a diagnosis other than sarcoidosis should be
considered. Identifying which nodal groups are involved may require other
radiographic studies in addition to the standard chest radiograph. The
subcarinal, tracheal bifurcation, or inferior tracheobronchial groups of nodes
are considered enlarged if the azygoesophageal recess, on the PA view, is
clearly visualized throughout its extent and displaced laterally to the right
in the cephalad portion (Bein et al. 1978). Subcarinal nodes are more
easily detected with tomography or after barium swallow which reveals
posterior displacement of the barium-filled esophagus (Bein et al. 1978).
Although anterior mediastinal nodes are hidden behind the sternum on the
PA chest radiograph, they may be identified on the frontal film if
mediastinal lines are properly interpreted. Lateral deviation of the anterior
pleural reflection indicates anterior mediastinal adenopathy. This sign is

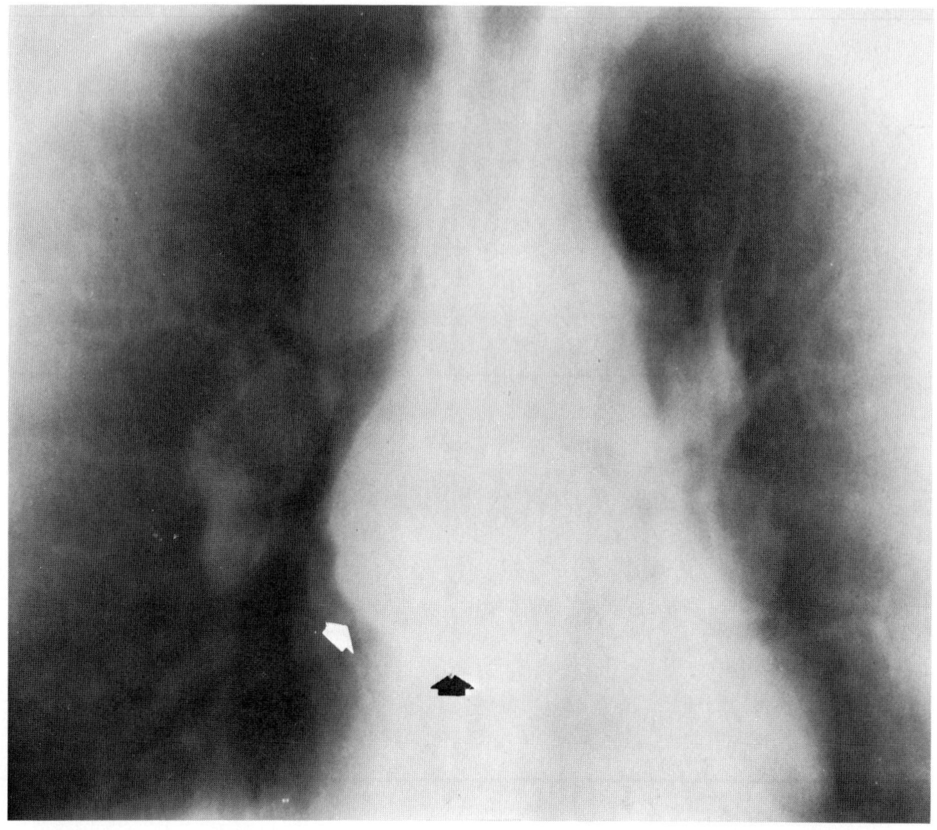

Figure 2 AP tomogram defines typical bilateral hilar and paratracheal adenopathy and less frequent subcarinal adenopathy (arrows). Narrowing of the left main stem bronchus by the lymphadenopathy. (From Bein et al. [1978] © 1978, American Roentgen Ray Society.)

often misinterpreted as suggesting adenopathy in the paratracheal location. On the lateral chest radiograph, increased density anterior to the great vessels and retrosternally indicates involvement of nodes in the anterior paratracheal and the left anterior mediastinal groups. This involvement may not be appreciated because of overlapping by the ascending aorta and the soft tissues of the axilla (Berkman and Javors 1976). However, these two nodal groups may be better defined with lateral tomography or computed tomography.

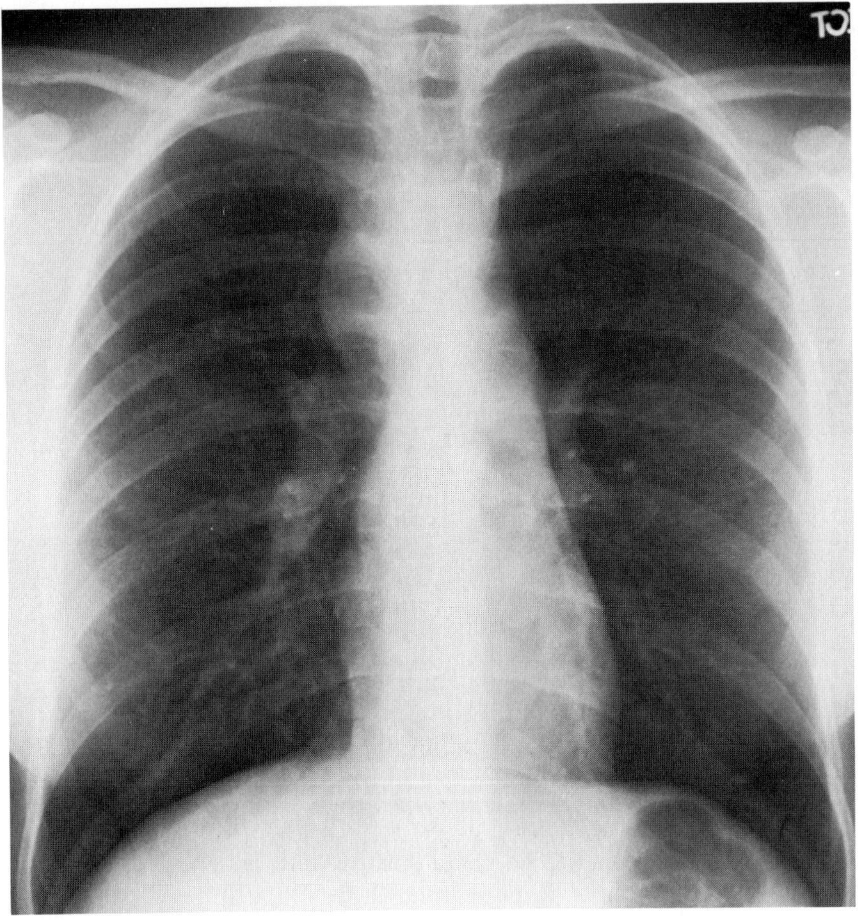

Figure 3a   Atypical nodal distribution in stage 1 sarcoidosis.   Asymmetric paratracheal adenopathy with a large lymph node on the right.

Lymph nodes may be readily identified by computed tomography (CT) in regions of the chest thought to be atypical for sarcoidosis, such as the anterior mediastinum (Karasick 1979, Putman et al. 1977).   CT scans may readily confirm the presence of hilar and paratracheal adenopathy.   The distribution of enlarged nodes in patients with sarcoidosis as seen by CT is somewhat different from the classical description.   This difference is primarily due to the limitations of conventional methods to image these mediastinal and hilar regions.

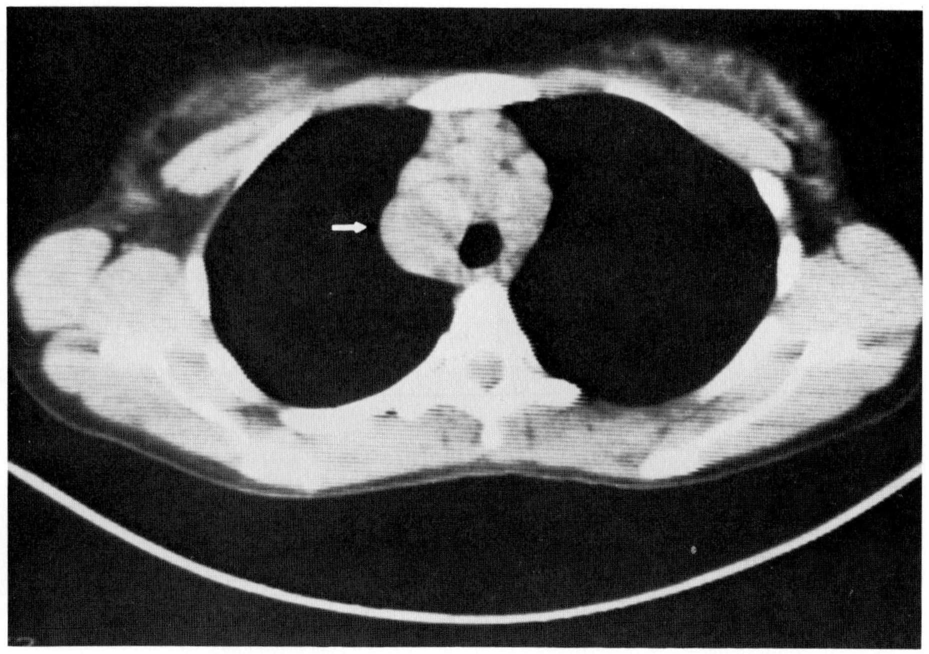

Figure 3b Computed tomography image through the upper mediastinum reveals bilateral paratracheal and anterior mediastinal lymphadenopathy (arrows).

The differential diagnosis for stage 1 sarcoidosis includes Hodgkin's lymphoma, primary tuberculosis, coccidioidomycosis, brucellosis, and metastatic involvement of nodes due to bronchogenic carcinoma (Sharma 1975). Paratracheal node enlargement seldom, if ever, occurs without concomitant enlargement of hilar nodes in sarcoidosis. This bilaterally symmetrical hilar and paratracheal lymph node enlargement contrasts sharply with the nodal enlargement of primary tuberculosis, which tends to be unilateral and less sharply demarcated. It is also in contrast to the node enlargement that characterizes Hodgkin's lymphoma (Fraser and Pare' 1978). Hodgkin's lymphoma, a frequent source of difficulty in the differential diagnosis, is more likely than sarcoidosis to involve the more centrally situated nodes around the tracheal bifurcation in addition to those nodes in Althe hila. When Hodgkin's lymphoma involves the hilar nodes it tends to be unilateral, or bilateral but asymmetric. The mass of nodes in Hodgkin's lymphoma tends to merge with the cardiovascular silhouette. Retrosternal nodes are common in Hodgkin's lymphoma but

rare in sarcoidosis. An additional contrasting feature is that in sarcoidosis
the onset of diffuse lung disease is commonly associated with a decrease
in nodal size or at least a cessation of growth (Fraser and Pare' 1978).
The occurrence of mediastinal nodes in the absence of hilar or paratracheal
nodes would favor the diagnosis of lymphoma or metastatic neoplasm.

Involvement of lymph nodes by sarcoidosis seems to be self-limiting.
Sixty to 80% of patients in the stage 1 category show resolution of the
lymphadenopathy within 6 months to 2 years (Dunbar 1978). After
returning to normal size, lymph nodes rarely enlarge again (Schabel et al.

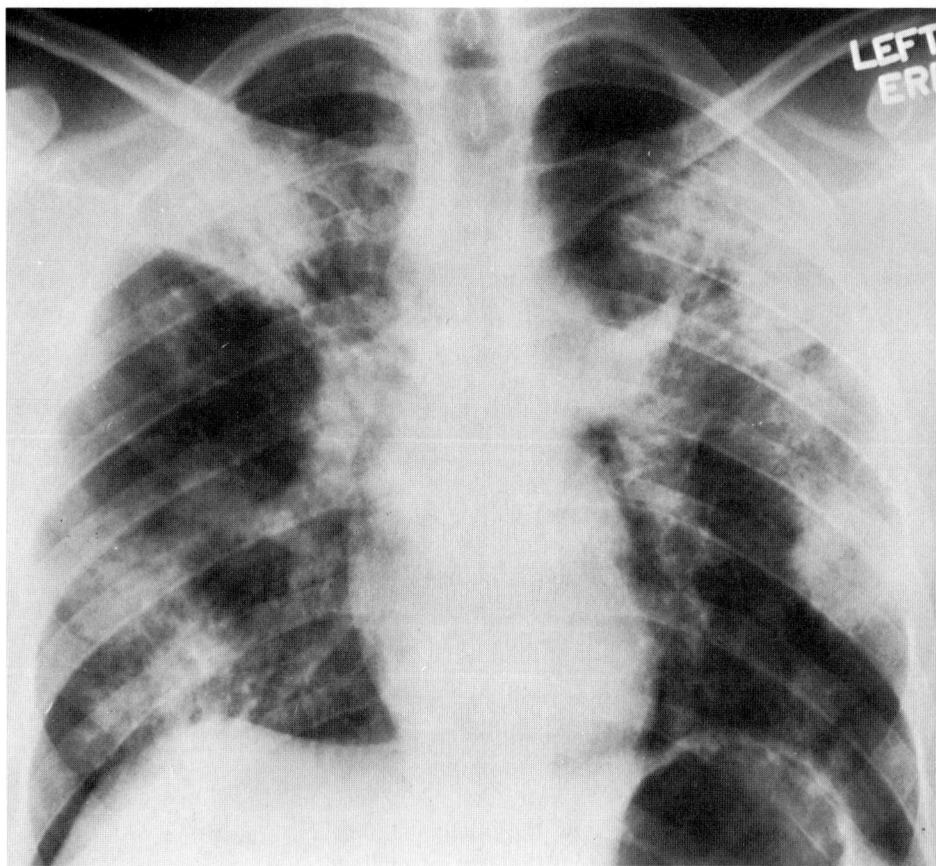

Figure 4a Stage 2A sarcoidosis showing bilateral hilar and right paratracheal adenopathy in addition to an acinar pattern of parenchymal
involvement. Fluffy ill-defined opacities are scattered throughout the
lung fields.

1978). The remaining patients with stage 1 sarcoidosis either have a stationary radiographic appearance or gradually advance to stage 2.

The radiographic and histological findings in stage 1 sarcoidosis are not closely associated. Granulomata and interstitial pneumonitis were found in all lung biopsies of 19 patients with stage 1 radiographic findings reported by Winterbauer and Hutchinson (1980). Only six of these patients had normal pulmonary function tests. These observations indicate that parenchymal involvement is present histologically in stage 1 disease.

C. Stage 2

The initial chest radiograph in 25–30% of all patients with sarcoidosis indicates both bilateral hilar lymph node enlargement and diffuse pulmonary disease, which characterizes stage 2A disease (Fig. 4a, b). The development

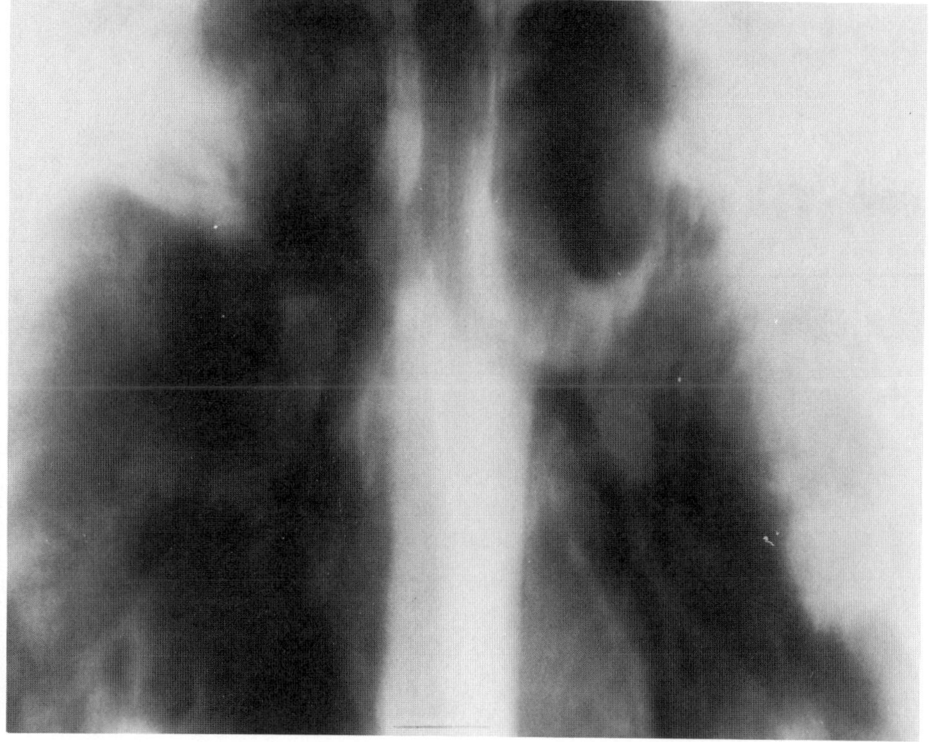

Figure 4b AP tomogram demonstrates air bronchograms within several of the upper lobe acinar consolidations. Bilateral hilar and paratracheal adenopathy are present.

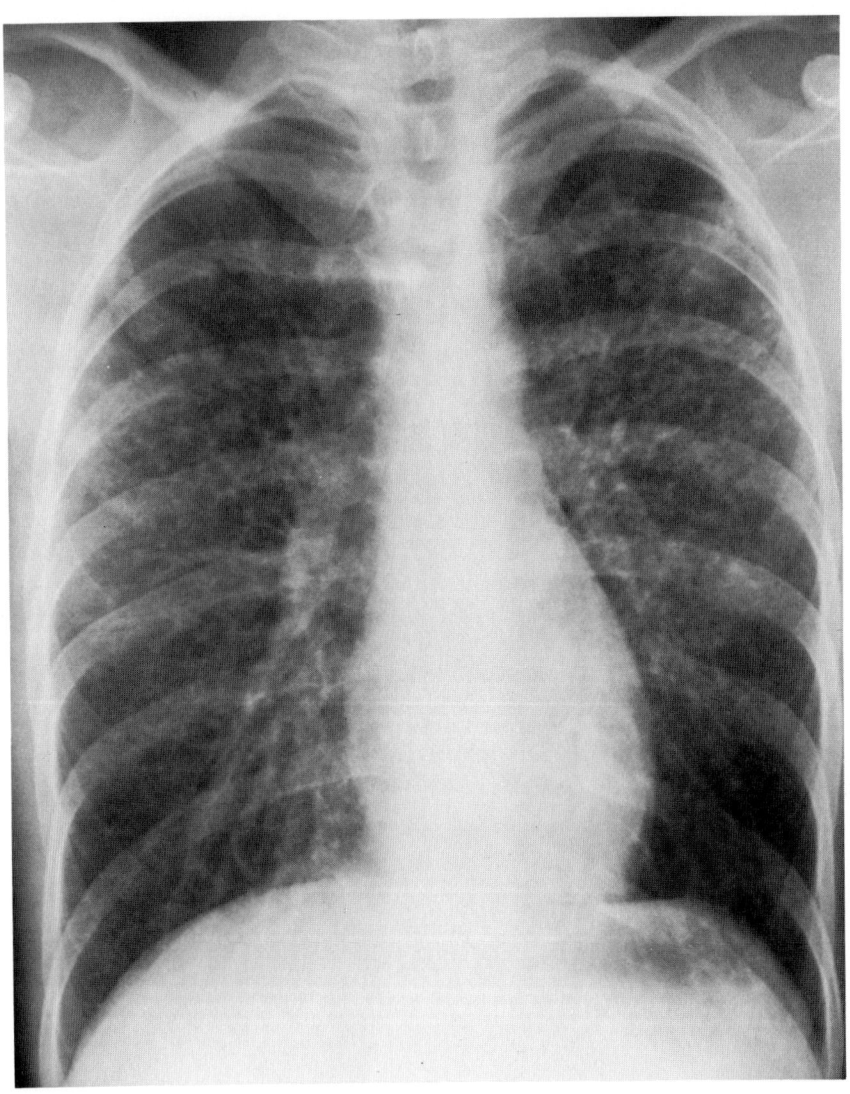

Figure 5 Stage 2B sarcoidosis reveals a diffuse reticulonodular pattern without adenopathy.

of each process, however, may follow a different temporal course. Diffuse pulmonary disease may become radiographically detectable when hilar node enlargement is regressing or nodal regression may occur several years after the development of detectable parenchymal involvement. The mediastinal adenopathy may regress asymmetrically. Although in chronic sarcoidosis retraction secondary to fibrosis may produce sufficient hilar deformity to suggest lymph node enlargement, there is no evidence to indicate that hilar lymph node enlargement develops subsequent to pulmonary parenchymal disease.

Approximately 25% of all patients with sarcoidosis present with radiological pulmonary disease without lymphadenopathy, i.e., stage 2B disease (Fig. 5) (Dunbar 1978, Ellis and Renthal 1962, Scadding 1961). Parenchymal abnormalities are noted on radiographs of the chest in 63% of all sarcoid patients (Kirks and Greenspan 1973). Three basic patterns are recognized: reticulonodular, acinar, and large nodular. Most patients develop more than one pattern of pulmonary involvement. Kirks et al. (1973) found that 95 patients developed 157 radiographic patterns including fibrosis with the three aforementioned categories. Pulmonary involvement is usually diffuse and evenly distributed throughout the lungs. Occasionally it is not symmetrical during the phases of development or resolution. Although the parenchymal abnormalities will usually show signs either of resolution or of developing fibrosis within 2–3 years, it may remain apparently nonprogressive for long periods of time. During this nonprogressive phase there may be minimal functional defects or symptoms. Albeit unusual, the disease may still resolve substantially with only minor radiographic residues and no clinical disability, regardless of how long the parenchymal abnormality has been present.

III. Parenchymal Patterns

A reticulonodular pattern is the most common parenchymal abnormality noted, although reticular and nodular patterns may occur separately. The reticulonodular pattern was noted in 80 to 95 patients with roentgenologic parenchymal lung disease in the study by Kirks et al. (1973). The reticulation may be in the form of a very fine or a very coarse network. The mixed reticulonodular pattern consists of fine linear densities and small nodules from 3 to 5 mm in diameter (Fig. 6). A pure miliary pattern is included in this group and was seen in two patients (Kirks et al. 1973). An example of the miliary pattern is shown in Figure 7. This reticulonodular pattern is due to noncaseating granulomatous nodules and associated interstitial inflammatory infiltrates. The chest radiograph is of limited usefulness until the parenchymal abnormalities are large enough to be

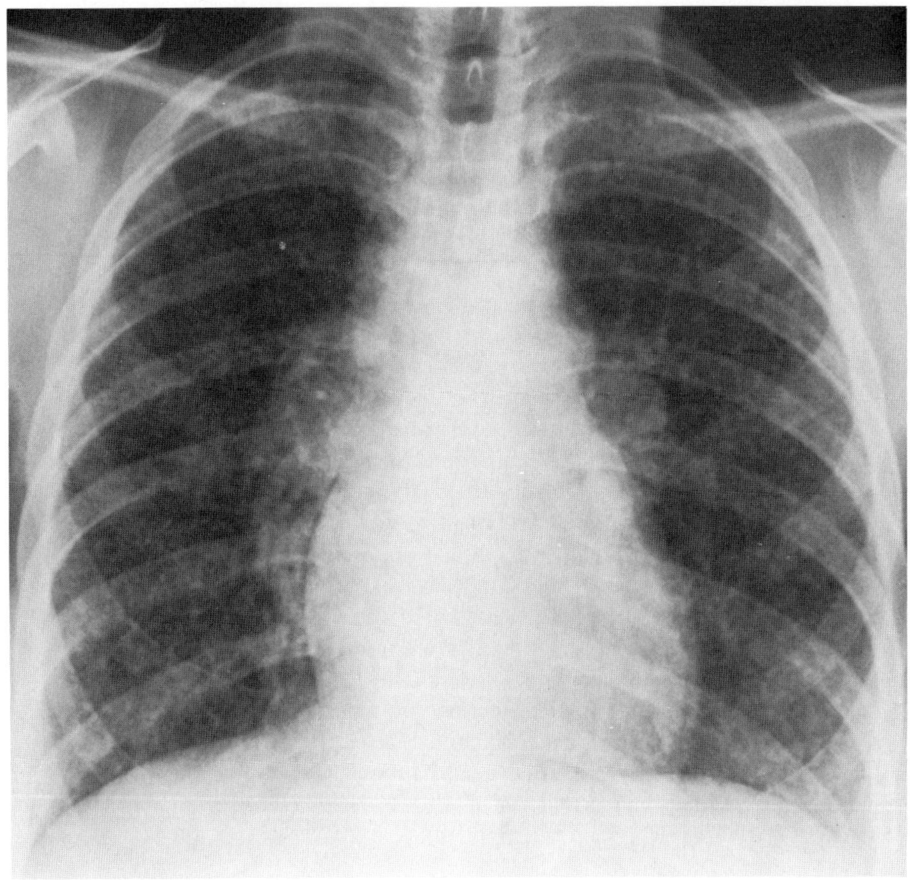

Figure 6 Stage 2A sarcoidosis with a diffuse nodular pattern ranging from 3 to 5 mm in size. Bilateral symmetrical hilar and paratracheal adenopathy is present.

radiographically detectable. Otherwise, the lung fields will appear to be clear even when there is impaired diffusing capacity. Diffuse thickening of the interstitial septae seen in profile appears as a linear or reticular opacity on the chest radiograph. When seen *en face* such interstitial septae will appear as a nodular opacity, as will a focal granuloma of at least 3 mm in diameter.

An acinar pattern was noted during the course of the disease in 32 of the 95 patients noted above (Kirks et al. 1973). The acinar pattern is characterized by coalescence, segmental or lobar distribution, fluffy margins,

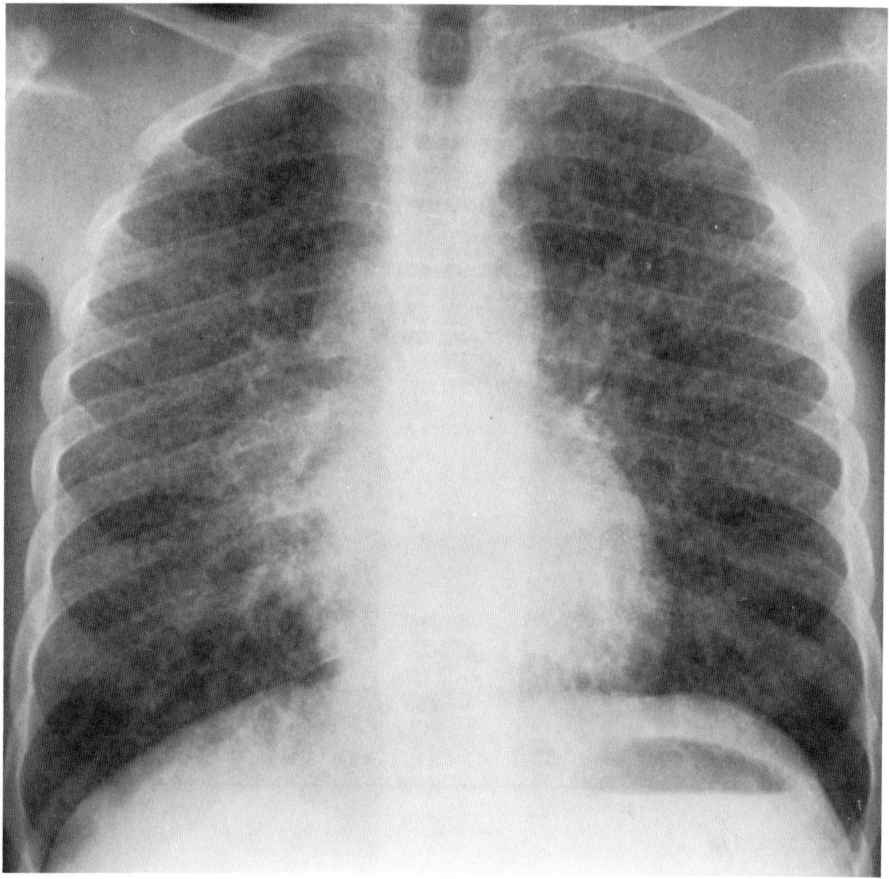

Figure 7   Stage 2A sarcoidosis with a miliary (fine nodular) pattern in addition to bilateral hilar and right paratracheal adenopathy.

air bronchograms, and acinar nodules. Large segmental consolidation and scattered, hazy consolidations with irregular borders were the most commonly noted abnormalities in this group. In most acinar filling diseases, the radiographic shadows are confluent and the individual acinar rosettes cannot be easily discerned. These acinar rosettes consist chiefly of indistinct fine opacities of up to 7 mm in diameter.

Based on pathologic correlation, it appears that the acinar pattern represents a secondary, nonspecific response of the lung to the primary interstitial injury (Sahn et al. 1974). The acinar pattern may be a result of alveolar filling with mononuclear cells as opposed to noncaseating granulomas, which are located in the interstitium. Chest radiographs will show eventual clearing in one-third of patients with the chronic acinar pattern; one-third will persist with little change during the course of follow-up; and one-third will progress to fibrotic changes. The acinar pattern, with or without lymphadenopathy, appears at times to progress rapidly to the fibrotic pattern and indicates very active disease. The acinar pattern may be associated with high levels of serum lysozyme and angiotensin 1-converting enzyme activity (Littner et al. 1977). These possible correlations will be discussed in another section of the book.

The large nodular pattern was noted in three of the 95 patients studied radiographically by Kirks et al. (1973). The chest radiographs revealed round to oval lesions, 5–40 mm in diameter. An example of this abnormality is shown in Figure 8. Although this pattern is widely distributed in the lungs, it is particularly concentrated in the central zones

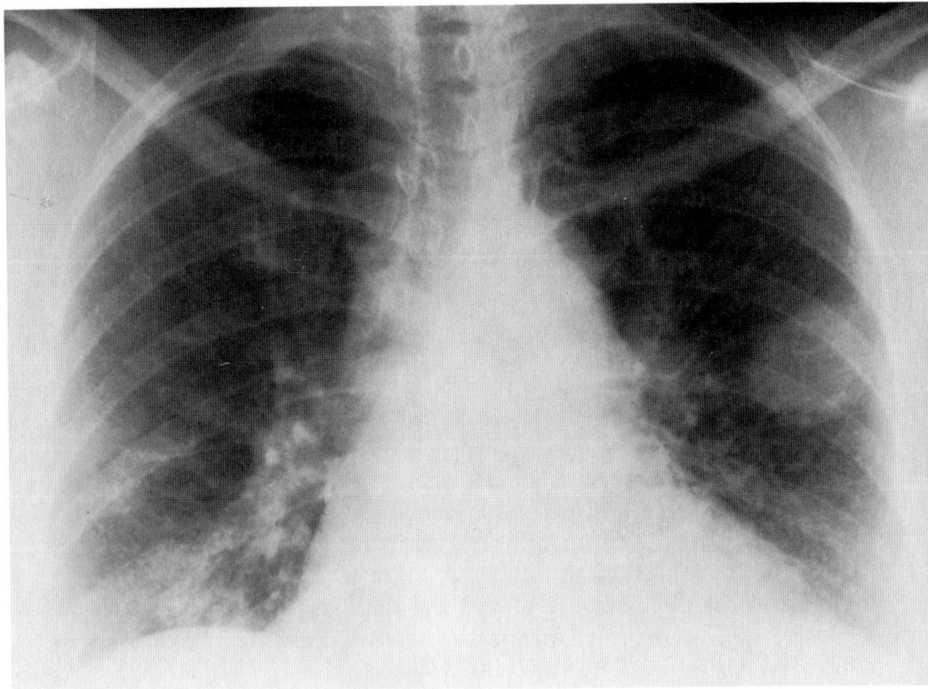

Figure 8 Stage 2A sarcoidosis with multiple large nodules scattered throughout the pulmonary parenchyma. Mediastinal widening due to lymphadenopathy.

where it tends to be confluent and may cavitate. Individual nodules present with a hazy or fluffy outline. The "soft" margin at times appears as a halo around the central density. The radiographic appearance suggests a far worse condition than is evident from the mild clinical manifestations. These large nodular or "cannonball" lesions may disappear rapidly with or without steroid therapy. The differential diagnosis includes metastatic disease, pulmonary lymphoma, and septic emboli (Kirks and Greenspan 1973). Rarely, a solitary lung nodule may be present.

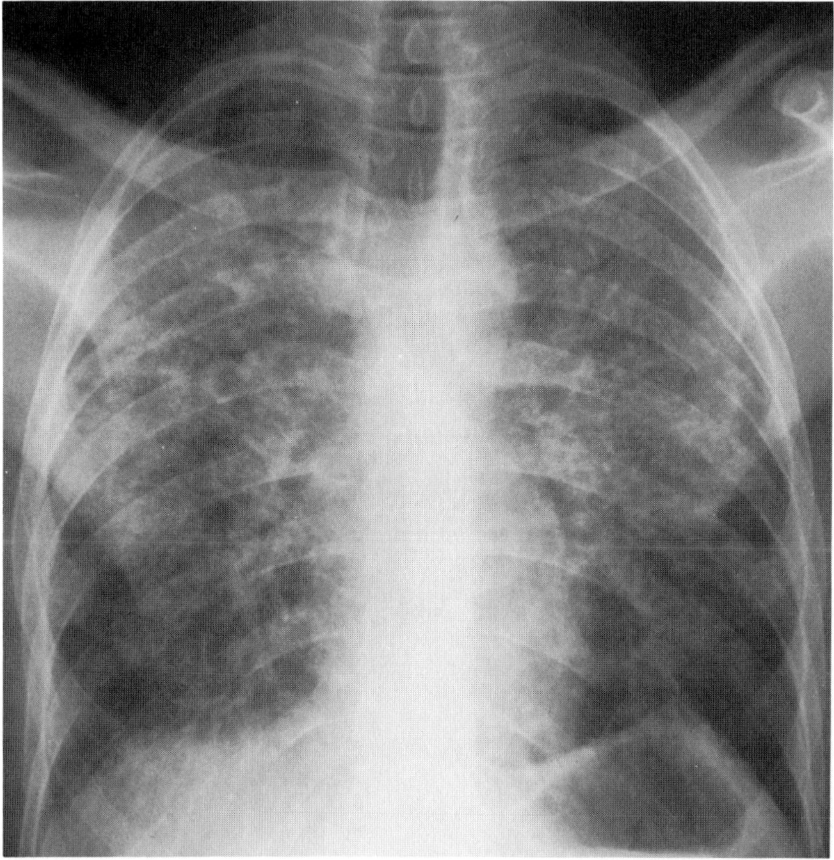

Figure 9a Initial chest radiograph reveals diffuse parenchymal involvement predominantly in the midlung zones, the degree of which makes evaluation of hilar adenopathy difficult.

A. Stage 3

The fibrotic pattern was noted in 42 of the 95 patients in the study of
Kirks et al. (1973). If the typical parenchymal disease does not resolve,
fibrosis will eventually result which, if sufficiently severe, may lead to
pulmonary insufficiency and right heart failure. The transition to interstitial fibrosis is subtle and the early changes of fibrosis are difficult to
appreciate radiographically. Radiological indication of such a transition is
shown in Figure 9a and b. On the basis of chest radiography alone, the
presence of fibrosis can be deduced only by the occurrence of well-defined

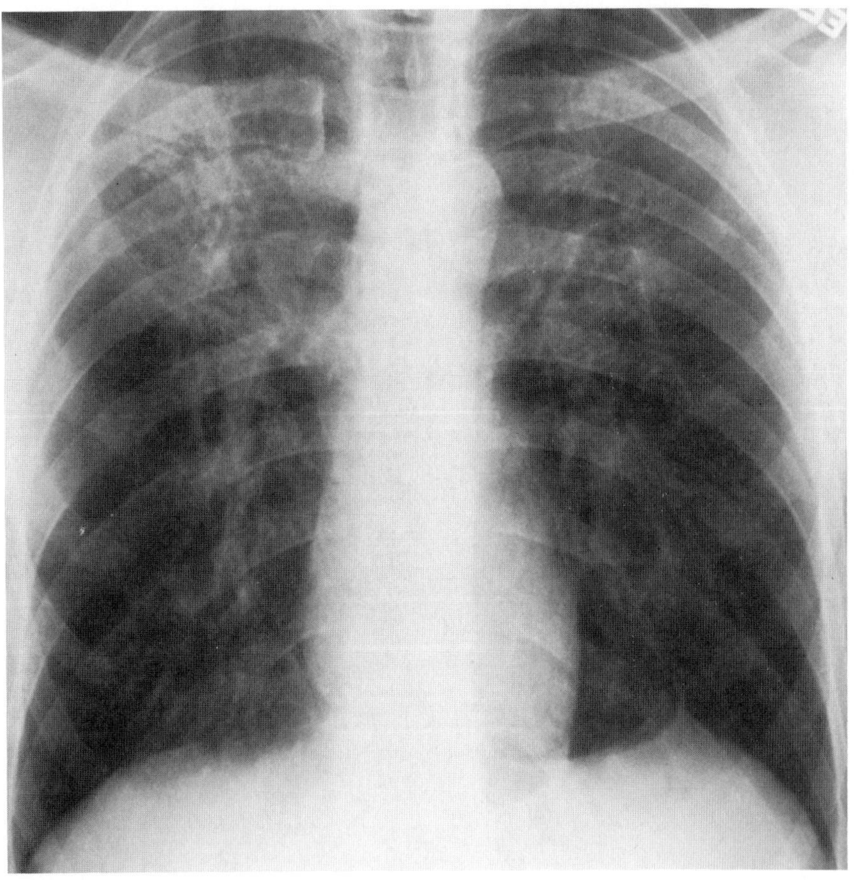

Figure 9b Two years later the patient progressed to a fibrotic pattern
with coarse reticulation, bilateral upper lobe volume loss, and retraction.

structural changes in the lung, such as emphysema, bleb or bulla formation, lobar or segmental atelectasis, and bronchiectasis (McCort and Pare' 1954). These structural changes occur as the result of fibrous tissue replacement of sarcoid granulomas. Without tissue diagnosis, this pattern is indistinguishable on the chest radiograph from scarring by tuberculosis, fungal disease, or pneumoconiosis.

The radiographic criteria for diagnosis of stage 3 disease are the presence of linear opacities that persist unchanged for as long as 6 months and are associated with decreased lung volume. An example of this is shown in Figure 10. The fibrotic parenchymal changes range from minimal

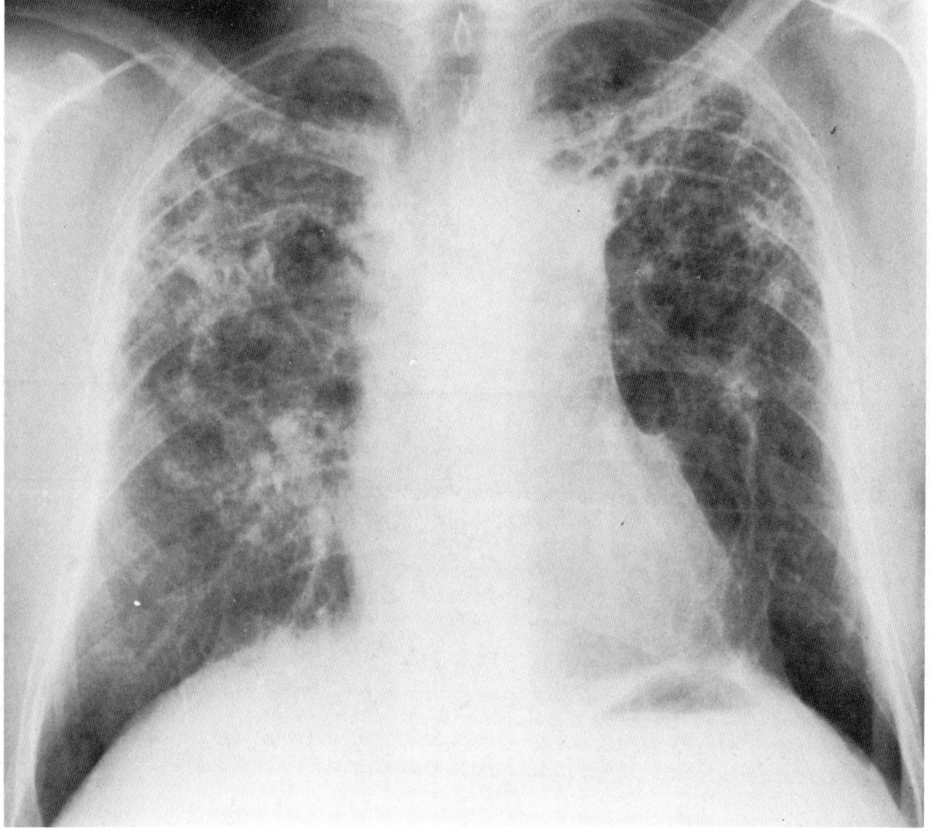

Figure 10 Stage 3 sarcoidosis with pulmonary fibrosis predominantly in the upper lobes with cystic changes. Superior retraction of the hila and apical volume loss is present.

linear scarring to more classic conglomerate densities of the upper lobes
with associated hilar retraction and extensive bullous change (Fig. 11).

Occasionally, a fine focal fibrosis develops. Patients without recorded
hilar adenopathy have an increased tendency to develop fibrosis. A high
proportion of patients developing fibrosis show a rather characteristic
radiographic appearance. In the early stage, mottled opacities are densest in
the middle and adjacent upper lung zones with relative sparing of the lower
lung zones and apices. Irregular linear shadows extend outward from the
hila. When fibrosis is established, retraction occurs. This is noted in 20%
of patients with sarcoidosis (Freundlich et al. 1970). Retraction occurs

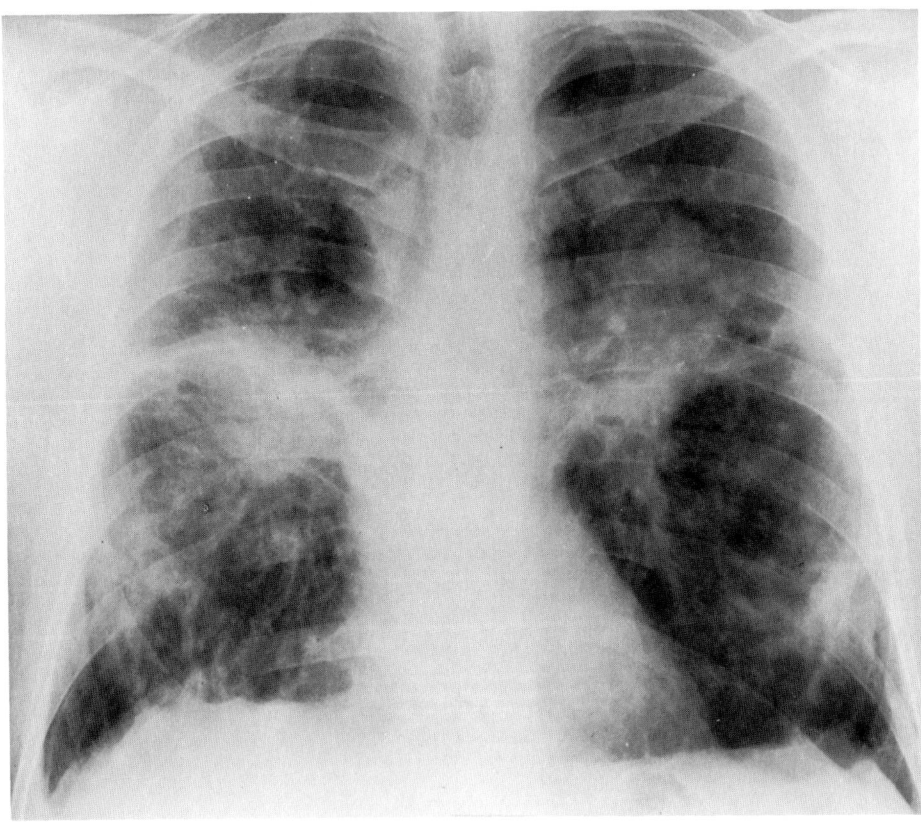

Figure 11 Progressive massive fibrosis in end-stage sarcoidosis. Conglomerate masses in midlung zones are retracted toward the hila,
resembling silicosis.

superiorly and posteriorly with distortion of fissures, hila, vessels, and bronchi.

Later in the disease process, the mottling tends to disappear. The linear shadows become more prominent and there may be localized dense shadows, presumably a confluence of fibrosis. Not all patients with developing fibrosis show the middle zone pattern. In a few, a widespread granulomatous infiltration appears to undergo focal fibrosis without confluence or evident distortion of macroscopic lung architecture. An even rarer development is airway obstruction with grossly over-distended lungs, suggestive of emphysema.

This fibrotic pattern has an important prognostic implication since patients with this pattern are especially susceptible to develop severe complications including respiratory failure, cor pulmonale, pneumothorax, mycetoma formation, or fatal intercurrent infection (McCort and Pare' 1954). Once this pattern of interstitial fibrosis has developed, it either stabilizes or progresses, but does not regress.

IV. Computed Tomography of Parenchymal Disease

Although lung changes associated with sarcoidosis may be demonstrated by chest radiography and computed tomography is usually not necessary, CT may provide a more critical assessment of these changes in some cases. Nodular, cavitary, and diffuse parenchymal disease are easily visualized by CT. In some instances, CT scans identify areas of unexpected involvement. It has been reported that findings from CT images correlate more closely with pulmonary function test abnormalities than do those from standard radiographs (Putman et al. 1977).

CT has also clarified interpretation of plain film findings. For example, linear opacities on chest radiographs have been verified as interstitial changes based on the course honeycombed pattern seen on CT images (Solomon et al. 1979). Small isolated granulomas of the lung, not visualized on chest radiographs, may be demonstrated by CT as round opacities 3–4 mm in diameter. These opacities are seen either along the anterior or posterior subpleural convexity of the lung field. Bullae appear as areas of low attenuation, devoid of blood vessels, and without a clear wall. In difficult cases, CT provides reliable information about the lung parenchyma and allows more sensitive follow-up of established abnormalities.

V. Gallium Scanning

Although gallium scanning will be discussed more extensively in another section, some mention of it will be made here in relation to radiological changes in sarcoidosis. Because gallium-67 citrate concentrates in metabolically active soft tissue lesions, it can be used to identify areas of pathology of the lung. Increased pulmonary uptake of gallium has been reported for a large number of neoplastic and inflammatory conditions. Hence, the nonspecificity of abnormal gallium deposition has limited its usefulness in differential diagnosis. However, it may be helpful for determining the degree of activity of a known disease process, the response to treatment, the spatial extent of the disease, and the presence of radiographically unsuspected disease foci (Siemsen et al. 1976).

The uptake of gallium by lung tissue of patients with sarcoidosis was noted by Langhammer et al. (1972) and by McKusick et al. (1973) who reported increased uptake in the mediastinum in patients with stage 1 sarcoidosis. Heshiki et al. (1974) reported gallium accumulation in hilar lymph nodes in eight patients with sarcoidosis who had normal chest radiographs. Uptake is less marked in patients with recent onset of adenopathy than in patients with asymptomatic adenopathy of long duration (Israel et al. 1976). Patients whose parenchymal disease is clearly apparent from their chest radiographs also exhibit consistent and striking gallium uptake. In fact, gallium scanning is more sensitive than chest radiography in showing pulmonary involvement (Nosal et al. 1979). In 20–25% of patients with sarcoidosis the spatial extent of the increased gallium deposition was substantially larger than the extent of the radiographic abnormality (Siemsen et al. 1976). This difference may indicate that gallium is detecting abnormal lung tissue before the appearance of radiographically discernible changes. No difference in gallium uptake was apparent for patients with stage 2A or 2B disease (Israel et al. 1976). Gallium uptake was suppressed by corticosteroid therapy (Heshiki et al. 1974, Israel et al. 1976, McKusick et al. 1973). The more frequent occurrence of gallium accumulation in acute as opposed to chronic sarcoidosis may indicate that uptake of gallium is related to the activity of the disease (Higasi 1969). This possible relationship is discussed in another chapter.

VI. Childhood Sarcoidosis

Sarcoidosis is relatively uncommon in children. It is diagnosed in symptomatic patients at a considerably later stage than in adults. Siltzback and Greenberg (1968) suggested that clinically silent intrathoracic sarcoidosis, detectable only by chest radiography, may remain unrecognized until symptoms appear, or may develop and resolve spontaneously during adolescence without detection. In a recent series of childhood sarcoidosis reported by Merten et al. (1980) radiographic abnormalities associated with pulmonary sarcoidosis were observed in 24 (92%) of 26 patients. Lymph node enlargement involving the major thoracic nodal groups was observed

in every patient. Bilateral hilar adenopathy was noted in all cases.
Bilateral paratracheal adenopathy with hilar adenopathy is more common
in children (88%) than in adults (33%) (Kirks et al. 1973). Pulmonary
parenchymal involvement was radiographically demonstrated during the
course of the disease in 63% of children (Merten et al. 1980). The
degree of pulmonary involvement shown on the chest radiograph at the
time of diagnosis is not always indicative of ultimate prognosis. The
prognosis in children is more favorable than in adults (Kendig and
Brummer 1976).

VII. Unusual Manifestations

A. Calcification

Calcification in lymph nodes occurs in about 5% of cases of sarcoidosis
(Dunbar 1978, Rabinowitz et al. 1974, Scadding 1970). Usually it is a
late manifestation associated with advanced pulmonary disease and, in

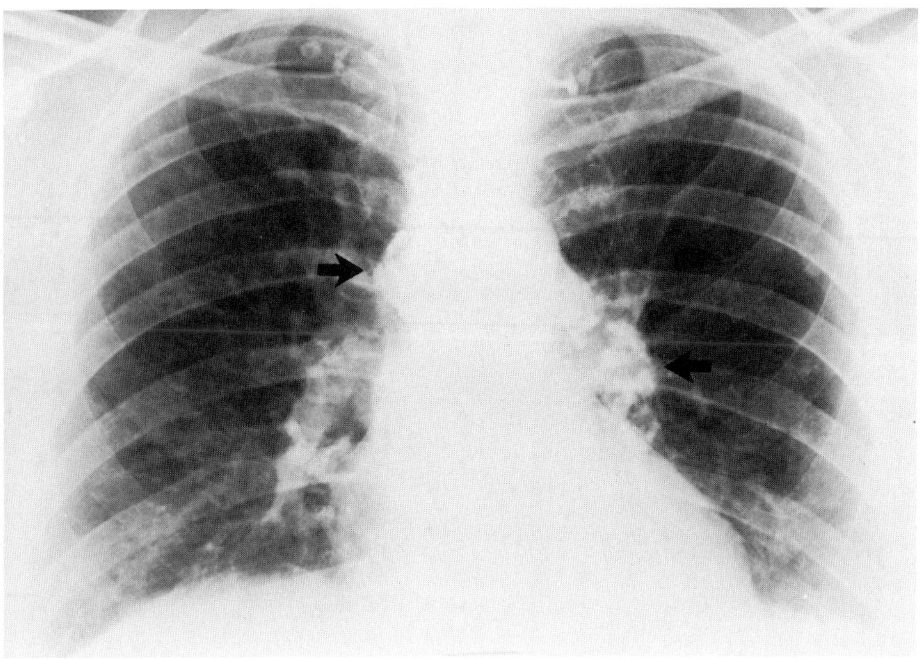

12a

Figure 12 PA (a) and lateral (b) chest radiographs shows egg shell calcification in hilar, paratracheal, and anterior mediastinal lymph node groups
(arrows). (From McLoud et al. [1974].)

some instances, with steroid therapy. Calcific deposits occur in areas where
lymph node enlargement occurred earlier, and is, therefore, predominantly
located in the hilar and paratracheal groups of nodes (Scadding 1970). The
calcification may be solid, although curvilinear deposition outlining the
periphery of the lymph nodes occurs, resembling the classic egg shell
calcification previously described for silicosis (McLoud et al. 1974)
(Fig. 12a, b). Calcification occurs in areas of ischemic fibrous tissue
(Scadding 1970). This usually follows the conversion of nonresolved
granulomas into areas of fibrosis and, therefore, accounts for its close
association with chronic pulmonary disease. Figure 13a and b shows

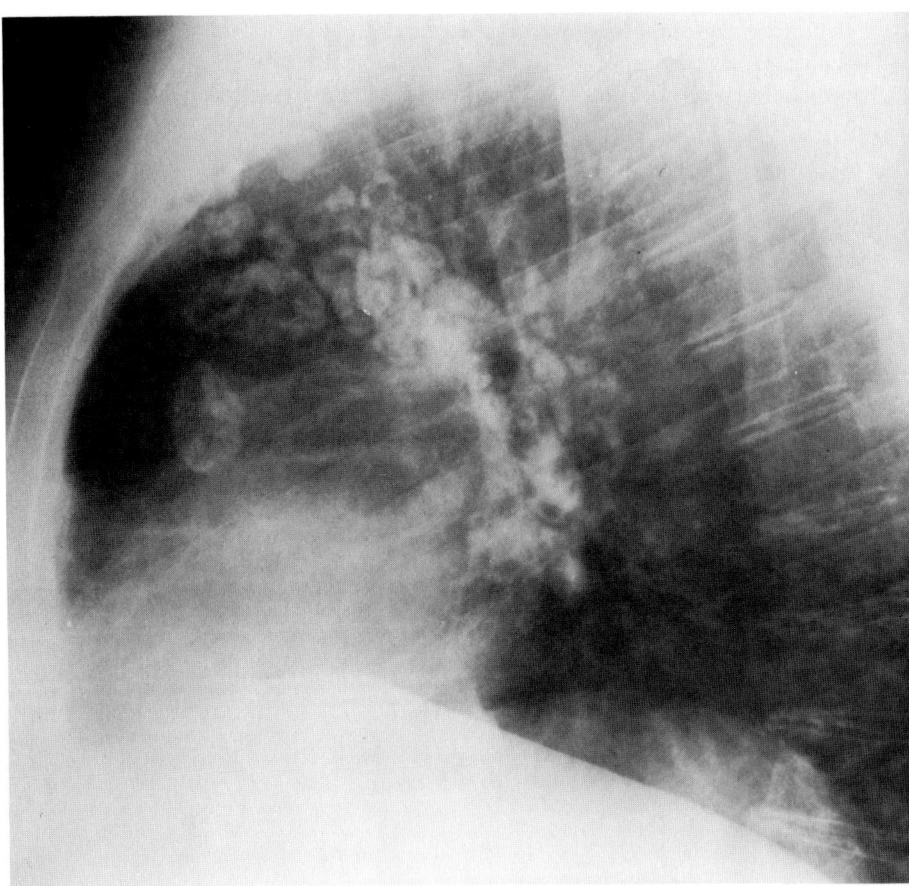

12b

calcification associated with fibrosis, in this case also involving the mediastinum. The reason for the rare calcification of the enlarged lymph nodes in sarcoidosis is not clear. This is in contrast to the other granulomatous infections that commonly calcify. Minimal calcific deposits can easily be detected by CT. Recent observations with CT show that calcification of lymph nodes may well accompany sarcoidosis in its earlier stages. CT will be able to detect more calcified nodes, since it is many times more sensitive in detecting calcification than conventional radiography.

B. Pleural Effusion

Pleural involvement occurs in 0.7–4% of patients with sarcoidosis and thus is an unusual entity (Kirks and Greenspan 1973). This may consist of

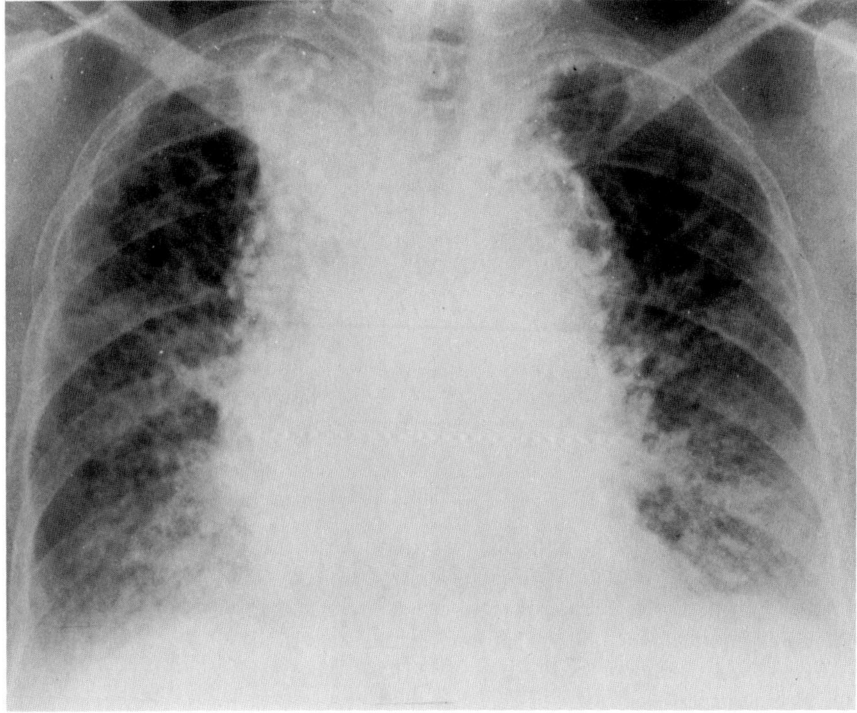

13a

Figure 13 (a and b) Marked widening of the mediastinum in stage 3 sarcoidosis with calcific fibrosing mediastinitis. Parenchymal fibrotic changes are also present. Superior vena cava syndrome was noted.

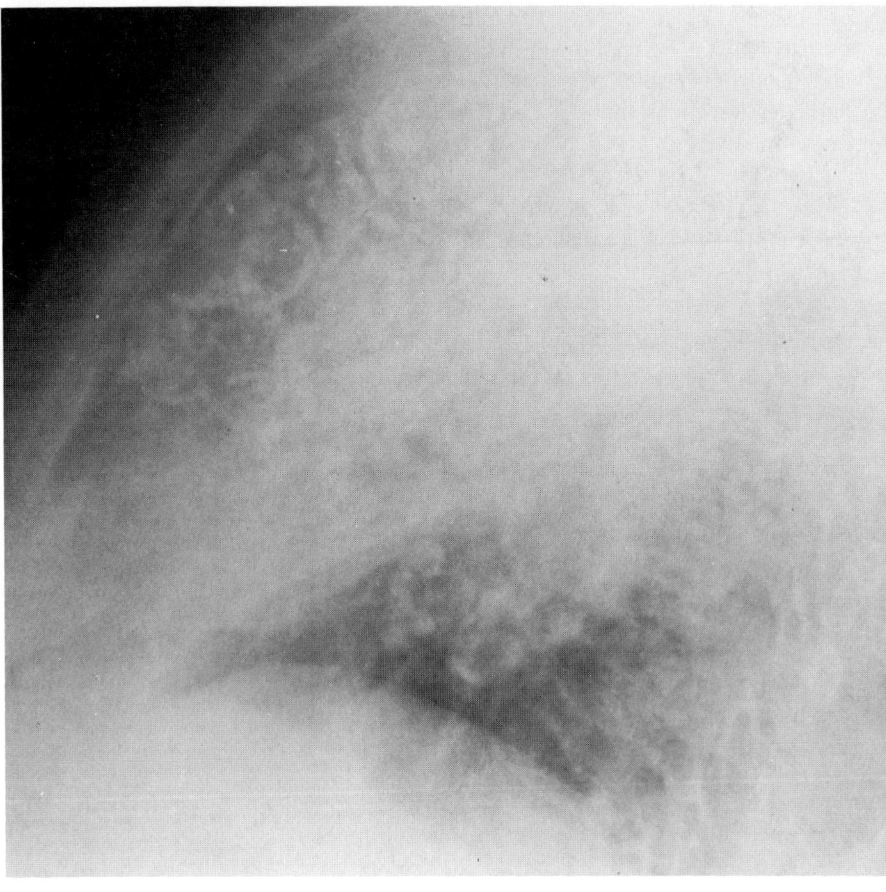

13b

extensive involvement of both the visceral and parietal pleura by granulomatous disease, with or without effusion (see Fig. 14 for a radiological
example). Extensive pleural disease can be present without chest radiographic abnormalities. Pleural disease is also associated with a diffuse
parenchymal component. Wilen et al. (1974) concluded that pleural
involvement appeared to be associated with progressive disease and may
represent part of the spectrum of dissemination of sarcoidosis. Pleural
effusions tend to clear in 4–8 weeks but some progress to chronic pleural
thickening. Tuberculosis, congestive heart failure, renal failure, fungal
disease, and neoplasia may also be the cause of pleural involvement in a
patient with sarcoidosis and must be excluded. Pleural sarcoidosis is not a

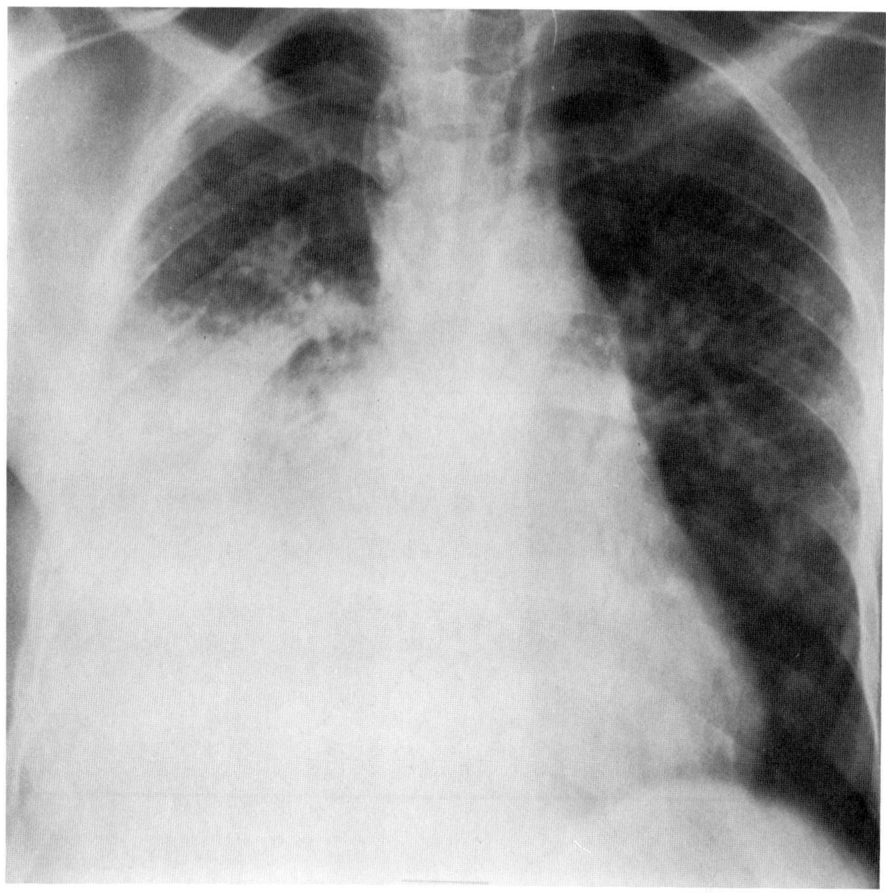

Figure 14 Large right pleural effusion with reticulonodular pattern. Bilateral paratracheal adenopathy is present. Pleural biopsy confirmed noncaseating granuloma, which was culture negative. (From Littner et al. [1977].)

diagnosis that can be made on the basis of radiographic findings alone, but must be established by biopsy demonstration of noncaseating granulomas.

CT is again changing the classic radiographic descriptions of sarcoidosis by demonstrating an increased incidence of pleural disease. Solomon et al. (1979) found at least minor pleural changes evident in 35% of patients with sarcoidosis by CT. They detected two small pleural effusions not suspected on chest radiography. By use of CT attenuation coefficient numbers and decubitus positioning, CT can differentiate among mobile pleural effusions, loculated effusions, and pleural thickening.

C. Cavitation

Cavitation is uncommon in sarcoidosis, occurring in 0.6–3% of reported series of cases (Mayock et al. 1963). Cavitation is found in sites of diffuse infiltrative sarcoidosis, the more chronic debilitating form of the disease. The pathogenesis is not clearly established, but may be related to the expulsion of hyaline material or ischemic necrotic tissue from the center of

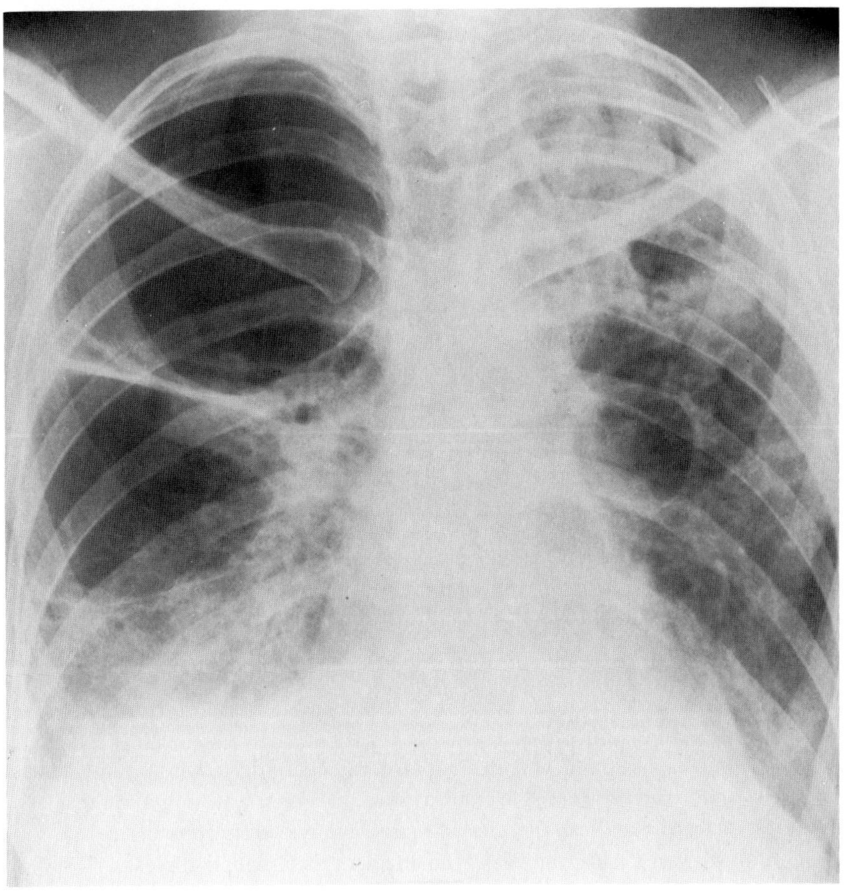

Figure 15a Stage 3 sarcoidosis with diffuse parenchymal fibrosis and large bullae, particularly in the right upper lobe.

large conglomerate sarcoid granulomas (Fraser and Pare' 1978). It is important to eliminate all other causes of cavitation before accepting sarcoidosis as the underlying etiology (Gorskee and Fleming 1970). The diagnosis is made by the exclusion of pulmonary tuberculosis and pathogenic

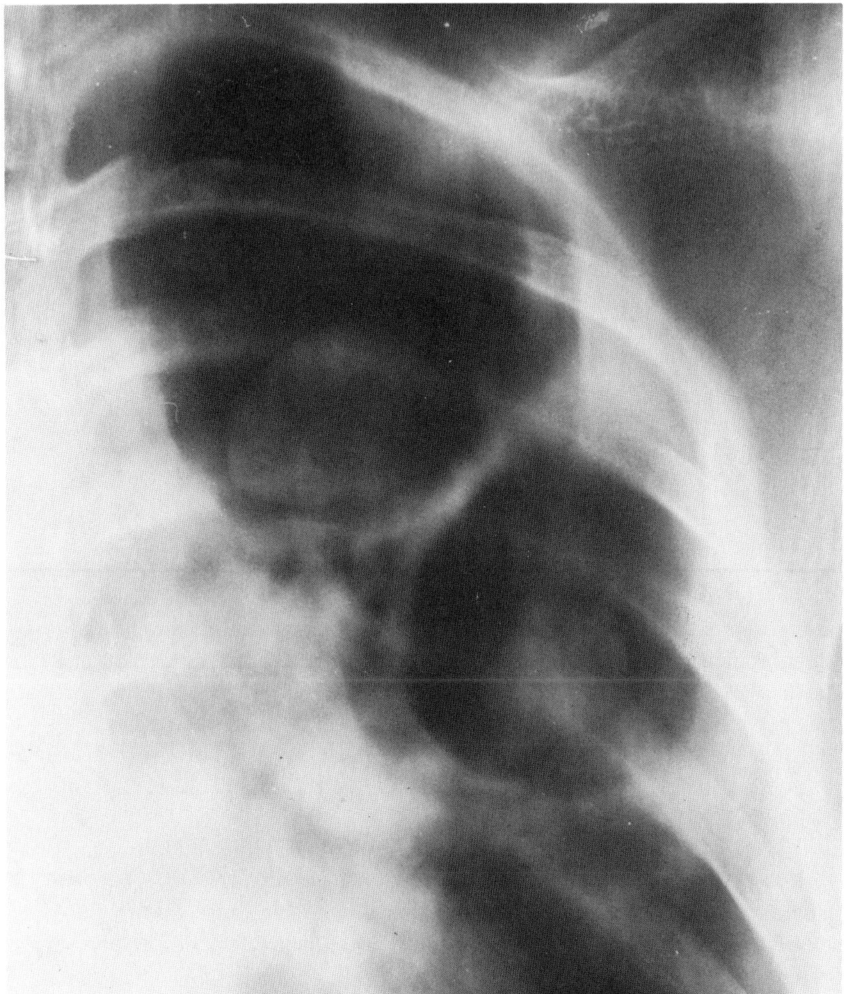

Figure 15b A tomogram of the same patient several years later shows the development of left upper lobe bullae containing mycetoma. The patient presented with hemoptysis at this time.

fungal diseases, e.g., histoplasmosis, blastomycosis, and coccidioidomycosis, as well as structural changes which can masquerade as cavities, for example, emphysematous bullae and bronchiectatic segments. With cavitating fungal infection associated with a pleural effusion the patient is usually very ill. This is in contrast to patients with uncomplicated cavitary sarcoidosis who are relatively asymptomatic and have associated adenopathy but lack an effusion (Gorskee and Fleming 1970). The series by Mayock et al. (1963) had a coexisting tuberculosis rate of 3.6% in 1254 cases and, with cavitation, tuberculosis must be excluded.

The natural history of the cavity in sarcoidosis is not known. Gorskee and Fleming (1970) found that cavities associated with sarcoidosis may remain unchanged for many years, may contain a mycetoma that may persist (Fig. 15a, b) or disappear. The distribution of the cavities is predominantly in the midlung zones. Routine tomography (Freundlich et al. 1970) and computed tomography (Putman et al. 1977) more readily identify cavities obscured by extensive parenchymal disease. It has been found that the larger the cavity the greater the incidence of associated mycetoma (Fraser and Pare' 1978). Aspergillus and candida are recognized fungi occurring in those mycetomas (Fraser and Pare' 1978). In this form they do not invade lung parenchyma but rather appear as secondary invaders at sites of preexisting disease. The appearance of a mycetoma therefore demonstrates nothing other than bronchial communication and possibly a decreased host resistance to the saprophytic fungus.

D. Atelectasis

Involvement of main, lobar, segmental, and large subsegmental bronchi in sarcoidosis is well recognized. Such patients are normally asymptomatic. Endobronchial sarcoidosis occurs often enough that blind biopsy of the tracheobronchial tree has been suggested as a diagnostic modality. Forty percent of stage 1 patients and 70% of stages 2 and 3 patients have positive transbronchial biopsies (Friedman et al. 1963). However, atelectasis is a rare manifestation, occurring in 1% of cases (Freundlich et al. 1970, Rabinowitz et al. 1974).

Occlusion of the bronchus may be caused by either endobronchial disease or extrinsic compression of the bronchus secondary to lymph node enlargement, although the latter is doubtful as a sole cause due to the infrequency of atelectasis contrasted to the frequency of lymphadenopathy (Freundlich et al. 1970). Bronchial narrowing is occasionally seen in the later stages of sarcoidosis and has a characteristic distribution; it affects the proximal portions of segmental and subsegmental bronchi or produces a long, smooth narrowing of the main bronchi. Endobronchial involvement that is sufficient to cause lobar or segmental atelectasis occurs, but is rare. An example is shown in Figure 16. The specific lesion causing bronchial obstruction must be documented by biopsy.

E. Laryngeal Sarcoidosis

Involvement of the larynx in sarcoidosis is rare, occurring in 1–2% of cases (Fraser and Pare' 1978). Although most cases are asymptomatic, there are isolated case reports of symptomatic patients (Firooznia et al. 1970). These patients exhibit dyspnea, hoarseness, and a nonspecific feeling of tightness. Airway obstruction can occur and may be severe enough to require tracheostomy (Carasso 1974).

F. Pulmonary Vascular Disease

The pulmonary vasculature, especially the small and medium-sized vessels, is frequently involved in sarcoidosis. Pathologically, the granulomas tend to

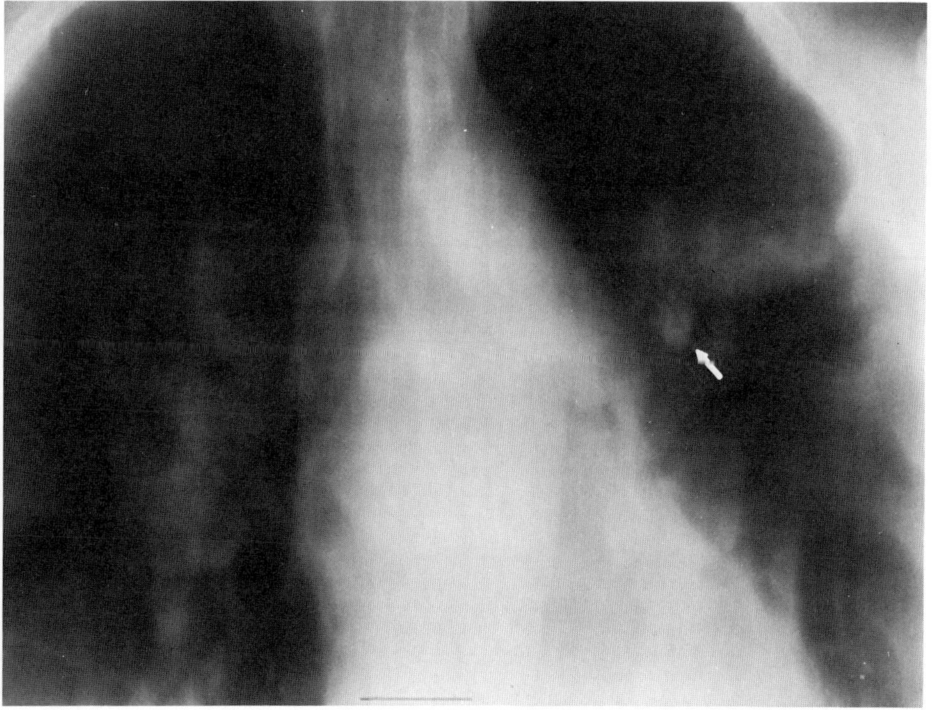

Figure 16 An AP tomogram reveals calcified endobronchial granuloma in the left upper lobe bronchus with distal atelectasis (arrow).

surround the blood vessels and cause a loss of alveolocapillary surface for gas transfer and a reduced diffusing capacity (Westcott and DeGraff 1973). Less frequently, granulomas infiltrate the vessel walls and, rarely, lead to intimal involvement or vascular thrombosis. The radiological detection of these changes is extremely difficult. When pulmonary hypertension is present central pulmonary vascular enlargement and peripheral vascular attenuation may also be present (Fig. 17). Westcott and DeGraff (1973) described a case of hilar lymphadenopathy which narrowed a major pulmonary artery and simulated pulmonary embolism both clinically and on radionuclide lung scan. The pathogenesis of pulmonary artery narrowing that is secondary to sarcoid lymphadenopathy may be similar to that described for bronchial narrowing.

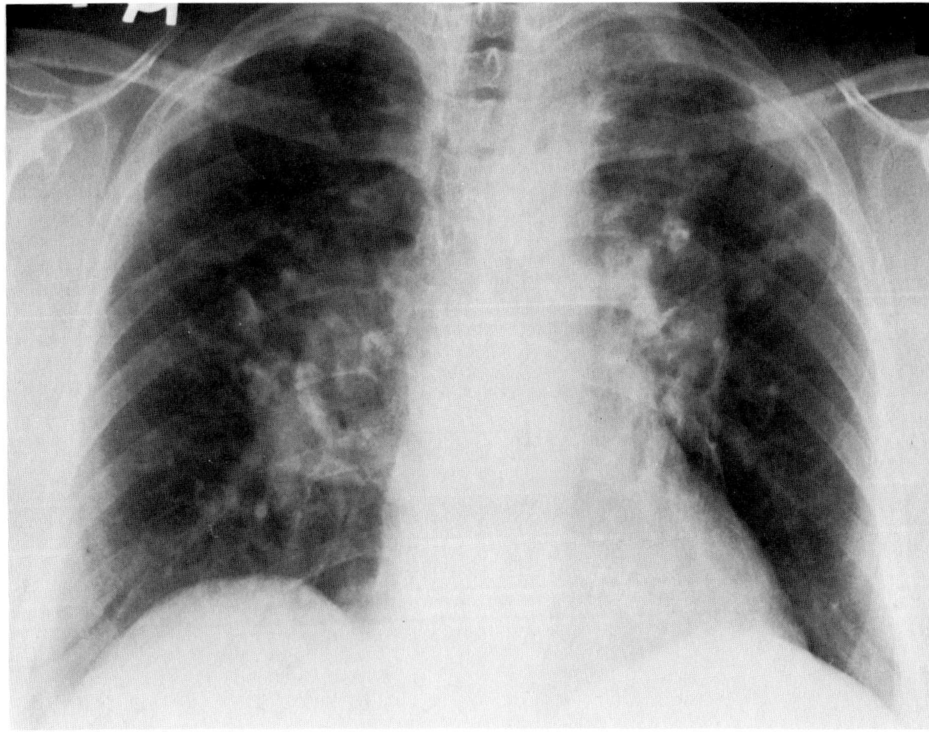

Figure 17 Pulmonary hypertension in sarcoidosis with central enlargement of the pulmonary vessels, peripheral vascular attenuation, and right-sided heart enlargement.

Sarcoidosis may also have an associated vasculitis or arteritis which differs from the pulmonary vascular involvement that occurs in the presence of interstitial disease. Vasculitis can occur without associated parenchymal involvement and is usually not radiographically detectable.

G. Cardiac Involvement

Myocardial involvement is common in sarcoidosis. Up to one-fourth of autopsy subjects with sarcoidosis have cardiac lesions (Silverman et al. 1978) and as many as one-half of living patients with sarcoidosis have been reported to have electrocardiographic abnormalities (Schuster et al. 1980).

Cardiomegaly has been reported radiologically without any other known predisposing etiology in 4–8% of patients with sarcoidosis (Fraser and Pare'

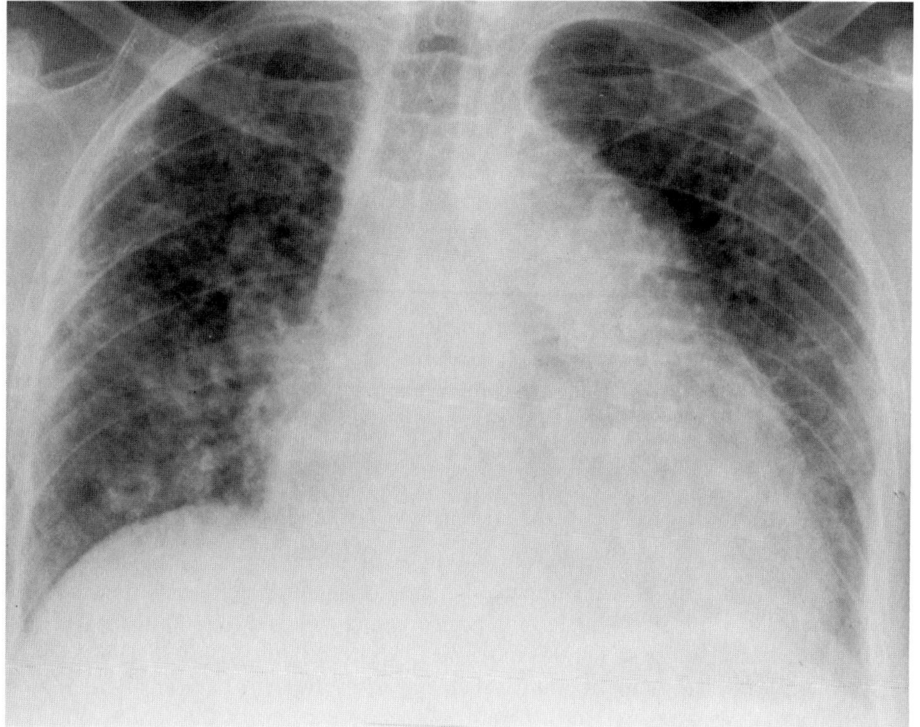

Figure 18 Cardiac involvement in sarcoidosis is demonstrated by cardiomegaly and arrhythmia on electrocardiogram. A coarse reticular fibrotic pattern is present.

1978, Kirks et al. 1973) (Fig. 18 for example). Heart disease in sarcoidosis may be due to direct myocardial involvement, usually manifest by arrhythmias, or it may be secondary to the lung disease (Mayock et al. 1963). Significant electrocardiographic abnormalities, such as right bundle branch block, may be the only indication of myocardial involvement by sarcoid granulomas (Tolbot et al. 1959). Valvular insufficiency may also occur. In one series of cases, all patients with myocardial disease had associated fibrotic parenchymal involvement, usually substantiated by clinical and electrocardiographic evidence of cor pulmonale. The cardiomegaly is predominantly an enlargement of the right ventricle. Serial chest radiographs are invaluable for evaluating changes in cardiac contour. Pericardial disease noted by chest radiographs or echocardiographic evaluation is infrequent. Cardiopericardial involvement is an indication for more aggressive treatment.

H. Pneumothorax

Spontaneous pneumothorax is reported in 1–3% of patients with sarcoidosis (Dunbar 1978, Kirks et al. 1973) (Fig. 19 for example). All of these patients had extensive pulmonary parenchymal involvement (Freundlich et al. 1970). Diffuse cystic changes called honeycomb lung are due to parenchymal infiltration by granulomas and subsequent fibrosis. The pathologic changes include transformation of the alveoli and bronchioles into small cystic dilatations and thickening of the interstitial septae. There is a tendency for the cysts to enlarge and this may eventually lead to rupture and spontaneous pneumothorax (Tolbot et al. 1959). These pneumothoraces are rarely under tension with mediastinal structures shifted toward the opposite hemithorax. However, development of a pneumothorax superimposed on already compromised pulmonary function may be a serious condition requiring immediate intervention.

VIII. Prognostic Indicators

As noted elsewhere in this book, two-thirds of patients with sarcoidosis recover completely or with minimal residual changes. Asymptomatic patients are more likely to have a benign course and those with symptoms are less likely to do so (Jones and Israel 1960, Smellie and Hoyle 1960). Patients with symptomatic multisystem organ involvement have an increased incidence of progression and, therefore, a worse prognosis. Regression of disease is most frequent in patients whose onset is with erythema nodosum; next in frequency are those with asymptomatic hilar adenopathy; and least frequent regressions occur in those having pulmonary involvement at the

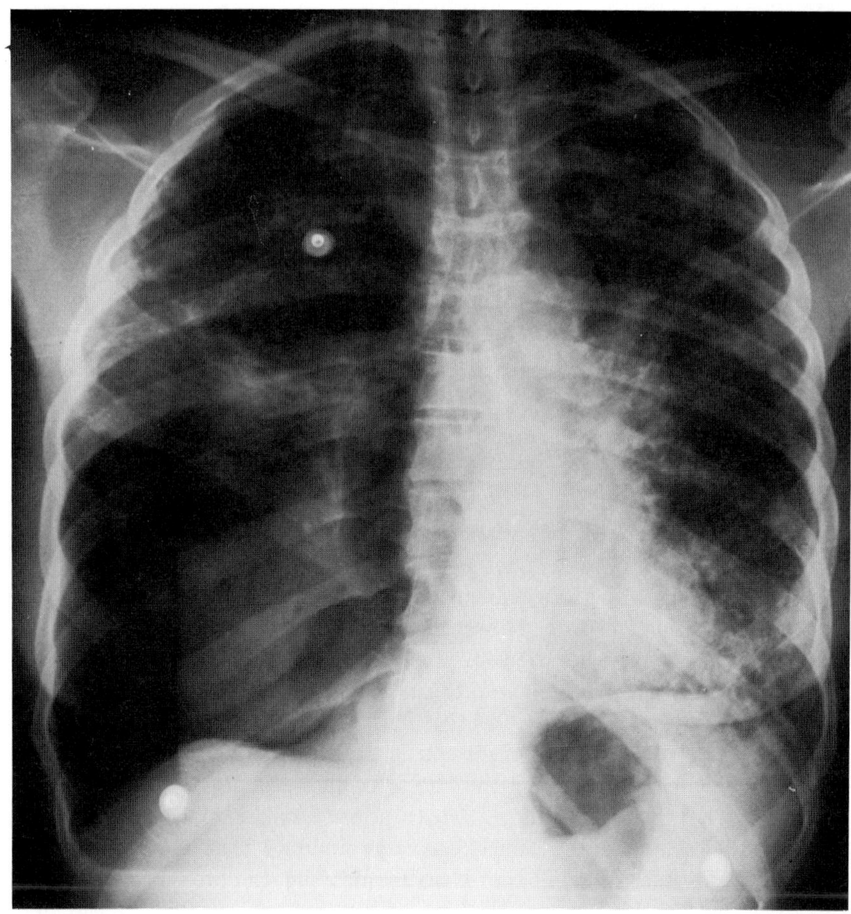

Figure 19 Spontaneous right tension pneumothorax in sarcoidosis with depression of the right hemidiaphragm and shift of the mediastinum to the left. Parenchymal opacities with a nodular component are present.

time of initial presentation (Scadding 1967). When the disease has been "active" for at least 3 years the prognosis is poorer and such patients rarely have complete resolution of disease (Stone and Schwartz 1966).

Radiographic appearance does not correlate well with functional impairment. In general, the usual interpretation of the chest radiograph does not provide enough specific information to suggest prognosis or even to determine the extent of pulmonary disability (Stone and Schwartz 1966).

Although more refined examinations such as pulmonary function tests should be performed to determine the exact patient status, certain specific radiographic features may be of some prognostic value. These include shrinkage of lung volume, appearance of multiple small bullae, and hilar retraction, changes characteristic of the fibrotic stage of sarcoidosis. Once present, they are permanent and usually associated with some degree of pulmonary impairment (Stone and Schwartz 1966). As mentioned elsewhere, a disparity may exist between the pulmonary diffusing capacity and the chest radiograph. Infiltrative pulmonary disease on chest radiography may be associated with normal pulmonary diffusing capacity, and a chest radiograph showing clear lungs may be associated with grossly abnormal diffusing capacity and changes in arterial gas tensions (Young et al. 1966).

IX. Summary

The radiological diagnosis of sarcoidosis can be made with a considerable degree of accuracy. The symmetry of the bilateral hilar lymph node enlargement along with the frequent association of paratracheal lymphadenopathy is characteristic. However, almost all lymph node groups within the thorax may be affected. In addition to the standard chest radiograph, barium swallow, conventional tomography, and computed tomography may more readily identify sites of lymph node enlargement.

Pulmonary parenchymal involvement is noted in two-thirds of patients with sarcoidosis during the course of their disease. The parenchymal involvement is often symmetrical. Three primary radiographic patterns are recognized: reticulonodular, acinar, and large nodular. The discrepancy between the extensive radiological changes and mild clinical symptoms is also of diagnostic significance. The unusual radiographic manifestations of sarcoidosis include lymph node calcification, pleural effusion, cardiomegaly, and atelectasis.

In patients with lymph node enlargement alone, one cannot predict which patients will progress and which will clear. Patients with lung disease demonstrated radiologically without lymph node enlargement have a higher incidence of progressing to pulmonary fibrosis. The irreversible fibrotic lung disease is most important in terms of prognosis. Patients with extensive fibrosis are particularly susceptible to develop severe complications including respiratory failure, cor pulmonale, pneumothorax, mycetoma formation, or fatal intercurrent infection. The morbidity and mortality in sarcoidosis is directly related to the involvement of the pulmonary parenchyma and more specifically to the ensuing complications.

Acknowledgment

The authors wish to express their appreciation to Dr. Laurence Hedlund for his editorial assistance in the preparation of this chapter.

References

Beekman, J. F., Zimmet, S. M. Chun, B. K., Miranda, A. A., and Katy, S. (1976). Spectrum of pleural involvement in sarcoidosis. *Arch. Intern. Med.,* **136**:323–330.

Bein, M. E., Putman, C. E., McLoud, T. C., and Mink, J. H. (1978). A reevaluation of intrathoracic lymphadenopathy in sarcoidosis. *Am. J. Radiol.,* **131**:409–415.

Berkman, Y. M., and Javors, B. R. (1976). Anterior mediastinal lymphadenopathy in sarcoidosis. *Am. J. Radiol.,* **127**:983–987.

Carasso, B. (1974). Sarcoidosis of the larynx causing airway obstruction. *Chest,* **65**:693–695.

Dunbar, R. D. (1978). Sarcoidosis and its radiologic manifestations. *CRC Crit. Rev. Diag. Imag.,* Dec:185–221.

Ellis, K., and Renthal, G. (1962). Pulmonary sarcoidosis: Roentgenographic observations on course of disease. *Am. J. Radiol.,* **88**:1070–1083.

Firooznia, H., Young, R., and Lee, T. (1970). Sarcoidosis of the larynx. *Radiology,* **95**:425–428.

Fraser, R. G., and Pare', J. A. P. (1978). *Diagnosis of Diseases of the Chest.* Philadelphia, Saunders, pp. 1665–1678.

Freundlich, I. M., Libshitz, H. I., Glassman, L. M., and Israel, H. L. (1970). Sarcoidosis. Typical and atypical thoracic manifestations and complications. *Clin. Radiol.,* **21**:376–383.

Friedman, O. H., Blaugrund, S. M., and Siltzbach, L. E. (1963). Biopsy of the bronchial wall as an aid in diagnosis of sarcoidosis. *JAMA,* **183**: 646–650.

Gorskee, K. J., and Fleming, R. J. (1970). Mycetoma formation in cavitary pulmonary sarcoidosis. *Radiology,* **95**:279–285.

Heshiki, A., Schatz, S. L., McKusick, K. A., Bowersox, D. W., and Soin, J. S. (1974). Gallium-67 citrate scanning in patients with pulmonary sarcoidosis. *Am. J. Radiol.,* **122**:744–749.

Higasi, T. (1969). Clinical evaluation of gallium-67 citrate scanning. *J. Nucl. Med.,* **10**:103–105.

Israel, H. L., Pask, C. H., and Mansfield, C. M. (1976). Gallium scanning in sarcoidosis. *Ann. NY Acad. Sci.,* **278**:514–516.

Jones, M., and Israel, H. L. (1960). Course and prognosis of sarcoidosis.
  Am. J. Med., **29**:84–93.
Karasick, S. R. (1979). Atypical thoracic lymphadenopathy in sarcoidosis.
  Am. J. Radiol., **133**:928–929.
Kendig, E. L., and Brummer, D. L. (1976). The prognosis of sarcoidosis
  in children. *Chest,* **70**:351–353.
Kirks, D. R., and Greenspan, R. H. (1973). Sarcoid. *Radiol. Clin. North
  Am.,* **11**:279–294.
Kirks, D. R., McCormick, V. D., and Greenspan, R. H. (1973). Pulmonary
  sarcoidosis. Roentgenologic analysis of 150 patients. *Am. J. Radiol.,*
  117:777–786.
Langhammer, H., Glaubitt, G., Grebe, S. F., Hampe, J. F., Haubold, V.,
  Hor, G., Kaul, A., Koeppe, P., Koppenagen, J., Roedler, H. D., and
  van der Schoot, J. B. (1972). Gallium-67 for tumor scanning. *J.
  Nucl. Med.,* **13**:25–30.
Littner, M. R., Schachter, E. N., Putman, C. E., Odero, D. O., and Gee,
  J. B. L. (1977). A clinical assessment of roentgenographically
  atypical pulmonary sarcoidosis. *Am. J. Med.,* **62**:361–368.
Mayock, R. L., Bertrand, P., Morrison, C. E., and Scott, J. H. (1963).
  Manifestations of sarcoidosis: Analysis of 145 patients with a review
  of nine series selected from the literature. *Am. J. Med.,* **35**:67–89.
McCort, J. J., and Pare', P. J. (1954). Pulmonary fibrosis and cor pul-
  monale in sarcoidosis. *Am. J. Radiol.,* **62**:496–504.
McKusick, K. A., Soin, J. S., Ghiladi, A., and Wagner, N. H. (1973).
  Gallium accumulation in pulmonary sarcoid. *JAMA,* **223**:688.
McLoud, T. C., Putman, C. E., and Pascual, R. (1974). Eggshell calcifica-
  tion with systemic sarcoidosis. *Chest,* **66**:515–517.
Merten, D. R., Kirks, K. R., and Grossman, H. (1980). Pulmonary
  sarcoidosis in childhood. *Am. J. Radiol.,* **135**:673–679.
Nosal, A., Schleissner, L. A., Michkin, F. S., and Lieberman, J. (1979).
  Angiotensin-1-converting enzyme and gallium scan in noninvasive
  evaluation of sarcoidosis. *Ann. Intern. Med.,* **90**:328–331.
Putman, C. E., Rothman, S. L., Littner, M. R., Allen, W. E., Schachter, E.
  N., McLoud, T. C., Bein, M. E., and Gee, J. B. L. (1977). Com-
  puterized tomography in pulmonary sarcoidosis. *Comput. Tomog.,*
  1:197–209.
Rabinowitz, J. G., Ulreich, S., and Soriano, C. (1974). The usual
  unusual manifestations of sarcoidosis and the "hilar haze"—A new
  diagnostic aid. *Am. J. Radiol.,* **120**:821–831.
Sahn, S. A., Schwartz, M. I., and Lakshminarayan, S. (1974). Sarcoidosis:
  The significance of an acinar pattern on chest roentgenogram.
  Chest, **65**:684–687.

Scadding, J. G. (1961). Prognosis of intrathoracic sarcoidosis in England. A review of 136 cases after five years observation. *Br. Med. J.,* **2**:1165–1172.

Scadding, J. G. (1967). *Sarcoidosis.* London, Eyre and Spottiswoode, pp. 81, 166, 190.

Scadding, J. G. (1970). The late stages of pulmonary sarcoidosis. *Postgrad. Med. J.,* **46**:530–536.

Schabel, S. I., Foote, G. A., and McKee, K. A. (1978). Posterior lymphadenopathy in sarcoidosis. *Am. J. Radiol.,* **129**:591–593.

Schuster, E. H., Conrad, G., Morris, F., Fisher, M. L., Carliner, N. H., Plotnick, G. D., and Greene, H. L. (1980). Systemic sarcoidosis and electrocardiographic conduction abnormalities. *Chest,* **78**:601–604.

Sharma, O. P. (1975). *Sarcoidosis: A Clinical Approach,* 1st ed. Springfield, Charles C Thomas, p. 30.

Siemsen, J. K., Grebe, S. F., Sargent, E. N., and Wentz, D. (1976). Gallium-67 scintigraphy of pulmonary diseases as a complement to radiography. *Radiology,* **118**:371–375.

Silverman, K. J., Hutchins, G. M., and Bulkley, B. H. (1978). Cardiac sarcoid: A clinicopathologic study of 84 unselected patients with systemic sarcoidosis. *Circulation,* **58**:1204–1211.

Siltzbach, L. E., and Greenberg, G. M. (1968). Childhood sarcoidosis—A study of 18 patients. *N. Engl. J. Med.,* **279** 23:1239–1245.

Smellie, H., and Hoyle, C. (1960). The natural history of pulmonary sarcoidosis. *Q. J. Med.,* **29**:539–558.

Solomon, A., Kreel, L., McNicol, M., and Johnson, N. (1979). Computed tomography in pulmonary sarcoidosis. *JCAT,* **3**:754–758.

Stone, D. J., and Schwartz, A. (1966). A long-term study of sarcoid and its modification by steroid therapy. *Am. J. Med.,* **41**:528–540.

Tolbot, F. J., Katz, S., and Matthews, M. J. (1959). Bronchopulmonary sarcoidosis. Some unusual manifestations and the serious complications thereof. *Am. J. Med.,* **26**:340–355.

Westcott, J. L., and DeGraff, A. C., Jr. (1973). Sarcoidosis, hilar adenopathy and pulmonary artery narrowing. *Radiology,* **108**:585–586.

Wilen, S. B., Rabinowitz, J. G., Ulreich, S., and Lyons, H. A. (1974). Pleural involvement in sarcoid. *Am. J. Med.,* **57**:200–209.

Winterbauer, R. H., and Hutchinson, J. F. (1980). Use of pulmonary function tests in the management of sarcoidosis. *Chest,* **78**:640–647.

Young, R. L., Kurmholz, R. A., and Harkleroad, L. E. (1966). A physiologic roentgenographic disparity in sarcoidosis. *Dis. Chest.,* **50**:81–86.

3

Pulmonary Function in Sarcoidosis

M. HENRY WILLIAMS, JR.

Albert Einstein College of Medicine
Bronx, New York

I. Introduction

During the past 50 years a large number and a wide variety of pulmonary function studies have been carried out on patients with sarcoidosis. Although there is some disagreement about the details, there is general consensus that any aspect of lung function may be abnormal in this disease and that the type and degree of abnormality relate to the location and the extent of the pathology. Although there is a relationship between functional changes and the extent of involvement on the x-ray film of the chest, there are notable discrepancies. It is well known that microscopic evidence of disease is frequently present in the lungs of patients with sarcoidosis in whom the x-ray films of the chest are normal. Pathology is more commonly reflected in abnormality of pulmonary function, particularly of diffusion, but even the most sensitive test may fail to detect the morphological changes.

For example, patients with stage I sarcoidosis (bilateral hilar adenopathy with normal x-ray film of the chest) frequently have abnormalities of pulmonary function, but even more frequently show microscopic disease on lung biopsy if sufficient tissue is available for examination. In contrast,

there are occasional patients with extensive abnormalities on the roentgenogram but with little symptomatology and normal pulmonary function.
This is a form of sarcoidosis in which localized visible lesions are not
associated with diffuse microscopic disease in other portions of the lung so
that function remains intact.

Although abnormal pulmonary function is common in sarcoidosis in
early stages, it is usually not associated with significant disability and it is of
little consequence to the patient. Functional abnormalities can be at
least partially reversed by corticosteroid therapy and, as will be discussed
later in this chapter, this may be one indication for such treatment
although it is not absolutely clear that maintenance of maximal lung
function is of great importance to the eventual outcome of the disease.
It also appears that early pulmonary function abnormalities may progress
very slowly with time, and spontaneous improvement, at least to normal
levels, is unusual.

This review will first consider studies of lung volume, diffusion, and
compliance, reflecting the pathological changes in the interstitium. Measurement of both small and large airway function will then be considered, and
this will be followed by studies of the pulmonary circulation and of
ventilation/perfusion relationships. Finally, the course of sarcoidosis with
respect to alterations of lung function and the acute and long-term impact
of corticosteroid therapy will be reviewed.

II. Functional Abnormalities

A. Lung Volumes, Diffusion, and Compliance

Since the earliest report of studies of lung function in 1940 (Bruce and
Wassen 1940) and the classical study of Baldwin and associates (1949) on
pulmonary fibrosis, it has been well known and amply confirmed that
sarcoidosis is frequently associated with reduction of lung volumes. This
familiar pattern of restrictive lung disease, always present when the x-ray
film of the chest reveals a diffuse abnormality, may even be present in the
absence of pronounced radiographic changes. Diffuse interstitial involvement is even more commonly reflected in reduction of the diffusing capacity,
the most common abnormality of pulmonary function in sarcoidosis
(Kanagami et al. 1961). Studies of the oxygen diffusing capacity (Kent
and Spence 1964, McClement et al. 1953, Riley et al. 1952, Williams 1953)
and of the carbon monoxide diffusing capacity measured by steady state
techniques at rest and exercise (Marshall et al. 1958, Renzi and Dutton
1974, Svanborg 1961) and by the single breath method (Boushy et al.
1965, Emergil et al. 1969, Lewis et al. 1965, Marshall and Karlish 1971,

Sharma et al. 1966a, 1966b, Young et al. 1968) have amply confirmed the frequency with which diffusion is impaired in sarcoidosis.

Figure 1 depicts a large number of measurements obtained in five different studies (Boushy et al. 1965, Emergil et al. 1969, Lewis et al. 1965, Sharma et al. 1966b, Young et al. 1968) of vital capacity and of diffusing capacity by single breath and steady state carbon monoxide techniques. It is clear that although vital capacity is commonly reduced, there is much more reduction of diffusing capacity. These results are highlighted by the frequent finding of a reduced diffusing capacity and, less commonly, of reduced vital capacity in patients with hilar adenopathy without abnormality of the lungs on x-ray film of the chest (DeRemee and Anderson 1974, Marshall and Karlish 1971, Miller et al. 1976, Sharma et al. 1966a, Ting and Williams 1965).

The data on five series of such patients are shown in Table 1. The variability is striking and not explained. The very low prevalence of impaired diffusion in the British series of Marshall and Karlish (1971) contrasts with the other data, particularly those of Svanborg (1961) and Sharma and associates (1966b). Possibly the British investigators selected patients with less extensive disease. The finding of impaired diffusion in patients with stage I sarcoidosis fits very nicely with the discovery of pathologic tissue on transbronchial biopsy in a large percentage of such patients (Poe et al. 1979). Huang and associates (1979) actually found granulomata and interstitial pneumonitis in all patients with normal pulmonary function studies and with normal x-ray films.

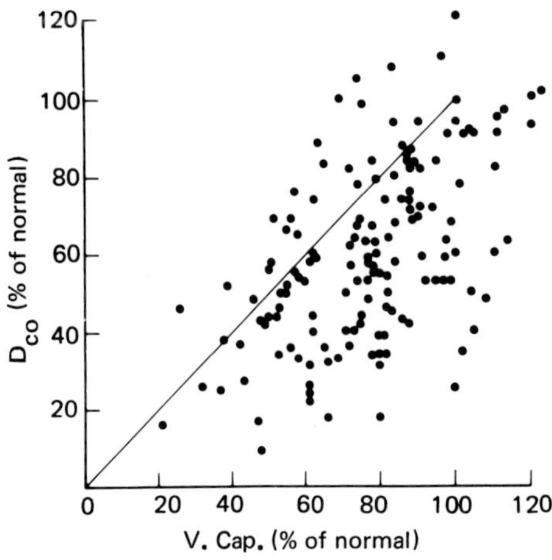

Figure 1 Relationship of diffusing capacity (D_{co}) to vital capacity (V. Cap.), both expressed as percentage of normal, in patients who had not received corticosteroid therapy, from five reports in the literature (Boushy et al. 1965, Emergil et al. 1969, Lewis et al. 1965, Sharma et al. 1966b, Young et al. 1968).

Table 1 Stage I Sarcoidosis

Reference	Percentage abnormal		No. of patients studied
	D_{co}	Vital capacity	
Svanborg (1961)	73	73	11
Marshall and Karlish (1971)	5	—	44
DeRemee and Anderson (1974)	19	0	21
Sharma et al. (1966a)	78	28	18
Miller et al. (1976)	55	20	25

Virtually all of these studies have shown that as disease becomes more evident on the x-ray film of the chest, impairment of diffusion and of vital capacity become more common. Miller and associates (1976) found a significant reduction of diffusing capacity and of vital capacity in stage II sarcoidosis as compared to stage I disease.

In more detailed studies of diffusion, Young and associates (1968) reported that a low D_{co} could be ascribed to reduction of either the membrane component (D_m) or the pulmonary capillary volume (V_c). However, Saumon and associates (1976) found that the D_m was the only abnormality in patients with either normal lungs or minimal changes on x-ray film of the chest, whereas V_c was reduced in subjects with roentgenographic evidence of interstitial disease. Hamer (1963) also described reduced D_m in many subjects with normal x-ray films and vital capacity, whereas V_c was also reduced in more advanced disease. In the latter study, the more extensive abnormalities were related to the duration of known radiographic abnormalities, and a similar relationship between impairment of diffusion and duration of disease was reported by Ting and Williams (1965). However, no such correlation between duration of disease and impairment of function has been found by others (Marshall and Karlish 1971, Young et al. 1968). It is possible that such a relationship is spurious since patients with mild disease and little impairment of function may never be studied or followed, whereas patients with more severe illness, persistent radiographic abnormalities, and symptoms are more apt to receive continuing attention and to have pulmonary function studies.

The diffuse interstitial involvement of the lung is also reflected in reduction of pulmonary compliance (Lewis et al. 1965, Lyons 1958, Marshall et al. 1958, Marshall and Karlish 1971, Sellers and Siebens 1965, Ting and Williams 1965). In general, as with diffusion, there is a significant relationship between the reductions of compliance and of vital capacity, but the compliance seems to be more affected (Lewis et al. 1965, Marshall and Karlish 1971, Ting and Williams 1965). Although in many cases the reduction of compliance is no more than would be predicted from reduction of lung volume (Lyons 1958, Marshall et al. 1958), the entire effect cannot be explained by reduction of volumes and there is undoubtedly a change in the elastic properties of the lung (Stone et al. 1953). Reduction of compliance, accompanied by resting hyperventilation (see below), may be an important cause of dyspnea in sarcoidosis, but DeRemee and Andersen (1974) found a closer relationship of shortness of breath to expiratory slowing from airway obstruction.

A number of attempts have been made to correlate functional abnormalities with morphological changes in the lung (Carrington et al. 1976, Huang et al. 1979, Snider and Doctor 1964, Young et al. 1967, 1968). By and large, the best correlation of the amount of interstitial disease, reflected in numbers of interstitial cells or alveolar wall thickness, is with reduction of diffusing capacity (Snider and Doctor 1964, Young et al. 1968). The degree of interstitial infiltration also correlates well with overall functional impairment (Carrington et al. 1976). Patients with beryllium disease have been reported to have slightly more physiological impairment and more interstitial pathology than patients with sarcoidosis having similar x-ray films (Carrington et al. 1976). However, pathologic-physiologic correlation may be difficult in studies such as these since a lung biopsy may not accurately reflect the overall pathology. A detailed morphometric study by Divertie and associates (1976), which included seven patients with sarcoidosis, rejected the hypothesis that thickening of the alveolar wall-blood gas barrier was responsible for impaired diffusion in sarcoidosis, in keeping with current concepts that ventilation/perfusion inhomogeneities and reduction of the number of functioning capillaries in the lung are responsible for most, if not all, of the reduced diffusing capacity measured in patients with diffuse interstitial disease of the lung.

Although emphasis has been placed on the contention that impairment of diffusion as well as reduction of lung volumes and of compliance are extremely common in sarcoidosis, much more so than are abnormalities on the x-ray film of the chest, there are rare examples of the opposite phenomenon in which pulmonary function is normal despite rather extensive radiographic changes. Young and associates (1966) reported five patients with sarcoidosis who had marked abnormalities on x-ray film of the chest but normal diffusion. In addition, other cases of nodular alveolar sarcoidosis, often mimicking carcinoma of the lung, have been found to have normal pulmonary function, including diffusion (Romer 1977, Williams 1953). Although these giant, confluent alveolar infiltrates may produce striking changes on the x-ray films, it is likely that the intervening paren-chyma is normal so that functional impairment is minimal or absent.

B. Airways

Although the abnormalities of pulmonary function discussed above reflect pathologic changes in the interstitium and have long been thought to be characteristic of sarcoidosis, it is now apparent that there is also frequent involvement of the airways. As might be expected, the prevalence of airway involvement bears a direct relationship to the sensitivity of the tests employed. In an increasing order of prevalence, there is an increase of airway resistance, reduction of expiratory flow rates, and abnormalities of small airway function reflected in closing volume and frequency dependence of compliance.

Coates and Comroe (1951) reported abnormalities in sarcoidosis consistent with airway obstruction, and they attributed this to pathologic involvement of the airways. Snider and Doctor (1964) reported elevation of airway resistance in six of 21 patients with sarcoidosis, all of whom had parenchymal infiltration on the chest roentgenogram, and Ting and Williams (1965) reported that three of 23 patients with reduced compliance had an increased airway resistance. Thus, large airway involvement sufficient to cause elevation of the airway resistance occurs in sarcoidosis, but much less frequently than do alterations reflecting parenchymal damage.

Miller and associates (1973) reported reduction of expiratory flow rates in the majority of patients with sarcoidosis associated with fibrosis whom they studied, and they pointed out that this was all the more significant because the increased lung recoil in these patients should have caused an increase of expiratory flow rate. Even in patients with stage I sarcoidosis, without abnormalities on the x-ray film of the chest, some reduction of expiratory flow rate is common. Eight of 18 such patients studied by Sharma and associates (1966a) had reduction of expiratory flow. Miller and associates (1976) reported a significantly higher prevalence of reduction of the maximal midexpiratory flow rate in patients with stage II as compared to stage I sarcoidosis.

More recent studies involving tests of small airway function have revealed an even higher frequency of abnormality. Levinson and associates (1977) studied 18 patients with restrictive lung disease of whom only two had had a decreased conductance, but multiple tests of small airways function revealed one or more abnormalities in all individuals. Specific conductance was reduced in two, eight of the patients had a reduction in frequency-dependence of compliance, and all but two had an increased closing volume. Radwan and associates (1978) studied 25 patients with stage I and II sarcoidosis who had normal spirograms. Only one had an increased airway resistance, approximately one-third had reduced flow rates at low lung volumes, and almost one-half had an increased alveolar nitrogen on the single breath test. In both of these studies, the abnormalities could not be ascribed to smoking. Thus, pathologic changes in the airways consisting of granuloma and fibrosis may be present in most patients with sarcoidosis. Rarely these changes are associated with sufficient narrowing of the large airways to cause increased airway resistance, and slightly more frequently with enough involvement to cause reduction of expiratory flow rates.

Nonetheless, obstructive disease can be the predominant feature of sarcoidosis. In a study of 107 patients, DeRemee and Andersen (1974) ascribed exertional dyspnea to expiratory slowing, and Benatar and Clark (1974) reported a patient with severe airway obstruction with a maximum midexpiratory flow rate of 0.11 L/sec due to sarcoidosis. Dines and associates (1978) described five patients with stage I sarcoidosis who had severe obstructive disease of the airways with evident expiratory slowing and, in four of them, exertional dyspnea. The large airway obstruction was ascribed to mucosal granulomata with lesions that are generally visible on bronchospy. Airway obstruction by a granulomatous lesions may lead to atelectasis.

In all likelihood, granulomatous changes in large airways are responsible for the development of cystic changes of the lungs, a common finding in advanced sarcoidosis (Miller et al. 1977). These bullae are important because they may become infected, notably with aspergillus, and this may lead to significant hemoptysis.

Thus, sarcoidosis is frequently associated with measurable abnormality of small airway function, although this is usually of little clinical significance. Extensive involvement with obstruction of large airways may be associated with significant dyspnea, and localized changes may lead to the development of bullae and important adverse effects.

C. Circulation and Ventilation/Perfusion Relationships

In view of the widespread distribution of granuloma and fibrosis in the lungs of patients with sarcoidosis, it is not surprising to find that there are frequently abnormalities of the pulmonary circulation. Pulmonary vascular obstruction leading to pulmonary hypertension is most commonly encountered in patients with diffuse pulmonary fibrosis, and Battesti and associates (1978) described chronic cor pulmonale in 6 of 20 patients with chronic pulmonary sarcoidosis. However, pulmonary hypertension may be largely due to pulmonary arteritis with little evidence of parenchymal involvement. Levine and associates (1971) reported such a patient who died of progressive pulmonary hypertension largely due to pulmonary vascular disease without striking interstitial fibrosis, indicated by a vital capacity which was 76% normal.

In an important study of the pulmonary circulation, Emirgil and associates (1971) studied 15 patients with pulmonary fibrosis secondary to sarcoidosis. Ten of these patients had a mean pulmonary artery pressure of 31 mmHg or higher. In all of them the diffusing capacity was less than 50% of normal, suggesting that widespread involvement of the small vessels by granuloma and fibrosis produced both pulmonary hypertension and reduction of diffusion surface in the alveolar capillary bed. This is similar to other types of interstitial lung disease, and in marked contrast to primary pulmonary vascular disease in which diffusion impairment may be minimal or absent (Williams et al. 1969). There was a surprisingly good correlation between pulmonary hypertension, elevated pulmonary vascular resistance, and reduction of diffusing capacity, but little correlation of pulmonary hypertension with vital capacity. Hence, interstitial pathology may cause pulmonary restriction without involvement of the pulmonary vascular bed and vice versa.

In addition, Emirgil and associates (1969) pointed out the absence of a correlation of blood gas abnormalities with pulmonary hypertension, in contrast to the positive relationship that exists in chronic obstructive lung disease. In the latter condition, pulmonary hypertension is much more the result of hypoxemia, whereas in sarcoidosis it is caused by the anatomical changes in the pulmonary circulation.

More subtle abnormalities of the circulation are evident in other patients without diffuse disease and pulmonary hypertension. Renzi and associates (1974) found that 18 of 20 nonsmokers with sarcoidosis had abnormalities of ventilation and perfusion when studied by measurements of regional lung function with xenon. In this study, xenon scans were abnormal in 18 of 20 subjects, four of whom had normal x-ray films. There was more evidence of abnormality at the apices than at the bases, and there was a general correlation between the extent of abnormality of ventilation/perfusion ratios with reduction of the diffusing capacity.

Weitzenblum and associates (1977) studied 26 subjects with xenon. In stages I and II of sarcoidosis, there was some increase of ventilation in relationship to lung volume. The normal gradient of ventilation from apex to base was preserved and perfusion was distributed normally in these subjects. In stage III sarcoidosis with diffuse interstitial disease of the lung on the x-ray film, ventilation distribution was normal but there were areas of reduced perfusion, particularly at the bases. As in the previous study (Renzi et al. 1974), the extent of abnormalities correlated with reduction of the diffusing capacity.

The overall effect of these ventilation/perfusion abnormalities has long been recognized as an increased alveolar-arterial (A-a) oxygen tension gradient (Kanagami et al. 1961, Kent and Spence 1964, McClement et al.

1953, Riley et al. 1952, Svanborg 1961, Williams 1953). In Svanborg's (1961) classical study, there was widening of the A-a gradient in all stages of sarcoidosis, and this increased with the amount of parenchymal disease on the x-ray film of the chest. Nonetheless, the arterial PO_2 was usually 70 mmHg or higher, both at rest and during exercise, even in patients with extensive interstitial fibrosis (Fig. 2). Thus, although abnormalities are present, hypoxemia is only a problem in advanced disease, and then uncommonly.

In addition to the increased A-a gradient for oxygen, the ventilation/perfusion disturbance causes an increase of the physiologic dead space (Kanagami et al. 1961, Kent and Spence 1964, McClement et al. 1953, Riley et al. 1952, Williams 1953). This, in turn, requires an increase of the total ventilation for maintenance of a normal Pa_{CO_2}. Despite this abnormality, the Pa_{CO_2} is actually reduced as noted below. There is some suggestion that lung damage due to sarcoidosis is associated with less abnormality of pulmonary function than is the case in other interstitial disease. It has already been mentioned that beryllium disease is associated with more functional impairment than sarcoidosis (Carrington et al. 1976). Vale (1971) compared eight cases of sarcoidosis to eight cases of interstitial lung disease due to other causes but with similar x-ray films of the

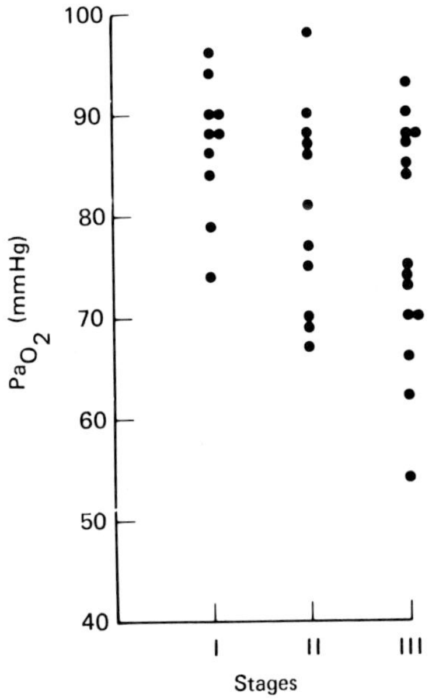

Figure 2 Arterial PO_2 in patients with sarcoidosis in stage I (hilar adenopathy without abnormality of the x-ray film of the chest), stage II (pulmonary infiltrates), and stage III (pulmonary fibrosis) (Svanborg 1961).

chest. In this study, there was less impairment of pulmonary function
for the patients with sarcoidosis than for those with other types of interstitial lung disease.

D. Control of Ventilation

One very common feature of sarcoidosis, mentioned in most studies, is the
frequency of resting hyperventilation reflected in an arterial PCO_2 that is
less than normal. The hypocapnia is particularly notable in the face of the
increased respiratory work resulting from airway obstruction and reduced
compliance, and of the increased physiologic dead space resulting from the
ventilation/perfusion abnormalities discussed above. The mechanisms responsible for the increased respiratory drive that must be present have been
discussed by Kornbluth and Turino (1980). They pointed out there is
little evidence of increased respiratory sensitivity to carbon dioxide or to
hypoxia in patients with diffuse interstitial disease, and they likened the
hyperventilation to the effects of external elastic loading which causes
immediate increase of respiratory work, presumably via vagally mediated
mechanoreceptors in the lungs or chest wall. It is also possible that
reflex stimuli from the diseased lung, long held to be the cause of hyperventilation in diffuse interstitial disease, play a role.

III. Course and Effect of Steroids

It is frequently stated in medical texts and journals that sarcoidosis is a
chronic progressive disease. This statement needs careful evaluation. It
has already been noted, and repeatedly documented, that pathologic changes
are very poorly reflected in the appearance of the x-ray film of the chest.
Measurements of lung function, although in general worse in patients with
severe abnormalities on x-ray examination, often correlate poorly with
radiographic changes but are probably more representative of the anatomical
changes in the lungs. The course of sarcoidosis is probably reflected better
in measurements of pulmonary function than in radiographic changes.
There are many ways in which sarcoidosis may appear to progress
when, in fact, the pathologic lesions remain dormant. Narrowing of a large
airway may lead to gradual development of a bulla without any changes in
the airway lesion. Sustained elevation of pulmonary vascular resistance
from damage to the pulmonary circulation may lead to gradual enlargement
of the right ventricle and signs of cor pulmonale without any further
damage to the lung. Patients, particularly those who smoke, may develop
slowly worsening airway obstruction with increasing dyspnea, and the
sustained effects of increased work of breathing imposed by stiff lungs and

increased airway resistance may lead to worsening dyspnea without any change in the pathology. In fact, as will be discussed, it appears that in most patients, once the disease is established, there is very little further change in pulmonary function with the passage of time although there is a tendency toward some gradual deterioration. It is difficult to disassociate even this small change from the effects of aging or from additional insults to the lung.

There have also been reports of spontaneous remission, generally referable to improvement of radiographic findings or of symptoms. However, it has been frequently noted that reduction in size of pulmonary infiltrates is associated with little or no change of vital capacity or diffusing capacity and that sizable granulomata have simply been replaced by less visible but equally significant pulmonary fibrosis. Onal and associates (1977) described three such patients with marked improvement of roentgenograms and of symptoms, and although in two there was measurable improvement of vital capacity, in one there was no change of either vital capacity or diffusing capacity. As will be noted, similar findings have been described in a number of patients treated with corticosteroids.

As mentioned previously, it is difficult to predict the course of sarcoidosis from studies of pulmonary function. Data are conflicting on whether patients with the longer duration of the disease do indeed have more abnormality of function (Hamer 1963, Marshall and Karlish 1971, Ting and Williams 1965, Young et al. 1968), and the problem of selection in interpreting such analyses has already been noted. It does appear that if improvement is to occur, particularly by x-ray, this is more likely to happen soon after onset of the disease. The weight of pathologic and physiologic evidence suggests that once the lung is involved by sarcoidosis there will never be complete return to normal even if there is some evidence of improvement.

Boushy and associates (1965) reported serial studies of pulmonary function over a period of 41 months in 18 patients with sarcoidosis. Although several patients showed improvement of symptoms and of radiographic changes, particularly of hilar adenopathy, none had improvement of pulmonary function. In 23 patients followed over a 6-year period without steroid therapy, Sharma and associates (1966b) found little change of vital capacity and diffusing capacity, although there was a slight improvement of one or both tests in some patients and slight worsening in others. More recently, Colp and associates (1976) analyzed the courses of these and other patients over a 15-year interval and reported a decrease of diffusing capacity, but little change of vital capacity, with the passage of time. In their study, about 10% of patients developed new lesions associated with worsening of pulmonary function after the initial presentation. However, the usual pattern of the illness was an abrupt onset without progression and without the development of new lesions in the lungs or elsewhere. In a similar vein, Emirgil and associates (1969) described 16 patients followed for 12 years, emphasizing that, if pulmonary function were to worsen, it almost always did so within 2 years of the onset of illness. Although there was slight worsening of pulmonary function thereafter in some patients, others showed slight improvement of diffusing capacity and vital capacity.

There is ample evidence that the abnormalities of pulmonary function can be favorably affected by corticosteroid therapy. Riley and associates (1952) reported that ACTH caused substantial improvement of vital capacity, maximal breathing capacity, and arterial oxygen tension, as well as in the chest roentgenograms of three patients with sarcoidosis. There was less improvement of ventilation/perfusion abnormalities, as measured by the A-a oxygen gradient, and no increase of the diffusing capacity during exercise. Relapse occurred after cessation of treatment. McClement and associates (1953) described some physiologic improvement in five of their patients with sarcoidosis treated with corticosteroids and noted, from serial biopsies, that therapy was associated with conversion of granulomata to fibrosis. Stone and associates (1953) described deterioration of pulmonary function in four of seven patients treated with corticosteroids.

Wigderson and associates (1959) reported dramatic resolution of extensive radiographic densities following corticosteroid therapy, associated with some improvement of diffusing capacity and vital capacity but, nonetheless, severe residual abnormality of lung function. Two similar cases were reported by Onal and associates (1977) and subsequent series have contained other examples of this phenomenon. Thus modular radiologic abnormalities of sarcoidosis may rarely regress spontaneously or, more often, respond markedly to corticosteroid therapy. Although there may be improvement of lung function with or without treatment, severe abnormality of function may persist, reflecting the transformation of visible granulomatous disease into less apparent pulmonary fibrosis.

Smellie and associates (1961) found only slight improvement of pulmonary function in 11 patients with sarcoidosis treated with corticosteroids, despite substantial improvement of roentgenograms, and Young and associates (1970) found little difference in pulmonary function after 6 months of steroid therapy compared to a control group. In both these studies, however, there was minimal impairment of lung function to start with and, in the second study, not all of the patients studied at the outset were restudied at 6 months so that it is not entirely certain that there was no improvement.

Sharma and associates (1966b) described the effects of corticosteroid therapy in 20 patients with sarcoidosis and emphasized that although, as previously noted, spontaneous improvement was rare, there was improvement after therapy. Most important, although therapy for sarcoidosis had no consistent effect on patients with mild impairment of pulmonary function (D_{co} greater than 65% normal), all but one of the 13 patients with severe impairment improved after therapy. Although the improvement was substantial in some instances, in most there was continued impairment of pulmonary function. These findings were confirmed by a more extensive analysis by Colp and associates (1976) and by the data published by Emirgil and associates (1969). Data from four large series on corticosteroid therapy are shown in Figure 3. Although there was little more improvement than worsening in patients with an initial vital capacity of 60% of normal or higher, those with more impairment of pulmonary function generally showed substantial improvement both of vital capacity and of diffusing capacity. Thus, measurable improvement is to be expected only in patients with relatively severe impairment of pulmonary function. Evident from Figure 3 is the tendency for vital capacity to improve more consistently than the diffusing capacity, a phenomenon frequently noted in the literature. Although, as previously noted, the diffusing capacity is apt to be more severely reduced than the vital capacity in sarcoidosis, more improvement occurs in the latter with steroid therapy.

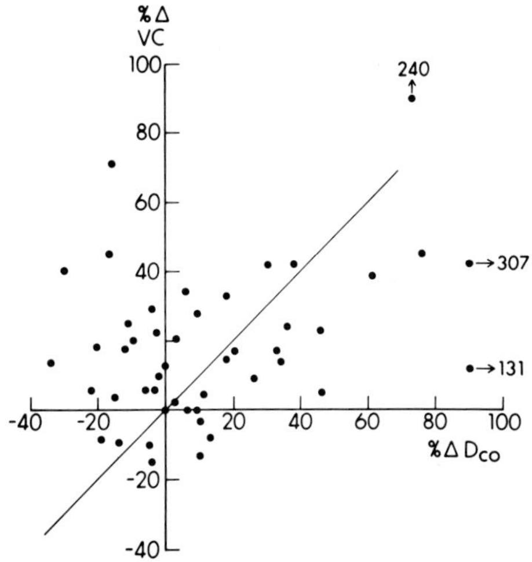

Figure 3 Relationship between the change of vital capacity and change of diffusing capacity after steroid therapy from four reports in the literature (Block and Light 1973, Emergil et al. 1969, Sharma et al. 1966b, Smellie et al. 1961).

For this reason, measurement of only the vital capacity may be a sufficient guide to the institution and continuation of corticosteroids.

There is little dispute that severe involvement of the lungs, particularly if reflected in impairment of pulmonary function, can be favorably affected by corticosteroid therapy. It is also clear that for at least 2 years, and generally longer, cessation of therapy is apt to be followed by worsening of lung function (Colp et al. 1976, Emergil et al. 1969, Johns et al. 1974, 1976). It is uncertain whether such prolonged therapy is warranted to maintain functional improvement. Clearly, symptomatic patients who can be improved by treatment should be, but the ultimate outcome has not been proven to be better in patients with impaired pulmonary function who received prolonged courses of steroid therapy. The general impression of those who have treated and studied patients for many years is that if pulmonary function is impaired, or if it worsens during observation, corticosteroid therapy is warranted (Colp et al. 1976, Emergil et al. 1969, Johns et al. 1976, Miller et al. 1977). If there then is improvement, treatment should be continued as long as and in as high a dosage as necessary to maintain optimal pulmonary function. Fortunately, for most patients such an effect can be achieved with relatively small doses of prednisone, less than 15 mg per day. There is some evidence that this can also be achieved by alternate day therapy, particularly after an initial period of intensive treatment (Block and Light 1973, Selroos and Sellergren 1979). The exact dosage and time required to induce improvement has not really been studied but certainly substantial improvement, perhaps the full effect, can be achieved by 2 weeks of 30–40 mg of prednisone per day. It is possible that these results occur earlier and could occur with smaller doses.

In an effort to provide a therapeutic effect on the lungs without inducing systemic effects, Dr. Charlotte Colp and I studied the effect of steroid aerosol (beclomethasone diproprionate) in six patients who had been maintained on systemic steroids for several months to years. In these patients, the dosage of prednisone was gradually reduced until it was discontinued. All patients revealed reduction of vital capacity and usually of diffusing capacity (Fig. 4). They were then given 400 μg of steroid aerosol daily for 2 weeks or longer. In one patient there was partial reversal of the deterioration of pulmonary function but the others failed to improve. Reinstitution of prednisone therapy led to improvement in five patients.

To evaluate the effects of the topical agents more rigorously, we performed a controlled study on four untreated patients. Each patient was given steroid aerosol and placebo for a 2-week period in a double-blind, randomized crossover fashion. None of the patients showed significant improvement on aerosol, but at the end of the trial three of them showed substantial improvement after 2 weeks of treatment with 30 mg of oral prednisone (Fig. 5).

These meager data suggest that steroid aerosols are not effective for primary treatment of sarcoidosis. This is in keeping with reports of development or recurrence of allergic alveolitis in patients with asthma controlled with steroid aerosol (Paterson et al. 1975), indicating that although the aerosol has a beneficial effect on the airways it fails to reach the steroid-responsive disease in the alveoli. However, more extensive experience is necessary to evaluate the effect of these agents, perhaps in larger doses, in maintaining improvement already induced by oral prednisone.

As is the case with interstitial disease, it is now apparent that obstruction resulting from airway lesions is also apt to improve with corticosteroids, although perhaps to a lesser extent. Dines and associates (1978) reported improved expiratory flow rates in a patient with airway obstruction related to sarcoidosis, as did Benatar and Clark (1974). The latter study is interesting in that after therapy expiratory flow rate became

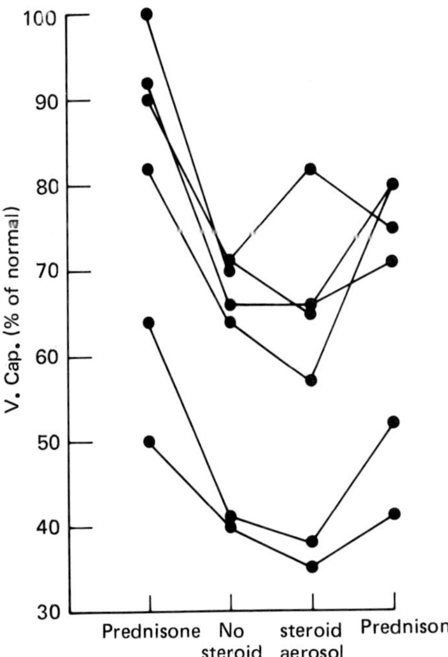

Figure 4 In six patients who had been treated with steroids for several months to years, prednisone was gradually discontinued with a substantial fall of vital capacity. Steroid aerosol then resulted in improvement in one patient, but reinstitution of prednisone caused improvement in five patients. Measurement of the diffusing capacity revealed similar but smaller effects.

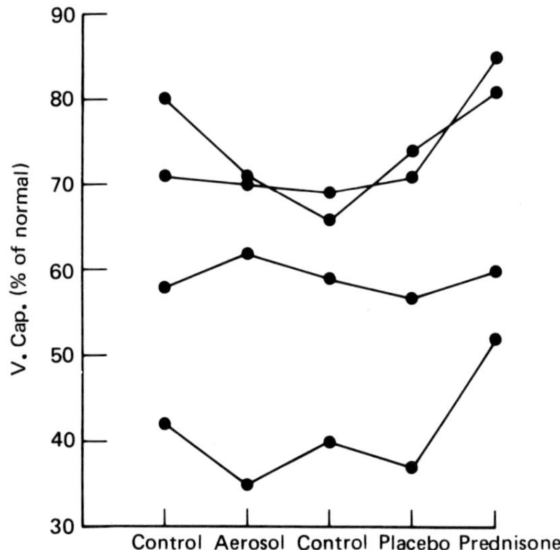

Figure 5   Randomized, double-blind crossover trial of the effect of 2
weeks of steroid aerosol compared to placebo on the vital capacity in four
patients with sarcoidosis. Control measurements were obtained before
each agent was started, and there was no evidence of an effect from the
active drug. At the end of the trial, the patients were given prednisone
with substantial improvement of vital capacity in three of four patients.
There were similar effects on the diffusing capacity.

dependent upon the density of impaired gas, suggesting a differential effect
on small and large airways. In addition, treatment was associated, as
expected, with reduction of lung recoil, so that the increased expiratory
flow rate, shown to increase in relation to lung recoil, had to be the
result of increased airway diameter. Data from three reports in the
literature on the effects of corticosteroids on maximal midexpiratory flow
rate are shown in Figure 6. It appears that although trivial changes
occurred in many individuals, substantial improvement was associated with
steroid therapy in some. Twenty-nine percent of patients had a greater
than 20% increase of maximum midexpiratory flow. Clearly then, as with
interstitial disease, substantial improvement may occur following corticosteroid therapy. The only way to learn whether steroid therapy will
benefit the individual patient is to study the effect on pulmonary function.

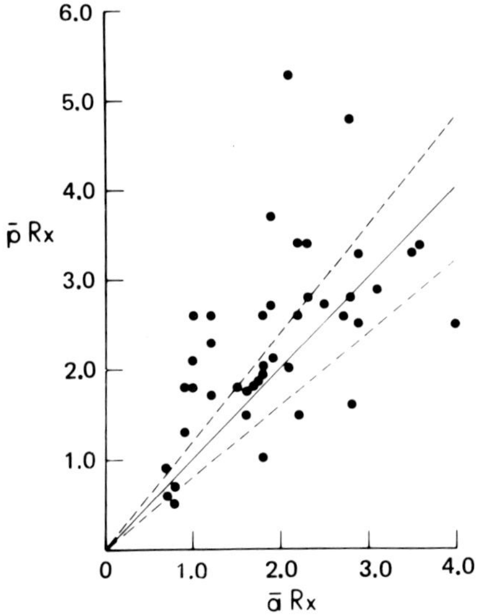

Figure 6 Maximal midexpiratory flow rate (MMF) in liters per second before (ā) and after (p̄) corticosteroid therapy (Boushy et al. 1965, Emergil et al. 1969, Sharma et al. 1966b). The line of identify (solid line) is shown along with 20% improvement or worsening (broken lines).

IV. Summary

Sarcoidosis is a disease which usually, if not always, involves the lung with varying degrees of granulomatosis and fibrosis. This is reflected in abnormalities of pulmonary function which vary with the degree and location of the pathology. Interstitial disease frequently causes reduction of diffusing capacity and, almost as often, of lung compliance and lung volumes. These reductions in lung function only infrequently cause significant dyspnea, despite the associated hyperventilation. Severe interstitial disease causes restriction of the pulmonary vascular bed which may lead to pulmonary hypertension, proportional to the reduction of diffusing capacity. Rarely this is severe enough to cause cor pulmonale. Airway involvement, as reflected in abnormal tests of small airways, is also commonly present. This is infrequently so extensive as to cause reduction of expiratory flow rates and rarely severe enough to cause increased airway resistance and dyspnea.

   These pathologic abnormalities frequently cause disturbance of ventilation/perfusion ratios due to variable involvement of airways and of circulation in different parts of the lungs. This leads to widening of the A-a gradient for oxygen in many patients but, in part because of the reflex hyperventilation reflected in hypocapnia, rarely produces significant hypoxemia.

Sarcoidosis usually develops to its fullest extent soon after onset, and progressive impairment of pulmonary function is infrequent. If patients are left untreated, pulmonary function is not apt to improve. Severe abnormalities are more likely to improve after steroid therapy than are minor abnormalities, but lung function practially never returns to normal. Steroids are probably indicated in patients with marked impairment of pulmonary function just to maintain maximal function, but they usually have to be given for 2 years or longer and there is no proof that the treatment actually has a beneficial impact on the course of the disease. The use of steroids is adequately guided by measurement of vital capacity.

References

Baldwin, E. deF, Cournand, A., and Richards, D. W., Jr. (1949). Pulmonary insufficiency. II. A study of thirty-nine cases of pulmonary fibrosis. *Medicine,* **28**:1–25.

Battesti, J. P., Georges, R., Basset, F., and Saumon, G. (1978). Chronic cor pulmonale in pulmonary sarcoidosis. *Thorax,* **33**:76–84.

Benetar, S. R., and Clark, T. J. H. (1974). Pulmonary function in a case of endobronchial sarcoidosis. *Am. Rev. Respir. Dis.,* **110**:490–496.

Block, A. J., and Light, R. W. (1973). Alternate day steroid therapy in diffuse pulmonary sarcoidosis. *Chest,* **63**:495–500.

Boushy, S. F., Kurtzman, R. S., Martin, N. D., and Lewis, B. M. (1965). The course of pulmonary function in sarcoidosis. *Ann. Intern. Med.,* **62**:939–955.

Bruce, T., and Wassen, E. (1940). Clinical observations on the course and prognosis of lymphogranulomatosis benigna Schaumman, particularly in regard to pulmonary lesions. *Acta Med. Scand.,* **104**:63–104.

Carrington, C. B., Gaensler, E. A., Mikus, J. P., Schachter, A. W., Burke, G. W., and Goff, A. M. (1976). Structure and function in sarcoidosis. *Ann. NY Acad. Sci.,* **278**:265–283.

Coates, E. O., and Comroe, J. H. (1951). Pulmonary function studies in sarcoidosis. *J. Clin. Invest.,* **30**:848–852.

Colp, C., Park, S. S., and Williams, M. H., Jr. (1976). Pulmonary function follow-up of 120 patients with sarcoidosis. *Ann. NY Acad. Sci.,* **278**:301–307.

DeRemee, R. A., and Andersen, H. A. (1974). Sarcoidosis. A correlation of dyspnea with roentgenographic stage and pulmonary function changes. *Mayo Clin. Proc.,* **49**:742–745.

Dines, D. E., Stubbs, S. E., and McDougall, J. C. (1978). Obstructive disease of the airways associated with stage I sarcoidosis. *Mayo Clin. Proc.,* **53**:788–791.

Divertie, M. B., Cassan, S. M., O'Brien, P. C., and Brown, A. L., Jr. (1976). Fine structural morphometry of diffuse lung diseases with abnormal blood-air gas transfer. *Mayo Clin. Proc.,* **51**:42–47.

Emirgil, C., Sobol, B. J., and Williams, M. H., Jr. (1969). Long-term study of pulmonary sarcoidosis. The effect of steroid therapy as evaluated by pulmonary function studies. *J. Chronic. Dis.,* **22**:69–86.

Emirgil, C., Sobol, B. J., Herbert, W. H., and Trout, K. (1971). The lesser circulation in pulmonary fibrosis secondary to sarcoidosis and its relationship to respiratory function. *Chest,* **60**:371–378.

Hamer, N. A. J. (1963). Changes in the components of the diffusing capacity in pulmonary sarcoidosis. *Thorax,* **18**:275–287.

Huang, C. T., Heurich, A. E., Rosen, Y., Moon, S., and Lyons, H. A. (1979). Pulmonary sarcoidosis. Roentgenographic, functional and pathologic correlations. *Respiration,* **37**:337–345.

Johns, C. J., Zachary, J. B., and Ball, W. C., Jr. (1974). A 10-year study of corticosteroid treatment of pulmonary sarcoidosis. *Johns Hopkins Med. J.,* **134**:271–283.

Johns, C. J., Macgregor, M. I., Zachary, J. B., and Ball, W. C., Jr. (1976). Extended experience in the long-term corticosteroid treatment of pulmonary sarcoidosis. *Ann. NY Acad. Sci.,* **278**:722–731.

Kanagami, H., Katsura, T., Shiraishi, K., Baba, K., Ogata, K., Tanaka, M., and Munakata, K. (1961). Clinical aspects of sarcoidosis with emphasis on pulmonary function tests. *Jap. J. Chest. Dis.,* **20**: 853–862.

Kent, D. C., and Spence, W. (1964). Physiologic abnormalities in pulmonary sarcoidosis. *Dis. Chest.,* **46**:680–691.

Kornbluth, R. S., and Turino, G. M. (1980). Respiratory control in diffuse interstitial lung disease and diseases of the pulmonary vasculature. *Clin. Chest Med.,* **1**:91–102.

Lewis, B. M., Kurtzman, R. S., Martin, N. D., and Boushy, S. F. (1965). Effects of sarcoid on the lungs. *Arch. Intern. Med.,* **115**:330–335.

Levine, B. W., Saldana, M., and Hutter, A. M. (1971). Pulmonary hypertension in sarcoidosis. *Am. Rev. Respir. Dis.,* **103**:413–417.

Levinson, R. S., Metzger, L. F., Stanley, N. N., Kelsen, S. G., Altose, M. D., Cherniack, N. S., and Brody, J. S. (1977). Airway function in sarcoidosis. *Am. J. Med.,* **62**:51–59.

Lyons, H. A. (1958). Pulmonary compliance in granulomatous disease of the lung. *Am. J. Med.,* **25**:23–30.

Marshall, R., and Karlish, A. J. (1971). Lung function in sarcoidosis. *Thorax,* **26**:402–405.

Marshall, R., Smellie, H., Balis, J. H., Hoyle, C., and Bates, D. V. (1958). Pulmonary function in sarcoidosis. *Thorax,* **13**:48–58.

McClement, J. H., Renzetti, A. D., Himmelstein, A., and Cournand, A. (1953). Cardiopulmonary function in the pulmonary form of Boeck's sarcoid and its modification by cortisone therapy. *Am. Rev. Tuber.,* **67**:154–171.

Miller, A., Teirstein, A. S., Jackler, I., Chuang, M., and Siltzbach, L. E. (1973). Airway function in chronic pulmonary sarcoidosis with fibrosis. *Am. Rev. Respir. Dis.,* **109**:179–189.

Miller, A., Chuang, M., Teirstein, A. S., and Siltzbach, L. E. (1976). Pulmonary function in stage I and II pulmonary sarcoidosis. *Ann. NY Acad. Sci.,* **278**:292–300.

Miller, A., Teirstein, A. S., and Chuang, M. (1977). The sequence of physiologic changes in pulmonary sarcoidosis: Correlation with radiographic changes and response to therapy. *Mt. Sinai Med.,* **44**:852–865.

Onal, E., Lopata, M., Lourenco, R. V. (1977). Nodular pulmonary sarcoidosis—Clinical roentgenographic, and physiologic course in five patients. *Chest,* **72**:296–300.

Paterson, I. C., Cooke, N. J., Murray, K., Crompton, G. K., and Grant, I. W. B. (1975). Pulmonary eosinophilia after substitution of aerosol for oral corticosteroid therapy. *Br. J. Dis. Chest,* **69**:217–222.

Poe, R. H., Israel, R. H., Utell, M. J., and Hall, W. J. (1979). Probability of a positive transbronchial lung biopsy result in sarcoidosis. *Arch. Intern. Med.,* **139**:761–763.

Radwan, L., Grebska, E., and Koziorowski, A. (1978). Small airways function in pulmonary sarcoidosis. *Scand. J. Respir. Dis.,* **59**:37–43.

Renzi, G., and Dutton, R. E. (1974). Pulmonary function in diffuse sarcoidosis. *Respiration,* **31**:124–136.

Renzi, G., Anthonisen, N. R., Grassino, A., Knight, L., and Martin, R. R. (1974). Regional lung function in sarcoidosis. *Scand. J. Respir. Dis.,* Suppl. **85**:64–74.

Riley, R. L., Riley, M. C., and Hill, H., McD. (1952). Diffuse pulmonary sarcoidosis: Diffusing capacity during exercise and other lung function studies in relation to ACTH therapy. *Bull. Johns Hopkins Hosp.,* **91**:345–370.

Romer, F. K. (1977). Sarcoidosis with large nodular lesions simulating pulmonary metastases. An analysis of 126 cases of intrathoracic sarcoidosis. *Scand. J. Respir. Dis.,* **58**:11–16.

Saumon, G., Georges, R., Loiseau, A., and Turiaf, J. (1976). Membrane diffusing capacity and pulmonary capillary blood volume in pulmonary sarcoidosis. *Ann. NY Acad. Sci.,* **278**:284–291.

Sellers, R. D., and Siebens, A. A. (1965). The effects of sarcoidosis on pulmonary function, with particular reference to changes in pulmonary compliance. *Am. Rev. Respir. Dis.,* **91**:660–664.

Selroos, O., and Sellergren, T. L. (1979). Corticosteroid therapy of pulmonary sarcoidosis. (A prospective evaluation of alternative day and daily dosage in stage II disease). *Scand. J. Respir. Dis.,* **60**: 215–221.

Sharma, O. P., Colp, C., and Williams, M. H., Jr. (1966a). Pulmonary function studies in patients with bilateral sarcoidosis of hilar lymph nodes. *Arch. Intern. Med.,* **117**:436–439.

Sharma, O. P., Colp, C., and Williams, M. H., Jr. (1966b). Course of pulmonary sarcoidosis with and without corticosteroid therapy as determined by pulmonary function studies. *Am. J. Med.,* **41**:541–551.

Smellie, H., Apthrop, G. H., and Marshall, R. (1961). The effect of corticosteroid treatment on pulmonary function in sarcoidosis. *Thorax,* **16**:87–90.

Snider, G. L., and Doctor, L. (1964). The mechanics of ventilation in sarcoidosis. *Am. Rev. Respir. Dis.,* **89**:897–908.

Stone, D. J., Schwartz, A., Feltman, J. A., and Lovelock, F. J. (1953). Pulmonary function in sarcoidosis. Results of cortisone therapy. *Am. J. Med.,* **15**:468–483.

Svanborg, N. (1961). Studies on the cardiopulmonary function in sarcoidosis. *Acta Med. Scand.,* Suppl. **366**.

Ting, E. Y., and Williams, M. H., Jr. (1965). Mechanics of breathing in sarcoidosis of lung. *JAMA,* **192**:619–624.

Vale, J. R. (1971). Respiratory function in sarcoidosis and other interstitial lung diseases with similar radiological appearance. *Scand. J. Respir. Dis.,* **52**:3–12.

Weitzenblum, E., Moyses, B., Hirth, C., Meunier-Carus, J., Methlin, G., and Oudet, P. (1977). Regional pulmonary function in sarcoidosis. *Scand. J. Respir. Dis.,* **58**:17–26.

Wigderson, A., Williams, M. H., Jr., Zohman, L. R., and Childress, W. G. (1959). Impaired diffusion in pulmonary sarcoidosis. *NY State J. Med.,* **59**:2420–2423.

Williams, M. H., Jr. (1953). Pulmonary function in Boeck's sarcoid. *J. Clin. Invest.,* **32**:909–913.

Williams, M. H., Jr., Adler, J. J., and Colp, C. (1969). Pulmonary function studies as an aid in the differential diagnosis of pulmonary hypertension. *Am. J. Med.,* **47**:378–383.

Young, R. C., Jr., Carr, C., Shelton, T. G., Mann, M., Ferrin, A., Laurey, J. R., and Harden, K. A. (1967). Sarcoidosis: Relationship between changes in lung structure and function. *Am. Rev. Respir. Dis.,* **95**: 224–238.

Young, R. L., Krumholz, R. A., and Harkleroad, L. E. (1966). Physio-
    logical roentgenographic disparity in sarcoidosis. *Dis. Chest.,* **50**:
    81–86.
Young, R. L., Lordon, R. E., Krumholz, R. A., Harkleroad, L. E., Branam,
    G. E., and Weg, J. G. (1968). Pulmonary sarcoidosis: Pathophysio-
    logic correlation. *Am. Rev. Respir. Dis.,* **97**:997–1008.
Young, R. L., Harkleroad, L. E., Lordon, R. E., and Weg, J. G. (1970).
    Pulmonary sarcoidosis. A prospective evaluation of glucocorticoid
    therapy. *Ann. Intern. Med.,* **73**:207–212.

Part Two

EPIDEMIOLOGY AND GENETICS OF SARCOIDOSIS

4

Worldwide Distribution and Epidemiology of Sarcoidosis

ALVIN S. TEIRSTEIN

The Mount Sinai Medical Center
New York, New York

MARVIN LESSER

Mount Sinai School of Medicine
New York, New York
and Bronx Veterans Administration Hospital
Bronx, New York

I. Introduction

Epidemiology is the study of the distribution of disease among population groups (MacMahon and Pugh 1970). The study subjects may be classified by age, sex, race, nationality or geographic location, climatic and other environmental factors, and occasionally, by a specific biologic marker such as blood and HLA type. By analysis of epidemiologic patterns, one hopes that profiles of subjects may emerge which are of value in identifying etiologic agents, specific population groups which are at particular risk for contracting a disease, and/or public health measures for prevention of illness (Lilienfeld 1976). Although voluminous epidemiologic data have been gathered concerning sarcoidosis, and a few special features of patient cohorts with sarcoidosis have been identified, there has been no significant contribution by epidemiologic study to our understanding of this disease.

In this chapter, the frequency of age, sex, race, family, and HLA typing in sarcoidosis will be discussed. It will be shown that none of the existing data support a significant role for any of these factors in the etiology or diagnosis of sarcoidosis. Simply stated, sarcoidosis is a common disease which occurs at any age, in both men and women of all races, and

"

is distributed worldwide. The major portion of this chapter will be devoted to an encyclopedic review of the reports of prevalence and incidence of sarcoidosis in the six continents.

II. Worldwide Distribution of Sarcoidosis

The accuracy of the multitude of published studies reporting the frequency of sarcoidosis by country of origin varies. In a few reports, accurate prevalence data have been achieved. In most, the data reflect an individual experience at a single hospital or clinic. Prevalence data are often a faulted extrapolation from such an anecdotal study. Incidence data are rarely obtained, existing only in those few countries where the population is small and the majority of the citizens have been subjected to mass radiographic investigations. Furthermore, studies such as the autopsy review in Malmo, Sweden (Hagerstrand and Linell 1963) strongly suggest that even in countries with well-developed case-finding techniques, the true prevalence of sarcoidosis far exceeds that uncovered in the best epidemiologic surveys. From this postmortem investigation and others, it has been proposed that sarcoidosis occurs from four to ten times more frequently than the number of patients with proven disease would suggest. Presumably, most individuals contract sarcoidosis in a relatively asymptomatic form, never consult a physician or have a chest radiograph performed, and experience a complete remission or benign course without the diagnosis ever being established.

Prevalence of disease is the actual number of patients with a given disease at any single point in time. The prevalence rate equals the number of patients with the disease divided by the total number of persons in the study population, usually reported per 100,000 population. *Incidence* is the number of patients contracting a disease during a specified time period, usually 1 year, and may be reported as the number of patients contracting the disease in 1 year divided by the total population (Lilienfeld 1976). It is quite clear that both prevalence and incidence data are completely dependent on the sophistication and diligence of the investigators performing the screening surveys and on the diagnostic techniques available to them.

In sarcoidosis, there is no readily available worldwide diagnostic test. Most reports of disease frequency rely on the finding of chest radiographic surveys. In many patients, the diagnosis is accepted without histological proof or a positive Kveim test. Even when a biopsy is obtained, the histological finding of noncaseating epithelioid granulomas is not conclusive in establishing the diagnosis of sarcoidosis and must be buttressed by the presence of a compatible clinical picture or a positive Kveim test. Early reports of the diagnostic significance of elevated levels of serum angiotensin-converting enzyme (SACE) have been succeeded by numerous studies noting elevated SACE levels in patients with a variety of other nonsarcoidal diseases. In addition, a false negative SACE occurs in from 20% to 45% of patients with sarcoidosis.

To date, the test that best approaches the high sensitivity and specificity required for an acceptable diagnostic procedure is the intracutaneous Kveim test. An international Kveim trial employing a single, validated test suspension, known as Chase-Siltzbach type I suspension, was undertaken in a study of 2400 subjects in 37 countries on six continents (Siltzbach 1967a). Among 1200 subjects eventually diagnosed as having sarcoidosis, the result of the Kveim test was similar regardless of nationality. A number of parallel studies were made in the same patients using the type I suspension in parallel with validated test antigens made from spleens and lymph nodes obtained from patients in England, Australia, and Finland. It was found that any of these four test suspensions could be used interchangeably for the diagnosis of sarcoidosis throughout the world.

Unfortunately, at this time no Kveim test suspension is available commercially and each batch must be produced by individual investigators with meticulous attention to validation. Furthermore, Kveim tests require a high level of patient compliance and physician involvement because biopsy and histological analysis are necessary 4–6 weeks after injection (Siltzbach 1976). Finally, although remarkably specific, even validated Kveim antigen gives false negative results in approximately 20% of patients with proven sarcoidosis, with the test most often positive in the early stages of the disease and less positive as the disease becomes chronic (Siltzbach 1961).

Thus, all data concerning the frequency of sarcoidosis in population groups are subject to the vagaries of diagnostic criteria, with some investigators requiring organ biopsy or a positive Kveim test for diagnosis while others accept a "typical clinical picture" as sufficient.

Therefore, the reader must recognize that in the following presentation of the worldwide distribution of sarcoidosis, the data rarely reflect the true prevalence or incidence of the disease. However, these data do demonstrate that with a careful search the disease may be found almost everywhere, and in a few instances it occurs in unexplained high concentrations, while in still fewer localities there is little or no sarcoidosis.

As stated, epidemiologic data gathered from around the world dealing with the frequency and geographic patterns of sarcoidosis are difficult to compare because of variable methods of data collection and differences in recognition and classification of the disease. In Europe, for example, where mass radiographic surveys have been carried out and repeated regularly to encompass a major and representative portion of the general population, extensive information on frequency, geographic distribution, and racial differences often allow detailed comparisons not only within countries but also between countries. Such intensive efforts have also led, secondarily, to a heightened awareness among physicians and subsequently increased detection rates outside screening studies.

In the United States, on the other hand, in the absence of mass screening surveys of the general population (except for one study conducted in New York City), epidemiologic data dealing with sarcoidosis come primarily from studies of military personnel, patients attending Veterans Hospitals, and case-matched comparisons with controls or patients with other diseases. Although these studies have provided information about the prevalence and geographic features of the disease in restricted groups, they have not given reliable estimates for the country as a whole.

Epidemiologic data from much of the rest of the world, with a few exceptions, come largely from case reports or descriptions of symptomatic individuals in which prevalence rates are calculated by relating the number of such patients seen at hospitals or clinics. Obviously, these estimates overlook the more numerous silent cases within the unstudied population and, therefore, cannot be readily used in comparisons with data obtained by mass screening. In addition, in many countries the frequency is under-estimated because of a general lack of familiarity with the varied roentgeno-graphic and clinical patterns of intrathoracic and extrathoracic sarcoidosis.

A. Europe

The first mass screening survey conducted anywhere in the world that reported epidemiologic data in sarcoidosis was performed in Switzerland during World War II. Through the use of chest fluroscopy, a total of 516,879 Army personnel were evaluated between March 1943 and March 1944 with the detection, and subsequent confirmation, of definite sar-coidosis in 67 individuals (13 per 100,000 surveyed) (Schönholzer 1947). This study led to the recognition, for the first time, that most sarcoidosis patients have involvement predominantly of the lungs or mediastinal lymph nodes and that the majority of these affected individuals are asymptomatic. Within the next few years, a number of other screening studies were performed throughout most of the countries in Europe leading to an accumulation of data that has better characterized the epidemiologic features of sarcoidosis there than on any other continent (Table 1).

Scandinavia

In Sweden, mass radiographic screening surveys have been conducted since 1945, and all discovered sarcoidosis patients have been registered separately in the annual statistics since 1952 (Bauer and Wijkstrom 1963). Generalized surveys carried out in large parts of the country from 1945 to 1953, and again from 1953 to 1960, yielded data suggesting prevalence rates of 55 per 100,000 and 64 per 100,000 respectively, the highest numbers for any country in Europe, even when compared with more recent data from some of the other European countries. The higher prevalence rate noted during the second survey was attributed to greater awareness and recognition of the disease by medical personnel rather than to a true increase in the frequency of the disease.

Since both surveys detected only those patients with obvious intra-thoracic abnormalities at a given time, the calculated prevalence rates obviously underestimated the total number of diseased individuals in the general population. Therefore, information that may more accurately reflect the overall prevalence of sarcoidosis in Sweden comes from the city of Malmo (population 230,000), where autopsies were conducted during the

Table 1 Reported Prevalence of Pulmonary Sarcoidosis in Some European Countries

Country	Prevalence/ 100,000	Reference
Sweden	64	Bauer and Wijkstrom (1963)
Denmark	52.9	Levinsky et al. (1976)
Federal Republic of Germany	43.3	Levinsky et al. (1976)
German Democratic Republic	41.1	Levinsky et al. (1976)
Irish Republic	40.0	Levinsky et al. (1976)
Norway	26.7	Riddervold (1963)
Czechoslovakia	23	Levinsky et al. (1976)
The Netherlands	21.6	Urie and Ter Brugge (1963)
Great Britain	20	James and Brett (1963)
Switzerland	16.3	Sommer (1963)
Yugoslavia (Slovenia)	11.9	LaGrasta (1963)
France	9.5	Turiaf et al. (1963)
Italy (Milan)	9	Giobbi et al. (1971)
Scotland	8.2	Douglas (1963)
Finland	4.6	Patiala et al. (1963)
Poland (Silesia)	2.5	Zierski (1971)
Hungary (Budapest)	1.26	Mandi and Vezendi (1971)
Spain	0.04	Zapatero (1971)

years 1957 to 1962 on 6707 individuals (approximately 60% of all deaths).
A diagnosis of sarcoidosis was accepted only when typical sarcoid granulomas
were found to be widespread in several groups of lymph nodes and/or in
the lungs, liver, spleen, or other organs. Of the total number examined,
evidence for sarcoidosis was found in 43 individuals, giving a prevalence
rate at 641 per 100,000, approximately 10 times higher than that detected
by mass screening (Hagerstrand and Linell 1963). Interestingly, only three
of the 43 patients were known to have sarcoidosis during life.

In Norway, a mass radiographic screening survey of 1,448,148
individuals during the years 1954–1958 revealed a prevalence rate for
intrathoracic sarcoidosis of 26.7 per 100,000 examined (Riddervold 1963),
about one-half that for Sweden. In Finland, a screening survey of
1,450,000 individuals (total population 4,477,000) during 1960 and 1961
revealed a much lower prevalence rate of 4.6 per 100,000 (Patiala et al.
1963). More recently, screening surveys of the total population of Finland
have revealed a prevalence rate of 7.5 per 100,000 and an incidence of 5.3
per 100,000, again confirming, for reasons that seem factual rather than
accidental, that sarcoidosis is much less common in Finland than in any
other country in Scandinavia (Levinsky et al. 1976). Interestingly, pulmonary tuberculosis is more prevalent in Finland than in Sweden, Norway,
or Denmark.

In Denmark, an annual incidence for sarcoidosis was estimated to be
5 per 100,000 individuals on the basis of data recorded in the National
Registry during the years 1962 through 1965 (Horwitz et al. 1967). The
incidence rates were the same for males and females and were identical for
the urban and rural populations. There were variations from county to
county but without a consistent geographical pattern. More recent data,
presented at the Seventh International Conference on Sarcoidosis, revealed
a prevalence of 52.9 per 100,000 and an incidence of 5 per 100,000 for
sarcoidosis in Denmark (Levinsky et al. 1976), a prevalence only slightly
less than that found in Sweden.

Great Britain and Ireland

In Ireland, information about the frequency of sarcoidosis in the southern
part of the country comes from a survey of 383,000 predominantly urban
individuals from Dublin during the years 1958, 1959, 1960, and 1962,
where a prevalence of 33 per 100,000 inhabitants was found (Logan 1963).
During the years of the survey, there was no apparent increase in the
prevalence. In Northern Ireland, a survey of 1,448,000 individuals during
the years 1945–1962 revealed a lower prevalence of 10.3 per 100,000
(Milliken 1963). More recently, mass chest radiographic screening involving

over one-third of the population of the Irish Republic revealed a prevalence of intrathoracic sarcoidosis of 40 per 100,000 persons examined (Levinsky 1976). Other data obtained from the majority of tuberculosis clinics and from almost all hospitals revealed a diagnosis of definite or probable sarcoidosis in 822 individuals, giving a prevalence of 27 per 100,000 (Levinsky et al. 1976). In both of these surveys there was a higher frequency of sarcoidosis noted in males than in females, an observation that is at variance with that seen for most other countries in Europe.

In Great Britain, a chest radiographic survey of 3,323,910 individuals during 1958 revealed a prevalence of intrathoracic sarcoidosis of 20 per 100,000 (James and Brett 1963). Although the prevalence rate was similar for men and women, it was higher among women of childbearing ages (39 per 100,000) and among Irish women (200 per 100,000) and Irish men (120 per 100,000) surveyed in London. In a more detailed study to determine the true annual incidence of all forms of sarcoidosis in the civilian population, a survey of four areas of Great Britain (Cornwall and Plymouth, East Anglia, Sheffield and neighboring towns, and northeastern and eastern Scotland), conducted between 1961 and 1966 revealed an incidence of 2.7 per 100,000 for males and 3.8 per 100,000 for females (Baldry et al. 1969). All cases in which sarcoidosis was diagnosed or suspected were reviewed by a central panel whose opinion was accepted for the purpose of the survey. The highest incidence was present in both sexes in the 24–34 age group with the exception of Sheffield, the only highly industrialized area, where a high incidence was found among women in the 15–24 age range and a very low incidence was found in both men and women over the age of 45. The overall incidence was found to increase from north to south in both sexes but the range of variation was much smaller in women than in men. In a clinical study of 83 patients with sarcoidosis from southeast London (36 of West Indian origin and 47 Caucasians), it was observed that the age at onset of the disease was later in West Indians, and that they presented more often with respiratory symptoms or evidence of multiorgan dissemination (Honeybourne 1980). Erythema nodosum, on the other hand, was found more commonly among the Caucasians.

In Scotland, a mass radiographic survey from 1958 to 1961 of 1,709,000 individuals revealed a prevalence of 8.2 per 100,000 inhabitants (Douglas 1963). However, the five centers involved in the survey reported higher prevalence rates with each successive year of the survey, strongly suggesting an increasing recognition of the radiographic pattern of sarcoidosis by survey personnel. Thus, the overall prevalence figure probably was underestimated.

Continental Europe

In the Netherlands, a mass screening survey between 1952 and 1962 of
4,591,377 individuals over the age of 16 (about one-half the total
population) revealed a prevalence of 21.6 per 100,000 examined (Orie and
Ter Brugge 1963). Since the yearly detection rate remained relatively
constant during the 10 years of the study, the results probably reflect an
efficient system of recognition and reporting.

In the Federal Republic of Germany, data presented at the Seventh
International Conference on Sarcoidosis in 1976 representing the total
population revealed an overall prevalence in the country of 43.3 per
100,000 examined (Levinsky et al. 1976). Since an estimated prevalence
for the same 10 areas of the country for the years 1961–1962 was 8 per
100,000 (Levinsky et al. 1976), the increase to 43.3 was viewed by the
investigators as indicating a true increase in the frequency of the disease
rather than simply reflecting better methods of detection and reporting.
In a screening survey of the younger members of the German Federal
Army, the prevalence rate was found to be the highest (49.8 per 100,000
persons examined) in Bavaria, the southernmost part of the country
(Levinsky et al. 1976).

In the German Democratic Republic, a survey of 3,017,558 individuals
in Leipzig from 1960 to 1962 revealed a prevalence of 13.3 per 100,000
(Lindig 1963). For the country as a whole, surveys conducted from 1959
through 1968 revealed an increase in prevalence from 2.4 in 1959 to 33.4
in 1968 with a corresponding increase in incidence from 2.1 to 8.1 during
the same period (Zaumseil 1971). By 1968, 5784 sarcoidosis patients
were registered in the German Democratic Republic (2391 males and 3393
females) with no differences in frequency among rural and urban populations.
In 1975, the numbers had risen to a prevalence of 41.1 per 100,000 and an
incidence of 9.6 per 100,000 (Levinsky et al. 1976). As with the data
from the Federal Republic of Germany, the significant increase in both
prevalence and incidence from 1960 to 1975 has been interpreted as
suggesting an increase in the numbers of diseased individuals rather than
solely reflecting improved recognition and better diagnosis. Comparison of
data from the 15 different regions of the country revealed variations in
incidence figures during the 1975 survey ranging from 5.9 per 100,000 to
12 per 100,000, with the highest incidence occurring in the southern parts
of the country (Levinsky et al. 1976), a geographic pattern similar to that
found in the Federal Republic of Germany.

In Switzerland, a radiographic screening survey of 3,160,000 individuals
revealed a prevalence of 16.3 per 100,000 inhabitants (Sommer 1963). A
survey in Geneva of 560,057 individuals during the years 1966–1975
revealed a very similar prevalence of 16.6 per 100,000 (Press 1977), but with
marked, unexplained, annual variations ranging from maximums of 25 in

1968 and 29.17 in 1974 to minimums of 10 in 1966 and 7.8 in 1975. Ninety-four percent of the patients detected were under the age of 40. The higher frequency in men (59%) was attributed to the fact that more of the people who registered for screening were working individuals.

In Czechoslovakia, a mass radiographic survey of 3,436,000 individuals reported in 1963 revealed an overall prevalence rate of 3.4 per 100,000, but with variations from district to district ranging from 0 to 20.7 per 100,000 (Levinsky and Altmann 1963). A follow-up survey through 1975 revealed an overall prevalence of 23 per 100,000 and an incidence of 2.3 per 100,000 (Levinsky 1976), but again, with variations in the 112 districts as in the first study, ranging from 0 to 32 per 100,000 people (Levinsky et al. 1977). Since seven of the 10 districts reporting the higher rates (over 6 per 100,000) adjoined districts with a 0 incidence, the differences in rates suggest variation in recognition and reporting, particularly since in the earlier study it was noted that the physicians reporting the highest numbers of patients had a special interest in sarcoidosis (Levinsky and Altmann 1963).

In Poland, a single mass screening survey originated in the urban region of Silesia where, in 1967, a radiographic study of 614,000 individuals over the age of 15 revealed a prevalence of 2.5 per 100,000 examined (Zierski 1971). A questionnaire survey of 14 of the country's 22 District Chest Clinics (representing a population of 18 million) between 1963 and 1967 detected 315 sarcoidosis patients. When this number was apportioned according to districts, prevalence rates ranging from 0.52 to 5.22 per 100,000 were observed suggesting lack of uniform methods of diagnosis and notification (Zierski 1971). An additional 136 sarcoidosis patients had been previously diagnosed through 1962 among students attending the University Academic Centers at Warsaw, Zabrze, and Gliwice and among 19,516 patients seen at Medical Academy Hospitals of Tuberculosis and Lung Diseases (Jaroszewicz 1963). More recent data compiled from studies of sarcoidosis patients listed at chest clinics, hospitals, and sanatoriums throughout the country, and thought to be relevant to the frequency in the general population, revealed an overall incidence of sarcoidosis of 7.1 per 100,000 population in 1973 and 7.7 per 100,000 for 1974, with the highest frequency in the 30–40 age group (Jaroszewicz et al. 1977). A slight female predominance was noted.

In Hungary, a radiographic survey in Budapest from 1966 to 1968 of 1,000,000 individuals yielded an incidence of 1.26 per 100,000 (Mandi and Vezendi 1971). During the same period an additional 38 sarcoidosis patients were diagnosed in institutions. By combining these numbers, Mandi and Vezendi (1971) estimated that the overall incidence in Budapest during that time was between 2.5 and 3 per 100,000. A screening survey in Debrecen between 1961 and 1968 of more than two-thirds of the adult population each year revealed an overall incidence of 4 per 100,000 surveyed (Mandi and Vezendi 1971). For the country in general, in the absence of screening surveys, epidemiologic data come from reports of individual sarcoidosis patients, including 287 diagnosed from areas dispersed throughout the country and 315 seen at 50 major tuberculosis institutions through 1968 (Mandi and Vezendi 1971, Mandi and Kelemen 1963).

In Italy, a survey of 3,564,464 individuals in the Milan district by miniature roentgenograms from 1956 to 1968 revealed a prevalence of 9 per 100,000 (Giobbi et al. 1971). In the absence of other surveys, data come from individual authors' observations of sarcoidosis patients including 89 who were diagnosed in Puglia and 8 in Lucania, giving an estimated prevalence of 2.5 and 1.2 per 100,000 respectively (Muratore 1963). At the tuberculosis Dispensary Clinic in Lecce, fluoroscopic examination of 6728 patients between 1961 and 1962 failed to detect any cases of sarcoidosis (Muratore 1963). Limited data suggest that sarcoidosis occurs more commonly in the northern part of the country, unlike the geographic trend seen in the Federal Republic of Germany and the German Democratic Republic. This observation is supported by the reports from important southern research centers in Naples, Catania, Palermo, and Bari, which failed to see as many patients with sarcoidosis as their sister institutions to the north (Mariani 1977).

In the Soviet Union, radiographic screening surveys revealed a prevalence of intrathoracic sarcoidosis of 2.3 per 100,000 in Leningrad, 1.1 per 100,000 in Moscow, 3.8 per 100,000 in Talin, and 2.1 per 100,000 in Riga (Levinsky 1976). In Middle-Slovakia, an area with 1,400,000 inhabitants, survey chest roentgenograms for tuberculosis control revealed a prevalence of sarcoidosis of 14.9 per 100,000 in 1971 and 27.7 per 100,000 in 1975 (Kemka and Halak 1977). With the detection of about 50 new cases every year in the district, the incidence for 1971 was estimated to be 3.5 per 100,000 inhabitants with variation in the different districts ranging from 0.65 to 15.2 per 100,000. In Lettish, an annual incidence of 3.09 per 100,000 females and 2.04 per 100,000 males was calculated following the detection of sarcoidosis in 292 women and 192 men during the years 1958 to 1975 (Magalif and Brencsone 1977). In contrast to the higher incidence in adult females over adult males, the incidence rate for boys was four to five times higher than for girls in the 10–19 age range. In the 20–29 age group, the incidence was higher in males, but the ratio was smaller in comparison with the younger group (Magalif and Brencsone 1977).

In Yugoslavia, mass screening surveys for tuberculosis control have been applied to larger cities, industrial centers, and some rural areas. In the Republic of Slovenia, in the course of fluoroscopic screening sarcoidosis was registered separately. Among 277,016 individuals examined in 1961,

33 patients with sarcoidosis were recognized, giving a prevalence of 11.9 per 100,000 (La Grasta 1963). Responses from questionnaires sent to 21 special hospitals and clinics reported additional identification of 207 patients with sarcoidosis, 56% proven by histology (La Grasta 1963).

In France, the only survey was performed in 1963 and involved 607,292 individuals, including 97,799 students. Of those surveyed, 58 patients with sarcoidosis were detected, yielding a prevalence of 9.5 per 100,000 (Turiaf et al. 1963).

In Spain, a mass radiographic screening survey for tuberculosis control in 1965 and 1966 involving 4,350,869 individuals revealed two patients with diagnosed sarcoidosis, giving a prevalence of 0.04 per 100,000, the lowest frequency reported in Europe (Zapatero 1971). However, a study by questionnaire surveying 160 doctors revealed 248 known patients with sarcoidosis, 109 of them confirmed by histology (Zapatero 1971). Therefore, the prevalence of sarcoidosis is undoubtedly greater than that reported by the early mass survey.

In Romania, 70 sarcoidosis patients (52 confirmed histologically) were recognized over a 19-year period through 1968 (Daniello and Centea 1971), and an additional 92 patients were detected through 1976, suggesting a prevalence of 3.3 per 100,000 inhabitants (Levinsky et al. 1976). In this group of patients, 47% had extrapulmonary sarcoidosis, most frequently involving bones.

For the other countries in Europe, few epidemiologic data are available. In Greece, a total of 32 patients with sarcoidosis had been recognized up to the time of the Fifth International Conference on Sarcoidosis in 1968 (Lazarou 1971). In Portugal, questionnaire responses from institutions and physicians identified 34 patients with sarcoidosis who had been discovered between 1929 and 1963 (Villar 1963). In Turkey, 75 histologically confirmed sarcoidosis patients were recorded up to 1976 (Levinsky et al. 1976). In Bulgaria, a prevalence of 4.3 per 100,000 and an incidence of 1.4 per 100,000 were calculated from limited data (Levinsky et al. 1976).

B. Africa

In Africa, few countries have reported cases of sarcoidosis and none have performed radiographic screening surveys. Epidemiologic data, therefore, come from case reports or small series of patients collected by questionnaire or review of hospital records.

In Zambia, 18 natives with roentgenographic changes suggestive of sarcoidosis were detected among a group undergoing preemployment physical examinations (Fietcher 1966). In western Africa, 4 sarcoidosis patients have been diagnosed in Nigeria and 20 (4 proven by histology) in the Ivory Coast (Delormas et al. 1971). In Egypt, a review of medical records from the University Hospitals of Cairo University (capacity 3000 beds) revealed that 29 patients with sarcoidosis had the diagnosis confirmed by organ biopsy between 1952 and 1962 (Gomaa 1963). The first reported cases from Ethiopia were 6 patients with sarcoidosis recognized in 1977. A subsequent review of the archives of the pathology department of the Faculty of Medicine, Addis-Ababa University, revealed that 23 additional patients with sarcoidosis had been diagnosed on the basis of skin or lymph node biopsies in 1976 and 1977 (Tsega et al. 1978).

In South Africa, a review published in 1961 of records of the five teaching hospitals revealed clinical and histological evidence of sarcoidosis in 18 individuals from the Caucasian population (total 3,500,000), and 30 from the African population (total 10,500,000) (Van Lingen 1961). Only 5 cases had been reported previously in the South African medical literature (Van Lingen 1961). At the Groote Schuur Hospital, 110 patients with sarcoidosis were seen between 1969 and 1975 (Benatar 1977), and an additional 44 cases during 1976 and 1977 (Benatar 1980). Of the 110 patients, 71 were colored, 25 were black, and 14 were white, giving a calculated minimum incidence of sarcoidosis in the Cape Peninsula of 23.2 per 100,000 blacks, 11.6 per 100,000 coloreds, and 3.7 per 100,000 whites. Extrathoracic sarcoidosis was noted more frequently in blacks than in whites, with the coloreds occupying an intermediate position. The blacks had a high incidence of deforming arthritis and skin lesions (Benatar 1977). Another report of 18 patients with sarcoidosis among the Bantu also emphasized the high frequency of gross skin lesions and destructive arthritis in blacks (Morrison 1974).

C. Asia

In Israel, from 1956 to 1962, 70 cases of histologically confirmed sarcoidosis were detected, giving a mean annual incidence of 0.5 per 100,000 (Rakower 1963). The prevalence obtained from radiographic screening was three times higher at 1.6 per 100,000 inhabitants. The peak incidence of sarcoidosis occurred in the 20–39 age group with a sex distribution of three males to one female, a ratio unlike that for most other countries. There was no difference in incidence rates between the European and Afro-Asian immigrants. However, the incidence rate was five times higher in Jerusalem than in Tel Aviv, and almost four times higher than in Haifa.

In Japan, a total of 94 patients with sarcoidosis were recognized by 1960, compiled from data obtained by questionnaires distributed to 325 medical school clinics and to 458 other institutions (Nobechi 1961). Of the 94 confirmed cases, four were diagnosed between 1921 and 1945, 26 between 1946 and 1955, and 64 between 1956 and 1960. A radiographic survey in 1953 of 50,000 individuals and another in 1958 of 70,000 individuals failed to detect a single case of sarcoidosis (Nobechi 1961). However, five subsequent surveys conducted throughout the nation between 1963 and 1972 revealed intrathoracic sarcoidosis in 2079 individuals (1425 confirmed by histology), giving an overall average annual incidence of 0.3 per 100,000 surveyed with values of 0.44, 0.24, and 0.13 for northern, central, and southern Japan respectively (Hosoda et al. 1976a). There was an almost equal male–female ratio, with the highest incidence in the 20–29 year-old age group. By 1976, the total number of patients with sarcoidosis had reached nearly 5000 and the calculated annual incidence had risen to 0.5 per 100,000 inhabitants (Hosoda et al. 1980). A higher prevalence for sarcoidosis (16 of 30,000 examined) has been reported from the Furano Basin in the central mountainous district of Japan (Hiraga et al. 1977).

In 1979, a review of six nationwide epidemiologic surveys (Yanagawa 1979) of sarcoidosis identified 5038 cases (2359 male and 2679 female) through 1977 and led to the following conclusions:

1. The incidence rates steadily increased until 1972, after which the rates have been constant.

2. The age distribution in males peaked at 20–29, while in females there was a high peak at 20–29 and a lower peak at 50–59 years.

3. The incidence rates were higher in the northern part of Japan, where the age of the patients shifted toward the younger group.

4. More than half of the cases reported were discovered by x-ray health examinations.

5. There was a marked seasonal variation in the onset of the cases discovered by health examinations, onset being most frequent in June or July.

6. The frequency of hilar lymphadenopathy and lung mottling decreased in the older group, while the incidence of eye and skin lesions increased with age.

In India, the first patient with sarcoidosis was reported in 1959 (Hosoda 1976b). An additional 27 patients with sarcoidosis (18 confirmed histologically) were detected among 44,110 new patients seen at the Vallchbai Patel Chest Institute between 1957 and 1974 (Hosoda 1976). Most of the patients had been referred because of complaints of chest diseases or failure to respond to antituberculosis treatment.

In Thailand, until 1974 only eight known patients with sarcoidosis had been recognized (Hosoda 1976b). Mass screening surveys for tuberculosis between 1963 and 1971 of 1,764,229 individuals failed to detect anyone with sarcoidosis.

In Singapore, one case of sarcoidosis was reported in 1964 and two were reported in 1973. Radiographic surveys of 248,740 individuals between 1957 and 1970 and 243,885 between 1959 and 1970 failed to detect a single case of sarcoidosis (Hosoda et al. 1976b).

In Malaysia, data obtained from questionnaires sent to chest clinics of general hospitals and through a search of records at the Institute for Medical Research, revealed evidence of suspected sarcoidosis in 13 individuals (Hosoda et al. 1976b). Investigation of the clinical and histopathologic material confirmed the diagnosis in eight, all detected between 1960 and 1973.

In the Republic of China (Taiwan), seven sarcoidosis patients had been reported by 1975 (Hosoda et al. 1976b). Further studies reviewed 35,000 70-mm microfilms taken from 1967 to 1968 and another 70,000 micro-films taken from 1972 to 1973, but both failed to detect hilar adenopathy suggestive of sarcoidosis in anyone in either survey (Hosoda et al. 1976b). In the Peoples' Republic of China (mainland China), the first case report of sarcoidosis appeared in 1958, describing a 13-month-old girl who pre-sented with fever, hilar adenopathy, and splenomegaly (Hosoda et al. 1976b). The diagnosis was made from histological sections of the spleen following splenectomy. Two additional Chinese patients with sarcoidosis have been reported, a 24-year-old woman born in Hong Kong and diagnosed in New York City, and a 33-year-old woman born in Hangchow and diagnosed in Taiwan.

In all, 11 Chinese patients with sarcoidosis have been reported (Nandi et al. 1981). To these, the authors added 4 additional Hong Kong Chinese, 3 female and 1 male. They were asymptomatic and the diagnoses were based on the radiographic pattern of bilateral hilar lymphadenopathy and were confirmed by mediastinoscopy. The geographic distribution of the 15 Chinese patients is 1 from the Phillipines, 1 from Shanghai, 1 from New York, 2 from Taiwan, 3 each from Malaysia and Singapore, and the recent 4 from Hong Kong. The total of 15 patients among the huge population of ubiquitous Chinese emphasizes the low prevalence of sarcoidosis in this major nationality. That these data reflect true prevalence in questionable when one considers that the four newly discovered patients were all encountered during a 1-year period.

In the Republic of South Korea, the first patient with sarcoidosis was detected in 1974 (Han et al. 1974). A radiographic survey of 46,844 inhabitants which was seeking to uncover tuberculosis and was reported at the Seventh International Conference on Sarcoidosis failed to detect anyone with roentgenographic changes that could be attributed to sarcoidosis (Hosoda et al. 1976b). Furthermore, questionnaires sent to main hospitals, and a search through records of the major medical institutions and their Departments of Thoracic Medicine and Pathology in the Seoul district, failed to detect any proven cases of sarcoidosis (Hosoda et al. 1976b).

In the Phillipines, six cases have been reported in the literature (Hosoda et al. 1976b). No cases have been diagnosed in large hospitals such as Veterans Memorial Hospital, V. Luna Hospital, San Lazaro Hospital, and the University of Santo Toman Hospital (Hosoda et al. 1976b).

D. North America/United States

In the United States, with the exception of New York City, less epidemiologic data is available regarding sarcoidosis than in Europe. Mass screening surveys that would allow calculations of prevalence and incidence rates in the general population have not been performed. The epidemiologic information that is available comes largely from studies of military personnel and patients attending Veterans Hospitals and from case-matched studies comparing series of clinically detected patients with sarcoidosis with controls or with patients suffering from other diseases.

One of the earliest military studies was the review of 300 consecutive patients with sarcoidosis who had biopsy or autopsy material on file at the Army Institute of Pathology (Ricker and Clark 1949). Of the total group, 278 were admitted to hospital because of sarcoidosis or for other presumed disease and were alive at the time of the study. In 22 patients, the diagnosis was detected at autopsy. Of the 42 patients who were asymptomatic, the diagnosis was made incidental to routine clinical examination or at autopsy. Most patients were symptomatic. Overall, 93% of the blacks reported symptoms as compared to 76% of the whites, and an appreciably greater number of blacks complained of weight loss and low-grade fever.

Of the 300 patients, 271 were in the Army. Of this group, 172 (63%) were black and 99 (31%) were white. By applying these numbers to the estimated Army population during the period from January 1943 to June 1946, the incidence for sarcoidosis was found to be 8.7 per 100,000 blacks and 0.5 per 100,000 whites per year. These numbers were the first to establish clearly the predominance of sarcoidosis in blacks—17 to 1 in this instance—in the United States (Table 2).

Two additional studies that showed a higher incidence of sarcoidosis in blacks were performed in the United States Navy and Marine Corps. In the first study, a total of 303 patients with sarcoidosis were detected during the years 1954 through 1958 (Gundelfinger and Britten 1961). The annual incidence rate was found to be 47.8 per 100,000 for blacks and 5.0 per 100,000 for whites, a 10 times higher incidence in blacks. In the second study, 134 patients with sarcoidosis were detected between 1958 and 1971 among 1,216,425 recruits who entered the Navy between 1958 and 1969 (Sartwell and Edwards 1974). Of the 134 patients, 65 were discovered by chest roentgenograms. In 43 individuals the roentgenogram was taken for

Table 2 Incidence of Sarcoidosis in Military and Veterans Administration Studies/100,000 by Race

Study group	Black	White	Ratio	Reference
U.S. Army (1943–1946)	8.7	0.5	17:1	Ricker and Clark (1949)
U.S. Veterans (1949–1954)	40.1	3.3	12:1	Cummings et al. (1956)
U.S. Navy (1954–1958)	47.8	5.0	10:1	Gundelfinger and Britten (1961)
U.S. Navy (1958–1969)	81.8	7.6	10:1	Sartwell and Edwards (1974)

investigation of clinical findings and in 22 of them the roentgenogram was part of the routine examination before discharge from service. In addition to these 65 patients, an additional 44 individuals were detected because of symptoms or signs. Overall, symptoms led to the diagnosis in 41% of the blacks and 28% of the whites. With the number of blacks and whites screened at entry to the service as denominators, the incidence rates were 81.8 for blacks and 7.6 for whites, revealing, as in the first United States Navy study, an attack rate of 10:1 in favor of blacks. The higher incidence rates reported in the second study probably reflect the fact that some of the patients with sarcoidosis were detected by screening, whereas in the first Navy study, and subsequent Army and Veterans Administration investigations, nearly all patients were detected because of clinical complaints (Table 2).

In a study of patients attending Veterans Administration hospitals, 1,194 patients with sarcoidosis were seen in 172 Veterans Administration hospitals between 1949 and 1954 (Cummings et al. 1956). Ninety percent of these were less than 44 years of age and 60% were less than 34 years old. Overall, the hospitalization rate for sarcoidosis for black World War II veterans was 40.1 per 100,000 and for white veterans 3.3 per 100,000, giving a comparative ratio of 13:1.

Military and Veterans Administration hospital studies have also evaluated the geographic distributions of the birthplaces of patients with sarcoidosis (Table 3). In the early Army study (Ricker and Clark 1949), where data were available, it was observed that 78% of the patients (79 of 101) came from the southeastern states. In the Navy and Veterans Administration hospital studies, it was also noted that most of the sarcoidosis patients came from the south Atlantic and east south central states (Cummings et al. 1956, Gundelfinger and Britten 1961, Sartwell and Edwards 1974). This geographic pattern led to the famous postulate that sarcoidosis might be caused by fine sandy soil or pine tree pollen found in the southern part of the country (Gentry et al. 1955, Cummings et al. 1956).

In contrast, a review of 177 patients with sarcoidosis seen at the Mayo Clinic from 1940 through 1951 failed to suggest a different geographic pattern than that seen for the total clinic registration (Carr and Gage 1954). In addition, a case-match comparison of 240 sarcoidosis patients diagnosed between 1961 and 1965 in New York City with an equal number of tuberculous and nontuberculous control patients failed to reveal an association of sarcoidosis with past residence in southern states (Terris and Chaves 1966). Similarly, a comparison of 420 male patients with sarcoidosis at the United States Veterans hospitals between 1960 and 1964 with 420 male control patients matched for race, age, and hospital attributes also failed to reveal a different geographic distribution of sarcoidosis for whites and blacks by either birthplace or later residence (Keller 1971, 1973) (Table 3).

Table 3 Distribution of Sarcoidosis According to Birthplace

I. Studies suggesting geographic differences		
Study group	Area of highest incidence	Reference
U.S. Army (1943–1946)	Southeastern states	Ricker and Clark (1949)
U.S. Veterans (1949–1954)	South Atlantic and Southeast Central states	Cummings et al. (1956)
U.S. Navy (1958–1969)	South Atlantic and Southeast Central states	Gundelfinger and Britten (1961), Sartwell and Edwards (1974)
II. Studies suggesting no geographic differences		
Study group	Method of study	Reference
Mayo Clinic (1940–1951)	Compared with total Mayo Clinic patients	Carr and Gage (1954)
New York City (1961–1965)	Matched controls	Terris and Chaves (1966)
U.S. Veterans (1960–1964)	Matched controls	Keller (1973)

The explanation for the apparently higher incidence of sarcoidosis among individuals from the South, as suggested by military and Veterans Administration hospital studies, but not confirmed by case-match comparison, appears to be that at the time of these studies, more blacks lived in the South than in later studies. When population density statistics for 1935 (the approximate date of birth for patients in the studies emanating from the Army and Navy) for whites and blacks from various parts of the country are applied to data obtained from sarcoidosis patients diagnosed in Veterans Administration hospitals between 1958 and 1964, the distribution among blacks and whites for the 1935 population statistics is as follows: Northeast 42.5 per 100,000 blacks and 3.0 per 100,000 whites; North-central 35.8 for blacks and 2.7 for whites; South 46.8 for blacks and 3.9 for whites; and West 26.7 for blacks and 2.0 for whites (Israel 1971, Keller and Dunner 1967). Thus, by these statistical methods the incidence of sarcoidosis based on black-white population densities for 1935 is similar for all parts of the country without selective localization to the Southeast. In addition, the ratios for the various parts of the country confirm the 12–14 times higher frequency among blacks.

Besides noting racial and geographical differences, military and Veterans Administration hospital studies have also reported that more patients with sarcoidosis come from rural environments (Michael et al. 1950, Dublin 1961, Cummings 1959). When this observation was subjected to the scrutiny of case-matched comparison, as was done with geographic distribution, it was confirmed that more sarcoidosis patients than controls or tuberculosis patients report having been born in rural areas or having spent a larger portion of their lifetime in rural areas before the onset of their disease (Terris and Chaves 1966, Buck 1961). However, as yet, no specific environmental or occupational factors that might relate the rural background to the etiology of sarcoidosis have been identified.

The only mass radiologic survey conducted in the United States that provided data concerning sarcoidosis was performed in New York City as part of a tuberculosis control program (Robins et al. 1962). During the years 1956–1962 a total of 449,605 individuals had chest radiographs performed in nine different districts. Sarcoidosis was found in 174 individuals. The diagnosis was based primarily on roentgenographic evaluation, although confirmation was made by biopsy or Kveim test in over 50% of the patients. In this survey, an overall prevalence rate of 39 per 100,000 was found, with a range from 64 per 100,000 in those districts where more than 40% of the population were nonwhite to 17 per 100,000 where fewer than 19% were nonwhite.

During the years 1958–1962, the New York City Department of Health kept a register of all sarcoidosis cases examined in its chest clinics.

Of the 291 registered cases, 73% were black, 16% were white, and 10.3% were of Puerto Rican origin (Robins et al. 1962).

Canada

Limited epidemiologic data are available from Canada. Three small mass radiographic surveys of a total of 77,000 individuals in British Columbia and Ontario during the years 1960 and 1961 revealed a prevalence for sarcoidosis of 10.5 per 100,000 (Pollak 1963). Sarcoidosis, in contrast to tuberculosis, appears to be rare among Eskimos and Indians: No cases were detected among 1200 individuals with abnormal chest roentgenograms from the Eastern Arctic region evaluated at the Mountain Sanatorium in Hamilton over a 12-year period, or among 31,183 individuals (20,313 roentgenograms) from the Foothills Region surveyed in 1961. The only three known patients with sarcoidosis among Indians were diagnosed at the Coqualeetza Indian Hospital in Sardis, British Columbia, in 1962 (Pollak 1963).

Jamaica

One hundred patients with sarcoidosis have been reported from Jamaica, West Indies, among a population of 2.1 million (Lowe 1980). With the exception of one East Indian woman, all of the individuals were black or of mixed blood. Surprisingly, 62% of the group were males, and most patients of both sexes were over 40 years of age (Buck 1961). No attempt was made to determine prevalence rates because of inadequate data.

E. South America

Sarcoidosis has been reported rarely in most countries in South America, probably because of a lack of intense case-finding techniques. When efforts have been made to detect the disease by screening or by questionnaire in a few countries, patients with sarcoidosis have been identified with some frequency.

In Argentina, a screening survey of 695,312 individuals in Buenos Aires for tuberculosis control between 1954 and 1962 led to the diagnosis of sarcoidosis in seven patients, giving a prevalence of 1 per 100,000 (Purriel et al. 1963). However, another screening survey for tuberculosis control involving 130,000 individuals in Rosario failed to detect a single patient with sarcoidosis. In response to a questionnaire sent to 699 physicians who treated patients with pulmonary diseases, 89 reported a total of 100 patients with sarcoidosis in Argentina (Purriel et al. 1963).

In Brazil, a tuberculosis control survey conducted in Sao Paulo from 1953 through 1963 revealed one instance of sarcoidosis among 52,861 individuals examined. A review of 111,870 hospital admissions in the same city during the years 1961 and 1962 failed to detect a single patient with sarcoidosis, and a review of 210,000 patients examined at the Research Institute, Clemente Ferreira, between 1960 and 1963 yielded two patients. A survey of 1,500,000 industrial workers between 1947 and 1963 revealed one patient with sarcoidosis (Purriel et al. 1963).

In Uruguay, radiographic screening of 1,077,180 individuals between 1952 and 1957 failed to reveal a case of sarcoidosis, whereas another survey of 1,838,913 individuals between 1951 and 1962 yielded eight cases of sarcoidosis. Throughout the country, 90 patients with sarcoidosis were reported up to 1963, giving a crude prevalence of 2.4 per 100,000 (Purriel et al. 1963).

Among the other countries in South America without screening surveys, two cases of sarcoidosis have been reported in Chile, one in Bolivia, and none from Peru, Ecuador, Colombia, and Venezuela (Purriel et al. 1963).

F. Australia and New Zealand

In Australia, a radiographic screening survey of 1,571,011 individuals in the state of Victoria between 1959 and 1962 revealed 145 sarcoidosis patients (9.2 per 100,000), diagnosed by radiographic evidence alone (Marshman 1963). The frequency was highest in people between the ages of 15 and 40 and there was no definite sex relationship. One case of sarcoidosis has been reported in an Austrailian aborigine (Webling 1978).

In New Zealand, mass radiographic surveys in Auckland (376,380 individuals), Wellington (306,547 individuals), and Christ Church (396,353 individuals) yielded overall prevalence rates of 6.13, 24.3, and 18.4, respectively (Reid 1963). The disparities in the data were attributed to differences in selecting the study groups and to variable methods of making a definitive diagnosis. Among approximately 31,200 Maoris surveyed, three patients with sarcoidosis were found.

III. Epidemiology

A careful reading of the reports relating to the worldwide distribution of sarcoidosis reveals many references to additional epidemiologic data. The Germans emphasize the preponderance of patients residing in southern Germany, while the Italians report the opposite. While stressing local geographic differences, the Japanese also note a peak age incidence from 20 to 30 years and a higher frequency among females. In the United States, reports of regional distribution of sarcoidosis are heavily laden with statistics regarding race. Thus, other epidemiologic data, in addition to geographic distribution, have been emphasized in sarcoidosis. The final section of this chapter will discuss sex, age, race, geography, family, and HLA type in sarcoidosis.

IV. Age

The youngest person with sarcoidosis was a 28-month-old child reported by Posner (1942). At autopsy, the patient was found to have involvement of all organs with noncaseating epithelioid granulomas "typical" of sarcoidosis. Acid-fast bacilli and fungi were absent. Because of the extreme youth of this patient and the well-recognized nonspecificity of noncaseating granulomas, the diagnosis is open to question. However, there are numerous reliable reports of the frequency of sarcoidosis in children.

Kendig (1974) reviewed 104 cases in patients 15 years old or younger and later added nine new patients. The distribution of organ involvement in children is similar to that in adults. However, it has been suggested that disabling disease may be more common among children (Kendig and Brummer 1976). The frequency in children is difficult to assess since in most countries physicians refrain from using routine chest radiography in the young. An interesting report of a comparison of 45 Japanese children and 40 children from the state of Virginia emphasizes the impact of mass radiography in detecting sarcoidosis (Kendig and Yasutaka 1980). In Japan, school children received an annual chest roentgenogram at the time of the report, while in the United States, radiographic examination was performed only when clinically indicated. Understandably, 42 of the 45 Japanese children were asymptomatic at the time of the diagnosis while only five of the 40 Americans were without symptoms. Otherwise, the two national groups were quite similar. It is apparent that sarcoidosis occurs with moderate frequency in children and must be considered when the primary care physician or pediatrician encounters a child of any age presenting with lymphadenopathy, pulmonary infiltrates, iritis, or fever.

Sarcoidosis has also been reported in patients above the age of 60 years. Cowdell cites a patient of Leitner who was 80 years old (Cowdell 1954) and Mayock's oldest patient was 74 years old (Mayock et al. 1963). In the group of 2765 patients seen at Mount Sinai Hospital in New York, the oldest patient was 72 at the time of diagnosis. The extremes notwithstanding, unquestionably most patients with sarcoidosis present between the ages of 20 and 40 years. Of Mayock's 145 patients, 41% were in their third decade. Israel reported that 88 patients were between 21 and 30 years, and 35 were between 31 and 40 years among a total of 160 (Israel and Sones 1958). A peak incidence between the ages of 25 and 35 was demonstrated by Rudberg-Roos (1962) among 296 patients. The age of onset has no relation to the clinical presentation, prognosis, or geographic location.

V. Sex

Most large series report a greater frequency of sarcoidosis in females than males (Mayock et al. 1963, Israel 1971, Rudberg-Roos 1962). Unfortunately, such data are open to some question since most of these reports emanate from the clinics of large cities. Study of other clinics in the same institutions, treating diseases other than sarcoidosis, might yield a similar predilection for females. For example, a recent review of 104 consecutive patients referred to the sarcoidosis clinic at The Mount Sinai Hospital in New York revealed that 70% were female and 30% were male (Teirstein et al. 1981). Investigation of the sex distribution among patients attending other clinics specializing in diseases not thought to exhibit any sexual preponderance revealed the same female preponderance found in the sarcoidosis clinic. The simultaneous study of 110 patients with sarcoidosis attending the private practice suites of the same physicians who attend the clinic patients at The Mount Sinai Hospital revealed that the distribution of sarcoidosis was approximately the same in both sexes. From this study, it is apparent that in some institutions more women attend clinics than men, thus challenging the validity of data derived from clinic populations, which show a sexual predilection in sarcoidosis.

VI. Race

When confronted with a chest radiograph which exhibits mediastinal lymphadenopathy, the viewer frequently asks, "Is the patient black?" The predominance of sarcoidosis among blacks, approximately 10–17 times the prevalence among whites in the United States, is based on the excellent studies performed among military personnel, Veterans Administration patients, and patients attending the clinics of large urban medical centers cited previously. Unfortunately, this apparent racial predisposition has become so integral a part of our knowledge of sarcoidosis that some physicians mistakenly consider the race of the patient to be of diagnostic significance. This view has also been communicated to patients. Many white patients, when informed of the diagnosis of sarcoidosis, respond querulously, "I thought sarcoidosis occurred only in blacks."

   In the above study comparing the sex distribution among patients attending The Mount Sinai Hospital Sarcoidosis Clinic and the private physicians' offices, racial distribution was also recorded (Teirstein et al. 1981). Not surprisingly, the sarcoidosis clinic population was 57% black and 31% white, while the private office population was 81% white and 16% black. Once again, comparing the racial distribution in the sarcoidosis clinic with that of the clinics serving patients with diseases with no known relation to race demonstrated a similar preponderance of blacks over whites. It is obvious that black females comprise the largest group of patients attending the Mount Sinai Hospital clinics, a fact that probably holds true for most clinics located in, or near, large urban ghettos in the United States. It should be remembered that sarcoidosis has been reported with increasing frequency in Japan and in heavy concentration in Sweden, that is, among Orientals and Caucasians. Although the remarkable frequency of sarcoidosis among blacks reported in the military and Veterans populations in the United States is irrefutable, the racial origin of patients, even in the United States, is of little or no diagnostic value.

VII. HLA Typing in Sarcoidosis

The search for a genetic predisposition for sarcoidosis has led several investigators to study the frequency of HLA types in patients with sarcoidosis. In two studies (Kueppers et al. 1974, Hedfors and Moller 1973), the overall distribution of HLA antigen was no different from that of controls. Persson (1975) reported that individuals with sarcoidosis and HLA-B7 were more likely to be symptomatic. Neville and associates (1980) confirmed the lack of HLA specificity in sarcoidosis but emphasized that white sarcoidosis patients with HLA-B8 are likely to have arthritis and/or erythema nodosum. They proposed that the link between erythema nodosum and B8 may explain the variable frequency with which erythema nodosum occurs among different population groups around the world.

At the Seventh International Conference on Sarcoidosis, Al-Arif and co-workers (1980) reported a frequency of sarcoidosis 5.5 times greater in black patients with HLA-Bw15 than in those lacking that antigen. This finding was particularly interesting because Bw15 is significantly increased in black patients with tuberculosis. Most recently, a study of HLA frequency in 164 health control subjects, 50 patients with persistent pulmonary fibrosis due to sarcoidosis, and 37 patients whose sarcoidosis cleared spontaneously, revealed that those subjects who experienced spontaneous resolution of sarcoidosis had a greater frequency of B8 than either the group with chronic sarcoidosis or the control group (Smith et al. 1981). Despite these interesting studies, to date, no significant correlation between the occurrence or the clinical pictures of sarcoidosis and HLA type has been conclusively demonstrated.

VIII. Familial Sarcoidosis

Sarcoidosis does appear to occur with noteworthy frequency among members of the same family, although there are no controlled studies to lend statistical significance to that observation. Two major reviews of the prevalence of familial sarcoidosis have been published. Jorgenson (1965) reported 54 instances of familial sarcoidosis, and the British Thoracic and Tuberculosis Association research committee (1973) noted 121 patients among 59 families. This latter group included 4 pairs of monozygotic twins and 1 dyzygotic twin set, 28 pairs of siblings, 22 parent-child combinations, and 7 husband-wife pairs. This report reviewed an additional 174 previously reported cases of familial sarcoidosis and emphasized the preponderance of monozygotic over dizygotic twins, females over males, and mother-child over father-child sets.

Sporadic reports of familial sarcoidosis continue to appear, tempting some investigators to speculate on the possible role of the genetic and environmental factors shared by these families that might offer insight into the etiology of sarcoidosis (James et al. 1974). The several instances of husband and wife pairs would support a common causative environmental factor, but would seem to militate against genetic theories. We have seen one instance of a wife who did not have sarcoidosis but whose first husband contracted a fatal case of the disease. Within a few years of her remarriage, her second husband also developed sarcoidosis. We have dubbed her "Sarcoid Mary." While there is no conclusive support for any genetic or environmental theory in the etiology of sarcoidosis, the apparent clustering of patients within families remains an attractive area for further study in causation.

IX. Geographic Distribution

As can be seen from the review of the world distribution of sarcoidosis, the disease has been reported throughout the six continents. In many locations where a significant prevalence of sarcoidosis has not been encountered, modern diagnostic and case-finding techniques have not been applied; one may predict that in the future the disease will be recorded in these countries with increasing frequency. For example, reports of isolated instances of sarcoidosis among black Africans are now beginning to appear. The paucity of reports from this continent has been particularly confusing in light of the great prevalence of sarcoidosis among blacks in the United States, whose forebears were, in great measure, black Africans. It is probable that this discrepancy is related to inadequate case-finding rather than to true prevalence. On the other hand, several excellent studies dedicated to uncovering lung disease by mass radiographic surveys have yielded evidence supporting the claim that sarcoidosis is rare among Canadian Indians, Eskimos, Southeast Asian populations, and New Zealand Maoris. These data tend to support the role of genetic differences or geography in the etiology of sarcoidosis.

Migration from the country of origin to a foreign location also has been implicated in the causation of sarcoidosis. Silzbach (1967b) noted an increased frequency of sarcoidosis among Puerto-Rican-born subjects living in New York City, and James et al. (1956) reported a similar increased prevalence in Irish-born females and males residing in London. Other than speculation about the stresses of settling in an alien environment, no explanation has been offered for these observations.

An extensive review of the clinical features of sarcoidosis from five cities, London, Paris, Tokyo, Los Angeles, and New York, revealed an extraordinary similarity in sex, age, thoracic and extrathoracic manifestations, and prognosis (Siltzbach et al. 1974). In these cities, the disease occurred in women only slightly more frequently than in men, 70% of the patients were between the ages of 20 and 40 years, initial chest radiographs revealed bilateral hilar lymph node enlargement with clear lung fields in 69–88% of the patients, and parenchycmal interstitial infiltrations accompanyed lymphadenopathy in 30–49%. In all, abnormal chest radiographs were reported at presentation in 88–93% of the patients. Clinically evident extrathoracic sarcoidosis was noted with similar frequency in the five cities, and the overall percentages of involvement at presentation were 28% with peripheral lymph nodes, 22% with ocular sarcoidosis, and 18% with cutaneous lesions. The Kveim test was positive in 79% of the patients studied, ranging from 54% in Tokyo to 92% in New York. Interestingly, the tuberculin skin test was positive in 34% of the combined group, ranging from 45% positive in London to only 15% positive in Los Angeles. While the study comprised patient cohorts derived from five of the larger cities in the developed world, this study is particularly noteworthy since the racial prevalence was dissimilar among the five groups; white (Paris and London), Oriental (Tokyo), and predominantly black (Los Angeles and New York). This study has now been extended to include 11 cities, and the major epidemiologic similarities throughout the urban world have been confirmed (James et al. 1976).

In the absence of an accurate denominator for calculating prevalence data in sarcoidosis, it is difficult to assess the overall prognosis of the disease. Early reports indicated that approximately two-thirds of all patients with diagnosed sarcoidosis will experience eventual cure, spontaneously or with therapy, and from 5 to 15% will die of their disease (Longcope and Freiman 1952, Sones and Israel 1960, Teirstein et al. 1971). With data indicating that many more patients contract and recover from sarcoidosis without diagnosis than are uncovered by physicians, it is obvious that the true prognosis is far better than one would conclude from early reports. Certain ethnic and geographic differences in the manifestations and course of sarcoidosis have been emphasized. Erythema nodosum, an explosive form of sarcoidosis accompanied by bilateral hilar lymphadeno-

pathy and often with ankle swelling and arthralgias, is rare among the
Japanese and quite common in Puerto Rican, Irish, and Swedish females.
Teirstein and Siltzbach (1974) reported 47% Puerto Rican, 34% white, and
only 18% blacks among 100 patients presenting with erythema nodosum
as the initial manifestation of sarcoidosis. A greater frequency of extrathoracic involvement in sarcoidosis has been recorded among black patients
when compared with whites. However, deaths due to sarcoidosis—usually
from pulmonary insufficiency, hemorrhage from aspergillomas, hypercalcemia
and renal failure, or cardiac sarcoidosis—occur with equal frequency among
blacks and whites (Teirstein et al. 1976, Teirstein and Siltzbach 1971).

X. Conclusion

1. Sarcoidosis is a common disease occurring worldwide with varying
   incidence and prevalence.

2. Sarcoidosis is especially common among the black population in
   the United States. However, it is also quite common among the
   American white population, among Scandinavians, particularly from
   Sweden, and among Japanese.

3. Eskimos, Canadian Indians, New Zealand Maoris, and Southeast
   Asians rarely contract the disease.

4. Sarcoidosis is most common in the 20–40 age group. However,
   young children and the aged may have the disease.

5. There is a slightly greater prevalence of sarcoidosis among women
   than among men.

6. Although certain geographic locations appear to have a high
   prevalence of sarcoidosis, and a few a low prevalence, there is no
   etiologically significant geographic pattern.

7. Familial sarcoidosis is common and has been emphasized in support
   of theories of environmental and genetic predisposition for
   sarcoidosis.

8. Careful review of all epidemiologic factors and the worldwide
   distribution of sarcoidosis fails to shed light on the etiology of
   sarcoidosis and is of little value in diagnosis.

References

Al-Arif, L., Goldstein, R. A., Affronti, L. F., Janicki, B. W., and Foellmer,
    J. W. (1980). HLA antigens and sarcoidosis in a North American

black population. *Proceedings of the VIIIth International Conference on Sarcoidosis,* Cardiff, Wales, Alpha Omega, pp. 206-212.

Baer, R. B. (1960). Familial sarcoidosis. *Arch. Intern. Med.,* **105**:60-68.

Baldry, P. E., Sutherland, I., and Scadding, J. G. (1969). Geographical variations in the incidence of sarcoidosis in Great Britain: A comparative study of four areas. *Tubercle,* **50**:211-231.

Bauer, H. J., and Wijkstrom, S. (1963). The prevalence of pulmonary sarcoidosis in Swedish mass radiography surveys. Sundbybeerg, Sweden, Centre of Mass Chest Radiography of the Royal Swedish Medical Boards, pp. 112-114.

Benatar, S. R. (1977). Sarcoidosis in South Africa—A comparative study in whites, blacks, and coloureds, *S. Afr. Med. J.,* **52**:602-606.

Benatar, S. R. (1980). A comparative study of sarcoidosis in white, black and coloured South Africans. *Proceedings of the VIIIth International Conference on Sarcoidosis.* Cardiff, Wales, Alpha Omega, pp. 508-513.

British Thoracic and Tuberculosis Association (1973). Familial association in sarcoidosis. *Tubercle,* **54**:87-98.

Buck, A. A. (1961). Epidemiologic investigations of sarcoidosis. *Am. J. Hyg.,* **74**:189-202.

Carr, D. T., and Gage, R. P. (1954). The geographic distribution of sarcoidosis. *Am. Rev. Tuberc. Pulmon. Dis.,* **70**:899-900.

Cowdell, R. H. (1954). Sarcoidosis: With special reference to diagnosis and prognosis. *Q. J. Med.,* **23**:29-55.

Cummings, M. M., Dunner, E., Schmidt, H., Jr., and Barnwell, J. B. (1956). Concepts of epidemiology of sarcoidosis. *Postgrad. Med.,* **19**:437-446.

Cummings, M. M., Dunner, E., and Williams, J. H., Jr. (1959). Epidemiologic and clinical observations in sarcoidosis. *Ann. Intern. Med.,* **50**: 879-890.

Daniello, L., and Centea, A. (1971). Epidemiological aspects of sarcoidosis in the North-West part of Romania. *Proceedings of the Vth International Conference on Sarcoidosis.* Praha, Universita Karlova, pp. 304-306.

Delormas, P., Coulibaly, N., and Pignot, F. (1971). Considerations upon sarcoidosis in Africa. *Proceedings of the Vth International Conference on Sarcoidosis.* Praha, Universita Karlova, pp. 240-241.

Douglas, A. C. (1963). Epidemiology of sarcoidosis in Scotland. Proceedings of the IIIrd International Conference on Sarcoidosis. *Acta Med. Scand.,* (Suppl. 425, 1964):118-122.

Dublin, T. D. (1961). Analysis of incidence and mortality data in the United States. *Am. Rev. Respir. Dis.,* **84**(suppl.):103-108.

Fietcher, G. H. (1966). Sarcoidosis in miners in the Republic of Zambia. *Cent. Afr. J. Med.,* **12**:29-30.

Gentry, J. T., Nitowsky, H. M., and Michael, M., Jr. (1955). Studies on the epidemiology of sarcoidosis in the United States: The relationship to soil areas and to urban-rural residence. *J. Clin. Invest.*, **34**: 1839–1856.

Giobbi, A., Casalone, G., and Pandiani, C. (1971). Epidemiology of pulmonary sarcoidosis in Milano district. *Proceedings of the Vth International Conference on Sarcoidosis.* Praha, Universita Karlova, pp. 244–249.

Gomaa, T. (1963). Sarcoidosis in Egypt (U.A.R.). Proceedings of the IIIrd International Conference on Sarcoidosis. *Acta Med. Scand.*, (Suppl. 425, 1964):161–162.

Gundelfinger, B. F., and Britten, S. A. (1961). Sarcoidosis in the United States Navy. *Am. Rev. Respir. Dis.*, **84**(suppl.):109–115.

Hagerstrand, I., and Linell, F. (1963). The prevalence of sarcoidosis in the autopsy material from a Swedish town. Proceedings of the IIIrd International Conference on Sarcoidosis. *Acta Med. Scand.*, (Suppl. 425, 1964):171–173.

Han, M. C., Ha, S. W., and Rhie, B. C. (1974). A case report of sarcoidosis with review of literature. *Korean J. Radiol.*, **10**:29–34.

Hedfors, E., and Moller, E. (1973). HLA antigens in sarcoidosis. *Tissue Antigens,* **3**:95–98.

Hiraga, Y., Hosoda, Y., and Zenda, I. (1977). A local outbreak of sarcoidosis in northern Japan. *Z. Erkrank. Atm.-Org.,* **149**:38–43.

Honeybourne, D. (1980). Ethnic differences in the clinical features of sarcoidosis in south-east London. *Br. J. Dis. Chest,* **74**:63–69.

Horowitz, O., Payne, P. G., and Wilbek, E. (1967). Epidemiology of sarcoidosis in Denmark. *Dan. Med. Bull.,* **14**:178–182.

Hosoda, Y., Hiraga, Y., Odaka, M., Yanagawa, H., Ito, Y., Shigematsu, I., and Chiba, Y. (1976a). A cooperative study of sarcoidosis in Asia and Africa: Analytic epidemiology. Proceedings of the VIIth International Conference on Sarcoidosis and Other Granulomatous Disorders. *Ann. NY Acad. Sci.,* **278**:355–367.

Hosoda, Y., Kosuda, T., Yamamoto, M., Hongo, O., Mochizumi, H., Mikami, R., Homma, H., Fumita, S., Ohira, I., Izumi, T., Kobara, Y., Yammato, H., Oshima, S., Teramatsu, T., Maekawa, T., Tsuji, S., Soon, C. P., Sodhy, T. S., Bovornkitti, S., Chakravarty, S. C., Yang, S. P., and Gomaa, T. (1976b). A cooperative study of sarcoidosis in Asia and Africa: Descriptive epidemiology. Proceedings of the VIIth International Conference on Sarcoidosis and Other Granulomatous Disorders. *Ann. NY Acad. Sci.,* **278**:347–354.

Hosoda, Y., Iwai, K., Odaka, M., Hiraga, Y., Ito, Y., Furuiye, T., Mikami, R., Yanagawa, H., Hashimoto, T., Shigematsu, I., and Chiba, Y. (1980). Recent epidemiological features of sarcoidosis in Japan.

Proceedings of the VIIth International Conference on Sarcoidosis. Cardiff, Wales, Alpha Omega, pp. 519-521.

Israel, H. L. (1971). Influence of race and geographic origin on incidence of sarcoidosis in the United States. *Proceedings of the Vth International Conference on Sarcoidosis.* Praha, Universita Karlova, pp. 235-237.

Israel, H. L., and Sones, M. (1958). Sarcoidosis, clinical observations in 160 cases. *Arch. Intern. Med.,* **102**:766-776.

James, D. G., and Brett, G. Z. (1963). Prevalence of intrathoracic sarcoidosis in Britain. Proceedings of the IIIrd International Conference on Sarcoidosis. *Acta Med. Scand.,* (Suppl. 425, 1964):115-117.

James, D. G., Thomson, A. D., and Willcox, A. (1956). Erythema nodosum as a manifestation of sarcoidosis. *Lancet,* **2**:218-221.

James, P. G., Piyasena, K. H. G., Neville, E., Walker, A. N., and Hamlyn, A. N. (1974). Possible genetic influences in familial sarcoidosis. *Postgrad. Med.,* **50**:664-670.

James, P. G., Neville, E., Siltzbach, L. E., Turiaf, J., Battesti, J. P., Sharma, O. P., Hosoda, Y., Mikami, R., Odaka, M., Villar, T. G., Djuric, B., Douglas, A. D., Middleton, W., Karlish, A., Blasi, A., Olivieri, D., and Press, P. (1976). A worldwide review of sarcoidosis. Proceedings of the VIIth International Conference on Sarcoidosis and Other Granulomatous Disorders. *Ann. NY Acad. Sci.,* **278**: 321-334.

Jaroszewicz, W. (1963). Tentative data concerning the frequency of pulmonary sarcoidosis in Poland. Proceedings of the IIIrd International Conference on Sarcoidosis. *Acta Med. Scand.,* (Suppl. 425, 1964): 138-139.

Jaroszewicz, W., Krychniak, W., Rudzinska, H., and Zych, D. (1977). Epidemiologie de la sarcoidose en Pologne. *Z. Erkrank. Atm. Org.,* **149**:15-18.

Jorgensen, G. (1965). Untersuchungen zur Genetik der Sakoidose. Gottingen, Habie Schrift.

Keller, A. Z. (1971). Hospital, age, racial, occupational, geographical, clinical and survivorship characteristics in the epidemiology of sarcoidosis. *Am. J. Epidemiol.,* **94**:222-228.

Keller, A. Z. (1973). Anatomic sites, age attributes, and rates of sarcoidosis in U.S. veterans. *Am. Rev. Respir. Dis.,* **107**:615-620.

Keller, A. Z., and Dunner, E. (1967). Inquiry into the epidemiological aspects of sarcoidosis. In *La Sarcoidose.* Paris, Masson, pp. 319-325.

Kemka, L., and Halak, O. (1977). Uber das Vorkommen von Sarkoidose bei radiofotografischen Reihenuntersuchungen. *Z. Erkrank. Atm.-Org.,* **149**:33-37.

Kendig, E. L., Jr. (1974). The clinical picture of sarcoidosis in children. *Pediatrics,* **54**:289-292.

Kendig, E. L., Jr., and Brummer, D. M. (1976). The prognosis of
    sarcoidosis in children. *Chest,* **70**:351–353.
Kendig, E. L., Jr., and Yasutaka, N. (1980). Sarcoidosis in Japanese and
    American children. *Chest,* **77**:514–516.
Kueppers, F., Mueller-Eckhardt, C., Heinrich, P., Schwab, B., and
    Brackerty, D. (1974). HLA antigens of patients with sarcoidosis.
    Tissue Antigens, **4**:45–58.
LaGasta, M. (1963). A report on the epidemiological situation of sar-
    coidosis in Yugoslavia. "Jordanovac" in Zagreb, University of
    Zagreb, Yugoslavia, pp. 143–144.
Lazarou, P. (1971). Prevalence of pulmonary sarcoidosis in Greece.
    Proceedings of the Vth International Conference on Sarcoidosis.
    Praha, Universita Karlova, p. 251.
Levinsky, L., and Altman, V. (1963). Prevalence of pulmonary sarcoidosis
    in Czechoslovakia. Proceedings of the IIIrd International Conference
    on Sarcoidosis. *Acta Med. Scand.,* (Suppl. 425, 1964):171–173.
Levinsky, L., Cummiskey, J., Romer, F. K., Wurm, K., Buss, J., Dorken,
    H., Steinbruck, P., Zaumseil, P., Jaroszewicz, W., Mandi, L., Szegedy,
    G., Centea, A., Burilkov, T., Blasi, A., Olivieri, D., Mariani, B.,
    Bisetti, A., Goldman, S., Djuric, B., Lazarous, P., and Celikoglu,
    S. I. (1976). Sarcoidosis in Europe: A cooperative study. Proceed-
    ings of the VIIth International Conference on Sarcoidosis and Other
    Granulomatous Disorders. *Ann. NY Acad. Sci.,* **278**:335–346.
Levinsky, L., Svandova, E., and Hyncica, V. (1977). The incidence of
    sarcoidosis in Czechoslovakia in the years 1971–1975. *Z. Erkrank.
    Atm.-Org.,* **149**:19–23.
Lilienfeld, A. M. (1976). Foundations of epidemiology. Oxford
    University Press, New York.
Lindig, W. (1963). Bericht über das Vorkommen von Lungensarkoidose
    im bezirk Leipzig. Proceedings of the IIIrd International Conference
    on Sarcoidosis. *Acta Med. Scand.,* (Suppl. 425, 1964):131–133.
Logan, J. (1963). Prevalence of sarcoidosis in the Irish Republic.
    Proceedings of the IIIrd International Conference on Sarcoidosis.
    Acta Med. Scand., (Suppl. 425, 1964):126.
Longcope, W. T., and Freiman, D. H. (1952). A study of sarcoidosis.
    Based on a combined investigation of 160 cases including 30
    autopsies from the Johns Hopkins Hospital and Massachusetts General
    Hospital. *Medicine,* **31**:1–132.
Lowe, M. V. (1980). Sarcoidosis in Jamaica. *Proceedings of the VIIIth
    International Conference on Sarcoidosis.* Cardiff, Wales, Alpha Omega,
    pp. 514–518.
MacMahon, B., and Pugh, F. F. (1970). *Epidemiology.* Boston, Little
    Brown.

Magalif, N. I., and Brencsone, R. B. (1977). Betrachtungen zur Sarkoidose-Inzidenz in der Lettischen SSR. *Z. Erkrank. Atm.-Org.,* **149**:44–46.

Mandi, L., and Kelemen, J. (1963). Sarcoidosis in Eastern-Hungary. Proceedings of the IIIrd International Conference on Sarcoidosis. *Acta Med. Scand.,* (Suppl. 425, 1964):135.

Mandi, L., and Vezendi, S. (1971). Epidemiology of sarcoidosis in Hungary. *Proceedings of the Vth International Conference on Sarcoidosis.* Praha, Universita Karlova, pp. 298–303.

Mariani, B. (1977). Epidemiological data on sarcoidosis in Italy. *Z. Erkrank. Atm.-Org.,* **149**:47–49.

Marshman, R. S. A. (1963). Prevalence of pulmonary sarcoidosis in the state of Victoria, Australia. Proceedings of the IIIrd International Conference on Sarcoidosis. *Acta Med. Scand.,* (Suppl. 425, 1964): 167–168.

Mayock, R. L., Bertrans, P., Morrison, C. E., and Scott, J. H. (1963). Manifestations of sarcoidosis. Analysis of 145 patients with a review of nine series selected from the literature. *Am. J. Med.,* **35**:67–89.

McGovern, J. P., and Merritt, D. M. (1956). Sarcoidosis in childhood. *Adv. Ped.,* **8**:97–135.

Michael, M., Jr., Cole, R. M., Beeson, P. B., and Olson, B. J. (1950). Sarcoidosis. *Am. Rev. Respir. Dis.,* **62**:403–407.

Milliken, T. G. (1963). Sarcoidosis in Northern Ireland. Proceedings of the IIIrd International Conference on Sarcoidosis. *Acta Med. Scand.,* (Suppl. 425, 1964):123–125.

Morrison, J. G. L. (1974). Sarcoidosis in the Bantu. *Br. J. Dermatol.,* **90**:649–655.

Muratore, F. (1963). Notes on sarcoidosis in Puglia and Lucania, Italy. Proceedings of the IIIrd International Conference on Sarcoidosis. *Acta Med. Scand.,* (Suppl. 425, 1964):136.

Nandi, P. L., Au, M. D., and Ong, F. B. (1981). Sarcoidosis among Chinese. *Chest,* **80**:74–79.

Neville, E., James, D. G., Brewerton, D. A., James, D. C. O., Cockburn, C., and Fenichal, B. (1980). HLA antigens and clinical features of sarcoidosis. *Proceedings of the VIIIth International Conference on Sarcoidosis.* Cardiff, Wales, Alpha Omega, pp. 201–205.

Nobechi, K. (1961). Epidemiology of sarcoidosis in Japan. *Am. Rev. Respir. Dis.,* **84**(suppl.):148–152.

Orie, N. G. M., and Ter Brugge, R. (1963). Prevalence of pulmonary sarcoidosis in The Netherlands. Proceedings of the IIIrd International Conference on Sarcoidosis. *Acta Med. Scand.,* (Suppl. 425, 1964):137.

Patiala, H., Riska, N., and Selroos, O. (1963). Sarcoidosis in Finland. Proceedings of the IIIrd International Conference on Sarcoidosis. *Acta Med. Scand.,* (Suppl. 425, 1964):110.

Persson, I., Ryder, L. P., Nielsen, L. S., and Svejgaard, A. (1975). The HLA A7 histocompatibility antigen in sarcoidosis in relation to tuberculin sensitivity. *Tissue Antigens,* **6**:50–53.

Pollak, B. (1963). Epidemiology of sarcoidosis in Canada. Proceedings of the IIIrd International Conference on Sarcoidosis. *Acta Med. Scand.,* (Suppl. 425, 1964):145.

Posner, I. (1942). Sarcoidosis: Case report. *J. Pediatr.,* **20**:487–495.

Press, P. (1977). Depistage de la sarcoidose par radiophotographie—Geneve, 1966–1975. *Z. Erkrank. Atm.-Org.,* **149**:24–32.

Purriel, P., Navarrete, E., and Piaggio, A. (1963). Epidemiology of sarcoidosis in South America. Proceedings of the IIIrd International Conference on Sarcoidosis. *Acta Med. Scand.,* (Suppl. 425, 1964): 152–155, 157–160.

Rakower, J. (1963). Epidemiology of sarcoidosis in Israel. Proceedings of the IIIrd International Conference on Sarcoidosis. *Acta Med. Scand.,* (Suppl. 425, 1964):163–164.

Reid, J. D. (1963). M. M. R. survey of sarcoidosis in New Zealand. Proceedings of the IIIrd International Conference on Sarcoidosis. *Acta Med. Scand.,* (Suppl. 425, 1964):169–170.

Ricker, W., and Clark, M. (1949). Sarcoidosis—A clinicopathologic review of three hundred cases, including twenty-two autopsies. *Am. J. Clin. Pathol.,* **19**:725–749.

Riddervold, L. (1963). Sarcoidosis in Norway. Proceedings of the IIIrd International Conference on Sarcoidosis. *Acta Med. Scand.,* (Suppl. 425, 1964):111.

Robins, A. B., Abeles, H., and Chaves, A. D. (1962). Prevalence and demographic characteristics of sarcoidosis. Bureau of Tuberculosis, the City of New York, Department of Health, New York, pp. 149–151.

Rudberg-Roos, J. (1962). The course and prognosis of sarcoidosis as observed in 296 cases. *Acta Tuberc. Scand.,* (Suppl.)**52**:1–40.

Sartwell, P. E., and Edwards, L. B. (1974). Epidemiology of sarcoidosis. *Am. J. Epidemiol.,* **99**:250–257.

Schönholzer, V. G. (1947). Morbus Besnier-Boeck-Schaumann und Armeedurchleuchtung. *Schweiz. Med. Wochenschr.,* **77**:585–588.

Siltzbach, L. E. (1961). The current status of the Nickerson-Kveim reaction. *Am. Rev. Respir. Dis.,* **84**(suppl.):89–93.

Siltzbach, L. E. (1967a). An international Kveim test study (1960–1966). *Proceedings of the IVth International Conference on Sarcoidosis.* Paris, Masson, pp. 201–213.

Siltzbach, L. E. (1967b). Geographic aspects of sarcoidosis. *Trans. NY Acad. Sci.,* **29**:364–374.

Siltzbach, L. E. (1976). Qualities and behavior of satisfactory Kveim suspensions. *Ann. NY Acad. Sci.,* **278**:665–669.

Siltzbach, L. E., James, D. G., Neville, E., Turiaf, J., Battesti, J. P., Sharma, O. P., Hosoda, Y., Mikami, R., and Odaka, M. (1974). Course and prognosis of sarcoidosis around the world. *Am. J. Med.,* **57**:847–852.

Smith, M. J., Turton, C. W. G., Mitchell, D. N., Turner-Warwich, M., Morris, L. M., and Lawler, S. D. (1981). Association of HLA B8 with spontaneous resolution in sarcoidosis. *Thorax,* **36**:296–298.

Sommer, E. (1963). Prevalenz der pulmonaler Sarkoidose in der Schweiz. Proc. IIIrd Int. Conf. on Sarcoidosis. *Acta Med. Scand.,* (Suppl. 425, 1964):142.

Sones, M., and Israel, H. L. (1960). Course and prognosis of sarcoidosis. *Am. J. Med.,* **29**:84–93.

Teirstein, A. S., Siltzbach, L. E., Berger, H. W., and Barthold, D. (1971). Causes of death in sarcoidosis: The significance of the presenting chest radiograph. *Proceedings of the Vth International Conference on Sarcoidosis.* Praha, Universita Karlova, pp. 541–545.

Teirstein, A. S., and Siltzbach, L. E. (1974). Sarcoidosis with accurately dated onset—A study of 100 patients with initial erythema nodosum. *Proceedings of the VIth International Conference on Sarcoidosis.* Tokyo, University of Tokyo Press, pp. 453–455.

Teirstein, A. S., Siltzbach, L. E., and Berger, H. (1976). Patterns of sarcoidosis in three population groups in New York City. *Ann. NY Acad. Sci.,* **278**:371–376.

Teristein, A. S., Siltzbach, L. E., Gabelman, M., and Lesser, M. (1981). Socioeconomic factors influencing epidemiologic data in sarcoidosis among a mixed ethnic urban population. *Proceedings of the IXth International Conference on Sarcoidosis and Other Granulomatous Disorders,* Paris. In press.

Terris, M., and Chaves, A. D. (1966). An epidemiologic study of sarcoidosis. *Am. Rev. Respir. Dis.,* **94**:50–55.

Tsega, E., Getahun, B., and Teklehaimanot, R. (1978). Sarcoidosis in Ethiopia. *Tubercle,* **59**:261–268.

Turiaf, J., Brun, J., and Meyer, A. (1963). Epidemiologic investigation on sarcoidosis in France. Proceedings of the IIIrd International Conference on Sarcoidosis. *Acta Med. Scand.,* (Suppl. 425, 1964):129.

Van Lingen, B. (1961). Sarcoidosis in South Africa. *Am. Rev. Respir. Dis.,* **84**(suppl.):162.

Villar, T. G. (1963). Sarcoidosis in Portugal. Proceedings of the IIIrd International Conference on Sarcoidosis. *Acta Med. Scand.,* (Suppl. 425, 1964):140–141.

Webling, D. D. (1978). Sarcoidosis in an Australian aboriginal. *Med. J. Aust.,* **1**:169–170.

Yanagawa, H., Hosoda, Y., Odaka, M., Mikami, R., Hashimoto, T., and Shigematsu, I. (1979). Recent epidemiological features of sarcoidosis in Japan. In *Sarcoidosis.* Tokyo, University of Tokyo Press, pp. 355–377.

Zapatero, J. (1971). Sarcoidosis in Spain. *Proceedings of the Vth International Conference on Sarcoidosis.* Praha, Universita Karlova, pp. 242–243.

Zaumseil, I. (1971). Sarcoidosis in the German Democratic Republic with a review of epidemiology, diagnostics and therapy. *Proceedings of the Vth International Conference on Sarcoidosis.* Praha, Universita Karlova, pp. 259–264.

Zierski, M. (1971). Epidemiological aspects of sarcoidosis in Poland. *Proceedings of the Vth International Conference on Sarcoidosis.* Praha, Universita Karlova, pp. 293–297.

5

Genetics and Familial Sarcoidosis

D. GERAINT JAMES

Royal Northern Hospital and St. Thomas' Hospital
London, England
and University of Miami School of Medicine
Miami, Florida

I. Epidemiologic Background

Sarcoidosis has a worldwide distribution, but it is more frequently recognized in sophisticated communities. Whenever tuberculosis is rampant sarcoidosis will be in eclipse, but as tuberculosis is brought under control so will sarcoidosis become more evident. It now seems that the same relationship holds for leprosy, and that sarcoidosis bobs to the surface not only in the wake of tuberculosis but also following the eradication of leprosy.

As the eradication of tuberculosis and leprosy in the Third World takes place, it is anticipated that sarcoidosis will be detected more frequently. It would be of great interest to know the incidence of sarcoidosis in the Caribbean and in Africa. Sarcoidosis is well recognized in the black population in the United States. It is also common in the West Indian population in Britain and in Martiniques living in France, but we do not know if there is the same preponderance in the home environments of these individuals. As more epidemiologic studies of this disease evolve, we may have better clues to "latent" sarcoidosis and to a better appreciation of factors contributing to familial sarcoidosis.

Table 1 Familial Occurrence of Sarcoidosis

Authors	Year	Relationship	Location
Martenstein	1923	Two sisters	Germany
Sellei and Berger	1926	Three sisters and two brothers	Vienna
Dressler	1938 1939	Two brothers Brother and sister	Switzerland
MacCormac	1940	Two sisters	London
Richter and Richter	1941	Two sisters	Germany
van Buchem	1946	Two brothers	Tilburg, Holland
Robinson and Hahn	1947	Two brothers Four brothers	Baltimore
Bickerstaff	1949	Two brothers	Ireland
Sherer and Kelly	1949	Identical twins	U.S.A.
Klingmuller	1951	Mother and son Two sisters	Germany
Gilg	1952	Identical twins	Copenhagen
Rodgers and Netherton	1954	Identical twins	Cleveland
van Zwanenberg and Barry	1955	Three brothers and a sister	England
Swirsky and Lowman	1955	Brother and sister	Connecticut
Moriarty	1956	Two sisters	England
Warin	1958	Mother and son Brother and sister	England
Kendig et al.	1959	Three sisters	Virginia
Baer	1960	Two brothers and two sisters	Texas
Kinoshita et al.	1966	Mother and two daughters	Japan
Beresford	1971	Mother and daughter Mother and son	England
Sharma et al.	1971	Three brothers and a sister	Los Angeles

Table 1 (Continued)

Authors	Year	Relationship	Location
Wiman	1973	Four families (21 members, 3 generations)	Sweden
Ito et al.	1974	Twelve families (23 members affected)	Japan
James et al.	1974	Five families (11 members affected)	London
Sharma et al.	1978	Sixteen families (33 members affected)	London and Los Angeles
Kendig	1976	One family (4 children)	Virginia
Israel and Washbourne	1980	Eight patients (7 black)	Philadelphia
Hosoda et al.	1980	Sixteen siblings (9 parent-child, 2 husband-wife)	Japan

II. Analysis of Familial Sarcoidosis

During the last 60 years almost 200 patients have been reported to have familial sarcoidosis (Table 1). In the small number of individuals reported, sarcoidosis seems to be more frequent in monozygotic than in dizygotic twins. We have reported a series of 16 families in whom 33 persons had sarcoidosis. Clinical and laboratory information are available for 31 of these patients (Table 2). The family relationships were brother-sister (6), sister-sister (5), mother-son (2), mother-daughter, uncle-niece, and husband-wife once each.

A. Age, Sex, and Race

The age at presentation of familial sarcoidosis is approximately the same as that of sporadic sarcoidosis (Table 2). About 70% of patients present with the disease before the age of 40 years. The incidence is higher in women than in men and there appears to be an equal incidence of familial sarcoidosis in blacks and whites. Four of the families were from the West Indies. Turiaf (personal communication, 1976) has also noted a greater

Table 2 Clinical Features of 31 Patients with Familial Sarcoidosis
Compared with Those of Sarcoidosis Overall

Feature	Sarcoidosis overall		Familial sarcoidosis	
	No.	%	No.	%
Women	500	61	21	70
Black	79	10	17	55
Age at presentation				
Under 40 years	604	74	22	71
Over 40 years	214	26	9	29
Total	818	100	31	100

incidence of familial sarcoidosis in French West Indians from Martinique; he
finds familial sarcoidosis in 1% of white Europeans but in 8% of Martiniques
living in Paris.

B. Mode of Onset

The mode of onset of familial sarcoidosis, as indicated by the appearance
of erythema nodosum, acute uveitis, or hilar adenopathy, was similar to
that of our overall series.

C. Intrathoracic Sarcoidosis

All patients with familial disease had intrathoracic changes, ranging from
bilateral hilar lymphadenopathy (stage 1) in 42%, hilar adenopathy with
pulmonary infiltration in 32% (stage 2), and late stage pulmonary infiltration in 26% of cases (Table 3).

Table 3 Stages of Intrathoracic Sarcoidosis in Familial Sarcoidosis
Compared with Sarcoidosis Overall

Stage	Sarcoidosis overall		Familial sarcoidosis	
	No.	%	No.	%
0	118	15	0	—
1	458	56	13	42
2	150	18	10	32
3	92	11	8	26
Total abnormal	818	100	31	100

D. Extrathoracic Sarcoidosis

The familial cases showed a pattern of multisystem involvement similar to that of our whole series (Table 4).

E. Investigations

The tuberculin skin test was negative in 20 of 26 patients (76%) with familial sarcoidosis, approximately the same percentage noted in sporadic sarcoidosis (Table 5). Likewise, the Kveim-Siltzbach skin test in familial sarcoidosis was similar to that of our overall series (Table 5).

F. Course and Prognosis

Intrathoracic changes in familial sarcoidosis cleared spontaneously in 8 patients and with corticosteroids in 12 patients, representing an expected resolution rate of 64%. In 6 patients the chest x-rays remained unchanged and in three patients there was progression to pulmonary fibrosis.

The overall mortality in familial sarcoidosis is what may be anticipated from sarcoidosis in general; one patient died directly due to sarcoidosis whereas two others had unrelated deaths (Table 5).

Table 4 Involvement of Tissues in Familial Sarcoidosis Compared with Sarcoidosis Overall

Feature	Sarcoidosis overall		Familial sarcoidosis	
	No.	%	No.	%
Involvement of				
Lungs	716	88	31	100
Erythema nodosum	251	31	3	10
Lymph nodes	225	27	8	26
Eyes	224	27	7	22
Skin (other than erythema nodosum)	147	21	5	16
Spleen	101	12	2	6
Parotid	52	6	3	10
Bone cysts	31	3	3	10
Nervous system	77	9	1	3
Total	818	100	31	100

Table 5 Features of Familial Sarcoidosis in 31 Patients Compared with Sarcoidosis Overall

	Sarcoidosis overall		Familial sarcoidosis	
Feature	No.	%	No.	%
Tuberculin skin test negative	488/702	70	20/26	76
Kveim-Siltzbach skin test positive	430/658	65	11/20	55
Corticosteroid therapy necessary	344	42	19/31	61
Mortality due to				
Sarcoidosis	25	3	1	3
Other causes	23	3	2	6

G. Discussion of Series

The most common family relationship in patients with sarcoidosis is that between a brother and sister, followed in frequency by a mother-offspring relationship. We have not observed it in a father-offspring relationship, which is exceedingly rare. Wiman (1973) noted a father-offspring relationship once. A husband-wife combination with sarcoidosis has been noted to occur at least once in most large series of patients with this disease. This relationship is too rare to point to an infective factor, but it may suggest a common environmental background.

The clinical, radiographic, and other features of the disorder are similar in familial and sporadic sarcoidosis.

We applied the methods of Hogben and Smith which allow for the truncated binomial distribution of recessives in affected families and compared this with the observed distribution expected on the basis of probability. This evidence suggests a recessive mode of inheritance for susceptibility to sarcoidosis (James et al. 1974).

The British Thoracic and Tuberculosis Association (1973) conducted a survey and found 59 families in Britain with more than one case of sarcoidosis. The most striking finding was the significant preponderance of like sex over unlike sex pairs among both siblings and parent-child associations. Their observed preponderance of monozygotic (4) over dizygotic (1) twin pairs concordant for sarcoidosis is also strongly suggestive of a genetic predisposition.

III. HLA Antigens in Sarcoidosis

We have studied the distribution of inherited histocompatibility (HLA) antigens in sarcoidosis patients with erythema nodosum, polyarthritis, uveitis, lupus pernio, and bone cysts. The HLA antigens were identified within 24 hours of venepuncture, using a modified two-stage lymphotoxicity micromethod and testing the lymphocytes of patients for 22 different antigens (Neville et al. 1980).

In a series of 107 patients with histologically proven sarcoidosis there was no overall alteration in frequency of HLA antigens (Table 6). However, B8 antigen was significantly associated with sarcoid arthritis and erythema nodosum occurring either singularly or in combination. Because of the linkage disequilibrium between A1 and B8, A1 was increased in association with arthritis. Of 52 patients with acute sarcoidosis B8 was present in 26 (50%; p = 0.02), but when those patients with either arthritis or erythema nodosum are removed from this group, only 5 of 21 (24%) show B8 antigen; that is, B8 may not be associated with acute sarcoidosis itself, but may be an accompaniment of arthritis and/or erythema nodosum. Similarly, when the same patients are excluded from the group who achieved chest x-ray resolution, B8 is found in only four of 22 (18%).

Of 55 patients with chronic sarcoidosis six (11%) were HLA-B13 (p = 0.002), and this association was also significant when chronic was compared with acute sarcoidosis (p = 0.034). B17 also occurred in six (11%) of the chronic sarcoid population, but this association did not achieve statistical significance.

Other studies in white patients indicate a normal overall distribution of HLA antigens in familial sarcoidosis (Turton et al. 1980), but clinical features were sometimes not selected (Kueppers et al. 1972, Hedfors and Möller 1973). In Sweden, HLA-B7 patients are more likely to be tuberculin-negative and to be symptomatic (Persson et al. 1975). In black patients in South Carolina there is a suggestion of an overall increase in HLA-B7 (McIntyre et al. 1977), but this is not confirmed in Washington where, instead, it has been noted that sarcoidosis occurs 5.5 times more frequently among Bw15 individuals when compared with those lacking that antigen. However, the presence of HLA-Bw15 does not correlate with specific disease manifestation. This increased expression of Bw15 was also observed in black patients with tuberculosis in Washington (Al-Arif et al. 1980).

The close link between HLA-B8 and erythema nodosum may explain in part the different frequencies with which erythema nodosum is observed in sarcoidosis populations around the world (James et al. 1976). In the three British series, erythema nodosum was reported in 31% while B8 was found in 29% of the population (Svejgaard 1977), whereas in Japan erythema nodosum was unusual (4%) and B8 was present in less than 2% of the general population (Aizawa 1977, Fukunishi 1977). Despite this good correlation in the series at either end of the scale, it is not as convincing

Table 6 HLA Antigens in Relation to Clinical Features in 107 Patients with Sarcoidosis

Manifestations of sarcoidosis	Patients studied		A1		B8			B7		B27	
	No.	%	No.	%	No.	%	p	No.	%	No.	%
Overall	107	100	40	37	43	40	—	33	31	9	8
Arthritis	9	8	6	66	8	89	0.002	0	—	1	11
Erythema nodosum	13	12	5	38	8	62	0.015	6	46	1	8
Erythema nodosum and arthritis	11	10	5	45	9	82	0.002	1	9	2	18
Acute anterior uveitis	21	20	7	33	5	24	—	10	48	1	5
Chronic anterior uveitis	31	28	11	35	8	26	—	9	29	2	6
Chest x-ray resolution	53/90	59	22	42	29	55	0.002	17	32	6	11
Lupus pernio	13	12	6	46	5	38	—	2	15	2	15
Bone	12	11	6	50	5	42	—	2	17	1	8
Mantoux negative	67/86	78	28	42	30	45	—	21	31	5	7

when compared with other series (Table 7). British Caucasians who have HLA-B8 and develop sarcoidosis are likely to express it with arthritis and/or erythema nodosum. Not all patients with these manifestations of sarcoidosis have B8 and not all with B8 will develop these lesions. Clearly, other factors are important and the search for them must continue.

Table 7 Frequency of Erythema Nodosum in Sarcoidosis Compared with HLA-B8 in Different Populations

City	Investigator	Year	Erythema nodosum No.	Erythema nodosum %	B8 in population[a] %
Stuttgart	Wurm	1958	218	10	19
Stockholm	Löfgren et al.	1961	33	25	24
Brussels	Lebacq	1964	25	25	14
New York	Siltzbach[b]	1968	33	11	16[c] 15[d]
Helsinki	Hannuksela et al.	1969	85	30	18
Hamburg	Behrend	1973	97	28	19
Paris	Turiaf et al.	1976	22	7	16
Los Angeles	Sharma[b]	1976	14	9	7[e]
Novi Sad	Djuric	1976	31	11	15
Geneva	Press	1976	13	11	18
Naples	Blasi et al.	1976	38	6	10
Tokyo	Hosoda et al.	1976	10	4	2[f]
Reading	Karlish	1976	134	32	29
Edinburgh	Douglas et al.	1976	167	33	29
London	James and Neville	1977	251	31	29

[a]All European figures after Svejgaard, 1977.
[b]Both American sarcoid series included a majority of blacks. (82% in Los Angeles and 47% in New York).
[c]New York blacks after Dausset et al. 1970.
[d]New York whites after Dausset et al. 1967.
[e]Los Angeles blacks after Albert et al. 1970.
[f]Combined data from Aizawa 1977 and Fukunishi 1977.

References

Aizawa, M. (1977). Data submitted to the HLA and disease registry in
  Copenhagen.

Al-Arif, O., Goldstein, R. A., Affronti, L. H., Janicki, B. W., and Foellmer,
  B. J. W. (1980). HLA antigens and sarcoidosis in a North American
  black population. In *Eighth International Conference on Sarcoidosis.*
  Edited by W. J. Williams and B. H. Davies. Cardiff, Wales, Alpha
  Omega, pp. 206–212.

Albert, E. D., Mickey, M. R., McNicholas, A. C., and Terasaki, P. I. (1970).
  *Seven New HLA Specificities and Their Distribution in Three Races in
  Histocompatibility Testing 1970.* Edited by P. I. Terasaki.
  Munksgaard, Copenhagen, pp. 221–230.

Baer, R. B. (1960). Familial sarcoidosis: Epidemiological aspects with notes
  on a possible relationship to the chewing of pine pitch. *Arch.
  Intern. Med.,* **105**:60.

Beresford, O. D. (1971). Familial sarcoidosis. *Jap. J. Chest Dis.,* **30**:297.

Bickerstaff, E. R. (1949). The familial aspects of sarcoidosis. *Br. J.
  Tuberc.,* **43**:112.

British Thoracic and Tuberculosis Association (1973). Familial association
  in sarcoidosis. *Tubercle,* **54**:87.

Buchem, R. S. P. van (1946). On morbid conditions of the liver and
  diagnosis of Besnier-Boeck-Schaumann disease. *Acta Med. Scand.,*
  124:168.

Dausset, J., Colombani, J., Legrand, L., and Fellows, M. (1970). *Genetics
  of the HLA System. Deduction of 480 Haplotypes in Histocompatibility Testing 1970.* Edited by P. I. Terasaki. Munksgaard,
  Copenhagen, pp. 53–57.

Dausset, J., Ivanyi, P., Colombani, J., Feingold, N., and Legrand, L. (1967).
  The Hu-1 System in Histocompatibility Testing, 1967. Edited by
  E. S. Curtoni, P. L. Mattiuz, and R. M. Iozi. Munksgaard,
  Copenhagen, pp. 189–202.

Dressler, M. (1938). Boeck'sche Krankheit der Lungen bei Geschwisern.
  Schweiz. Med. Wochenschr., **19**:417.

Dressler, M. (1939). Familiares Vorkommen des Besnier-Boeck'Schon
  Krankheit. *Schweiz. Med. Wochenschr.,* **19**:417.

Fukunishi, T. (1977). Data submitted to the HLA and disease registry in
  Copenhagen.

Gilg, I. (1952). Boeck's sarcoid in identical twins. *Acta Dermatovener.,*
  (Suppl.) **29**:108.

Hedfors, E., and Möller, E. (1973). HLA antigens in sarcoidosis. *Tissue
  Antigens,* **3**:95.

Hosoda, Y., Iwai, K., Odaka, M., Hiraga, Y., Ito, T., Furniye, T., Mikami, R., Yaragawa, H., Hashimoto, T., Shigematou, I., and Chiba, Y. (1980). Recent eipdemiological features of sarcoidosis in Japan. In *Eighth International Conference on Sarcoidosis*. Edited by W. J. Williams and B. H. Davies. Cardiff, Wales, Alpha Omega, pp. 519–521.

Israel, H. L., and Washbourne, J. D. (1980). Characteristics of sarcoidosis in black and white patients. Analysis of 162 recent cases. In *Eighth International Conference on Sarcoidosis*. Edited by W. J. Williams and B. H. Davies. Cardiff, Wales, Alpha Omega, pp. 497–507.

Ito, Y., Ogima, I., and Kinoshita, Y. (1974). Familial sarcoidosis in Japan. In *Proceedings of the Sixth International Conference on Sarcoidosis*. Edited by K. Iwai and Y. Hosoda. Tokyo, Tokyo University Press, pp. 30–33.

James, D. G., Piyasena, K. H. G., Neville, E., Walker, A. N., and Hamlyn, A. N. (1974). Possible genetic influences in familial sarcoidosis. *Postgrad. Med. J.*, **50**:664–670.

James, D. G., Neville, E., Silzbach, L. E., Turiaf, J., Battesti, J. P., Sharma, O. P., Hosoda, Y., Mikami, R., Odaka, M., Villar, T. G., Djuric, B., Douglas, A. C., Middleton, W., Karlish, A., Blasi, A., Oliveri, D., and Press, P. (1976). A worldwide review of sarcoidosis. *Ann. NY Acad. Sci.*, **278**:321.

Kendig, E. L., Peacock, R. L., and Ryburns, S. (1959). Sarcoidosis: Report of three cases in siblings under 15 years of age. *N. Engl. J. Med.*, **260**:962.

Kendig, E. L. (1976). Familial sarcoidosis. *Ann. NY Acad. Sci.*, **278**:400.

Kinoshita, Y., Ogima, I., and Aoki, S. (1966). 3 cases of sarcoidosis occurring in 2 generations of a family. *Jap. J. Clin. Med.*, **23**:190.

Klingmuller, G. (1951). Der Morbus Boeck in der Familie. *Derm. Wochenschr.*, **124**:119.

Kueppers, F., Brackertz, D., and Mueller-Eckhardt, C. (1972). HL-A antigens in sarcoidosis and rheumatoid arthritis. *Lancet*, 2:1425.

MacCormac, H. (1940). Schaumann's disease in two sisters. *Acta Med. Scand.*, **103**:152.

Martenstein, H. (1923). Knochveranderungen bei lupus pernio. *Z. Haut. Geschlechtskr.*, **7**:308.

McIntyre, J. A., McKee, K. T., Leadholt, C. B., Nercurio, S., and Lin, I. (1977). Increased HLA-B7 antigen frequency in South Carolina blacks in association with sarcoidosis. *Transplant. Proc.*, (Suppl.) I:173.

Moriarty, M. A. (1956). Sarcoidosis in siblings. *J. Irish Med. Assoc.*, **38**:7.

Neville, E., James, D. G., Brewerton, D. A., James, D. C. O., Cockburn, C., and Fenichal, B. (1980). HLA antigens and clinical features of sarcoidosis. In *Eighth International Conference on Sarcoidosis.* Edited by W. J. Williams and B. H. Davies. Cardiff, Wales, Alpha Omega, pp. 201–205.

Perrson, I., Ryder, I. P., Nielsen, L. S., and Svejgaard, A. (1975). The HL-A histocompatibility antigen in sarcoidosis in relation to tuberculin sensitivity. *Tissue Antigens,* **6**:50.

Richter, R., and Richter, W. (1941). Beitrag zur Klinik der Besnier-Boeck-Schaumannscher Erkrankung. *Derm. Wochenschr.,* **113**:797.

Robinson, R. C. V., and Hahn, R. D. (1947). Sarcoidosis in siblings. *Arch. Intern. Med.,* **80**:249.

Rodgers, R. J., and Netherton, E. W. (1954). Sarcoidosis in identical twins. *JAMA,* **156**:974.

Sellei, J., and Berger, M. (1926). Sarkoide Gescjwulste in eine Familie. *Arch. Derm. Syph. (Wien.),* **150**:47.

Sharma, O. P., Johnson, C. S., and Balchum, O. J. (1971). Familial sarcoidosis: Report of four siblings with acute sarcoidosis. *Am. Rev. Respir. Dis.,* **104**:255–257.

Sherer, J. F., and Kelly, R. T. (1949). Sarcoidosis in identical twins. *N. Engl. J. Med.,* **240**:328.

Svejgaard, A. (1977). Personal communication.

Swirsky, M. Y., and Lowman, R. N. (1955). Sarcoidosis in siblings. *N. Engl. J. Med.,* **252**:476.

Turton, C. W. G., Turner-Warwick, M., Morris, L., and Lawler, S. D. (1980). HLA in familial sarcoidosis. In *Eighth International Conference on Sarcoidosis.* Edited by W. J. Williams and B. H. Davies. Cardiff, Wales, Alpha Omega, pp. 195–200.

van Zwanenberg, D., and Barry, M. (1955). A case of sarcoidosis and 3 cases of atypical tuberculosis in one family. *Lancet,* **1**:483.

Warin, R. P. (1958). Familial sarcoidosis. *Br. J. Dermatol.,* **70**:250.

Wiman, L. G. (1973). Familial occurrence of sarcoidosis. In *Proceedings of the Sixth International Conference on Sarcoidosis.* Edited by K. Iwai and Y. Hosoda. Tokyo, Tokyo University Press, pp. 22–26.

Part Three

PATHOLOGY OF GRANULOMATOUS DISEASE OF THE LUNG

6

Pathology of Sarcoidosis, Granulomatous Vasculitis, and Other Idiopathic Granulomatous Diseases of the Lung

SOLON R. COLE

Hartford Hospital and
University of Connecticut
Health Center
Hartford, Connecticut

KENT J. JOHNSON
and PETER A. WARD

The University of Michigan Medical School
Ann Arbor, Michigan

I. Introduction

Many diseases that affect the lungs as well as other organ systems produce a granulomatous reaction characterized by the proliferation of epithelioid histiocytes and are commonly associated with Langhans' giant cell formation. Although the exact mechanism of the granuloma formation is not clearly understood, the etiologic agent is often easily established in the case of infectious diseases such as tuberculosis and histoplasmosis. In addition, the inhalation of organic dusts such as thermophilic actinomycetes may result in a lung hypersensitivity reaction which histologically manifests itself in part by the formation of epithelioid granulomas. Aspirated foreign material may also produce a granulomatous reaction which, although classically described as the foreign body type, is in fact often difficult to distinguish from other granulomatous reactions.

Eosinophilic granuloma of lung is yet another disease often characterized as granulomatous. The characteristic histiocyte associated with eosinophilic granuloma is not of the so-called epithelioid type. Although errors in diagnosis do occur, the histiocytic reniform nuclei of eosinophilic granuloma of lung more closely resemble those of the other histiocytoses than of the diseases related to the presence of epithelioid histiocytes. Other diseases, including parasitic and rheumatoid disease, may occasionally induce granulomatous reactions in the lung.

In addition to these diseases of known or suspected etiology, there exists a group of diseases, whose incidence ranges from common to rare, that are associated with granulomatous reactions in the lung. These include sarcoidosis, Wegener's granulomatosis, limited Wegener's granulomatosis, lymphomatoid granulomatosis, pulmonary allergic granulomatosis (Churg-Strauss disease), necrotizing sarcoidal angiitis, and bronchocentric granulomatosis. The etiology of these diseases is not understood and their clinical courses vary greatly from benign to often fatal outcomes. Although these diseases may ultimately prove to be unrelated and of diverse etiology, they are grouped in this chapter because of the histological features that they share, often presenting the pathologist with problems in differential diagnosis.

II. Sarcoidosis

A. Pathology

Based on autopsy analysis, Mallory (1948) found the incidence of sarcoidosis to be higher than that indicated by symptomatic patients who seek medical attention. Histologically, sarcoidosis is characterized by noncaseating miliary granulomas involving many organ systems, including lungs, lymph nodes, liver, spleen, skin, eye structures, salivary glands, upper respiratory tract, joints, nervous system, and male genitalia. The lungs, however, are most commonly involved by the process, closely followed by lymph nodes.

In the early forms of the disease, gross examination of the lungs from autopsy or surgical specimens reveals a fine miliary pattern not dissimilar from miliary tuberculosis. There appears to be some predilection for the upper lobes of the lungs with sparing of the bases. Specimens obtained at later stages of the disease reveal patchy scarring of the lung with no other distinguishing features. In these instances, it is only from evidence of previous biopsy material or from the occasional residual epithelial granuloma that the diagnosis of sarcoidosis can be established. End-stage findings in sarcoid lung disease involve fibrocystic or honeycombing changes. Small, thin-walled or emphysematous cysts are more common in end-stage sarcoidosis than in other forms of fibrocystic end-stage diseases (McCort and Pare 1954).

The early lesions of pulmonary sarcoidosis are composed of confluent, well-circumscribed epithelioid granulomas which have a predilection for peribronchial, subpleural, interlobular septal, and perivascular connective tissue, although they may be found in alveolar septa not adjacent to connective tissue structures (Figure 1). In addition, sarcoid granulomas may be seen in the submucosa of the bronchus and bronchial wall, as well as in peribronchial connective tissue. The frequent involvement of these structures accounts for the high diagnostic yield by transbronchial biopsy.

Histologically, sarcoidosis involves the pleura in approximately 35% of patients with sarcoidosis (Rosen et al. 1979), although clinical evidence of this involvement is uncommon (Chusid and Siltzbach 1974). The granulomas are usually confined to the connective tissue within the limiting elastic membrane of the pleura. In this manner they differ from the granulomas of necrotizing sarcoidal granulomatosis, which frequently involve the visceral pleura and may result in adherence of the visceral and parietal pleura (Liebow 1973).

Sarcoid granulomas involving the veins and arteries and especially the connective tissue adjacent to vessels are common (Figure 1) and are reportedly present in 42–92% of all cases of pulmonary sarcoidosis (Carrington et al. 1976, Rosen et al. 1977, 1979). The granulomas most commonly involve the adventitia, but elastic tissue layers may also be affected. Involvement of the vessel is seldom circumferential and is usually confined to a single or a few granulomas in one portion of the wall. Veins are more frequently involved than arteries. Occlusion of the vessels and thrombosis do occur but are uncommon. The involvement of blood vessels in sarcoidosis appears to be incidental to more widespread pulmonary disease without the predilection for arteries observed in the more angiocentric necrotizing sarcoidal granulomatosis. In addition, the extensive necrotizing features of the latter entity, which may also be angiodestructive, are not features of sarcoidosis.

The early sarcoid granulomas are composed largely of epithelioid histiocytes which are derived from macrophages (Papadimitriou and Spector 1971). These cells range in size from 20 to 50 μm. Some of these fuse to form epithelioid giant cells similar to the Langhans' giant cells seen in the granulomas of tuberculosis. A peripheral ring of lymphocytes is commonly seen around the sarcoid granuloma and a few lymphocytes may be present in the central portion of the granuloma. Significant extension of chronic inflammatory cells into the alveolar septa adjacent to the granulomas is uncommon. When present, other disease entities, especially extrinsic allergic alveolitis, should be considered. Plasma cells and eosinophils are not usually present in the granulomas of sarcoidosis. Necrosis of the early granulomas of sarcoid is common and is characterized by the presence of small foci of nuclear debris within the center of the granulomas (Carrington et al. 1976, Rosen et al. 1979). True caseous

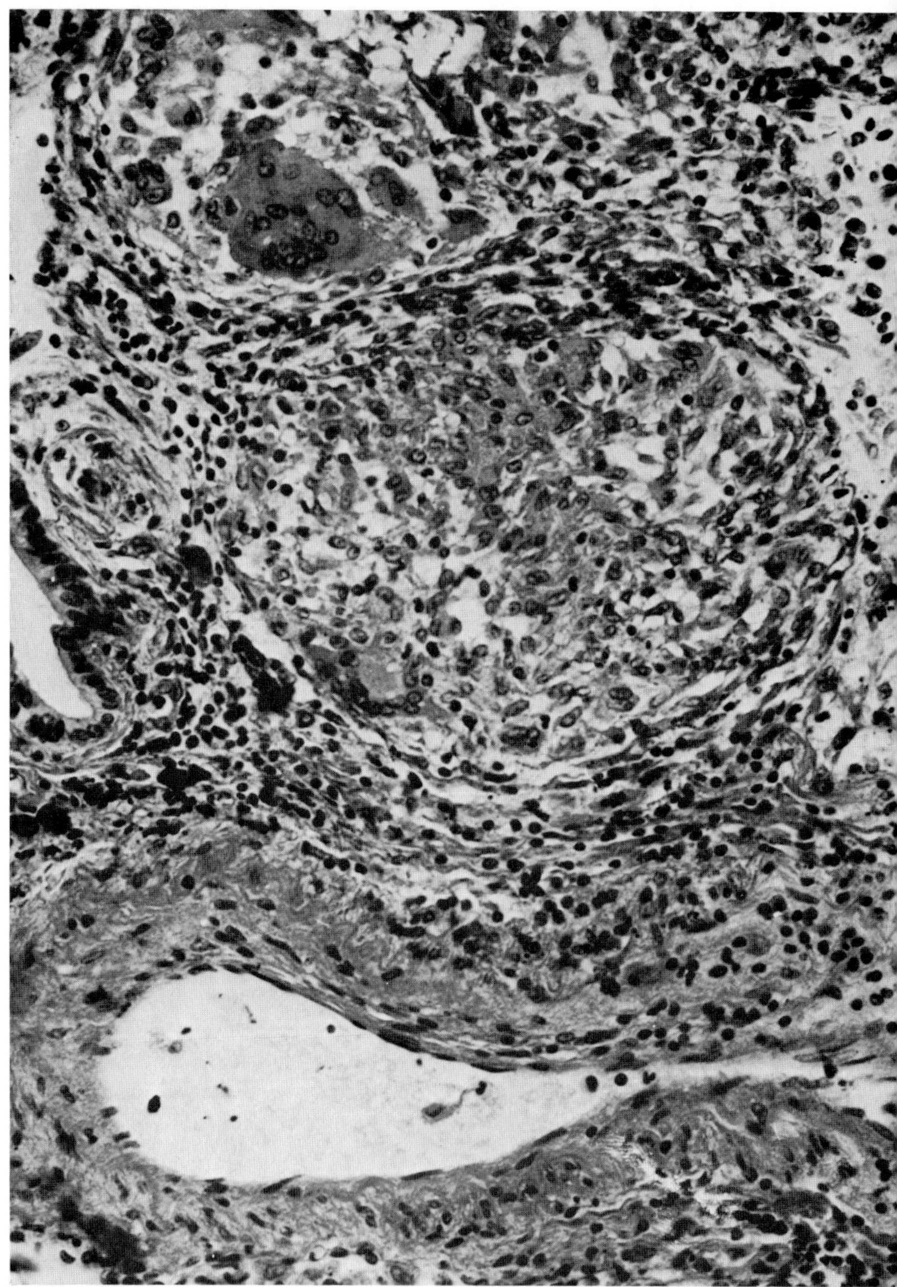

Figure 1   Sarcoidosis; noncaseating granulomas composed of epithelioid histiocytes and giant cells adjacent to a pulmonary artery (H&E × 16).

necrosis is not a feature of sarcoidosis. Cavitation, although reported (Hamilton et al. 1965, Tellis and Putnam 1977), is rare, but secondary infection of bronchiectatic and emphysematous cysts in the later stages of sarcoidosis may resemble cavitation.

During the development of the sarcoid granulomas, cystoplasmic structures, including vacuoles, asteroid bodies, Schaumann bodies, and birefringent crystals (Fig. 2), may be seen within the giant cells (Rosen et al. 1979, Azar and Lunardelli 1969, Uelinger 1964). These structures are not specific for sarcoidosis and are seen in a variety of granulomatous diseases of both infectious and noninfectious origin. They appear, however, to be less commonly seen in the granulomas produced by *Mycobacterium tuberculosis.*

The cytoplasmic vacuoles or centrospheres (Spencer 1977) of the giant cells are usually multiple and foamy in character. They may be centrally or peripherally located. *Asteroid bodies* are stellate-shaped cytoplasmic structures with deeply eosinophilic spokes radiating from a central core. *Birefringent crystals* may also be seen in the cytoplasm of some giant cells when the specimen is polarized. The crystals are usually irregular in configuration but may be round. X-ray diffraction studies suggest that these are composed largely of calcium salts. Concentrically laminated hematoxylin staining bodies, commonly called *Schaumann bodies,* are often seen in sarcoidosis. They are composed of calcium and iron salts. Schaumann bodies are frequently seen in other granulomatous diseases, including beryllium pneumonitis, in which case the large, concentrically laminated bodies are referred to as "conchoid bodies." The crystalline inclusions give a positive reaction with both iron and calcium stains. Extracellular Schaumann bodies are often seen in the fibrotic areas of healed sarcoidosis in the absence of active granulomas and are probably residual structures in areas of previously active granulomas.

Silver impregnation stains reveal abundant reticulin about the periphery and within the granulomas. Elastic tissue is not present within the granulomas and may be disrupted or destroyed in those involved structures that ordinarily contain elastin such as alveolar septa. As the granulomas mature, collagen is laid down about the periphery of the granuloma by the ingrowth of fibroblasts.

Although many microscopic features may suggest sarcoidosis, the epithelioid granulomas, especially in their earlier stages, are often indistinguishable from those of other idiopathic granulomatous diseases, tuberculosis, histoplasmosis, and other infectious diseases. In addition, sarcoidlike granulomas may be present in regional lymph nodes adjacent to sites involved by Hodgkin's disease as well as in lymph nodes draining other tumors. It is important to study the histology in light of the patient's clinical, laboratory, and radiographic findings. It is equally imperative that special stains for organisms, especially acid-fast organisms and fungi, as

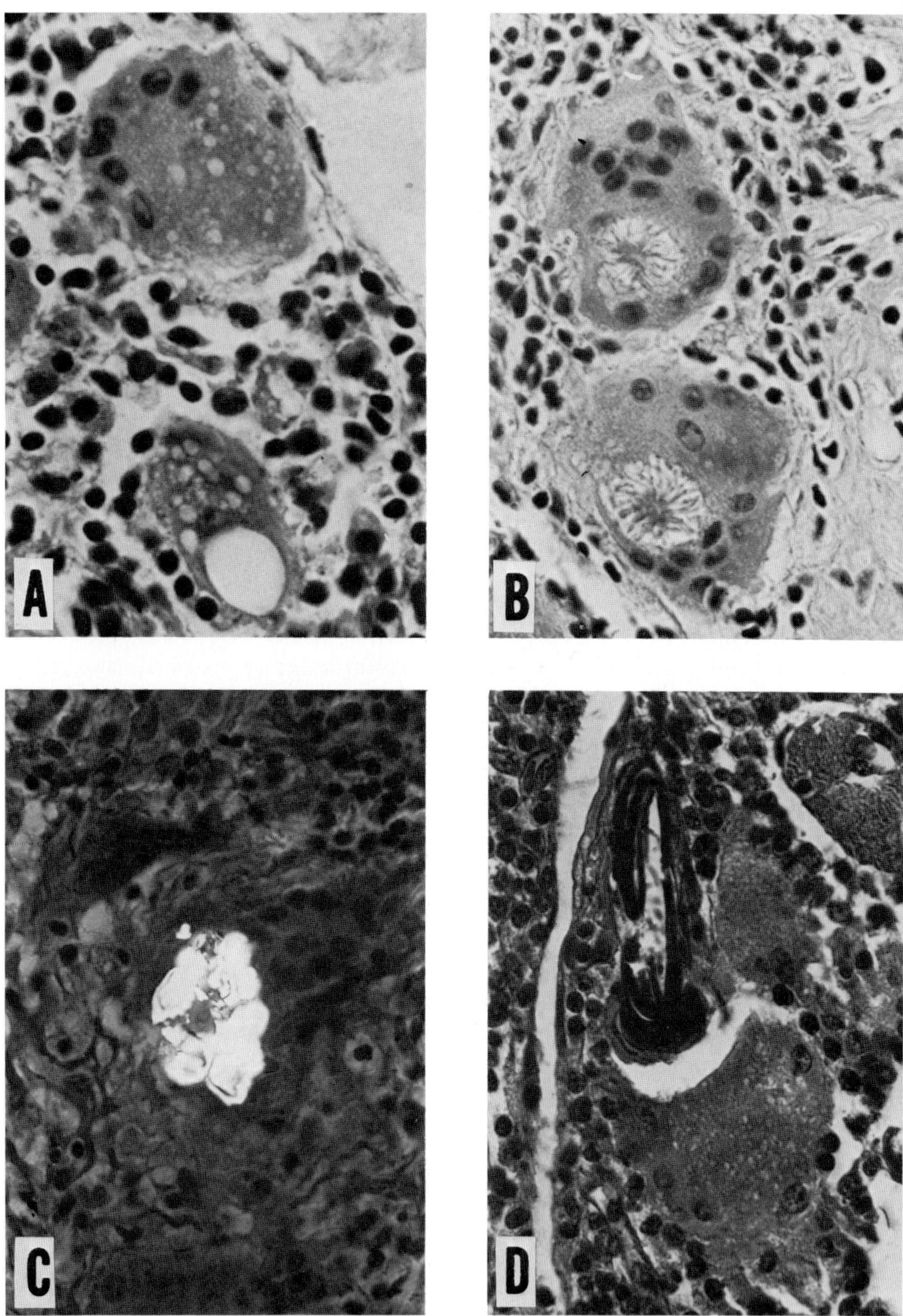

Figure 2 Sarcoidosis; giant cells containing vacuoles or centrospheres (A), asteroid bodies (B), birefringent crystals (C), and Schaumann bodies (D) (H&E X 40).

well as culture of tissues for pathogenic organisms, be performed in cases of granulomatous disease, unless the cause of the granulomatous reaction is clearly known.

Most patients with diagnosed sarcoid undergo clinical and radiological resolution of the disease over a period ranging from several months to a few years. A few develop a progressive form of the disease (Sones and Israel 1960, Siltzback et al. 1974) which may result in death. In those patients undergoing resolution, subsequent biopsy or material examined at autopsy has revealed changes ranging from complete resolution with no scarring to focal pulmonary scars without evidence of granulomatous inflammation. Hilar and mediastinal lymph nodes in these cases, although not enlarged, often contain patchy, highly collagenized scars. In chronic progressive cases, extensive pulmonary fibrosis often results. The pattern is that of extensive scar formation with adjacent cystic spaces, some of which are lined with cuboidal bronchiolar epithelium and appear bronchiectatic, while others remain thin-walled and emphysematous (McCort and Pare 1954). The process at this stage is not unlike that of the apical pulmonary scars with pericicatricial bullous emphysema, which is often observed on routine postmortem examination of the lung and in apical tissue in individuals undergoing spontaneous pneumothorax. Granulomas at this stage of the disease process may be infrequent or absent.

The end stage of this process differs from that of the diffuse fibrosing interstitial pneumonitis where the fibrosis is not patchy and the cystic areas are seldom thin-walled. The late stage of pulmonary sarcoidosis is often accompanied by hypertrophy and thickening of pulmonary arteries in a manner similar to that seen in other disease processes that reduce the pulmonary circulatory volume (McCort and Pare 1954). Calcification in sarcoidosis, which is occasionally observed radiographically (Rabinowitz et al. 1974, McLoud et al. 1974), is seldom observed histologically. In our experience, the terminal episode in end-stage fibrosis due to pulmonary sarcoidosis is a superimposed bronchopneumonia or pulmonary thromboembolism. Aspergillus fungus balls may also be seen in the cystic spaces of end-stage pulmonary sarcoid (Sepncer 1977). Histological involvement by the sarcoid process is, of course, not limited to the lungs. Lymph node involvement, involvement of the entire reticuloendothelial system, and involvement of many other organ systems is common.

B. Electron Microscopy

Several investigators have examined sarcoid granulomas with the electron microscope (Specter 1976, Greenberg et al. 1970, Soler et al. 1976). The sarcoid granuloma is divided into two zones. The central zone (Soler et al. 1976) consists of histiocytes, epithelioid histiocytes, giant cells (representing fused histiocytes), and occasional lymphocytes. Interdigitating complex cell processes with intercellular junctional complexes are common on ultrastructural examinations. The peripheral portion of the granuloma is more loosely arranged with less interdigitation of the cell processes where the cells appear more histiocytic and lymphocytes are more common. Junctional complexes between the cells are less common in this zone. In older lesions, abundant fibrohistiocytes and fibroblasts are present in the periphery of the granuloma. These are associated with abundant protocollagen as well as mature collagen.

Cell organelles within the histiocytes and epithelioid cells consist of abundant smooth and rough endoplasmic reticulum, mitochondria, and membrane-lined vesicles. Primary lysosomes appear to be present in a number of instances (Leake and Myrvik 1972). The giant cells are similar to those of the epithelioid cells but contain multiple nuclei and less endoplasmic reticulum. Large membrane-lined cytoplasmic vacuoles are present in the cytoplasm of some of the giant cells, and these correspond to the cytoplasmic vacuoles or centrospheres seen by light microscopy (Fig. 3). These appear to be autophagic vacuoles which contain osmiophilic myelin-like material as well as other cytoplasmic components. Some investigators (Uelinger 1964) have suggested that these cytoplasmic vacuoles are the early stage of what ultimately becomes the Schaumann body. Asteroid bodies by ultrastructural examination are composed of fibrillar structures resembling collagen, the central portion of which contains lysosomes and residual bodies (Vuletin and Rosen 1977, Jones et al. 1967). The latter finding gives further evidence for the evolution of the inclusion from the autophagic vacuole. Birefringent particles and Schaumann bodies appear ultrastructurally as dense, variably osmophilic, crystalline structures within the cytoplasm of the cell and have no other well-defined ultrastructural features.

C. Etiology and Immunopathology

It is considered likely that immune mechanisms are involved in the pathogenesis of sarcoidosis (Hedfors 1975, James et al. 1975). This hypothesis is based on the fact that other granulomatous diseases in both clinical and experimental settings are usually associated with an activation of the cell-mediated immune system (Epstein 1967). Although the immunologic aspects of sarcoidosis will be discussed in greater detail in another chapter of this book, cell-mediated immunity as it may relate to lung pathology will be reviewed briefly here.

One puzzling paradox of sarcoidosis is that immune studies have demonstrated a nonspecific depression of cell-mediated immunity rather than the expected activation. These patients usually have a consistent lymphopenia in their peripheral blood which is due to an absolute decrease in circulating T lymphocytes (Hedfors et al. 1974, Daniele and Rawlands 1976). Also, many of these patients have a diminished ability to express

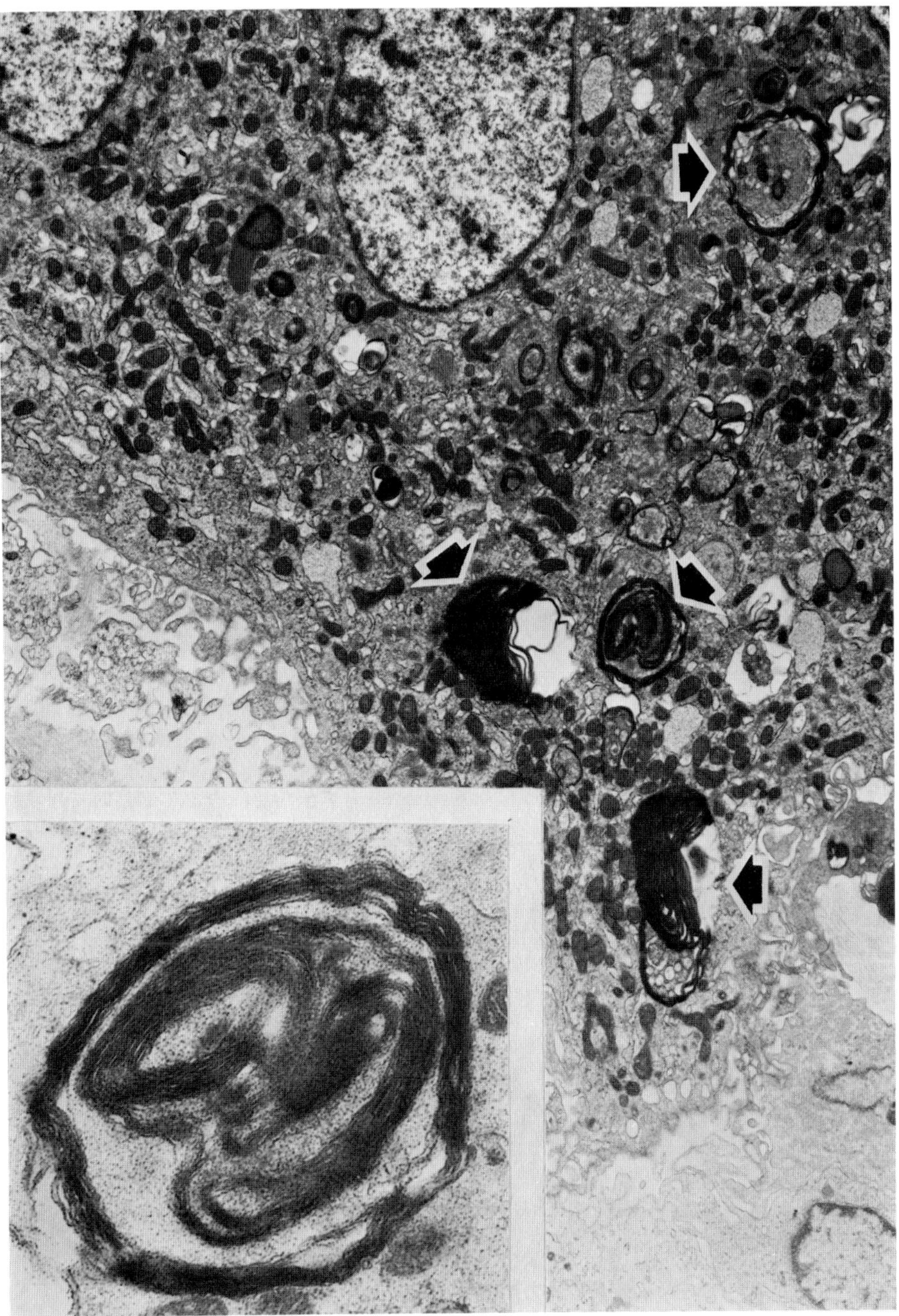

Figure 3 Electron micrograph of giant cell; membrane-lined cytoplasmic inclusions (arrows and inset) (uranyl acetate and lead citrate stain X 1900; insert X 4900).

delayed-type hypersensitivity as measured by decreased responsiveness to multiple antigens such as tuberculin, dinitrochlorobenzine, and *Candida,* in skin testing (Ceuppens and Stevens 1978). Lastly, various in vitro studies of lymphocyte function have shown that some groups of sarcoid patients, particularly those with chronic active disease, have diminished in vitro reactivity to mitogenic stimuli such as phytohemagglutinin A and concanavalin A (Goldstein et al. 1978).

In recent years, further research has suggested possible answers to these paradoxical findings. Multiple studies have shown that in spite of the inability of circulating lymphocytes to respond in vitro to the T-cell mitogens, there appears to be a spontaneous activation of T cells in vivo. Thus, nonstimulated lymphocytes from sarcoid patients show increased spontaneous DNA synthesis in vitro (Girard et al. 1971, Kantor et al. 1976). Associated spontaneous production of migration inhibition factor (MIF) may be responsible in part for the depression in delayed-type hypersensitivity seen in these patients. Studies by Yoshida and associates (1979) have shown that 60% of sarcoid patients studied have serum MIF activity. Patients with detectable circulating MIF show a diminution in reactivity in a variety of skin tests. The authors speculate that the circulating lympho-kine may be responsible for the cutaneous anergy seen in patients with sarcoidosis, since previous experimental studies have shown that the injection of preformed MIF into guinea pigs would render them anergic in delayed hypersensitivity testing (Yoshida and Cohen 1974).

Much interest in recent years has centered on the isolated cell populations in the specific organs affected by sarcoidosis. Thus, the technique of bronchopulmonary lavage has assumed major importance as a means of procuring leukocytes from the lower respiratory tract of patients with sarcoidosis. This technique allows one to compare leukocytes directly from the granulomatous tissues with those in the peripheral blood.

Initial lavage studies (Hunninghake et al. 1979) revealed that patients with sarcoidosis have a marked increase in the percentage of T lymphocytes in lung lavages when compared to lavage fluids from normal control subjects and also to lavage fluids from patients with idiopathic pulmonary fibrosis. The increase in lung T cells is in direct contrast to studies on the peripheral blood of the same patients, in which a consistent lymphopenia was demon-strated. In addition, more of the lung T lymphocytes are spontaneously activated when compared with those in the peripheral blood.

"Activation" has been defined by the ability of the cell to form rosettes with sheep red blood cells and also by the spontaneous secretion in cultures of a lymphokine, leukocyte inhibitory factor (LIF). Therefore, it has been suggested that there does appear to be a preferential localization of activated T lymphocytes in the lungs of sarcoid patients (Hunninghake et al. 1979). The mechanisms responsible for the localization are unknown.

Further studies by the same investigators (Hunninghake et al. 1980) have demonstrated that T lymphocytes from the lungs of patients with sarcoidosis secrete a factor that is chemotactic for monocytes. T lymphocytes obtained from bronchoalveolar lavage (BAL) fluids of patients without sarcoidosis do not show comparable production of chemotactic factor in vivo. Peripheral blood T lymphocytes from patients with sarcoidosis also secrete a chemotactic factor similar to that found in their culture fluids of bronchoalveolar layered cells, but in much lesser amounts. Thus, it appears likely that in sarcoidosis there is a higher concentration of this chemotactic factor in the lung compared with serum, which would theoretically create a concentration gradient to attract circulating monocytes to sites within the lung. Multiple studies have shown that the progenitors of alveolar macrophages are derived from bone marrow (Johnson et al. 1980), and it is tempting to postulate that in sarcoidosis the elaboration of monocyte chemotactic factor by the activated T lymphocytes within the lung is responsible for the increased number of macrophages in the lungs of these patients, and that the macrophages go on to form the characteristic granulomas.

Perhaps as a response to the elaboration of the monocyte chemotactic factor in patients with sarcoidosis, sera from these patients contain high levels of at least two natural regulators of chemotaxis (Maderazo et al. 1976, Campbell 1977). One of these regulators is chemotactic factor inactivator (CFI), which inactivates C5a and other chemotactic factors, including lymphokine-derived chemotactic factors (Maderazo et al. 1976). The other chemotactic inhibitor apparently present in the sera of these patients is a less well-defined cell-directed inhibitor, as described by Campbell (1977). The presence of abnormal levels of these inhibitors in sera from patients with sarcoidosis may simply reflect a secondary manifestation of an altered inflammatory system, although either inhibitor could theoretically influence the outcome of the granulomatous reaction.

Finally, there is a question of the role of humoral immunity in the pathogenesis of sarcoidosis. Many patients with sarcoidosis appear to have quantitative increases in gamma globulins, particularly IgG (Ceuppens and Stevens 1978). This would seem to indicate a hyperreactivity of the humoral system, either as a primary or as a secondary event in the disease. Similarly, there is evidence that at least in some stages of the sarcoidosis, circulating immune complexes are present in the serum.

There is evidence of the presence of circulating immune complexes, particularly in those patients with pulmonary sarcoid who have extra-pulmonary manifestations such as erythema nodosum or arthralgias accompanied by fever (Gupta et al. 1977), and malaise seen in acute sarcoidosis (Sjögren's syndrome) (Daniele et al. 1978). Some of the immune complexes appear to contain autoantibodies, directed against lymphocytes (Daniele et al. 1978).

Not surprisingly, in some studies rheumatoid factor activity has been reported in the sera of sarcoid patients (Oreskes and Siltzbach 1968). Evidence of immune complex deposition in the tissues of sarcoid patients is variable. Some studies have described the presence of immunoglobulin and complement in granulomas and in other lesions of sarcoid patients (Ghase et al. 1974, Ouismario et al. 1977), while others have not (Siltzbach 1964).

The cause of a generalized (presumably polyclonal) stimulation of the humoral system in sarcoid is unknown. However, recent studies by Hunninghake and Crystal (1981), again using lung lavage cells, may shed some light on this question. First, in BAL cells from untreated sarcoid patients, the number of IgG- and IgM-secreting cells is markedly increased when compared with BAL cells from normal controls. These data are in direct contrast to the picture with blood lymphocytes from the same sarcoid patients, since blood lymphoid cells, as contrasted to BAL lymphoid cells, secrete decreased levels of immunoglobulins (Katz and Fauci 1978). When purified "sarcoid" BAL T cells are co-cultured with blood lymphoid cells from normal individuals, the B lymphocytes are induced to undergo blast transformation accompanied by immunoglobulin secretion. On the other hand, co-culturing of blood T lymphocytes from the same sarcoid patients does not induce immunoglobulin secretion from B lymphocytes obtained from normal controls. Accordingly, these studies suggest that (a) there is a localized increase in immunoglobulin production at the site of the granulomatous reaction (lung) in the sarcoid lung, (b) no such systemic response occurs, and (c) the stimulation of the humoral immune system appears to be caused by the resident activated T lymphocytes obtained from sarcoid patients. The precise in vivo mechanisms of this stimulation are not yet defined.

III. Necrotizing Sarcoidal Granulomatosis

A. Clinical Presentation

Necrotizing sarcoid granulomatosis was first described by Liebow (1973) in the J. Burns Amberson lecture. Liebow reported 11 patients who had pulmonary lesions consisting of confluent sarcoidlike granulomas, a granulomatous vasculitis, and varying degrees of necrosis. The pulmonary histology appeared distinctive from that of sarcoidosis and from the other forms of pulmonary vasculitis. In this original study the lesions as seen by chest x-ray were usually bilateral and without hilar lymph node or extra-pulmonary involvement. These original patients were asymptomatic and followed a benign clinical course.

Subsequently, additional series have been reported (Saldana 1978, Churg et al. 1979, Koss et al. 1980). Although a few of these patients

may be asymptomatic when lung lesions are discovered on routine chest
x-ray examination, most present with cough, dyspnea, shortness of breath,
and fever. Additional symptoms include chest pain, hemoptysis, malaise,
and fatigue. Radiographically the patients usually present with bilateral,
noncavitary nodular or ill-defined densities in the lung. Unilateral and
solitary nodules are occasionally seen.

In the more recent series, hilar adenopathy was seen in approximately
one-half of the patients (Churg et al. 1979). Extrapulmonary involvement,
as indicated by clinical symptoms, is uncommon, but uveitis and central
venous system involvement have been reported (Churg et al. 1979, Breach
et al. 1980), and we have seen one case which presented as an intradural
mass in the cervical spinal canal with subsequent pulmonary disease (Singh
et al. 1981). Spontaneous remissions in the absence of treatment have
been reported (Churg et al. 1979), although other reports indicate treatment
may aid in the resolution of the disease (Koss et al. 1980). Because the
disease is uncommon or unrecognized, there are no large, controlled
therapeutic studies.

B. Pathology

Gross examination of the biopsy material reveals yellow nodular lesions
which occasionally show evidence of necrosis. Cavitation has not been
confirmed, although reports of cavitary sarcoid may be examples of
necrotizing sarcoidal granulomatosis (Tellis and Putnam 1977, Ohsaki et al.
1977). The nodular lesions are irregular in shape, have ill-defined borders,
and may be as large as 4 cm in diameter.

Histologically, necrotizing sarcoid granulomatosis exhibits three major
features: granulomas, vasculitis, and necrosis. The first major feature appears
to be confluent sarcoidlike granulomas which efface the architecture of the
lung. Like sarcoidosis, they appear to follow the bronchovascular bundles,
interlobular septa, and subpleural connective tissue. The granulomas, like
sarcoidosis, are well formed, contain giant cells, and are often ringed by
lymphocytes. The giant cells occasionally contain inclusions such as
vacuoles, asteroids, and Schaumann bodies. Such well-formed confluent
granulomas are not associated with other angiocentric granulomatoses such as
Wegener's granulomatosis and lymphomatoid granulomatosis (Liebow 1973).
The infiltrates in the latter two instances tend to be more polymorphonuclear and less granulomatous. Because of the granulomatous appearance
of this disease, special stains for organisms, as well as culture studies, should
be performed to exclude tuberculosis or fungus organisms.

Vasculitis is prominent in most cases and is usually evident in
routinely stained sections, although elastic tissue stains accentuate the
appearance of vascular involvement. Both arteries and veins are involved
by the process. The vessels often show circumferential and transmural

involvement. Veins usually contain inflammatory cells while arteries exhibit both inflammatory cells and granulomas. The muscle layer of arteries, as well as the external elastic lamina, often show the presence of granulomas although the internal elastic lamina usually remains intact (Fig. 4). The usual form of sarcoidosis often involves blood vessels but, unlike necrotizing sarcoid granulomatosis, it is usually restricted to the adventitia. Although transmural involvement by sarcoid granulomas may occur, occlusion and necrosis are uncommon (Rosen et al. 1977, Rosen et al. 1979).

Necrosis, which may be prominent, is another feature that distinguishes this entity from conventional sarcoidosis. It may be seen in the area of confluent granulomas and is of the coagulative type (Fig. 5). Necrosis may also be seen in the walls of some blood vessels. Microscopic foci of necrosis in the center of sarcoid granulomas are common (Rosen et al. 1979, Carrington et al. 1976), but not of the type or extent seen in necrotizing sarcoid granulomatosis. The necrosis of other angiocentric granulomatoses such as Wegener's granulomatosis and lymphomatoid granulomatosis is often more extensive and may resemble pulmonary infarction (Liebow 1973). The few reports of long-standing necrotizing sarcoid granulomatosis indicate that the lesions may become hyalinized and fibrotic, not unlike those of conventional sarcoidosis (Liebow 1973, Churg et al. 1979).

Electron microscopy reveals edematous swelling of the vascular endothelial cell basement membranes. Extracellular osmiophilic material is present in the interstitium (Fig. 6). Immunofluorescent studies (Koss et al. 1980) have revealed staining of the pulmonary granulomas with antisera to *Aspergillus.* However, *Aspergillus* has not been demonstrated in the lungs by either special stains or culture. Our immunofluorescent studies have shown some periarterial staining with IgG and IgA (Fig. 7). Intraalveolar material stained weakly with IgG and IgM. The areas of necrosis stained strongly for fibrin. Studies of T or B-lymphocytes revealed a normal peripheral distribution and normal transformation in the presence of plant mitogens.

C. Etiology and Immunopathology

The etiology of this entity, like that of sarcoidosis, is unknown. Part of the problem relates to the relatively few cases described in the literature and to the paucity of immunological and other parameters studied. The combination of necrosis and granulomatous inflammation may suggest an infectious etiology. However, no bacteria, fungi, or viruses have been identified (Koss et al. 1980). One patient in the Koss study had immunofluorescence studies done on lung tissue which revealed a strongly positive staining pattern for *Aspergillus fumigatus.* This finding suggests that perhaps

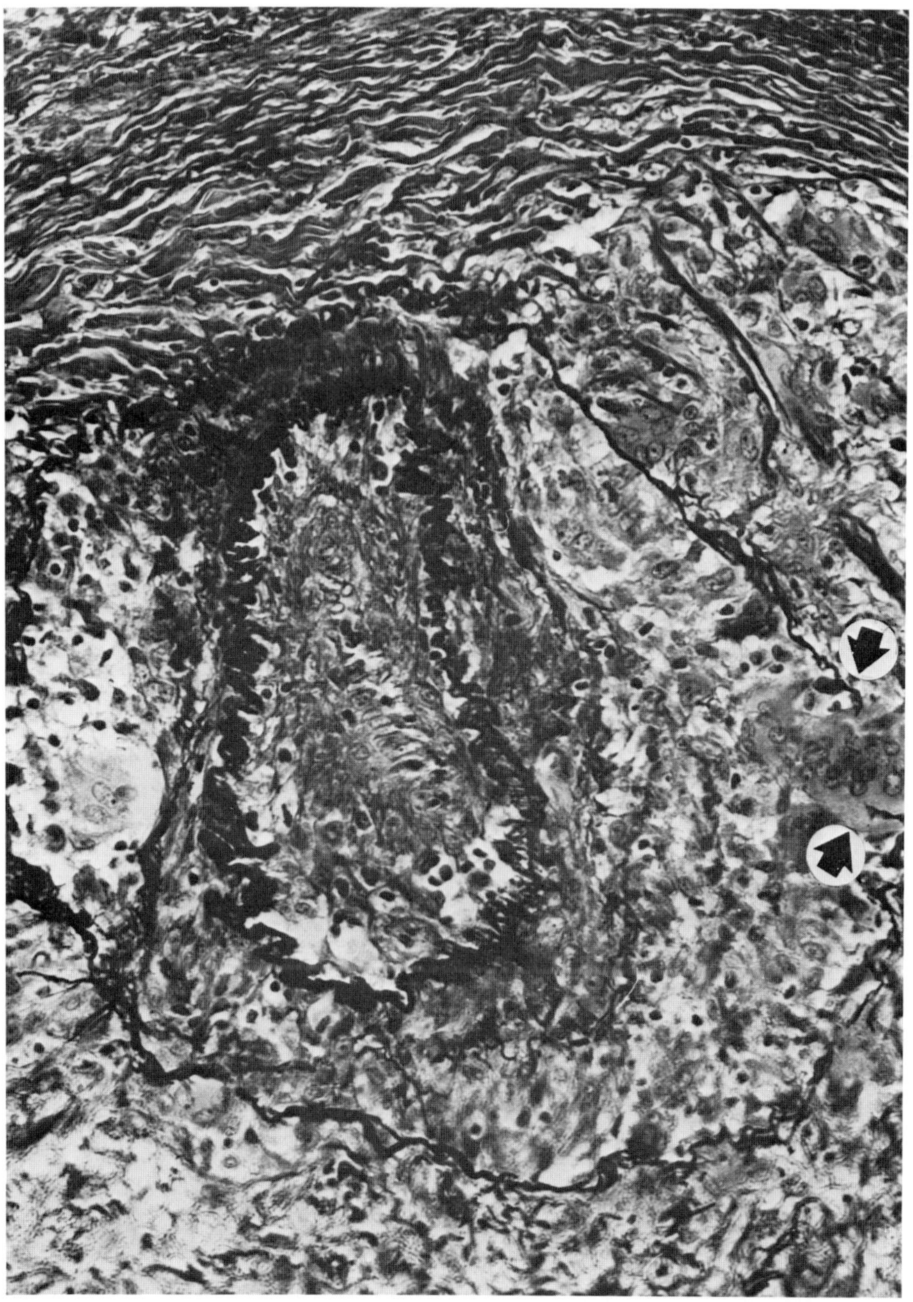

Figure 4 Necrotizing sarcoidal granulomatosis; pulmonary artery with transmural granulomatous vasculitis disrupting the external elastic lamina (arrows) (Verhoeff elastic tissue stain X 16).

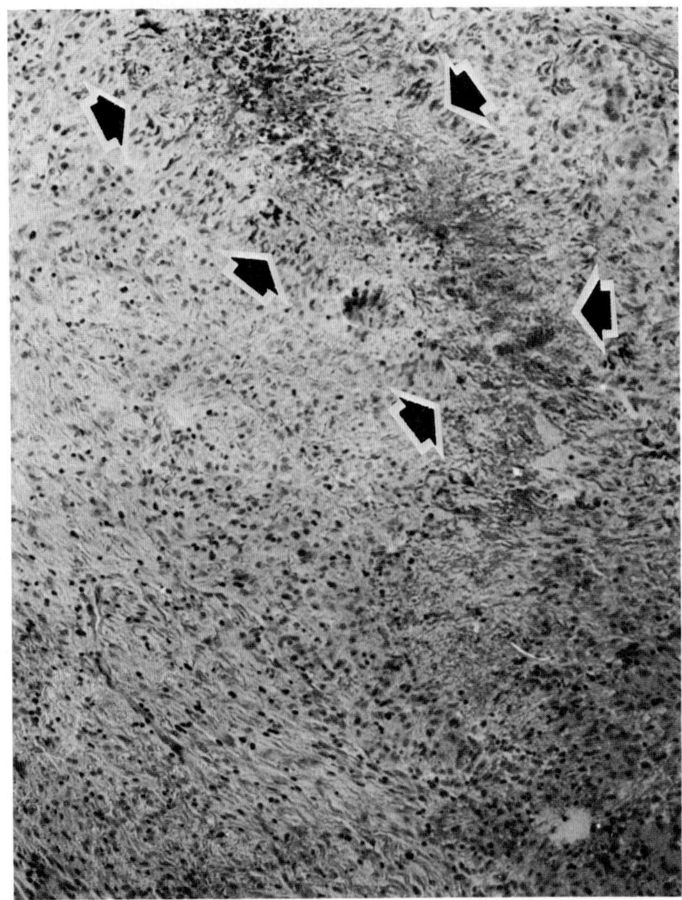

Figure 5 Necrotizing sarcoidal granulomatosis; confluent sarcoidlike granulomas with areas of extensive necrosis (arrows) (H&E X 6.3).

hypersensitivity to fungal antigens, particularly against *A. fumigatus,* may play a role in the development of the lesion.

Immunological screening tests have not usually been performed in these patients. In the one patient in whom these studies were carried out (Singh et al. 1981), T and B lymphocytes had a normal peripheral distribution and responded normally to mitogenic stimulation. However, the patient did have cutaneous anergy, and serum levels of IgG, IgA, and IgM were quantitatively elevated. No circulating immune complexes were found. Therefore, some of these immunologic parameters were consistent with

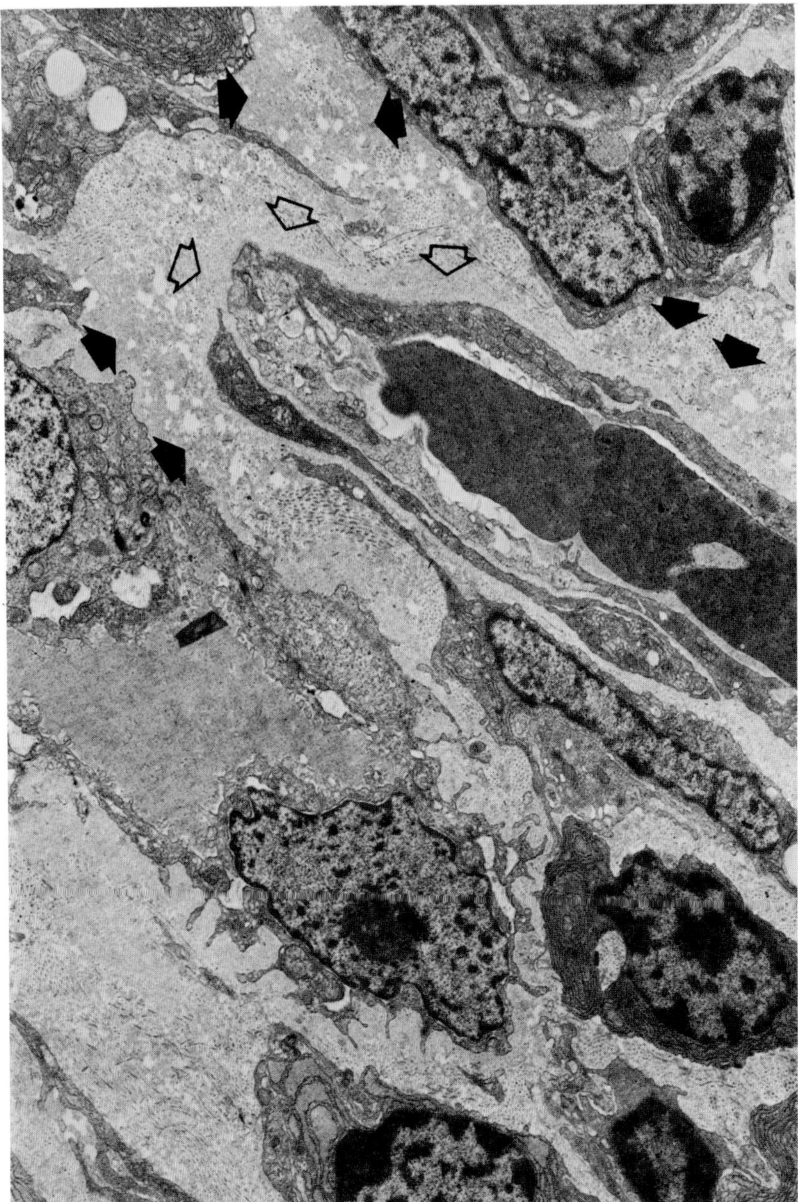

Figure 6 Necrotizing sarcoidal granulomatosis; electron micrograph demonstrating extracellular granular material (dark arrows) and swollen capillary basement membrane (hollow arrows) (uranyl acetate and lead citrate stain X 1900).

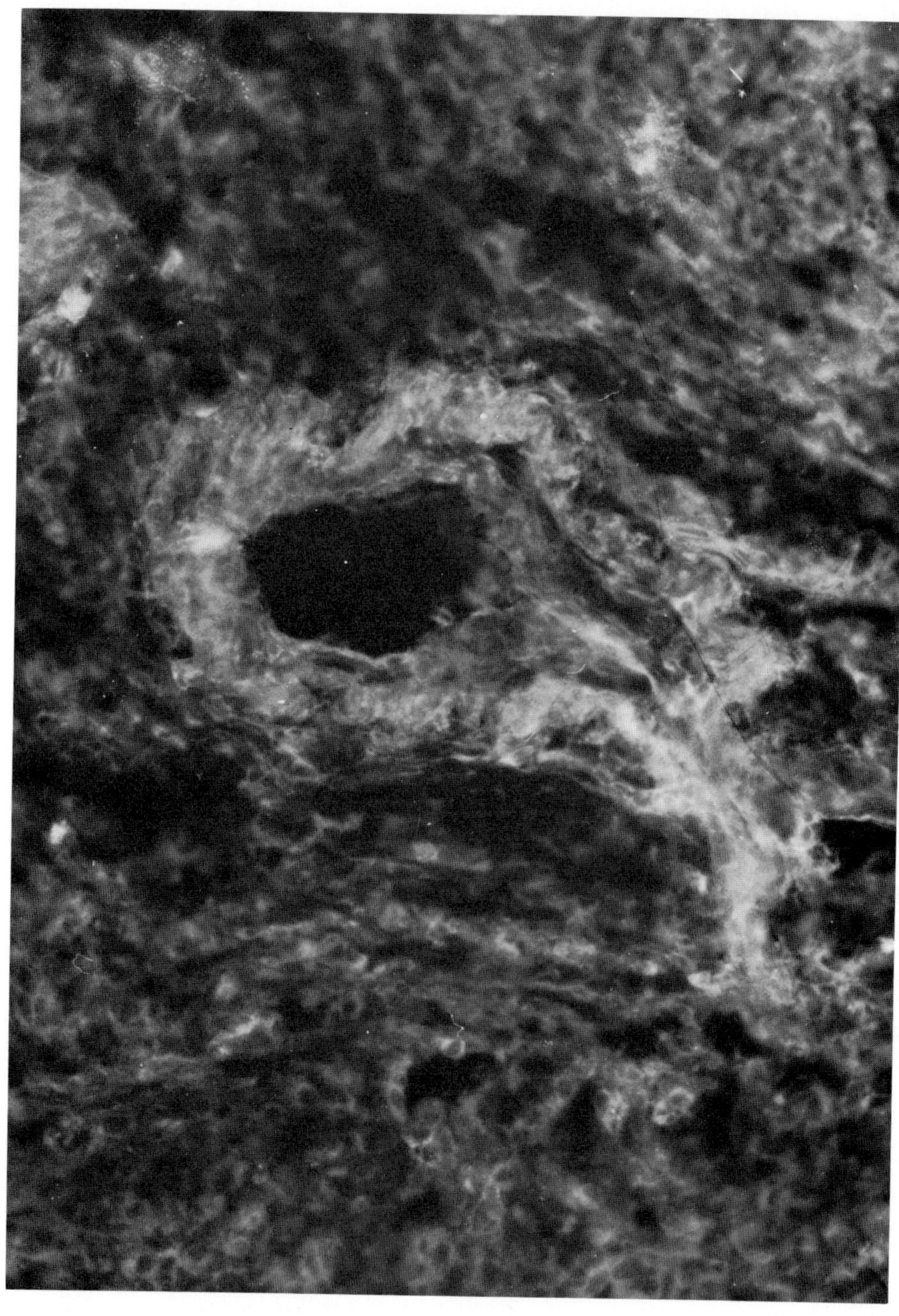

Figure 7 Necrotizing sarcoidal granulomatosis; immunofluorescent staining for IgG in a perivascular distribution (X 16).

those seen in the usual sarcoidosis, while others were not. Clearly, many more patients need to be studied, not only for these immunologic parameters, but also by immunofluorescence screening of tissue biopsies to assess the role of fungal antigens.

IV. Pulmonary Allergic Granulomatosis

A. Clinical Presentation

Pulmonary allergic granulomatosis is a term applied to the lung lesions of a systemic clinical syndrome consisting of asthma, peripheral eosinophilia, and pulmonary granulomatous vasculitis, first described by Churg and Strauss (1951). The clinical features and histopathological appearance of this syndrome bear some resemblance to both polyarteritis nodosa and Wegener's granulomatosis (Churg and Strauss 1951, Sokolov et al. 1962).

Most patients with this disease have a long history of severe asthma, which is the most common presenting complaint when pulmonary infiltrates and peripheral hypereosinophilia are discovered. The patients are often febrile and have a history of repeated pneumonia. Hayfever, various allergies, and upper respiratory complaints (Olsen et al. 1980, DeRemee et al. 1980) are common, but the necrotizing nasopharyngeal and sinus lesions of Wegener's granulomatosis are not present. Cutaneous lesions, which may be erythematous, macular, or pustular, are seen in a majority of patients (Strauss et al. 1951, Dickens and Winklemann 1978). Renal disease may be present but is uncommon. Other organ systems involved by the process include the heart, gastrointestinal system, liver, and the central and peripheral nervous systems (Fauci et al. 1978).

The majority of patients are found to have radiographic abnormalities. The infiltrates may be unilateral or bilateral, infiltrative and migratory, or multinodular (Chumbly et al. 1977). Cavitation, a feature of both Wegener's granulomatosis and lymphomatoid granulomatosis, is not present in pulmonary allergic granulomatosis. Hilar lymphadenopathy may be present but the lymph nodes are seldom significantly enlarged.

B. Pathology

On pathological examination pulmonary vascular thickening as well as pulmonary thrombi may be present. Patchy consolidation similar to that in pneumonia or, occasionally, nodular lesions may be observed (Churg and Strauss 1951). The nodular lesions are yellow and are generally smaller than the masses seen in the other angiocentric pulmonary vasculitides. Cavitation is not present.

Microscopically, the lesions of pulmonary allergic granulomatosis consist of a vasculitis involving small arteries and occasionally veins. In the parenchyma of the lung and usually adjacent to areas of vasculitis are small necrotic granulomas. These consist of a central area of necrosis, often surrounded by radially arranged epithelioid histiocytes and giant cells (Fig. 8). The necrotic debris is often intensely eosinophilic. The cellular infiltrate surrounding the granuloma consists largely of eosinophils, although lymphocytes, plasma cells and histiocytes may be present. This intense eosinophilia usually distinguishes pulmonary allergic granulomatosis (Liebow 1973) from the other pulmonary angiitides as well as from polyarteritis nodosa affecting the lung (Churg and Strauss 1951). The infiltrates in the arteries may be neutrophilic, but intense eosinophilia in the acute stage is a dominant feature. Necrotic granulomas centered on blood vessels similar to those in the parenchyma may be present. The elastic tissue of the vessel is often disrupted; this feature is best demonstrated by elastic tissue stains. Thrombosis of the affected vessel is common.

During resolution, fibrous nodules consisting of collagen and a few chronic inflammatory infiltrates develop adjacent to blood vessels and interlobular septa and within the lung parenchyma. Eosinophils, although often present, may be inconspicuous. It is in this healing stage when the nodules resemble, and may be indistinguishable from, those of healing polyarteritis nodosa (Fauci et al. 1978). Histological features of asthma are often present in the bronchi. These consist of increased mucus-secreting cells in bronchial epithelial lining and bronchial glands, thickening of the basement membrane, and eosinophilic infiltrates beneath the bronchial mucosa.

It should be emphasized that allergic granulomatosis, like polyarteritis nodosa, is a systemic disease. It differs significantly from polyarteritis nodosa in its predilection for the lungs, association with asthma, and significant tissue and peripheral eosinophilia. The lung is not the exclusive target in allergic granulomatosis; skin and subcutaneous tissues are often involved with necrotic eosinophilic granulomas, similar to those seen in the lungs. In this case the term "Churg-Strauss granuloma" has been applied (Dickens and Winklemann 1978).

Allergic granulomatosis also frequently involves the heart and pericardium. The kidneys may show interstitial eosinophilic infiltrates, but lesions of the glomeruli are uncommon. A few glomeruli may contain eosinophilic infiltrates and fibrin within the lumens of the capillary loops. Although hilar lymph node enlargement is seen by chest radiographs, histological alterations in the lymph nodes are nonspecific. A single case of sarcoidlike granulomas in lymph nodes was reported in the original series by Churg and Strauss (1951). Other organ systems, including the gastrointestinal tract, liver, spleen, and nerves, may also be involved by eosinophilic infiltrates and vasculitis.

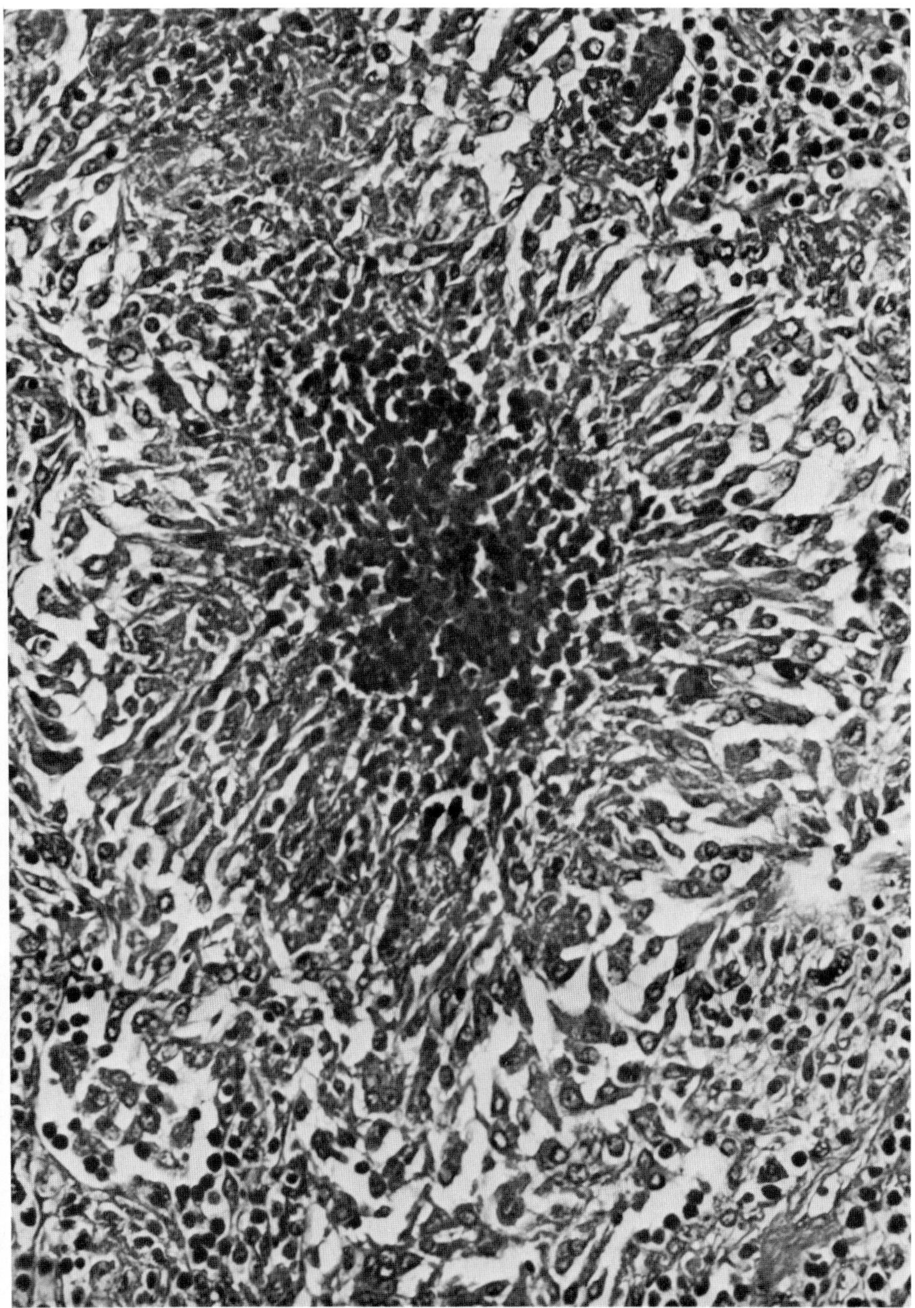

Figure 8 Pulmonary allergic granulomatosis; necrotizing granuloma with radiating epithelioid histiocytes (H&E × 16).

Untreated cases of allergic granulomatosis may result in death, usually occurring as a result of the vasculitis and, in particular, from coronary artery vasculitis. Pulmonary fibrosis may also result in death. Since the original series was described, corticosteroid therapy has proved to be effective in the control of the disease (Chumbley et al. 1977).

C. Etiology and Immunopathology

The etiology of this disease is unknown, although there is some evidence to suggest a hypersensitivity reaction. This hypothesis is based in part on the clinical history of induced atopy and elevated IgE levels associated with peripheral eosinophilia. Characteristically, cytotoxic agents and steroids bring about dramatic remissions.

V. Generalized Wegener's Granulomatosis

A. Clinical Presentation

Generalized Wegener's granulomatosis is characterized by destructive vasculitis with associated granuloma formation involving the upper respiratory tract, lungs, and kidneys. The disease was clinically recognized by Klinger (1931) and the pathology first described by Wegener (1936, 1939). Although the disease is reported in infants and in the aged, it is more common in the fourth and fifth decades. Although some reports indicate the disease to be more prevalent in men than women, others, including our series, suggest a more even distribution (Fauci and Wolf 1973, Israel et al. 1977). Common presenting symptoms include nasal crusting and bleeding. Many patients give a long history of sinusitis or rhinitis before the discovery of lung or renal involvement. Chest symptoms include cough, hemoptysis, and chest pain. Renal symptoms are present in the majority of patients but usually occur after the onset of respiratory symptoms. Low-grade fever, weakness, weight loss, and malaise may be presenting symptoms but are uncommon in the absence of respiratory symptoms. Maculopapular and ulcerative skin lesions may be present. Neurologic involvement, both central and peripheral, occurs in 25% of patients with systemic Wegener's granulomatosis (Fauci and Wolf 1973). Other organ systems may be involved to a lesser degree but seldom in the absence of the classic triad of upper respiratory tract, lungs, and kidneys. Anemia is common in these patients, but tissue and peripheral eosinophilia, although considered by some to be a usual feature in Wegener's granulomatosis (Spencer 1977, Fraser and Pare 1978), is uncommon in our experience and that of others (Liebow 1973).

Radiographically the disease often appears as multiple large, rounded lung opacities in a peripheral but random distribution. The lesions may show spontaneous regression and, in some patients, the nodules develop cavitation. Solitary pulmonary lesions may occur but are less common than the multinodular pattern (Israel and Patchefsky 1971). Occasionally, diffuse pneumonic infiltrates are seen.

Glomerulonephritis occurs in a majority of these patients, and untreated patients ultimately may die of uremia. Respiratory failure remains the second most common cause of death in systemic Wegener's granulomatosis.

B. Pathology

Examination of the upper respiratory tree on postmortem experiments reveals encrusted naso-labial folds with erosion or cavitation in the nasal region and perforation of the nasal septum. The sinuses may also be eroded and are often described as cloudy on x-ray examination of the nasal sinuses (McGregor and Sandler 1964).

The lungs reveal two gross patterns. One is that of circumscribed cavitary lesions, the contents of which vary from creamy to caseous (Fig. 9). The other pattern consists of lesions that are markedly hemorrhagic and may have a wedgelike configuration resembling a pulmonary infarct. The smaller lesions in the lung superficially resemble the small caseous granulomas of tuberculosis. The larger lesions may occupy entire lobes of lung. While the central portion of the lesion is often necrotic, lung tissue peripheral to the nodule may be consolidated in the pattern of a bacterial pneumonia. Fibrinopurulent exudate, as well as fibrous adhesions, may be present on the pleural surface, especially in those areas adjacent to subpleural cavitary lesions.

The histopathology of the lung lesions is variable in what is called classic, systemic, or generalized Wegener's granulomatosis. It is mandatory that an adequate sample of the diseased lung be obtained for examination, and presently the method of choice for obtaining tissue is open biopsy of the lung. Three histological features found in generalized Wegener's granulomatosis are vasculitis, necrosis, and a granulomatous reaction. Without these features, the diagnosis should be in some doubt.

Both gross examination and microscopic analysis reveal lesions of variable size. The larger lesions exhibit extensive necrosis which may resemble caseation necrosis, but more often the necrosis is composed of the ghost outline of cells, degenerating neutrophils, and nuclear debris (Fig. 10). About the periphery of the necrotic zones there is a variable infiltrate consisting of Langhans' giant cells, histiocytes, plasma cells, lymphocytes, and rare eosinophils (Liebow 1973, Townley et al. 1962).

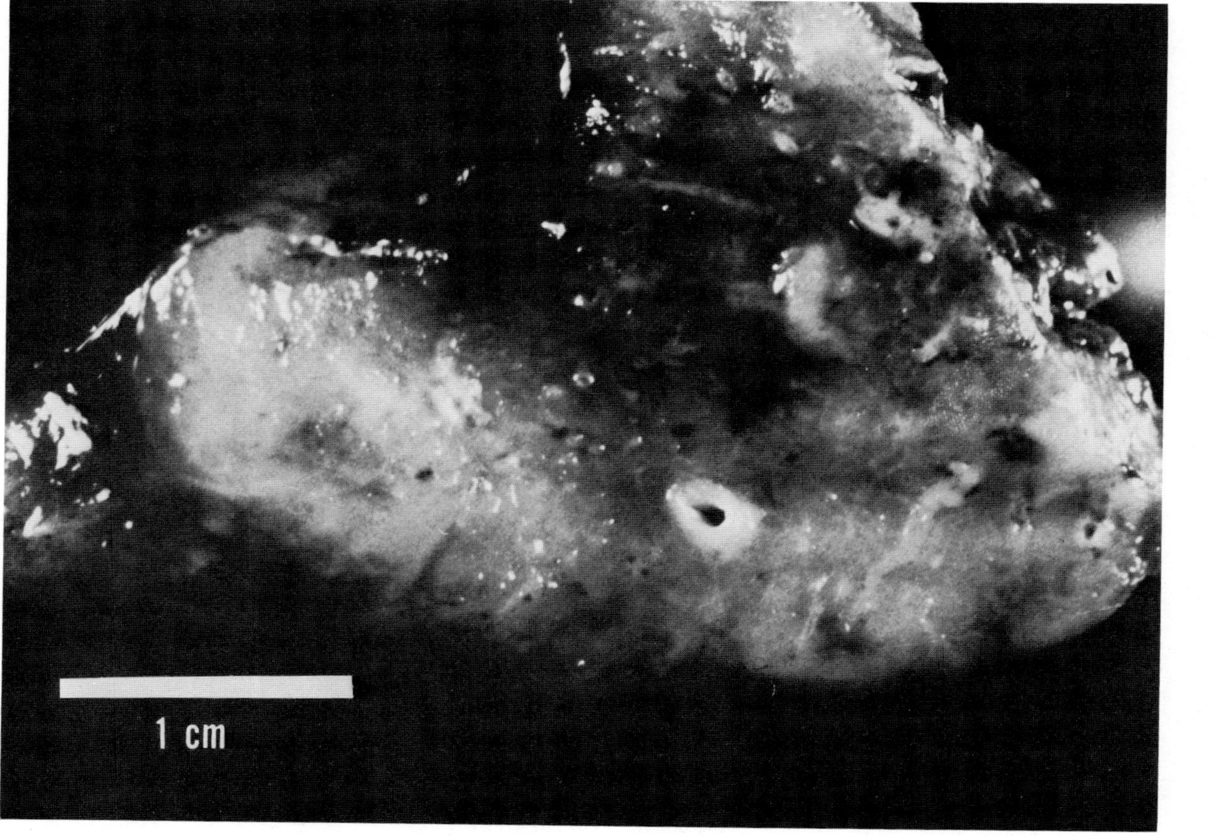

Figure 9 Wegener's granulomatosis; gross specimen of lung with nodular densities with central necrosis.

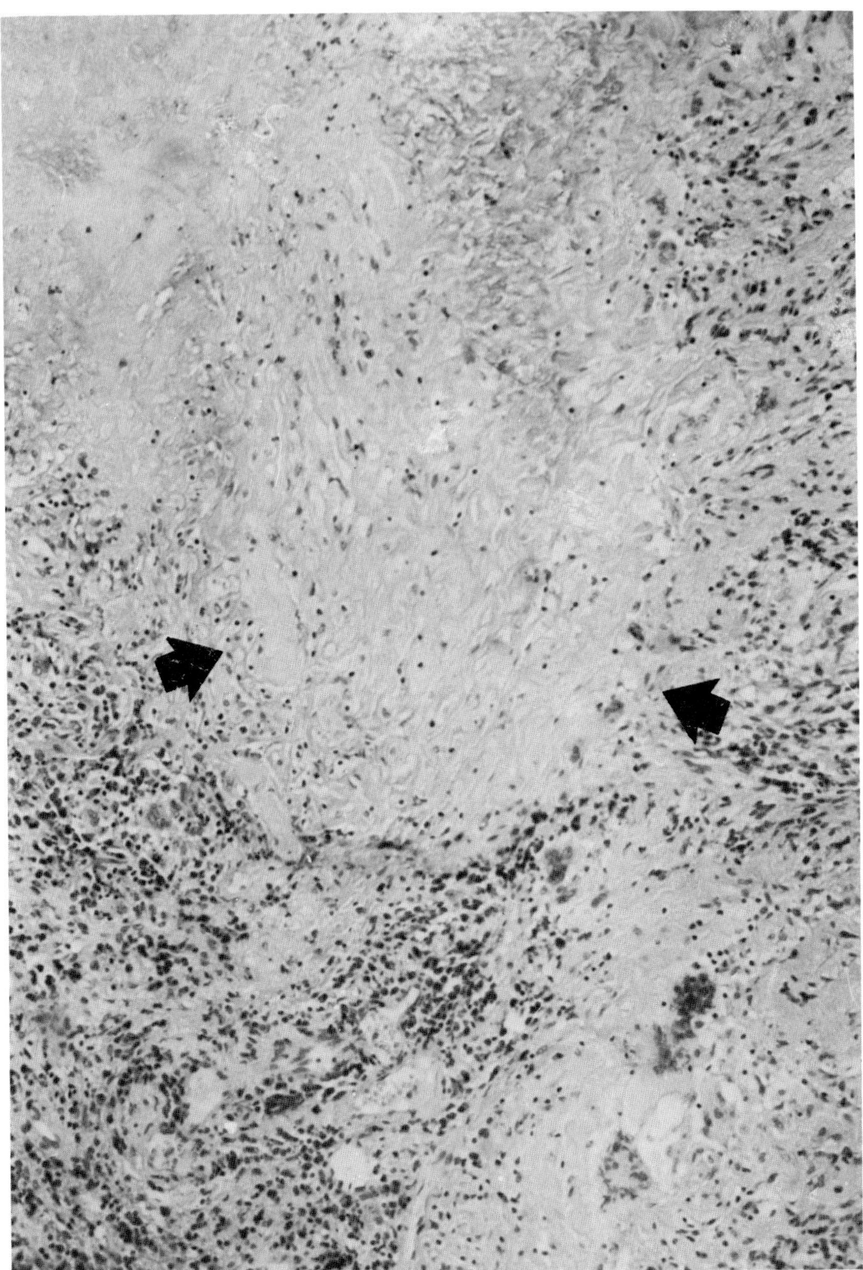

Figure 10 Wegener's granulomatosis; necrotic lung tissue (arrows) surrounded by chronic inflammatory cells including Langhans' giant cells (H&E × 6.3).

This combination of histological features often suggests tuberculosis or other infectious diseases which elicit a granulomatous response and for which both special stains and cultures should be routinely done.

Although vasculitis is often not apparent in the large lesions of patients with Wegener's granulomatosis, elastic tissue stains often reveal the outline of large vessels within the center of the areas of necrosis. The walls and lumens of these vessels are diffusely infiltrated with ghosts of inflammatory cells. These large necrotic areas are usually irregular in shape and randomly distributed throughout the lung parenchyma. They may occasionally be wedge-shaped and pleural-based and contain considerable numbers of red cells. In the latter instances, the lesions may be confused with pulmonary infarcts, as is occasionally the case in the radiological appearance of the disease. Around the periphery of the necrotic areas there may be a variable amount of fibrosis characterized by the proliferation of fibroblasts and deposition of collagen with the resulting eradication of lung tissue. Smaller nodules scattered throughout the lung or occurring as satellite nodules to the larger necrotic areas may show a vasculitis characterized by inflammatory infiltrates in the walls of small to medium-sized vessels. The cells in the infiltrate are usually composed of histiocytes and variable numbers of lymphocytes and plasma cells. Giant cells and necrosis may be absent. Such lesions are by themselves not diagnostic of Wegener's granulomatosis.

Smaller, necrotizing granulomatous lesions are often found in the walls of bronchi and in the walls of larger arteries (Fig. 11). These lesions are characterized by central, often fibrinoid, necrosis, Langhans' giant cells, and numerous epithelioid histiocytes oriented in a radial fashion around zones of necrosis (Liebow 1973). This latter feature helps distinguish the disease from tuberculosis and fungus granulomas. Ill-defined satellite epithelioid granulomas of the sarcoid type may be seen in the regions adjacent to the necrotizing granulomas as well as adjacent to the areas of extensive necrosis. Diffuse infiltrations of the alveolar capillaries, as well as alveoli filled with histiocytes, lymphocytes, and plasma cells, are seen in lung parenchyma adjacent to areas of necrosis (Fig. 12). Although capillaries and veins may be involved in the inflammatory process, the vascular infiltrates and necrotizing granulomatous infiltration seem to have a predilection for the larger arteries.

C. Electron Microscopy

Electron microscopic studies have revealed a variety of nonspecific ultra-structural alterations including vascular endothelial swelling and basement membrane thickening. Extracellular osmiophilic material is occasionally seen. No definite basement membrane densities have been described.

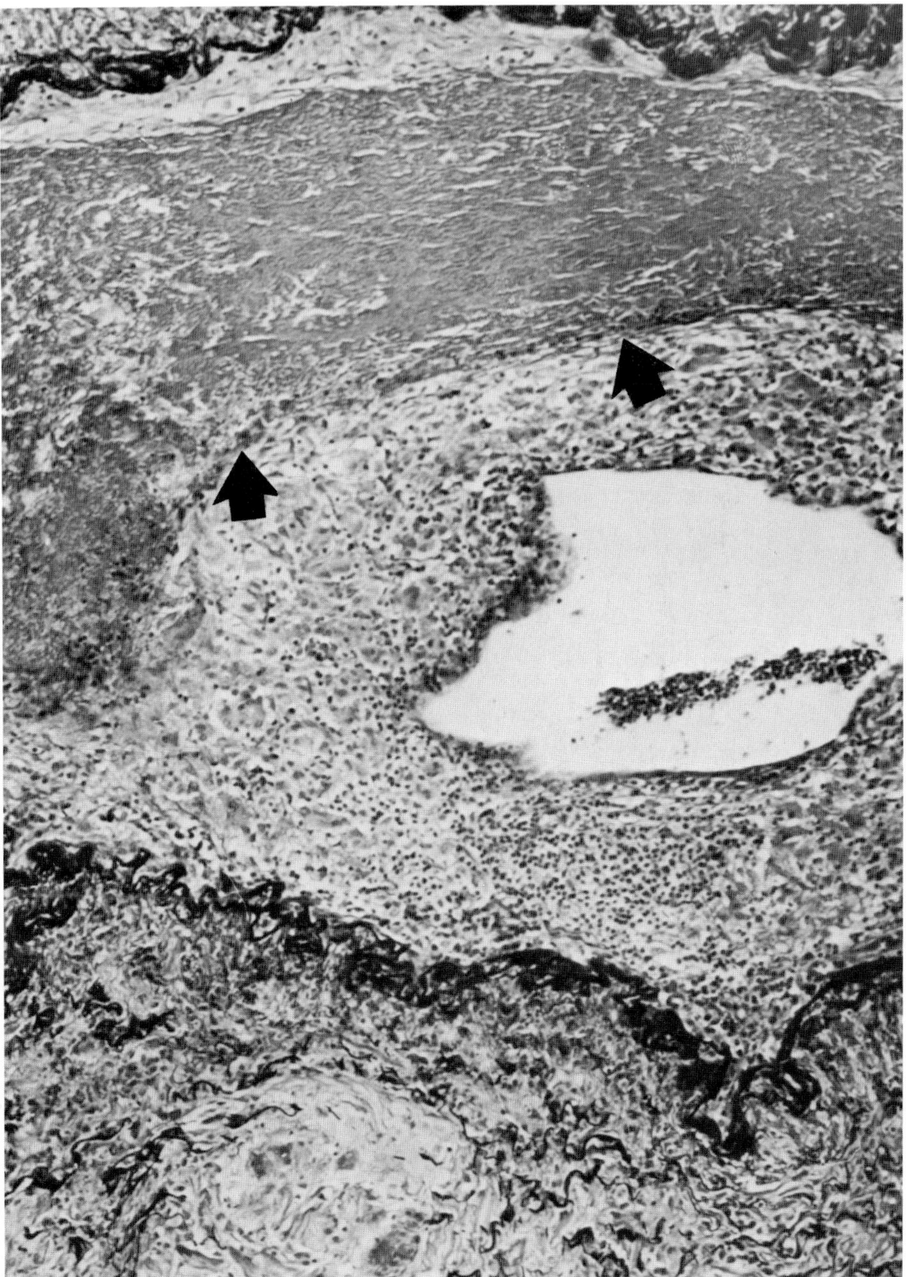

Figure 11 Wegener's granulomatosis; granulomatous vasculitis with necrosis (arrows) of the arterial wall (Verhoeff elastic tissue stain X 6.3).

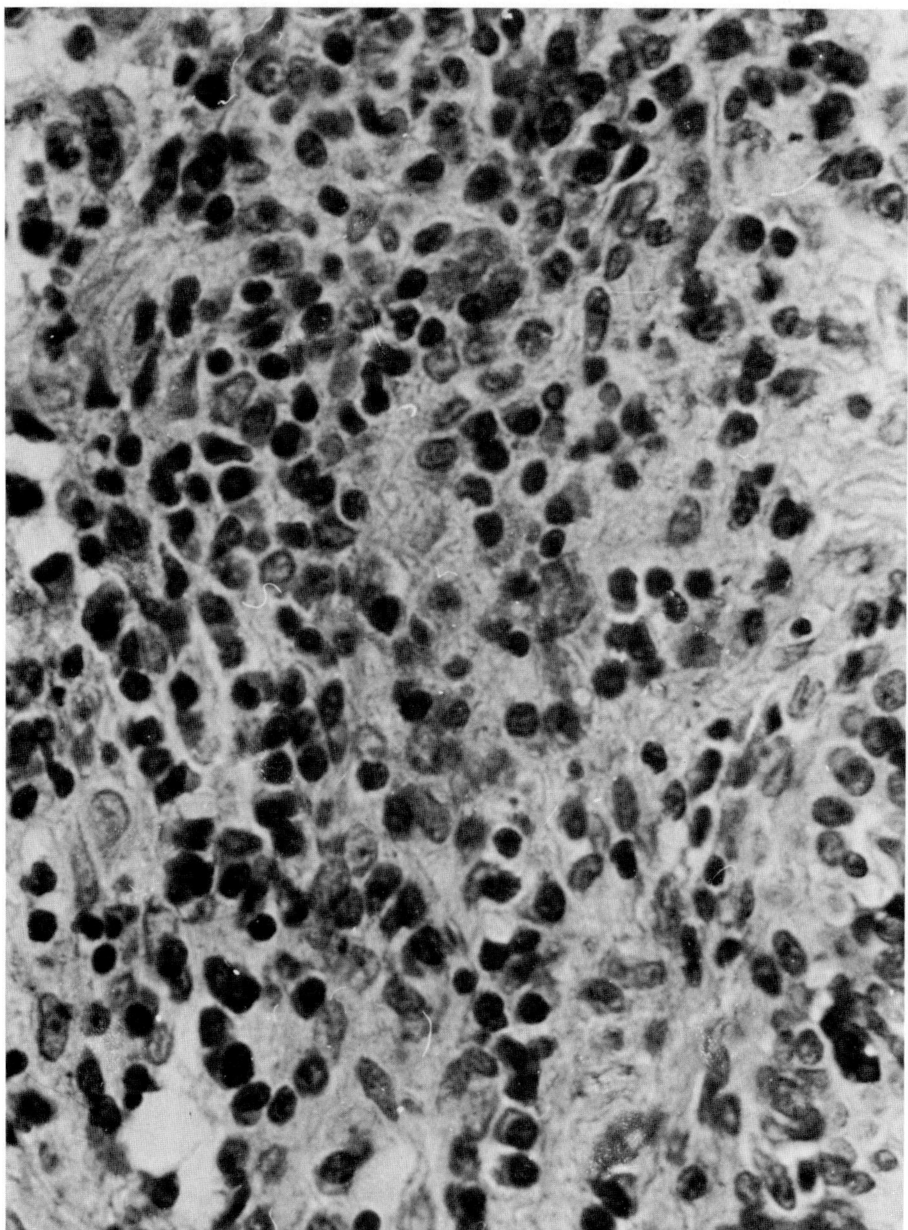

Figure 12   Wegener's granulomatosis; chronic inflammatory infiltrate consisting of histiocytes, lymphocytes, and plasma cells (H&E × 40). (This infiltrate should be compared with that in Figure 14.)

D. Extrapulmonary Disease

The lesions of the nose and sinuses also exhibit a necrotizing granulomatous inflammation, and considerable destructive necrosis may occur. Various inflammatory cells, including giant cells, are seen and, in general, the pathology is similar to that seen in the lungs. A vasculitis may be present but because of the nature of the area, ample biopsy tissue often is not available for examination.

Renal involvement is the hallmark of generalized Wegener's granulomatosis, and fulminant renal disease is considered the most serious complication (Wolff et al. 1974). Before the advent of cytotoxic drugs in therapy, particularly cyclophosphamide, renal failure was the main cause of death in these patients. In one such group of patients, the mean survival time from the onset of clinically evident renal disease was five months (Walton 1958). The urinary findings of proteinuria and macroscopic hematuria suggest an acute glomerulonephritis. However, unlike most acute glomerulonephritides, hypertension is usually not seen (Burkholder 1974).

Although both vascular (involving arteries and veins) and glomerular lesions may be present in renal biopsies, the classic picture is one of a focal and segmental necrotizing glomerulonephritis, which is extremely variable in severity (Fauci and Wolff 1973). Occasionally, necrotizing vasculitic lesions are present as well but this is much less common. Heptinstall (1974) comments that the renal lesion is identical to that seen in microscopic polyarteritis (hypersensitivity angiitis) except in those cases where granulomas are present in relation to blood vessels and glomeruli. Many cases, however, do not show any evidence of granulomas and it is rare that one is found in a renal biopsy specimen.

There is considerable overlap between the histopathology of granulomatous lung disease and that of vasculitis. Polyarteritis nodosa, a systemic disease, may affect the lungs (Rose and Spencer 1957), but it seldom presents with the classic triad found in systemic Wegener's granulomatosis. The lesions in the lung in polyarteritis nodosa are exclusively perivascular, and a granulomatous component is uncommon although necrosis may be found. The predominant inflammatory cell in the walls of vessels is the neutrophilic leukocyte, unlike that of classic Wegener's granulomatosis. Pulmonary allergic granulomatosis may also resemble systemic Wegener's granulomatosis clinically, but it is usually associated with a history of asthma and not with nasal and renal lesions. The lung lesions of pulmonary allergic granulomatosis are similar to the necrotizing granulomatous lesions and vasculitis of systemic Wegener's granulomatosis. However, pulmonary allergic granulomatosis, unlike systemic Wegener's granulomatosis, is usually associated with marked peripheral eosinophilia, marked tissue eosinophilia, and the absence of extensive areas of infarction necrosis.

Immunofluorescence findings have been variable. In some studies, no immunoglobulins were found in the kidney (Howell and Epstein 1976). However, IgG, IgM, and C3 are usually found in a granular pattern along glomerular capillary walls (Wolff et al. 1974). Fibrin has also been identified.

Ultrastructurally, the renal alterations are not specific. Electron-dense deposits have been described in paramesangial (Burkholder 1974) and subepithelial locations (Wolff et al. 1974). Fibrin in Bowman's space associated with proliferation of epithelial cells, increase in mesangial matrix, and focal loss of foot processes has also been described (Roback et al. 1969).

E. Etiology and Immunopathology

The cause and pathogenesis of Wegener's granulomatosis are unknown. One hypothesis is that Wegener's granulomatosis is due to some obscure type of infectious process. However, numerous studies have failed to find any evidence of a primary infectious agent with the exception of some chronic infections by *Staphylococcus aureus,* felt to be secondary to the tissue destruction (Fauci and Wolff 1973). Many patients have received empiric trials of antibiotics without effect. Treatment with corticosteroids and cytotoxic drugs has not "uncovered" an infectious agent (Israel and Pathchefsky 1971).

With an infectious etiology seemingly ruled out, speculation has for many years centered on the possible role of hypersensitivity or immune mechanisms. This has developed as a result of two general sets of observations. First, humans who develop drug sensitivity reactions to certain drugs, such as penicillin and sulfa drugs, occasionally develop granulomatous lesions, as well as the more usual vasculitis and glomerulonephritis (Godman and Churg 1954). Second, in early studies done many years ago, the injection of a crude foreign protein such as egg white into sensitized animals can lead locally in the early phase to vasculitic lesions (consistent with an Arthus reaction) and in the latter phases to development of granulomas (Goddard 1947). Unfortunately, this is where the matter has rested for many years, with no real progress having been made in identifying the causative antigen or antigens responsible for the lesions of Wegener's granulomatosis. Even with the advent of the use of purified antigens, no animal model has been identified that closely mimics the lesions seen in humans. In the classic model of acute serum sickness using a purified antigen (bovine serum albumin), vasculitis and a diffuse type of glomerulonephritis develop, but there is no evidence of a granulomatous reaction (Cochrane 1979). Also, with the exception of one report in the literature (Spector and Hessom 1969), the injection of preformed immune complexes has not led to the development of granulomas.

There is also a paucity of clinical evidence concerning the type of hypersensitivity reaction seen in Wegener's granulomatosis. There is no evidence to indicate a type I (anaphylactic) mechanism. These patients usually do not have an atopic history and there are no related clinical findings such as wheezing or elevated IgE levels as seen in allergic granulomatosis (Churg-Strauss). There is also no evidence implicating type II hypersensitivity (cytotoxic) reactions.

There is some evidence, albeit nonspecific, indicating a possible role for type III (immune complex) reactions. There is a high incidence of increased levels of rheumatoid factor (Wolff et al. 1974), with IgA in particular being elevated in the serum and secretions of many of these patients (Fauci et al. 1971, Shillitoe et al. 1974). In addition, there are occasional reports of these patients having circulating immune complexes, some of which have the ability to fix complement (Howell and Epstein 1976). This, coupled with the immunofluorescence findings of immune complexes in glomeruli and occasionally in vessel walls, lends support to an immune complex pathogenesis. However, these findings must be tempered with other data which have shown that many patients have no evidence of circulating immune complexes; cryoglobulins have not been found, and serology studies are usually normal. There is also no evidence to implicate autoimmune mechanisms. No antinuclear or anti-DNA antibody or LE cells have been identified (Wolff et al. 1974, Roback et al. 1969).

Lastly, there is the consideration of the possible role of type IV (delayed-type) hypersensitivity. The presence of granulomas is generally thought to be the hallmark of reactions involving cell-mediated immunity. However, no consistent evidence of cell-mediated immunity has been found in patients with Wegener's granulomatosis (Howell and Epstein 1976). There is one report of a group of patients with Wegener's granulomatosis with depressed cutaneous delayed hypersensitivity (Shillitoe et al. 1974). However, this study is compromised because many of these patients were on corticosteroid therapy which, by itself, can cause suppression of these reactions. Other studies in groups of patients with Wegener's granulomatosis have failed to find any defect in delayed hypersensitivity (Fauci and Wolff 1974).

VI. Limited Wegener's Granulomatosis

A. Clinical Presentation

In 1966 Carrington and Liebow (1966) described a disease process morphologically similar to systemic Wegener's granulomatosis but involving the lungs and not the nose or kidneys. These 16 cases were referred to as limited Wegener's granulomatosis; subsequently additional series of similar cases have been reported (Liebow 1973, Israel and Patchefsky 1971).

A significant number of patients are asymptomatic when the lung lesions are discovered by routine chest radiographic examination. However, most patients present with complaints of cough, hemoptysis, pleuritic chest pain, dyspnea, malaise, fever, weight loss, and painful skin lesions. Nasal crusting and sinusitis are absent, although occasionally patients complain of sore throats. Renal function tests and urinanalyses show no evidence of glomerulonephritis.

B. Pathology

Grossly the lesions may be irregular, round, or even wedge-shaped as in a pulmonary infarct. They are often yellow but may be hemorrhagic. The lesions may be necrotic and cavitary, although this finding is more common in generalized Wegener's granulomatosis. The histological findings in the lungs include vasculitis, necrosis, and granulomatous inflammation. The appearance is similar to the lung lesions of generalized Wegener's granulomatosis, although it is less extensive; it is not unlike the appearance of tuberculosis, for which it is often mistaken. Angiitis is invariably present and is best demonstrated in areas removed from those produced by necrosis. The vascular infiltrates include histiocytes, lymphocytes, and plasma cells. Eosinophils may be present but are seldom numerous (Liebow 1973). The areas of necrosis are usually of the coagulation or liquefaction type but may superficially resemble caseation necrosis. Multinucleated giant cells of the Langhans' type are frequently present around the areas of necrosis, although they are not as numerous as generally seen in the systemic form of the disease. Special stains for elastic tissue almost invariably reveal the remnants of a sizable, occluded vessel in the center of the necrosis. Satellite granulomas of the sarcoid type may occasionally be seen near the periphery of the areas of necrosis but are seldom as well circumscribed as those of sarcoidosis. Similar to those of generalized Wegener's granulomatosis, the lesions may be wedge-shaped, peripheral, and hemorrhagic, resembling a pulmonary infarct. Variable degrees of fibroblastic proliferation and fibrosis may be seen in the periphery of the lesions. Radially arranged histiocytes are often seen around the areas of necrosis. Fibrinoid necrosis with a granulomatous and giant cell reaction may be seen in the walls of bronchi and large vessels.

Electronmicroscopic studies in limited Wegener's disease are similar to those of the generalized form. Endothelial cells are often swollen. The basement membrane of the vascular endothelial cells is swollen, and interstitial edema is often prominent. Extracellular osmiophilic material is occasionally observed, but neither nodular nor diffuse deposits are seen in basement membranes.

C. Extrapulmonary Disease

The histological features of limited Wegener's disease in the lungs do not differ from those of the more generalized form, except by degree. It is the absence of clinical and pathologic features of upper respiratory involvement and glomerulonephritis that characterizes this disease. Although glomerulonephritis is not present in this form of the disease, biopsy and autopsy material may reveal a granulomatous vasculitis in the kidneys similar to that observed in the lungs. The skin lesions may show a granulomatous vasculitis but more commonly are of polymorphocellular infiltration and are occasionally associated with overlying ulceration.

The limited form of Wegener's granulomatosis is, in our experience, at least as common as the generalized form. This form of the disease is usually associated with a more benign course than is the generalized form (Liebow 1973, DeRemee et al. 1976, DeRemee et al. 1980). Spontaneous remissions have been reported as well as occasional cures by surgical excision of the lesion. However, recent advances in the use of cytotoxic immunosuppressive drugs have resulted in a higher success rate than with the other modalities of treatment.

VII. Lymphomatoid Granulomatosis

A. Clinical Presentation

Lymphomatoid granulomatosis was first described (Liebow et al. 1972) as an entity distinct from lymphomas, to which it bears histological similarity, and from limited Wegener's granulomatosis, to which it bears both clinical and histological similarities (Liebow et al. 1972). This series was expanded and reviewed in 1973 (Liebow 1973). The disease is characterized by pulmonary lymphoreticular infiltrates which are angiocentric and angiodestructive. There is a male predominance of the disease, and it affects all ages (Katzenstein et al. 1979). Pulmonary symptoms are present in at least 50% of the patients and include cough, shortness of breath, and chest pain. Constitutional symptoms of fever, malaise, and weight loss are frequent. Central nervous system involvement (Katzenstein et al. 1979, Pena 1977, Verity and Wolfson 1976) and skin rashes (Katzenstein et al. 1979) are each evident in approximately one-third of all patients. Neurologic symptoms include seizures, hemiparesis, ataxia, and confusion. Cranial and peripheral nerve involvement may also be present. Nasopharyngeal lesions may be present but seldom in the absence of central nervous system and pulmonary disease. Erythematous, macular, or nodular skin lesions may be the only presenting clinical symptom of some patients in whom the lung lesions are evident only by chest radiographs.

Chest radiographs characteristically reveal bilateral nodular infiltrates, usually peripheral, which are frequently mistaken for metastatic tumors. Less commonly the lesions appear indistinct and resemble pneumonias. Unilateral disease occurs only rarely. Cavitation may occur but is less common than in Wegener's granulomatosis. In addition, the lesions may change in configuration and size, although this feature is less common than in other angiocentric granulomatoses. Hilar lymph node enlargement is uncommon and when present should suggest lymphoma or other disease processes (Katzenstein et al. 1979).

Steroids and immunosuppressive agents have been used in the treatment of lymphomatoid granulomatosis, but the response to therapy and prognosis in these patients is less favorable than with other forms of angiocentric granulomatoses of the lungs. Most patients die from pulmonary disease although a significant number die from central nervous system involvement. Approximately 10% of lung disease that is initially diagnosed as lymphomatoid granulomatosis eventually becomes manifested as malignant lymphomas (Katzenstein et al. 1979, Cohen et al. 1979), including immunoblastic sarcoma (Reddic et al. 1978). Whether this represents a biologic potential of the disease entity or an incorrect initial diagnosis is not clear.

B. Pathology

Macroscopic examination of lung tissue reveals irregular but often rounded masses of firm, pinkish-white tissue which may be centrally cavitated. Secondary obstruction of adjacent bronchi may lead to pneumonic consolidation of the lungs peripheral to the lesion.

Microscopic examination reveals lymphoreticular infiltrates which are angiocentric, although veins may also be involved. The infiltrates consist largely of variable amounts of small lymphocytes and leukocytes, but plasma cells may also be present. As in generalized Wegener's granulomatosis and in the limited form of the disease, eosinophils are uncommon (Liebow et al. 1972). Necrosis centered about the artery is often present and may be cavitary (Fig. 13). Fibroblasts as well as a few acute inflammatory cells may be seen at the peripheral edge of the necrosis. Although the elements described here qualify the lesion as granulomatous, true epithelioid histiocytes with epithelioid giant cells are not a usual finding in this entity.

Since the disease may involve arteries adjacent to bronchi, involvement of the adjacent bronchus in the form of bronchiolitis obliterans is common (Liebow et al. 1972, Saldana et al. 1977). Obstructive pneumonia characterized by the intraalveolar accumulation of foamy macrophages peripheral to these areas of obstruction is seen occasionally.

The character of the cellular infiltrates varies considerably. The cells may be composed largely of small, mature lymphocytes, benign-appearing

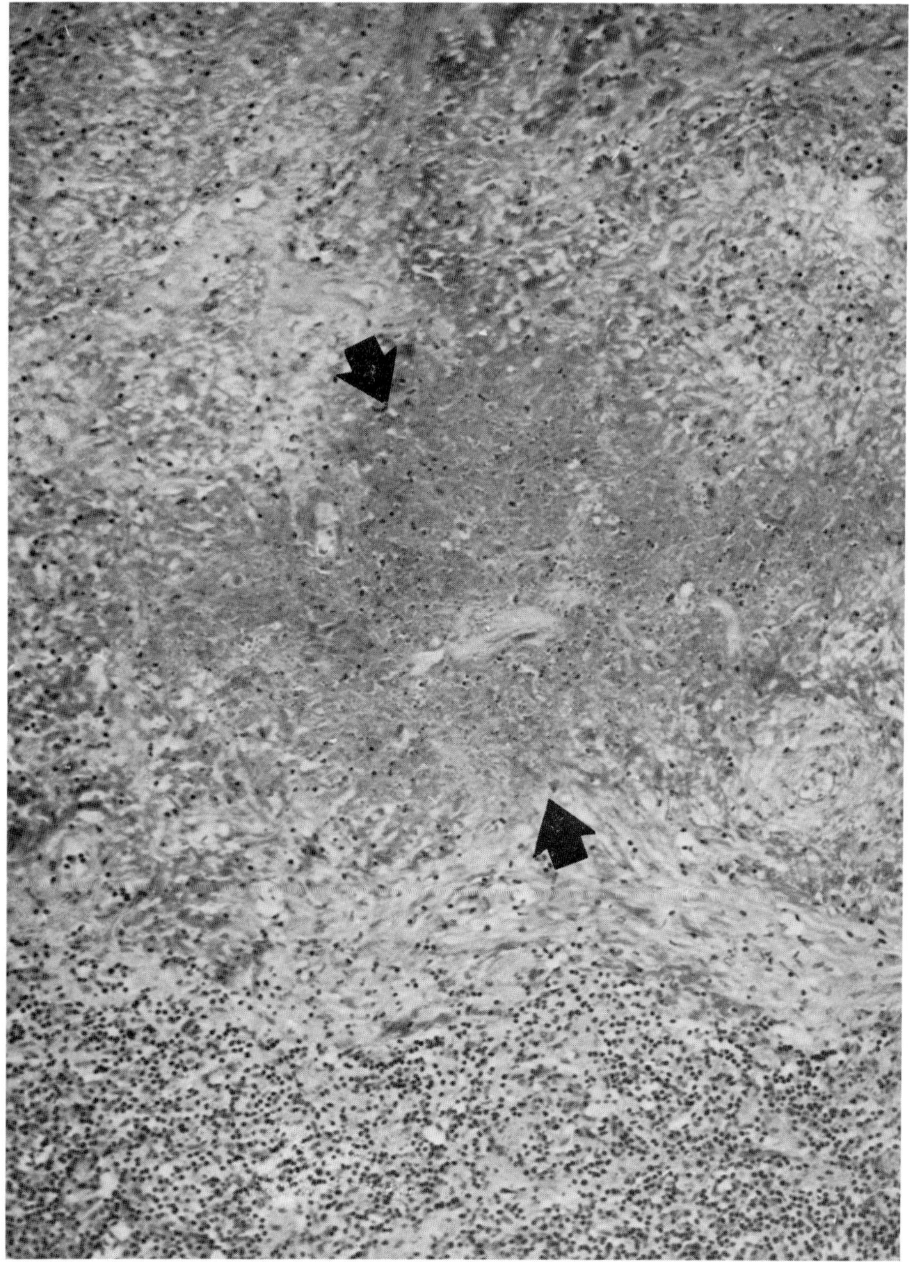

Figure 13 Lymphomatoid granulomatosis; necrotic lung tissue (arrow) centered around a pulmonary artery with peripheral chronic inflammatory infiltrates (H&E × 6.3).

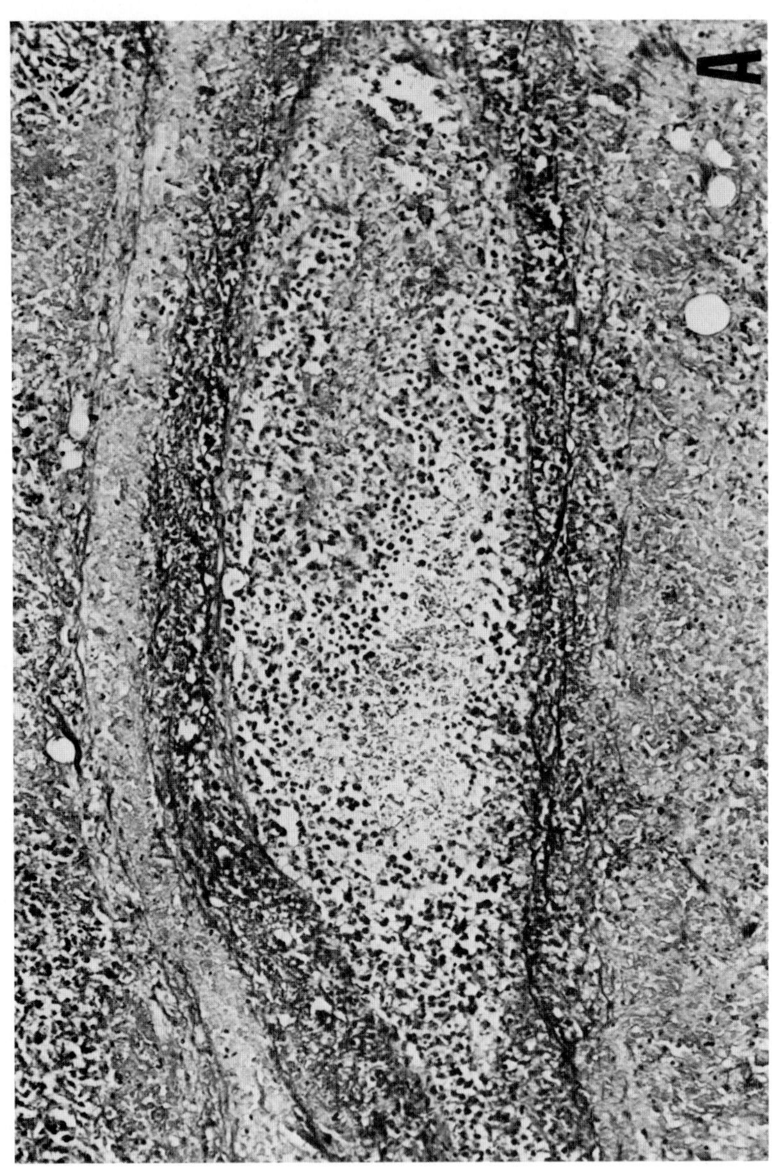

Figure 14 Lymphomatoid granulomatosis: (A) occlusion of an artery by cellular infiltrate without disruption of the elastic lamina (Verhoeff elastic tissue stain × 16); (B) pleomorphic cellular infiltrate including atypical histiocytes, lymphocytes, and plasma cells (H&E × 40).

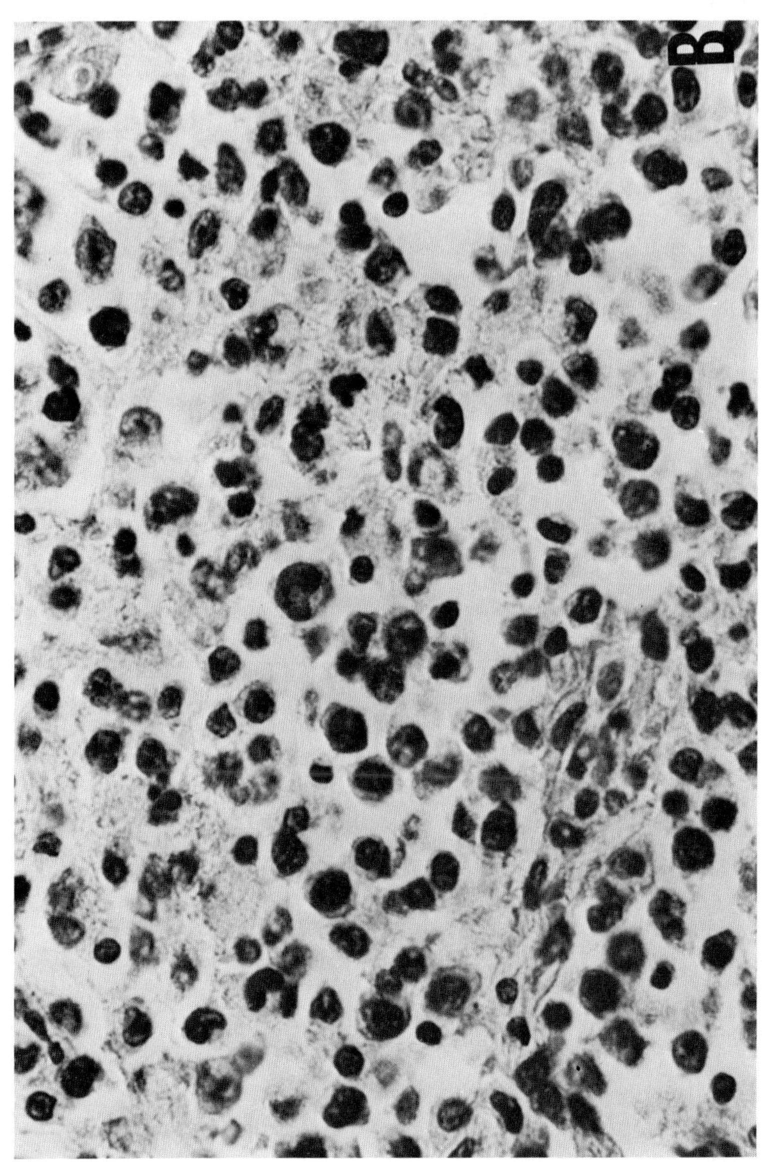

Figure 14 (Continued).

histiocytes, or a mixture of both. The term benign lymphocytic angiitis
has been applied by some investigators to these cases (Saldana et al. 1977,
Israel et al. 1977). In other cases the lymphocytes may be less mature
and in still others the histiocytes may be so bizarre as to suggest Hodgkin's
disease, a disease for which it is often mistaken (Fig. 14A, B). Mitoses
may be common. True Reed-Sternberg cells are not present. Some
investigators suggest a poorer prognosis in the less well-differentiated
infiltrates as well as a poorer response to chemotherapy (Saldana et al.
1977, Israel et al. 1977).

Elastic tissue stains indicate that the lymphoreticular cells infiltrate
the wall of the vessel and produce necrosis by obstruction (Fig. 14a, b).
Focal necrosis of the vessel wall and marked disruption of the vascular
elastic tissue fibers are not prominent in lymphomatoid granulomatosis when contrasted to the changes in generalized Wegener's granulomatosis,
limited Wegener's, and necrotizing sarcoidal angiitis. Untreated patients
with lymphomatoid granulomatosis continue to develop pulmonary
infiltrates and may die of pulmonary insufficiency due to extensive
parenchymal involvement. Some patients die with extensive fibrosis and a
few die of severe hemoptysis (Liebow 1973).

C. Extrapulmonary Disease

The histology of the skin lesions (Katzenstein et al. 1979, Kay et al. 1974)
is similar to that of the pulmonary lesions (Fig. 15) and consists of
angiocentric lymphoreticular infiltrates in the dermis. A few cases have
exhibited a giant cell response in the skin. The infiltrates in the brain are
also angiocentric and angiodestructive. Extensive involvement of the brain
with cavitation is responsible for death in approximately one-fourth of these
patients (Katzenstein et al. 1979, Pena 1977, Verity and Wolfson 1976).
The kidney is involved in approximately one-third of patients with
lymphomatoid granulomatosis (Katzenstein et al. 1979) and shows
lymphoreticular parenchymal infiltrates with no evidence of glomerulonephritis.
Other organs less commonly involved include tongue, nasal cavity, nasopharynx,
mesentery, skeletal muscle, small bowel, gallbladder, testes, and uvea.

The cause of lymphomatoid granulomatosis remains unclear. Whether
it represents viral infection, an autoimmune response, or a primary
malignant lymphoma remains unclear (Gross 1980).

VIII. Bronchocentric Granulomatosis

A. Clinical Presentation

Bronchocentric granulomatosis is a necrotizing granulomatous disease of the
lungs and is centered principally around bronchi and bronchioles. Along

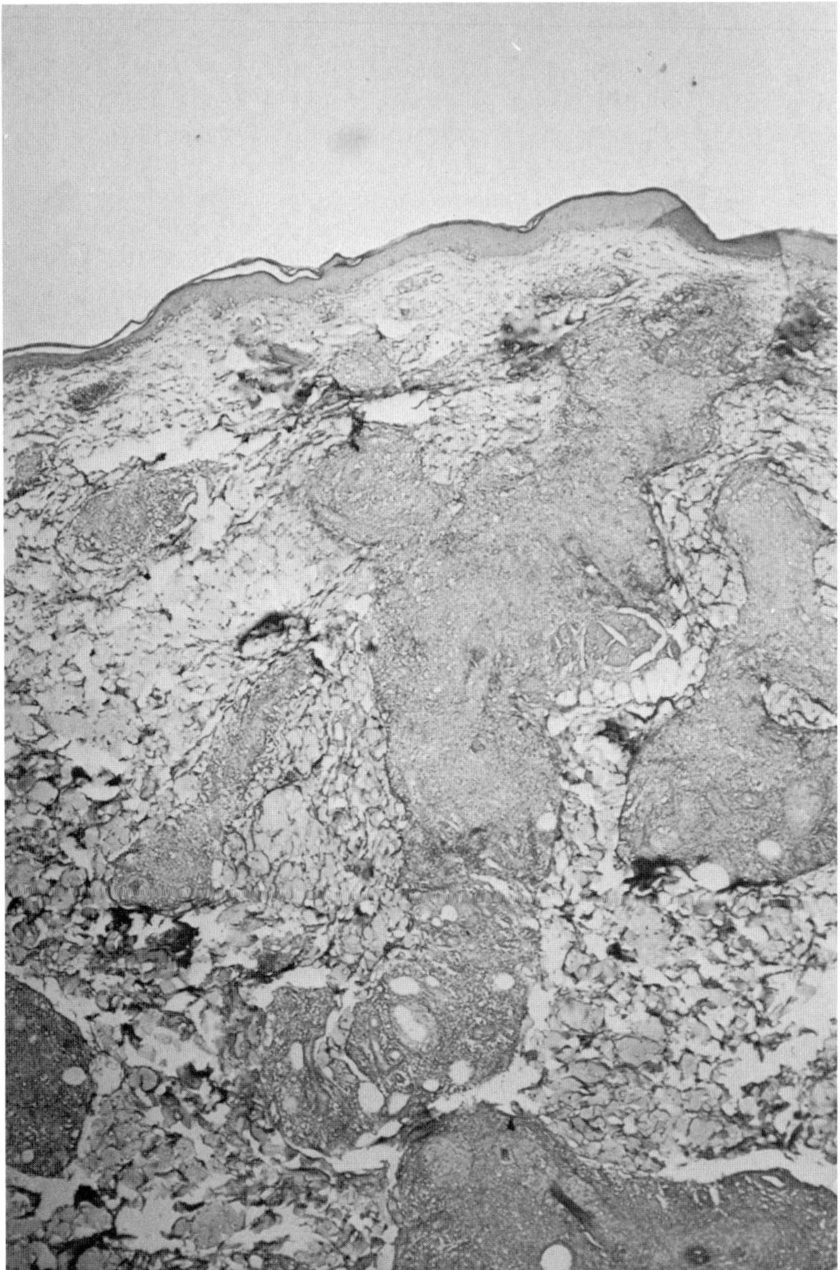

Figure 15 Lymphomatoid granulomatosis; skin with perivascular chronic inflammatory infiltrates in the dermis (H&E × 2.5).

with the limited form of Wegener's granulomatosis, necrotizing sarcoidal granulomatosis, and lymphomatoid granulomatosis, bronchocentric granulomatosis was first defined as a distinctive histopathologic entity by Liebow (1973). Patients often present with fever, cough, chest pain, and malaise. Approximately one-half of patients with bronchocentric granulomatosis have a history of chronic asthma and a few of these have multiple allergies. Peripheral eosinophilia of varying degree is present in only half of the reported cases and does not correlate well with the presence of asthma. Several studies (Katzenstein et al. 1975, Hanson et al. 1977) have shown that some patients have positive skin test and serum precipitins to *Aspergillus,* and *Aspergillus* has occasionally been cultured from the sputum of these patients. Extrapulmonary involvement by the granulomatous process has not been reported.

The radiographic appearance of the disease is variable. Most commonly it affects a single lobe, although multiple lobes may be involved and the process may be bilateral. The radiological appearance of mucoid impaction has been noted in a few cases, although multiple small nodules, large nodules, pneumonic consolidation, and infarction patterns have also been described. Bronchograms done in some cases have shown segmental obstruction.

B. Pathology

Examination of the gross specimens reveal the bronchi to be filled with an inspissated, yellow, caseous-like material which is unlike that of the more gelatinous mucoid impaction (Fig. 16). Although the central large bronchi may contain mucoid material, the yellow necrotic material is usually confined to segmental and more peripheral bronchi. The bronchi often appear dilated, and saccular areas may be present. Peripheral consolidation is a common feature and these areas are firm and yellow.

Microscopically, the necrotizing inflammatory process centers around and extends outward from involved bronchi and bronchioles. Unlike Wegener's granulomatosis, limited Wegener's, necrotizing sarcoidal granulomatosis, and lymphomatoid granulomatosis, bronchocentric granulomatosis is not angiocentric or angiodestructive, although blood vessels adjacent to involved bronchi may exhibit a secondary infiltration by the inflammatory process.

The lesions of bronchocentric granulomatosis are composed of necrotic granulomas surrounded by epithelioid histiocytes (Fig. 17). Superficially, the lesions may resemble those of Wegener's granulomatosis and the necrobiotic lesions of rheumatoid disease, tuberculosis, and other infectious processes. Careful examination usually reveals the bronchocentric nature of the process. The central necrotic portion of the lesion often

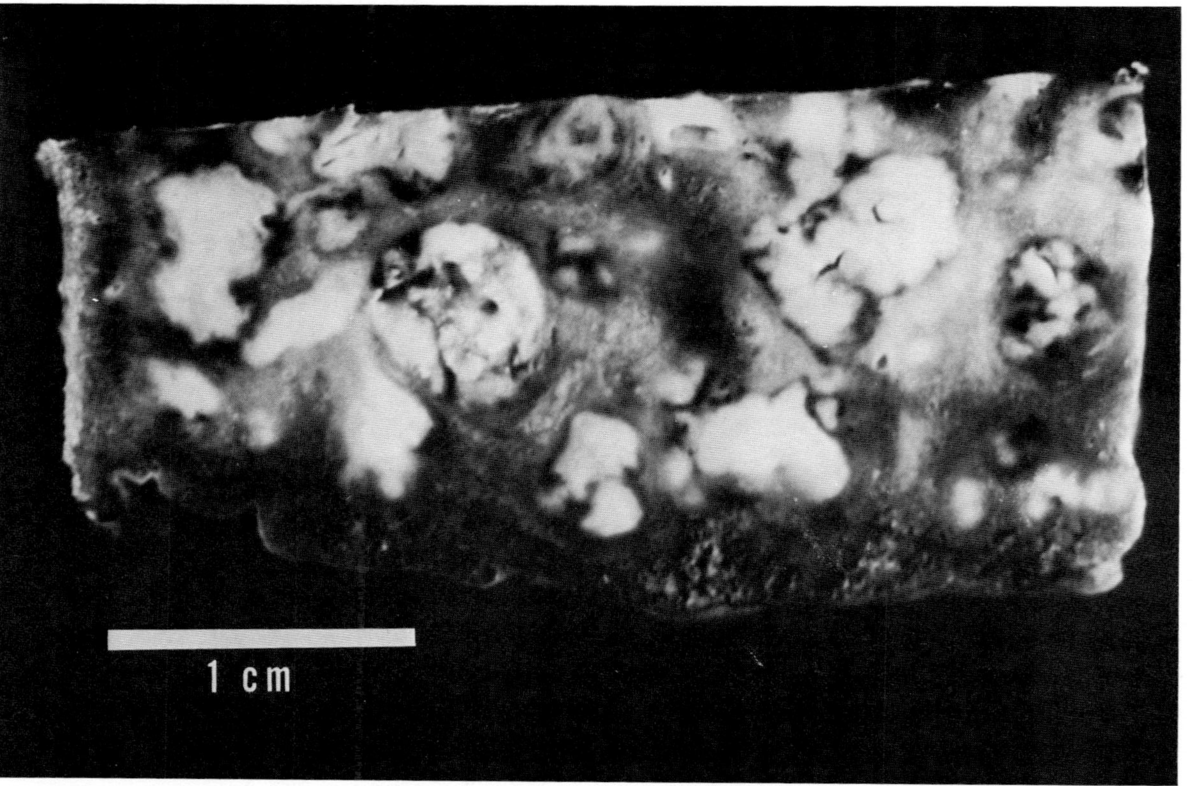

Figure 16 Bronchocentric granulomatosis; gross specimen of lung tissue revealing caseous-like material filling bronchi.

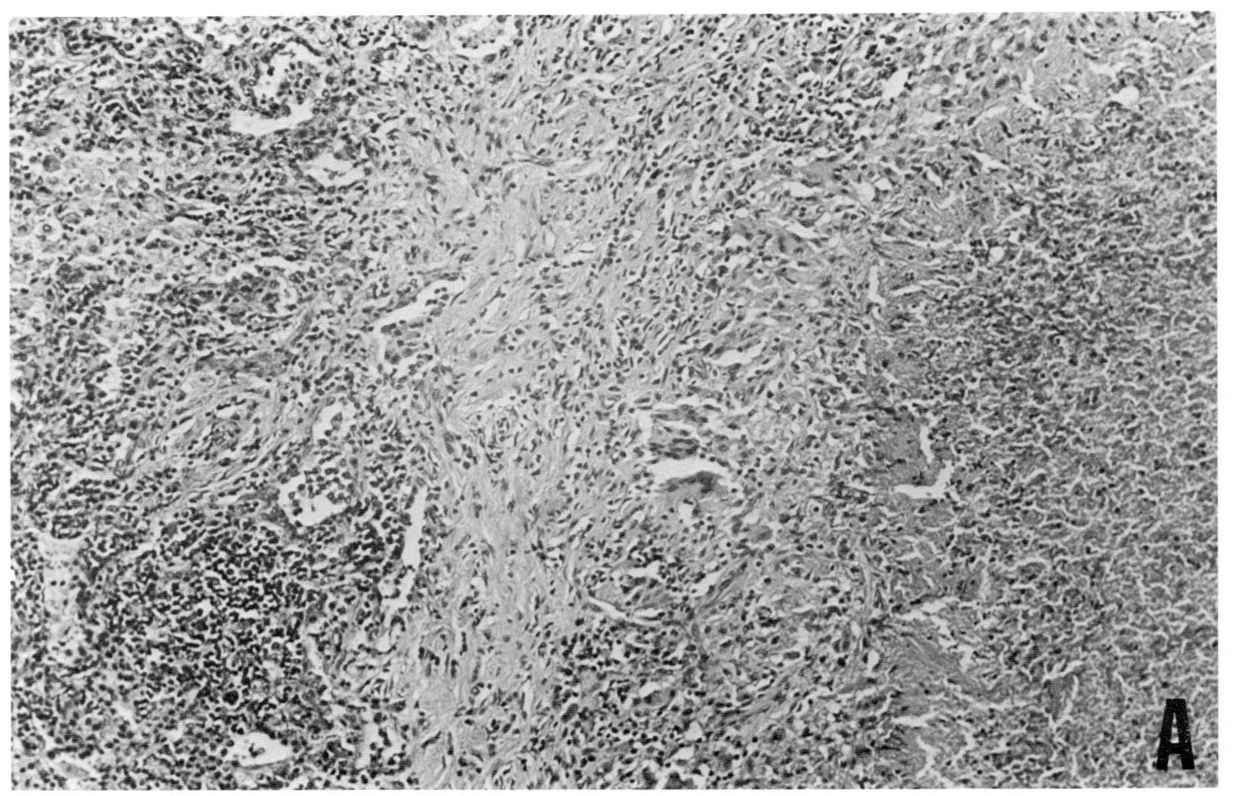

Figure 17 Bronchocentric granulomatosis: (A) Necrotic center of bronchus surrounded by palisading epithelioid histiocytes and giant cells. Chronic inflammatory infiltrates are peripherally located (H&E × 6.3). (B) Cartilagenous plates (arrows) of bronchi surrounded by chronic inflammatory infiltrates and undergoing resorption (H&E × 16).

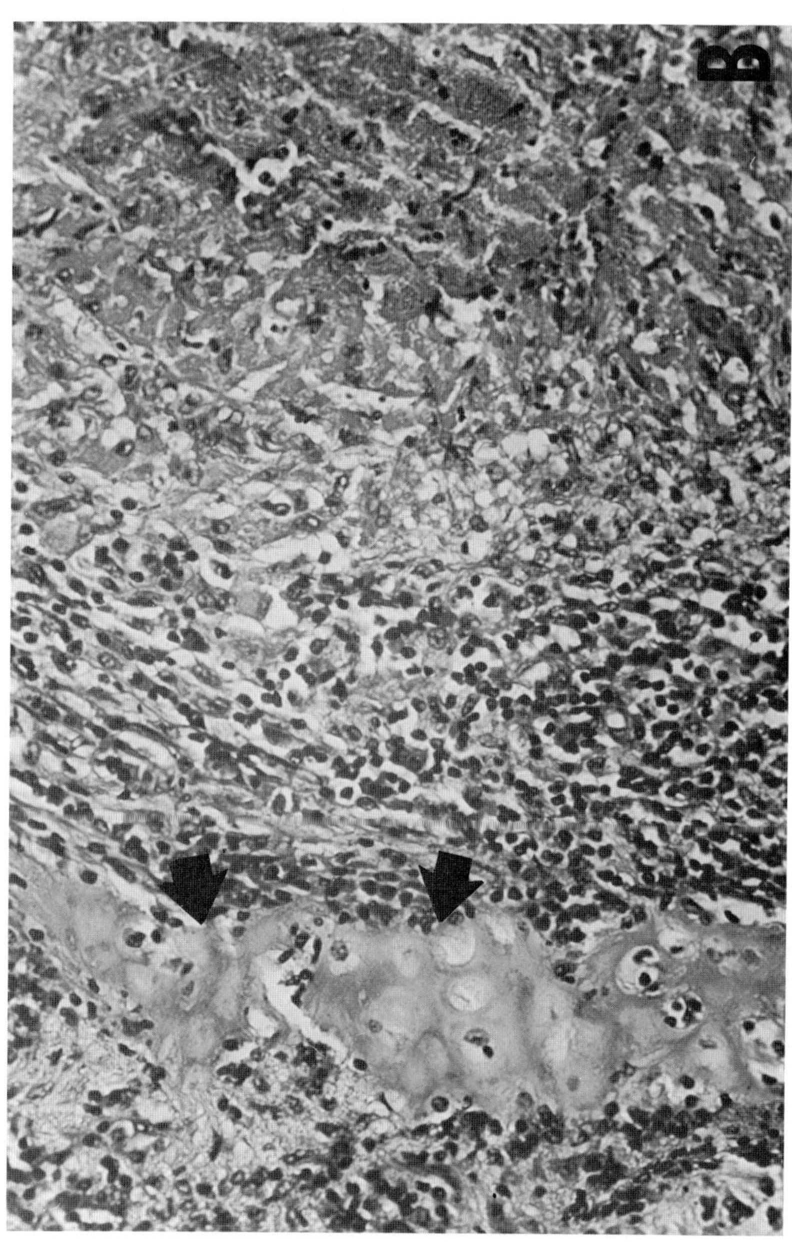

Figure 17 (Continued).

resembles the caseous necrosis of tuberculosis. In some cases the remnants
of eosinophils, neutrophils, and the ghost outline of other cells as well as
Charcot-Leydon crystals may be seen in the necrotic debris.

At the periphery of the necrotic areas, numerous epithelioid histiocytes
are arranged in a radial fashion around the necrotic center. These radially
arranged histiocytes are also seen in the Churg-Strauss granuloma of
pulmonary allergic granulomatosis and may occasionally be seen in
Wegener's granulomatosis. They are commonly seen in the pulmonary
necrobiotic lesions of rheumatoid disease. In addition to the epithelioid
histiocytes, giant cells of the Langhans' type may be present. Peripheral to
the epithelioid histiocytes are significant infiltrates of lymphocytes, plasma
cells, other histiocytes, and giant cells. Eosinophils in a few cases are
abundant, but more frequently are sparse. It is this latter inflammatory
process that may infiltrate adjacent blood vessels and simulate a vasculitis.

The inflammatory process in bronchocentric granulomatosis is not
associated with necrosis or destruction of the elastic lamina. The absence
of inflammation in those vessels not adjacent to a bronchus is of considerable diagnostic significance. The inflammatory infiltrates and granulomatous process may involve the cartilage of the bronchi. The cartilage
may show marked invasion by the inflammatory process with fragmentation,
destruction, and resorption of the cartilagenous plates (Fig. 17). Complete
destruction of the bronchi as well as the bronchioles by the necrotizing
process does occur.

In those cases in which histological landmarks have been destroyed,
the bronchocentric location may only be inferred by its location adjacent
to sizable pulmonary arteries. Special stains may, however, be of some help.
Elastic tissue stains may reveal the remains of elastic tissue in the bronchus,
and trichrome stains often reveal fragments of smooth muscle within
the inflammatory infiltrates of both bronchi and bronchioles. The degree
to which bronchi are involved is variable. While some bronchi are markedly
altered, other bronchi, usually larger bronchi, may show isolated necrotizing
granulomas within the wall of the bronchus. These too show central
necrosis and radially arranged epithelioid histiocytes. Occasional noncaseating, sarcoidlike granulomas in the walls of larger bronchi have been
reported (Katzenstein et al. 1975).

Special stains for organisms, including Gomori methenamine silver and
PAS stains, have revealed a few *Aspergillus* organisms in approximately
one-fourth of the reported cases of bronchocentric granulomatosis. This
finding is more common in patients with a history of asthma. Acid-fast and
other bacterial stains are usually negative. The resemblance of the process
to the necrobiotic lesions of rheumatoid disease may present a diagnostic
problem. Necrobiotic lesions are, however, not bronchocentric and are
not known to occur in the absence of rheumatoid disease or a strongly

positive rheumatoid factor. The lungs frequently exhibit obstructive pneumonia peripheral to the obstructed bronchi. This pneumonia is of the obstructive type and is characterized by foamy histiocytes filling the alveolar spaces. Spencer suggests that the long-term effect of the process is pulmonary fibrosis and peribronchial and periarterial fibrosis. There are few long-term follow-up studies on untreated cases of bronchocentric granulomatosis. Clinical studies indicate that some patients may undergo spontaneous resolution of the disease while others may respond promptly to corticosteroid therapy.

C. Etiology and Immunopathology

The pathogenesis of bronchocentric granulomatosis in asthmatic patients is likely related to hypersensitivity against *Aspergillus* fungal antigens. Allergic bronchopulmonary aspergillosis is a well-described complication of chronic asthma, particularly in Great Britain (Pepys and Simon 1973). This disease is caused by colonization of bronchial airways with *Aspergillus* with spores of the fungus diffusing through the bronchial wall and serving as antigens. The pathology is considered to be caused primarily by a combination of type I (anaphylactic) and type III (immune complex) immunologic reactions in lung (Johnson et al. 1979).

After inhalation of *Aspergillus* antigen, patients with allergic bronchopulmonary aspergillosis have an early, anaphylactic response with wheezing as well as a delayed response 4–6 hr later consisting of diffuse pulmonary infiltrates. Sera from these patients have elevated levels of IgE as well as precipitating antibodies to *Aspergillus* antigens. Immunofluorescent studies on lung tissue have shown peribronchial and interstitial deposition of IgG and IgM (Slavin et al. 1978). Histologically, there are many similarities between allergic bronchopulmonary aspergillosis and bronchocentric granulomatosis, and most investigators believe that bronchocentric granulomatosis in asthmatic patients is one manifestation of allergic bronchopulmonary aspergillosis (Katzenstein and Askin 1982).

The cause of bronchocentric granulomatosis in nonasthmatic patients is not known. Presumably, it is caused by the same type of hypersensitivity reaction seen in asthmatic patients, but the antigen or antigens responsible have not been identified.

IX. Comparative Features of Granulomatous Lung Diseases

It is clear from the descriptions given above that the final diagnosis of granulomatous lung disease represents the combination of clinical, pathologic, and radiographic findings. Depending on material obtained at

Table 1 A Comparison of the Usual Clinical, Radiological, and Pathological Features of the Seven Lung Granulomatous Diseases

Disease entity	Clinical features				X-ray appearance					Pulmonary pathology
	Cough, fever, dyspnea, chest pain	Asthma	Allergies	Peripheral eosinophilia	Nodular infiltrates	Diffuse infiltrates	Bilateral	Cavitation	Hilar adenopathy	Sarcoid granulomas
Sarcoid	++	0	0	0	++	+++	+++	0	+++	+++
Necrotizing sarcoid granulomatosis	+++	0	0	0	+++	++	+++	+	++	+++
Pulmonary allergic granulomatosis	+	+++	++	+++	+++	+++	++	0	+	++
Generalized Wegener's granulomatosis	+++	+	++	+	+++	+	+++	+++	+	+++
Limited Wegener's granulomatosis	+++	+	+	+	+++	++	+++	+++	+	+++
Lymphomatoid granulomatosis	+++	0	0	0	+++	+	+++	++	0	0
Bronchocentric granulomatosis	+++	+++	+++	++	++[c]	++[c]	++	++	0	+++

[a]Extensive necrosis is rare but microscopic necrosis is common.
[b]Lymphoreticular infiltrates are often histologically atypical.
[c]X-ray appearance is highly variable.
0 = never or not etiologically associated.
+ = uncommon.
++ = occasional.
+++ = frequent.

Table 1 (Continued)

| Pulmonary pathology | | | | | | Extrapulmonary involvement | | | | | | | |
| | | | | | | | Kidney | | | | | | |
Multinucleated giant cells	Granulomatous vasculitis	Extensive coagulative necrosis	Infarction necrosis	Lymphoreticular infiltrates	Tissue eosinophilia	Nasal sinuses	Glomerulonephritis	Vasculitis	Interstitial infiltrates	Skin	Central nervous system	Other organ systems	Prognosis
+++	+	+[a]	0	+	0	+	0	0	0	++	+	+++	1
+++	+++	+++	0	++	0	0	0	0	0	0	++	0	1
+++	+++	+++	0	++	+++	0	0	++	++	+++	0	+++	1
+++	+++	+++	+++	+++	+	+++	+++	+++	0	+++	+++	++	2
+++	+++	+++	+++	+++	0	0	0	++	0	+++	0	0	2
0	+++	+	+++	+++[b]	0	+	0	0	+++	+++	+++	+	3
+++	0	+++	0	+++	++	0	0	0	0	0	0	0	1

1. Spontaneous remission or good response to therapy.
2. Good response to therapy, poor prognosis without therapy.
3. Poor prognosis.

biopsy, it may not be possible to categorize definitively the findings into
what is an unequivocal diagnosis. This is particularly true for a disease
such as Wegener's granulomatosis. The data in Table 1 list the usual features
of each of the seven lung granulomatous diseases. The table emphasizes
the *usual* findings. In each individual clinical case, variations are found
when compared to comparison cases in the same diagnostic category.
However, consideration of the triad of data (clinical, pathological,
radiological) usually permits a reasonably definitive diagnosis that can
predict the clinical cause and response to therapy.

References

Azar, H. A., and Lunardelli, C. (1969). Collagen nature of asteroid bodies
of giant cells in sarcoidosis. *Am. J. Pathol.,* **57**:81–92.

Blatt, I. M., Holbrooke, S. S., Rubin, P., Furstenberg, A. C., Maxwell, J.
H., and Schull, W. J. (1959). Fatal granulomatosis of the respiratory
tract (lethal midline granuloma–Wegener's granulomatosis). *Arch.
Otolaryngol.,* **70**:707–757.

Breach, R. C., Corrin, B., Scopes, J. W., and Graham, E. (1980).
Necrotizing sarcoid granulomatosis with neurologic lesions in a child.
J. Pediatr., **97**:950–953.

Burkholder, P. M. (1974). *Atlas of Human Glomerular Pathology.*
Hagerstown, Maryland, Harper & Row, p. 366.

Campbell, P. B. (1977). Defective monocyte chemotaxis in sarcoidosis:
Possible relationship to a plasma factor. *Am. Rev. Respir. Dis.,*
116:251–259.

Carrington, C. B., and Liebow, A. A. (1966). Limited forms of angiitis
and granulomatosis of the Wegener's type. *Am. J. Med.,* **41**:497–527.

Carrington, C. B., Gaensler, E. A., Mikus, J. P., Schachter, A. W., Burke,
G. W., and Goff, A. M. (1976). Structure and function in sarcoidosis.
In *Proceedings of the VIIth International Conference on Sarcoidosis.*
Edited by L. E. Siltzback. *Ann. NY Acad. Sci.,* **278**:265–283.

Case Records of the Massachusetts General Hospital (Case 34). (1979).
N. Engl. J. Med., **301**:421–428.

Ceuppens, J., and Stevens, E. (1978). Immunological aspects of sarcoidosis.
Review. *Acta. Clinica Belgica.,* **33**(2):78–97.

Chumbley, L. C., Harrison, E. G., Jr., and DeRemee, R. A. (1977). Allergic
granulomatosis and angiitis (Churg-Strauss syndrome). Report and
analysis of 30 cases. *Mayo Clin. Proc.,* **52**:477–484.

Churg, J., and Strauss, L. (1951). Allergic granulomatosis, allergic angiitis,
and periarteritis nodosa. *Am. J. Pathol.,* **27**:277–301.

Churg, A., Carrington, C. B., and Gupta, R. (1979). Necrotizing sarcoid granulomatosis. *Chest,* **76**:406–412.

Chusid, E., and Siltzbach, E. (1974). Sarcoidosis of the pleura. *Ann. Intern. Med.,* **81**:190–194.

Cochrane, C. G. (1979). Immune-complex-mediated tissue injury. In *Mechanisms of Immunopathology.* Edited by S. Cohen, P. A. Ward, and R. T. McCluskey. New York, Wiley, pp. 29–48.

Cohen, M. L., Dawkins, R. L., Henderson, D. W., Sterrett, G. F., and Papadimitriou, J. M. (1979). Pulmonary lymphomatoid granulomatosis with immunodeficiency terminating as malignant lymphoma. *Pathology,* **11**:537–550.

Daniele, R. P., and Rawlands, D. F. (1976). Lymphocyte subpopulations in sarcoidosis: Correlation with disease activity and duration. *Ann. Intern. Med.,* **85**:593–600.

Daniele, R. P., McMillan, L. J., Dauber, J. H., and Rassman, M. D. (1978). Immune complexes in sarcoidosis. *Chest,* **74**:261–264.

DeRemee, R. A., McDonald, T. J., Harrison, E. G., Jr., and Coles, D. T. (1976). Wegener's granulomatosis. Anatomic correlates, a proposed classification. *Mayo Clin. Proc.,* **51**:777–781.

DeRemee, R. A., Weiland, L. H., and McDonald, T. J. (1980). Respiratory vasculitis. *Mayo Clin. Proc.,* **55**:492–498.

Dickens, C. H., and Winklemann, R. K. (1978). The Churg-Strauss granuloma. Cutaneous, necrotizing, palisading granuloma in vasculitis syndromes. *Arch. Pathol. Lab. Med.,* **102**:576–580.

Epstein, W. C. (1967). Granulomatous hypersensitivity. *Prog. Allergy,* **11**:36–88.

Fauci, A. S., and Wolff, S. M. (1973). Wegener's granulomatosis. Studies in eighteen patients and a review of the literature. *Medicine,* **52**:535–561.

Fauci, A. S., and Wolff, S. M. (1974). Immunological features of Wegener's granulomatosis. *Lancet,* **1**:688–689.

Fauci, A. S., Wolff, S. M., and Johnson, J. S. (1971). Effect of cyclophosphamide upon the immune response in Wegener's granulomatosis. *N. Engl. J. Med.,* **285**:1493–1496.

Fauci, A. S., Haynes, B. F., and Katz, P. (1978). The spectrum of vasculitis. Clinical, pathologic, immunologic, and therapeutic considerations. *Ann. Intern. Med.,* **89**:660–676.

Fraser, R. G., and Pare, J. A. P. (1979). *Diagnosis of Diseases of the Chest.* Volume III (2nd edition). Philadelphia, W. B. Saunders Company, p. 1665.

Ghase, T., Landrigan, P., and Asif, A. (1974). Localization of immunoglobulin and complement in pulmonary sarcoid granulomas. *Chest,* **66**:264–268.

Girard, J. P., Paupon, M. F., and Press, P. (1971). Culture of peripheral
    blood lymphocytes from sarcoidosis. Response to mitogenic factor.
    Int. Arch. Allergy, **41**:604–619.
Goddard, J. W. (1947). Granuloma in focal anaphylactic inflammation.
    Am. J. Pathol., **23**:943–965.
Godman, G. C., and Churg, J. (1954). Wegener's granulomatosis. Pathology
    and review of the literature. *Arch. Pathol.,* **58**:533–553.
Goldstein, R. A., Janicki, B. W., Mirro, J., and Faellmer, J. W. (1978).
    Cell mediated immune responses in sarcoidosis. *Am. Rev. Respir.
    Dis.,* **117**:55.
Greenberg, S. D., Gyorkey, F., Weg, J. G., Jenkins, D. E., and Gyorkey, P.
    (1970). The ultrastructure of the pulmonary granuloma in
    "sarcoidosis." *Am. Rev. Respir. Dis.,* **102**:648–652.
Gross, P. R. (1980). Lymphomatoid granulomatosis. *Cutis,* **25**:305–309.
Gupta, R. C., Keuppers, F., DeRemee, R. A., Huston, K. A., and McDuffie,
    F. C. (1977). Pulmonary and extrapulmonary sarcoidosis in relation
    to circulating immune complexes. *Am. Rev. Respir. Dis.,* **116**:
    261–266.
Hagerstand, I., and Linell, F. (1964). Epidemiology of sarcoidosis: The
    prevalence of sarcoid in the autopsy material from a Swedish town.
    Acta Med. Scand., **176**(425):171–174.
Hamilton, R., Petty, T. L., and Haiby, G. (1965). Cavitary sarcoidosis
    of the lung. *Arch. Intern. Med.,* **116**:428–430.
Hanson, G., Flod, N., Wells, I., Novey, H., and Galant, S. (1977).
    Bronchocentric granulomatosis: A complication of allergic broncho-
    pulmonary aspergillosis. *J. Allerg. Clin. Immunol.,* **59**:83–90.
Hedfors, E. (1975). Immunological aspects of sarcoidosis. *Scand. J.
    Respir. Dis.,* **56**:1–19.
Hedfors, E., Halm, G., and Petterson, D. (1974). Lymphocyte subpopula-
    tions in sarcoidosis. *Clin. Exp. Immunol.,* **17**:219–226.
Heptinstall, R. H. (1974). *Pathology of the Kidney,* Vol. II, 2nd ed.
    Boston, Little, Brown, pp. 621–622.
Howell, S. B., and Epstein, W. V. (1976). Circulating immunoglobulin
    complexes in Wegener's granulomatosis. *Am. J. Med.,* **60**:259–268.
Hunninghake, G. W., and Crystal, R. G. (1981). Mechanisms of hyper-
    gammaglobulinemia in pulmonary sarcoidosis. *J. Clin. Invest.,*
    67:86–91.
Hunninghake, G. W., Fulmer, J. D., Young, R. C., Jr., Gadek, J. E., and
    Crystal, R. G. (1979). Localization of the immune response in
    sarcoidosis. *Am. Rev. Respir. Dis.,* **120**:49–57.
Hunninghake, G. W., Gadek, J. E., Young, R. C., Kawanami, O., Ferrans,
    V. J., and Crystal, R. (1980). Maintenance of granuloma formation
    in pulmonary sarcoidosis by T lymphocytes within the lung. *N.
    Engl. J. Med.,* **302**(11):594–598.

Israel, H. L., and Patchefsky, A. S. (1971). Wegener's granulomatosis of lung. Diagnosis and treatment, experience with 12 cases. *Ann. Intern. Med.*, **74**:881–891.

Israel, H. L., Patchefsky, A. S., and Saldana, M. J. (1977). Wegener's granulomatosis, lymphomatoid granulomatosis and benign lymphocytic angiitis and granulomatosis of lung. Recognition and treatment. *Ann. Intern. Med.*, **87**:691–699.

James, D. G., Neville, E., and Walker, A. (1975). Immunology of sarcoidosis. *Am. J. Med.*, **59**:388–394.

Johnson, K. J., Ward, P. A., and Chapman, W. E. (1979). Immuno-pathology of the lung. A review. *Am. J. Pathol.*, **95**:795–844.

Johnson, K. J., Ward, P. A., Striker, G. S., and Kunkel, R. (1980). A study of the origin of pulmonary macrophages using the Chediak-Higashi marker. *Am. J. Pathol.*, **101**:365–374.

Jones, W., Williams, W., and Williams, D. (1967). "Residual bodies" in sarcoid and sarcoid-like granulomas. *J. Clin. Pathol.*, **20**:574–577.

Kantor, F. S., Dwyer, J. M., and Mangi, R. J. (1976). Sarcoid. *J. Invest. Dermatol.*, **67**:470–476.

Katz, P., and Fauci, A. S. (1978). Inhibition of polyclonal B-cell activation by suppressor monocytes by patients with sarcoidosis. *Clin. Exp. Immunol.*, **32**:554–562.

Katzenstein, A. L., Liebow, A. A., and Friedman, P. J. (1975). Broncho-centric granulomatosis, mucoid impaction and hypersensitivity to fungi. *Am. Rev. Respir. Dis.*, **111**:497–537.

Katzenstein, A. A., Carrington, C. B., and Liebow, A. A. (1979). Lymphomatoid granulomatosis. A clinicopathologic study of 152 cases. *Cancer*, **43**:360–373.

Katzenstein, A. A., and Askin, F. B. (1982). *Surgical Pathology of Non-Neoplastic Lung Disease.* Philadelphia, W. B. Saunders Company, p. 197.

Kay, S., Fu, Y., Minars, N., and Brady, J. W. (1974). Lymphomatoid granulomatosis of the skin. Light microscopic and ultrastructure studies. *Cancer*, **34**:1675–1682.

Klinger, H. (1931). Grenzformen der periarteritis nodosa. *Frankfurt Z. Pathol.*, **42**:455–480.

Koontz, C. H., Joyner, L. R., and Nelson, R. A. (1976). Transbronchial lung biopsy via the fiberoptic bronchoscope in sarcoidosis. *Ann. Intern. Med.*, **85**:64–66.

Koss, M. N., Hochholzer, L., Feigin, D. S., Garancis, J. C., and Ward, P. A. (1980). Necrotizing sarcoid-like granulomatosis. Clinical, pathologic and immunologic finding. *Hum. Pathol.*, **11**:510–515.

Leake, E. S., and Myrvik, Q. N. (1972). Osmiophilic structures in granuloma-tous macrophages and the problem of intracellular mycobacteria. *Am. Rev. Respir. Dis.*, **104**:132–133.

Liebow, A. A. (1973). The J. Burns Anderson Lecture: Pulmonary angiitis and granulomatosis. *Am. Rev. Resp. Dis.,* **108**:1–18.

Liebow, A. A., Carrington, C. B., and Friedman, P. J. (1972). Lymphomatoid granulomatosis. *Hum. Pathol.,* **3**:457–558.

Maderazo, E. G., Ward, P. A., Waronick, C. L., Kubik, J., and DeGraff, A. C., Jr. (1976). Leukotactic dysfunction in sarcoidosis. *Ann. Intern. Med.,* **84**:414–419.

Mallory, T. B. (1948). The pathology of pulmonary fibrosis, including pulmonary sarcoidosis. *Radiology,* **51**:468–476.

Maxwell, J. H., Schull, W. J., Blatt, I. M., Seltzer, H. H., Robin, P., and Furstenberg, A. C. (1959). Fatal granulomatosis of the respiratory tract (lethal midline granuloma-Wegener's granulomatosis). *Arch. Otolaryngol.,* **70**:707–757.

McCort, J. J., and Pare, J. A. P. (1954). Pulmonary fibrosis and cor pulmonale in sarcoidosis. *Radiology,* **62**:496–504.

McGregor, M. B. B., and Sandler, G. (1964). Wegener's granulomatosis. A clinical and radiological survey. *Br. J. Radiol.,* **37**:430–439.

McLoud, T. C., Putman, C. E., and Pascual, R. (1974). Eggshell calcification with systemic sarcoidosis. *Chest,* **66**:515–517.

Ohsaki, Y., Abe, S., Yahara, O., and Murao, M. (1977). Bilateral hilar adenopathy and cystic lung lesion. *Chest,* **71**:81–82.

Olsen, K. D., Carpenter, R. J., III, Deremee, R. A., Weiland, L. H. (1980). Nasal manifestations of allergic granulomatous and angiitis (Churg-Strauss syndrome). *Otolaryngol Head Neck Surg.,* **88**(1):85–89.

Oreskes, I., and Siltzbach, L. E. (1968). Changes in rheumatoid factor

Papadimitriou, J. M., and Spector, W. G. (1971). The origin, properties and fate of epithelioid cells. *J. Pathol.,* **105**:187–203.

Pena, C. E. (1977). Lymphomatoid granulomatosis with cerebral involvement. Light and electron microscopic study of a case. *Acta Neuropathol.,* **37**:193–197.

Pepys, J., and Simon, G. (1973). Asthma, pulmonary eosinophilia, and allergic alveolitis. *Med. Clin. North Am.,* **57**:573–591.

Quismorio, P. P., Jr., Sharma, O. P., and Chandor, S. (1977). Immunopathological studies on the cutaneous lesions in sarcoidosis. *Br. J. Dermatol.,* **97**:635–642.

Rabinowitz, J. G., Ulreich, S., and Soriano, C. (1974). The usual unusual manifestations of sarcoidosis in the "hilar-haze." A new diagnostic aid. *Am. J. Roentgenol.,* **120**:821–831.

Reddic, R. L., Fauci, A. S., Valsamis, M. P., and Mann, R. B. (1978). Immunoblastic sarcoma of the central nervous system in a patient with lymphomatoid granulomatosis. *Cancer,* **42**:652–659.

Roback, S. A., Herdman, R. D., Hoyer, J., and Good, R. A. (1969). Wegener's granulomatosis in a child. *Am. J. Dis. Child.,* **118**:608–614.

Rose, G. A., and Spencer, H. (1957). Polyarteritis nodosa. *Q. J. Med.,* **50**:43–82.

Rosen, Y., Moon, S., Huang, C. T., Gowin, C., and Lyons, H. A. (1977). Granulomatous pulmonary angiitis in sarcoidosis. *Arch. Pathol. Lab. Med.,* **101**:170–174.

Rosen, Y., Vuletin, J. C., Perschunk, L. P., and Silverstein, E. (1979). Sarcoidosis from the pathologist's vantage point. *Pathol. Annual,* **14**(1):405–439.

Saldana, M. J. (1978). Necrotizing sarcoid granulomatosis. Clinico-pathologic observations in 24 patients. *Lab. Invest.,* **38**:34 (abstract).

Saldana, M. J., Patchefsky, A. S., Israel, H. I., and Atkinson, G. W. (1977). Pulmonary angiitis and granulomatosis. The relationship between histological features, organ involvement, and response to treatment. *Hum. Pathol.,* **8**:391–409.

Shillitoe, E. J., Lehner, T., Lessof, M. H., and Harrison, D. F. N. (1974). Immunological features of Wegener's granulomatosis. *Lancet,* **1**:281–284.

Siltzbach, L. E. (1964). Significance and specificity of the Kveim reaction. *Acta Med. Scand. (Suppl.),* **425**:74–78.

Siltzbach, L. E. (1965). Editorial: Current thoughts on the epidermiology and etiology of sarcoidosis. *Am. J. Med.,* **39**:361–368.

Siltzbach, L. E., James, D. G., Neville, E., Turiaf, J., Battesti, J. P., Sharma, O. P., Husoda, Y., Mikami, R., and Odaka, M. (1974). Course and prognosis of sarcoidosis around the world. *Amer. J. Med.,* **57**:847–852.

Singh, N., Cole, S., Krause, P. J., Conway, M., and Garcia, L. (1981). Necrotizing sarcoidal angiitis with extrapulmonary involvement. Clinical, pathologic, ultrastructural and immunologic features. *Am. Rev. Respir. Dis.,* **124**:189–192.

Slavin, R. G., Fischer, V. W., Levine, E. A., Tsai, C. C., and Winzenberger, P. (1978). A primate model of allergic bronchopulmonary aspergillosis. *Int. Arch. Allergy Appl. Immunol.,* **56**:325–333.

Sokolov, R. A., Rachmaninoff, R., and Kaine, H. D. (1962). Allergic granulomatosis. *Am. J. Med.,* **32**:131–141.

Soler, P., Basset, F., Bernaudin, J. F., and Chretien, J. (1976). Morphology and distribution of the cells of a sarcoid granuloma: Ultrastructural study of serial sections. In *Proceedings of the VIIth International Conference on Sarcoidosis.* Edited by L. E. Siltzbach. *Ann. NY Acad. Sci.,* **278**:147–160.

Sones, M., and Israel, H. L. (1960). Course and prognosis of sarcoidosis. *Am. J. Med.,* **29**:84–93.

Spector, W. G. (1976). Epithelioid cells, giant cells and sarcoidosis. In *Proceedings of the VIIth International Conference on Sarcoidosis.* Edited by L. E. Siltzbach. *Ann. NY Acad. Sci.,* **278**:3–6.

Spector, W. G., and Hessom, N. (1969). The production of granulomata by antigen-antibody complexes. *J. Pathol.,* **98**:31–39.

Spencer, H. (1977). *The Lung.* Philadelphia, W. B. Saunders Company, p. 765.

Strauss, L., Churg, J., and Zak, F. G. (1951). Cutaneous lesions of allergic granulomatosis. A histopathologic study. *J. Invest. Dermatol.,* **17**:343–359.

Tellis, C. J., and Putnam, J. S. (1977). Cavitation in large multinodular pulmonary disease: A rare manifestation of sarcoidosis. *Chest,* **71**:692–793.

Topilsky, M., Siltzback, L. E., Williams, M., and Glade, P. R. (1972). Lymphocyte response in sarcoidosis. *Lancet,* **1**:117–120.

Townley, R. C., Martin, J. C., and Souders, D. R. (1962). Wegener's granulomatosis. *Am. Rev. Respir. Dis.,* **85**:576–582.

Uelinger, E. (1964). The sarcoid tissue reaction: The origin and significance of inclusion bodies. Differential diagnosis with particular delineation from tuberculosis. *Acta Med. Scand.,* **176**(425):7–13.

Verity, M. A., and Wolfson, W. L. (1976). Cerebral lymphomatoid granulomatosis. A report of two cases, with disseminated necrotizing leukoencephalopathy in one. *Acta Neuropathol.,* **36**:117–124.

Vuletin, J. C., and Rosen, Y. (1977). Nature of pseudo-fungal budding structures (Hamazaki-Wessenberg) bodies and asteroid bodies in sarcoidosis. *Am. J. Clin. Pathol.,* **68**:99 (abstract).

Walton, E. W. (1958). Giant-cell granulomatosis of the respiratory tract (Wegener's granulomatosis). *Br. Med. J.,* **2**:265–270.

Wegener, F. (1936). Uber generalisierte, septische Gefasserkrankungen. *Verh. Dtsch. Ges. Pathol.,* **29**:202–210.

Wegener, F. (1939). Uber eine eigenartige rhinogene Granulomatose mit besonderer Beteiligung des Arteriensystems und der Nieren. *Beitr. Pathol.,* **102**:36–68.

Wolff, S. M., Fauci, A. S., Horn, R. G., and Dale, D. C. (1974). Wegener's granulomatosis. *Ann. Intern. Med.,* **81**:513–525.

Yoshida, T., and Cohen, S. (1974). Lymphokine activity in vivo in relation to circulating monocyte levels and delayed skin reactivity. *J. Immunol.,* **112**:1540–1547.

Yoshida, T., Siltzbach, L. E., Masih, N., and Cohen, S. (1979). Serum-migration inhibitory activity in patients with sarcoidosis. *Clin. Immunol. Immunopathol.,* **13**:39–46.

Part Four

CELLULAR AND HUMORAL IMMUNITY ASSOCIATED WITH SARCOIDOSIS

7

Cell-Mediated Immunity in Sarcoidosis

ROSS E. ROCKLIN

New England Medical Center
Tufts University School of Medicine
Boston, Massachusetts

I. Introduction

Cell-mediated immunity is a term used to describe a type of immunological
response that is mediated by specifically sensitized thymus-derived lymphocytes (T lymphocytes). T lymphocytes have been shown to play a central
role in such clinically significant reactions as resistance to infection by a
variety of facultative intracellular microorganisms, allograft rejection, graft
vs. host disease, and destruction of neoplastic cells (Table 1). Cutaneous
delayed hypersensitivity, which is exemplified by the 24–48 hr cutaneous
inflammatory response resulting from the intradermal injection of antigen
in an appropriately sensitized host, may be thought of as a peripheral
manifestation of cell-mediated immunity. The cellular components involved
in this response include subclasses of T cells, macrophages, and cytotoxic
"killer" cells. In addition, there are subclasses of T cells that are
responsible for regulating both antibody production and various aspects of
the cellular-immune process.

As a prelude to reviewing known information about cell-mediated
immunity in sarcoidosis, this chapter will focus first on the general
mechanisms involved in the various expressions of cellular immunity, the

Table 1 Functions of T Lymphocytes

In vivo function	In vitro correlate
1. Cutaneous delayed hypersensitivity	Lymphokine production
2. Allograft rejection	Cytotoxicity of allogenic target cells
3. Resistance to infections (bacterial, viral, fungal)	Macrophage activation by lymphokines; cytotoxicity of viral-infected cells
4. Tumor surveillance	Cytotoxicity of tumor cells by T cells and NK cells
5. Helper function	Effect on antibody synthesis
6. Suppressor function	Regulation of antibody synthesis and other functions of cell-mediated immunity (lymphokines, proliferation, cytotoxicity)

differentiative history and function of T cells, and the biochemical basis for this responses. This information will then be applied to our current knowledge of cellular-immune function in patients with sarcoidosis. The reader is referred to additional sources for further information about cell-mediated immunity in general (Benacerraf 1976, Cantor and Boyse 1977, Moller 1974, Nelson 1976, Rheinherz and Schlossman 1980, Shearer and Schmitt-Verhulst 1977, Turk 1975).

II. Lymphocytes

A. Differentiation of T Cells

T lymphocytes are derived from the thymus gland, the only primary lymphoid organ in mammals. The thymus consists predominantly of lymphocytes, reticular cells, and macrophages. It is organized into lobules, each composed of a cortex and medulla. The cortex contains a dense accumulation of lymphocytes, whereas the medulla consists primarily of reticular cells in high concentration. Lymphocytes destined to differentiate within the thymus are derived during embryonic life from stem cells, located predominantly in the fetal liver and bone marrow. The mechanisms by which stem cells in the bone marrow become genetically programmed to migrate to and differentiate within the thymus gland are unknown. It is known, however, that during their stay in the thymus, a number of discrete differentiation steps occur which culminate in the elaboration from the thymus of fully mature and functionally competent T lymphocytes.

During their differentiation within the thymus gland, T cells acquire distinct alloantigens on their surface which distinguish them from both prethymic T cells and from T cells that eventually populate the peripheral lymphoid organs. For example, there is a surface antigen that is present only on thymocytes (TL) and not on peripheral T cells or bone marrow cells. In acute lymphatic leukemia of childhood, approximately 20% of patients have blast cells bearing this unique antigen. In addition, differentiating T cells also acquire cell surface markers that are subsequently found on all mature T cells. In the mouse, this T-cell marker is called theta, and similar antigens (T) have been identified on human thymocytes and T cells. Human T cells also acquire receptors to bind with sheep red blood cells (E). In addition to the alloantigens and E receptors acquired during differentiation, T cells also acquire other antigens on their surfaces that are found on thymocytes and are preserved during further differentiation only on sublcasses of peripheral T lymphocytes. At present, these alloantigens may be found on one subset of peripheral T cells but not on others, and therefore have been utilized as a means of functionally defining unique subclasses of peripheral T cells.

T lymphocytes also acquire the capacity to recognize self-antigens related to the major histocompatibility complex (MHC) and to distinguish them from nonself MHC determinants while in the thymus. During later stages of differentiation, this process becomes critical to many of the important functions ascribed to T lymphocytes. The precise mechanisms of differentiation of T cells within the thymus is unknown. However, there is substantial evidence suggesting that hormones (thymosin, thymopoietin) synthesized and secreted from reticular and epithelial cells within the thymus play an important role in this differentiation process.

Following their exodus from the thymus, immunocompetent T lymphocytes emigrate to other central lymphoid organs including lymph nodes and spleen. In addition, T cells recirculate from blood to lymph, and a number of these recirculating cells are designated memory cells. That is, they are capable of being stimulated years later following an immunologic experience, retain the "memory" of that past encounter, and respond to a subsequent exposure to that particular antigen. Each antigenic exposure serves to enlarge the pool of circulating memory cells capable of reacting to a given antigen.

B. T-Cell Diversity

Cells undergoing thymus-dependent differentiation mediate a wide range of immunologic activities. Until recently, these diverse functions of T cells have been attributed to a single pluripotent mature T cell. It has become apparent that T cells become "programmed" during differentiation to

express not all but only a limited range of functions. For example,
distinct subclasses of T cells express either helper activity or suppressor
function, but not both. Furthermore, T-cell subclasses destined to release
lymphokines are distinct from T cells that express killer cell activity. In
addition to their distinct functions, lymphocyte subclasses are also
identified by specific surface antigens present on the plasma membrane.
Cells capable of expressing helper activity possess surface antigens that are
distinct from those cells capable of functioning as suppressor or cytotoxic
lymphocytes.

Through the use of heteroantisera capable of detecting these unique
antigens, detailed studies of cellular interactions occurring between the
various T-cell subsets have been realized. At least four separate subclasses
of mouse T lymphocytes have been identified on the basis of three antigens
designated Ly 1, Ly 2, and Ly 3.

One subclass, the thymocyte, expresses all three distinct lymphocyte
differentiation antigens (Ly 1,2,3) on its surface as well as the TL and theta
antigens. This subclass of thymocytes is found almost exclusively in the
cortex of the thymus and is not found in the peripheral lymphoid tissue.
It is therefore considered to be an immature cell and probably the precursor
of all T lymphocytes.

A second subclass of T lymphocytes expresses all Ly antigens (Ly 1,
2,3), but during differentiation it has lost the TL antigen. This Ly 1,2,3
cell is the most abundant peripheral T cell, comprising about 50% of the
circulating T cells in the blood. During early neonatal existence, two
additional T-cell subclasses appear. One cell expresses exclusively the Ly 1
antigen while the other expresses the Ly 2 and Ly 3 antigens. The latter
cells comprise about 30% and 10%, respectively, of the remaining T
cells in the blood.

The Ly 1 T cell has been found to have the following functions:
(1) It is the helper cell for T-cell–B-cell interactions. (2) It proliferates in
response to allogenic stimuli. (3) It produces delayed-type hypersensitivity
reactions including the production of lymphokines. (4) It can collaborate
with certain other T cells resulting in the induction of cytotoxic lymphocytes
(Ly 2,3). The Ly 2,3 cell type has none of the functions attributed to
Ly 1 cells but is programmed to suppress both antibody and cell-mediated
immune responses as well as to mediate specific killer cell activity. The
precise function of Ly 1,2,3 T lymphocytes is unknown, but it has been
documented that these cells can be triggered by certain stimuli to further
differentiate into more mature Ly 1 or Ly 2,3 T cells. Similar kinds of
unique differentiation antigens and functional diversity have been found
with human T lymphocyte subclasses.

III. Delayed Hypersensitivity Reactions

A. General

Beginning 6–8 hr following the intradermal injection of antigen into an
appropriately sensitized host, one can detect an inflammatory response
characterized by erythema and induration. The erythema is caused by
increased vasodilatation accompanied by changes in vascular permeability.
The induration was formally thought to be caused by the cellular infiltrate,
but more recent evidence indicates that it is due to deposition of fibrin in
the lesion. The tissue changes become maximal by 24–48 hr after injection
and then gradually subside.

In addition to tissue changes, fever and localized lymphadenopathy
may accompany delayed hypersensitivity reactions. The onset of fever is
delayed 5–6 hr after injection of antigen into sensitized individuals and is
probably the result of the release of endogenous leukocyte pyrogen. Aside
from the contribution made by mononuclear cells, an inflammatory response
involving various components is also necessary for this reaction to take
place.

B. Histology

In a mild to moderate delayed hypersensitivity reaction, the earliest cellular
infiltrate consists of basophils, followed by neutrophils, and finally, mononuclear cells around the postcapillary venules. The mononuclear cells
consist of small to medium-sized lymphocytes and monocytes which appear
at 5–6 hr and reach a maximum number at 18–48 hr. At the time of
maximum reaction, the entire dermis is involved and mononuclear cells may
also be found in the epidermis. Necrosis of small blood vessels, muscle,
and connective tissue, as well as areas in the epidermis may occur to
varying degrees. The mononuclear cells in delayed hypersensitivity reactions
are primarily derived from the circulation. Over half of the cells have
characteristics of monocytes and the remainder are lymphocytes. Most of
the circulating mononuclear cells originate in bone marrow, although a few
may be derived from lymph nodes.

C. Cutaneous Basophil Hypersensitivity Reaction

The Jones-Mote or cutaneous basophil hypersensitivity reaction is a form
of delayed hypersensitivity associated with large numbers of infiltrating
basophils. Sensitization for this type of hypersensitivity may be induced
by antigen contained in incomplete Freund's adjuvant, with antigen-

antibody complexes or with very small amounts of antigen. This form of hypersensitivity is transient, lasting only 2–4 weeks. Upon reexposure to antigen, inflammation is maximal at 24 hr and tends to be more erythematous and less indurated than the typical delayed hypersensitivity lesion.

Histologically, approximately 50–70% of the cellular infiltrate is composed of basophils, the remainder being lymphocytes. In a typical tuberculin delayed hypersensitivity response, there are between 2–30% basophils in the cellular infiltrate. The role of the basophil in these reactions is unknown, but it is of interest that these cells accumulate at sites of tumor and allograft rejection as well.

D. Factors in the Development of Delayed Hypersensitivity

A number of factors determine whether or not sensitivity to a given protein antigen will develop. These include the chemical nature of the antigen itself, the route of administration, the presentation of antigen on the surface of living cells, the total dose administered, and the modification of antigen by complexing with antibody, combination with simple chemicals, and denaturation. The intradermal administration of antigen is far more effective than subcutaneous, intramuscular, or intravenous routes in inducing delayed hypersensitivity. The reasons why sensitization develops by one route and not by another are incompletely understood but may involve bypass of macrophage processing of antigen.

This brings up a relatively new concept of compartmentalization of T lymphocytes and macrophages. They may be functionally divided into peripheral and central compartments with the former containing macrophages that are capable of processing and presenting antigen to immunocompetent T cells. The central compartment contains suppressor cells. If antigen is injected intradermally or intraperitoneally, antigen processing by macrophages occurs and a delayed hypersensitivity and/or antibody response results. By other routes of administration, the peripheral compartment may be bypassed and suppressor cells preferentially activated, resulting in a diminished or absent response.

Sensitization most readily occurs to antigens on the surface of living cells. Therefore, sensitivity to tuberculin is elicited most strongly by living tubercule bacilli, less strongly by dead tubercule bacilli, and not at all by tubercular protein alone. The dose and chemical nature of the antigen are more effective in inducing delayed hypersensitivity than are large concentrations of antigen, which are more likely to induce antibody formation. Sensitization may also occur with small haptens such as dinitrochlorobenzene which have been complexed to peptides or proteins. For small haptens, a minimal size of complexing peptide is necessary for sensitization.

If haptens are complexed to smaller peptides, delayed hypersensitivity is not elicited. Also, the antigen to which sensitization may occur appears to include not only the hapten, but also part of the protein carrier as well.

Although, in general, carbohydrates by themselves elicit antibody responses and not delayed hypersensitivity, polysaccharides attached to proteins or peptides are capable of inducing delayed sensitivity. The development of sensitivity to various antigens is greatly improved by the use of adjuvants such as Freund's complete adjuvant (a water and oil emulsion containing killed mycobacteria). Many simple proteins, which by themselves are weak sensitizers, readily induce delayed hypersensitivity when combined with adjuvant.

E. Relationship of Delayed Hypersensitivity and Cell-Mediated Immunity

Cutaneous delayed hypersensitivity may be thought of as an in vivo model to study certain cell-mediated immune reactions. Cutaneous delayed hypersensitivity responses to certain specific antigens often reflect the host's cellular immune status or resistance to that antigen. For example, the cutaneous delayed hypersensitivity response of mice to killed microorganisms such as *Listeria monocytogenes* parallels the development of immunity to virulent strains of this bacterium. However, some studies in guinea pigs that were sensitized to extracts of *Mycobacterium tuberculosis* were subsequently shown to produce delayed hypersensitivity reactions to intradermal challenge with tuberculin but were not resistant to challenge with viable mycobacterium. In some human diseases, for example in patients with chronic mucocutaneous candidiasis, there is a marked susceptibility to candida infections even though cutaneous delayed hypersensitivity responses to candida antigens may be intact. Thus, cutaneous delayed hypersensitivity may not always reflect the actual state of immunity relative to host resistance. Nevertheless, there is considerable evidence that the cellular mechanisms underlying both delayed hypersensitivity and cell-mediated immunity are identical, and delayed hypersensitivity as such provides an invaluable tool for the study of the cellular basis of this reaction. In addition, the measurement of cutaneous delayed hypersensitivity is of great value clinically in the assessment of cell-mediated immune function as discussed below.

F. Molecular Basis for the Expression of Delayed Hypersensitivity/Cell-Mediated Immunity

As mentioned previously, the delayed hypersensitivity reaction is characterized by a tissue infiltration of mononuclear cells. The stimulus for these cells to accumulate at the reaction site is still not clearly understood but may involve a series of events initiated by soluble substances called lymphokines released by activated lymphocytes. When specifically sensitized lymphocytes are stimulated in vitro by antigen, they release a number of biologically active substances with effects on numerous inflammatory cells including macrophages, granulocytes, and a variety of other target cells. A partial list of these nonantibody lymphokines is shown in Table 2.

The small number of specifically sensitized lymphocytes responding to any given antigen elaborate chemotactic factors which recruit macrophages and other cell types to the site of the reaction. Once brought to the site of reaction, their surface properties and migration pattern is altered such that they remain at the site. Lymphokines such as the macrophage migration inhibitory factor (MIF) and leukocyte inhibitory factor (LIF)

Table 2 Lymphocyte Mediators (Lymphokines)

A. Mediators affecting macrophages
1. Migration inhibitory factor (MIF)
2. Macrophage activating factor (MAF)
3. Chemotactic factors for macrophages
4. Antigen-dependent MIF

B. Mediators affecting PMN leukocytes
1. Chemotactic factors
2. Leukocyte inhibitory factor (LIF)
3. Eosinophil stimulation promoter (ESP)
4. Histamine releasing factor

C. Mediators affecting lymphocytes
1. Mitogenic factors (interleukin-2)
2. Factors enhancing antibody formation (antigen-dependent and antigen-independent)
3. Factors suppressing antibody formation (antigen-dependent and antigen-independent)

D. Mediators affecting other cells
1. Cytotoxic factors–lymphotoxin (LT)
2. Growth inhibitory factors (? same as LT)
3. Osteoclastic factor (OAF)
4. Collagen-producing factor
5. Colony-stimulating factor
6. Interferon

E. Immunoglobulin-binding factor (IBF)

F. Procoagulant (tissue factor)

may serve such a purpose. These factors may also be involved in enhancing the function of the inflammatory cells so that they are more active metabolically and able to phagocytize and kill microorganisms or tumor cells.

This reaction may be amplified by mitogenic or growth factors that nonspecifically activate other lymphocytes so that these cells may produce more lymphokines. In addition, the lymphokines that activate monocytes/ macrophages (macrophage activating factor) result in the elaboration from these cells of soluble factors (monokines) that may further stimulate lymphocytes such that a positive feedback cycle is established. However, the reaction usually subsides because the supply of antigen becomes exhausted and/or the lymphokines/monokines become inactivated by regulatory proteins.

IV. Cell-Mediated Cytotoxicity

A. General

Another important role of cell-mediated immune reactions is to be able to recognize foreign or altered antigenic determinants on the surface of cells; as a consequence of this recognition effector mechanisms are generated that result in destruction of the foreign or "altered" cell. In addition to direct antibody and complement-mediated cellular destruction, lymphoid cells may utilize a variety of mechanisms to destroy foreign target cells. These mechanisms require intimate contact between two cells, a cell that can be damaged (the target cell) and a cell that is capable of administering such damage (the effector cell). Cell-mediated cytotoxic reactions are important in the rejection of allografts, destruction of autologous tissue that is infected by viruses, rejection of tumor cells, and in some autoimmune phenomena.

B. Types of Cytotoxic Reations

At least four types of cellular cytolytic effector mechanisms have been clearly delineated. In one, T lymphocytes are triggered by antigens on the surface of foreign cells to proliferate and differentiate into killer cells, which then have the capacity to lyse target cells bearing surface determinants in common with the sensitizing cell. In another, macrophages are activated by factors released from T lymphocytes (macrophage activating factor) to destroy foreign tissues. Unlike cytotoxic T lymphocytes, however, activated macrophages lyse cells nonspecifically. That is, once activated, macrophages will kill a variety of cell types independent of the original sensitizing foreign cell.

Another mechanism involves null lymphocytes (cells lacking typical T- or B-cell markers) bearing Fc receptors. Upon contact with IgG-coated target cells, these Fc-receptor-bearing cells will lyse the "sensitized" target cells. This mechanism is called antibody-dependent cytotoxicity and can also be performed by other cells bearing Fc receptors including granulocytes and monocytes.

Finally, null lymphocytes have the capacity to lyse tumor cells, but not normal tissues, in the absence of antibody or complement. This phenomenon has been termed natural killer (NK) cell activity. The precise determinants that NK cells recognize are not clearly understood. It is thought that NK activity, however, may be important in the destruction of small numbers of tumor cells which might arise endogenously in the host.

C. Antigenic Determinants Recognized by Cytotoxic Cells

The generation of cytotoxic T lymphocytes requires the cooperation of two distinct T-cell subclasses: cytotoxic precursor cells and helper cells. Although specific clones of cytotoxic lymphocytes are activated by interaction with HLA-A, B, and C series antigenic determinants on foreign cells, their differentiation into killer cells requires the participation of helper T cells that recognize and proliferate in response to distinct major histocompatibility complex determinants that are coded for in the HLA-D region.

Insight into the evolutionary and biologic significance of why the organism can readily generate cytotoxic lymphocytes has come from recent studies. Cytotoxic T lymphocytes are generated having specificity for autologous or syngeneic cells displaying non-MHC surface structures, including tumor-associated antigens, chemicals, and virus-associated cell surface determinants. An important aspect of these studies has been the demonstration that cytotoxic lymphocytes generated to neoantigens on the surface of autologous cells lyse targets bearing the neoantigens (virus or tumor) only in association with self-MHC surface determinants. The same neoantigens, when presented on cells not sharing MHC structures, are not lysed. It is clear, therefore, that cytotoxic lymphocytes reactive with modified autologous cells recognize not only the neoantigen but also self-MHC structures.

Clinically, cytotoxic lymphocytes reactive with altered self-determinants may not only be important with respect to viral infection and neoplasia, but these cells may also be involved in autoimmune phenomena. For example, it is known that cytotoxic lymphocytes reactive with altered self can initiate a number of autoimmune diseases in animals, including autoimmune encephalomyelitis, polyneuritis, and autoimmune orchitis. In humans, evidence exists that cytotoxic lymphocytes may be involved in the pathogenesis of diseases such as chronic active heaptitis and polymyositis.

Table 3 Evaluation of Cellular-Immune System

I. In vivo
   A. Delayed hypersensitivity skin tests
      1. Environmental-tuberculin PPD, *Candida albicans,* streptokinase-streptodornase, mumps, trichophyton
      2. Sensitize "de novo"–dinitrochlorobenzene
   B. Lymphoid histology
      1. Lymph node–paracortical areas
      2. Thymus–cortical and medullary structure

II. In vitro
   A. Blood lymphocytes
      1. Total small lymphocyte count (<1500 mm^3)
      2. E rosettes
      3. Anti-T cell sera (thymocytes, mature T cells, T_H, T_S)
      4. Ig-bearing cells
      5. EA rosettes
      6. EAC rosettes
      7. Ia antigens
   B. Lymphocyte proliferation
      1. Mitogens–phytohemagglutinin, concanavalin A, pokeweed
      2. Antigens–soluble, allogenic
   C. Lymphokines
      1. Macrophage MIF or activating factor
      2. Macrophage chemotactic factor
      3. Lymphotoxin
      4. Interferon
   D. T-cell-mediated cytotoxicity
      1. Allogenic
      2. Tumor cell
   E. Helper and regulatory cell function
      1. T-cell helper factors for antibody synthesis
      2. Suppressor cell factors for antibody synthesis and cell-mediated function of T cells
   F. Macrophage
      1. Biochemical
      2. Phagocytosis
      3. Killing–bacteria, tumor cells
      4. Chemotaxis

V. Evaluation of Cell-Mediated Immunity in Humans

As discussed above, cell-mediated immune reactions are complex and involve interactions between various subpopulations of T cells, B cells, and macrophages. Accordingly, any consideration of this system must include tests that can dissect and measure the function of the individual components. This evaluation can be separated into an in vivo assessment, which provides initial screening measures, and an in vitro component to dissect the individual cellular elements. In general, the in vivo assessment tends to provide qualitative information concerning the integrity of the system but is difficult to quantitate. In contrast, the in vitro assessment of T, B, or macrophage function is more quantitative, as well as yielding information about each component. Examples of the types of patients that may require an evaluation of cellular immunity include those with certain types of recurrent infections (fungal, viral, and mycobacterial), cancer, immunodeficiency (primary and acquired), and patients with organ transplants. A protocol summarizing the assessment of cell-mediated immunity is presented in Table 3. Further information concerning the evaluation of cell-mediated immunity can be obtained from other sources (Cerottini and Brunner 1974, Chess and Schlossman 1977, David and Rocklin 1978, Rose and Friedman 1980).

VI. Delayed-Type Hypersensitivity Skin Testing

The best in vivo screening procedure available to the clinician to evaluate cell-mediated immunity is still the 24–48 hr skin test reaction. Developing one or more positive cutaneous responses to environmental antigens (tuberculin purified protein derivative [PPD] , *Candida albicans,* streptokinase-streptodornase, mumps) and/or being newly sensitized to a contact allergen (dinitrochlorobenzene) usually indicates intact cellular immunity. The ability to express a positive delayed skin test response is dependent upon intact lymphocyte-macrophage interactions as well as certain components of the inflammatory response. Therefore, the demonstration of positive delayed skin test reactivity in a patient is ordinarily sufficient and the performance of in vitro lymphocyte or macrophage testing in such patients is usually unnecessary. Failure to respond to a battery of environmental antigens, or to be sensitized to a new antigen, is referred to as cutaneous anergy and is usually associated with depressed cellular immunity. There may also be lowered resistance to infection. However, it should be pointed out that individuals may be anergic without any apparent clinical abnormality such as history of recurrent infections, cancer, or autoimmune disease.

The use of a battery of skin test reagents statistically enhances the chances of obtaining one or more positive skin test responses. The initial skin testing should be carried out with environmental antigens. These antigens are derived from microorganisms present ubiquitously in the environment; most individuals develop some immunologic reaction to them. Such a battery might consist of tuberculin PPD, *Candida albicans,* streptokinase-streptodornase, trichophyton, and mumps antigen. One may also use certain fungal antigens which are endemic to an area including coccidioidin, histoplasmin, and blastomycosis. If the responses to environmental antigens are negative, the patient should be sensitized to a "new" antigen such as dinitrochlorobenzene. Normal subjects respond to at least two or more environmental antigens and can be sensitized to dinitrochlorobenzene 90–95% of the time.

The reasons for cutaneous anergy are varied and may be subdivided into nonimmunological conditions and diseases associated with immunological defects. Nonimmunological causes of anergy may include an inappropriate choice of antigens (use of endemic rather than ubiquitous antigens), poor technique (superficial or subcutaneous injection of antigen), lack of exposure (pediatric age group), accompanying skin conditions (eczema or lichenification), vaccination within the preceding 6–8 weeks (measles, influenza, yellow fever, polio), anticoagulant therapy, accompanying metabolic diseases (hypothyroidism, uremia, protein-calorie malnutrition), scurvy, immediate hypersensitivity reaction at the same site, immunosuppressive therapy (steroids, immuran, or cyclophosphamide), or surgery within 2 weeks. Anergy due to immunologic defects might include either a problem with the lymphocyte or macrophage. Causes related to lymphocytes may include inadequate numbers of cells, an intrinsic cell defect, redistribution of circulating cells (sampling error), lack of lymphokine production, serum factors that inactivate lymphokines, lymphocytic antibodies, hyperactive suppressor cells, or receptor blockade. Defects in the macrophage have not been as well defined, but may include similar problems that pertain to the lymphocyte described above.

VII. In Vitro Assessment of T-Cell Function

The tests that quantify lymphocytes and assess their function detect surface markers and measure their ability to proliferate, produce mediators, mount cytotoxic responses, and regulate immune responses. The enumeration of lymphocyte subpopulations (T cells and B cells) utilizes the observation that unique receptors are present on each cell type. Immunofluorescence techniques are used to identify immunoglobulin receptors on B cells, and rosetting techniques are used to identify T cells and B cells. In addition, techniques are now available to discern functionally distinct T-cell subpopulations. For example, T helper and delayed hypersensitivity effector cells can be identified by means of certain membrane structures such as an Fc receptor for IgM (Tu) and a unique differentiation antigen detected by monoclonal antisera. In contrast, a functionally distinct subpopulation of cytotoxic/suppressor T cells is identified by the presence of an Fc receptor for IgG (Tγ) and a differentiation antigen that does not cross react with the antigen on T helper cells.

Lymphocyte proliferative responses can be evaluated by using non-specific mitogenic stimulants such as phytohemagglutinin, concanavalin A, or pokeweed mitogen, and by specific stimuli such as soluble antigens. The nonspecific activation of lymphocytes measure both T-cell and B-cell function, although the kinetics of these responses differ. In contrast, specific antigenic challenge appears to measure only T-cell function. By using autologous as well as homologous serum in the cultures, one can also determine whether the patient's serum contains factors that may interfere with the proliferative response.

The elaboration of soluble mediators by lymphocytes indicates that these cells are capable of producing factors that alter the function of a variety of cells involved in cellular immune reactions. Some examples include migration inhibitory factor, leukocyte inhibitory factor, chemotactic factor, lymphotoxin, and lymphocyte mitogenic factor. Although the elaboration of these factors can be shown to correlate with in vivo delayed hypersensitivity in humans, they do not necessarily measure the function of a particular cell type (T or B cells).

The mixed lymphocyte culture and cytotoxicity tests measure responses to allogenic antigens on the surface of target cells and are indicators of T-cell function. The ability of T cells to regulate immunoglobulin synthesis or antibody production, as well as lymphocyte proliferation, has recently been appreciated to have clinical relevance. Excessive or diminished regula-tion of these immune responses can result in disorders in each system.

Whenever possible, more than one in vitro test of lymphocyte function should be used since each assay may measure a distinct subpopulation of cells. Furthermore, present evidence indicates that lymphocytes are com-partmentalized; that is, cells in the blood may be functionally different from those in lymph nodes or spleen. Therefore, sampling blood lympho-cytes alone may not yield representative results. An evaluation should include a quantitation of the numbers of T and B cells, proliferative responses to mitogens and specific antigens, measurement of at least one lymphocyte mediator, and a cytotoxic response. If any of the preceding functions are found to be abnormal, then assessment of suppressor cell activity would be indicated. It should be pointed out that the precise role of suppressor cells in disease is presently an area of active investigation and some of the data are still preliminary.

Because of their complexity, these in vitro assays are not routinely carried out in most clinical laboratories and are restricted at present to research centers that specialize in basic and applied investigation. Moreover, because of the nature of these assays, that is, because they are biologic phenomena and subject to considerable variation, the results should be interpreted with caution. Therefore, in an individual patient a negative result should be repeated to confirm abnormal cellular function. For this reason, these tests are more useful when applied to the study of groups or populations of patients with certain diseases rather than to individual patients. Although they are not usually diagnostic, these tests are clinically valuable in identifying certain pathogenic factors and in monitoring the results of therapy and the clinical course of patients with depressed cellular function.

VIII. Abnormalities of Cell-Mediated Immunity in Patients with Sarcoidosis

A. General

While numerous studies have documented an impairment of cell-mediated immunity in patients with sarcoidosis, the nature of this defect, like the etiology of the disease itself, remains an enigma. The apparent paradox in this disease that is likewise mystifying is why anergic sarcoid patients, while not responding to environmental antigens, are uniquely capable of

Table 4 Abnormalities in Cell-Mediated Immunity in Sarcoidosis

A. In vivo
  1. Partial or complete anergy to environmental (tuberculin PPD, mumps, SK-SD, trichophyton) and "new" (DNCB) antigens

B. In vitro
  1. Lymphocytopenia–decreased absolute numbers of T cells
  2. Imbalance in T-cell subsets–decreased T_H and increased $T_{S/C}$
  3. Depressed proliferative responses in some patients to mitogens, soluble antigens, and allogenic stimuli
  4. Depressed antigen or mitogen-induced lymphokine production
  5. Sarcoid sera inhibit proliferative responses of lymphocytes from normal subjects to mitogens and antigens
  6. Sarcoid monocytes inhibit lymphocyte proliferation
  7. Autoantibodies to T cells

mounting a cutaneous response to Kveim antigen. Of further interest is the
observation that the impairment in cell-mediated immunity present in this
disease is "mild" compared to primary immunodeficiency diseases (e.g.,
DiGeorge syndrome or severe combined immunodeficiency disease) or even
other acquired immunodeficiency diseases such as Hodgkin's disease. That
is, although many patients with sarcoidosis are anergic and have abnormal
lymphocyte function, they do not develop the recurrent infections by
facultative intracellular microorganisms that characterize these other
conditions. This raises the question of whether the defect in cell-mediated
immunity in this disease is in fact real or apparent. Some of these issues
will be addressed below. A summary of the cellular-immune abnormalities
reported in sarcoid patients is presented in Table 4. The interested reader
is referred to other reviews for further information (Daniele et al. 1980,
Faguet 1978, Geraint et al. 1978).

B. In Vivo Responses

As mentioned previously, it is particularly interesting that anergic sarcoid
patients respond to Kveim antigen. However, the significance of this
reaction is not entirely clear since there are marked differences between the
Kveim reaction and the classic delayed-type hypersensitivity skin reactions.
For example, the most obvious difference is in the kinetics of the two
reactions. The delayed-type hypersensitivity reaction begins at 8 hr, peaks
at 24–48 hr, and resolves by 96–120 hr. By contrast, the Kveim reaction
takes 4–6 weeks to develop. Furthermore, no specific antigen in the Kveim
preparation has been identified as the inducing agent in this response, and
no convincing data have been generated to persuade one to believe that
sarcoid lymphocytes are actually sensitized to this material. Therefore,
despite the fact that Kveim reactions are characterized histologically by
mononuclear cell infiltrates, how these cells are recruited to the skin site,
the nature of the stimulus, and the reaction itself remain the subjects of
much controversy.

Traditionally, anergy in sarcoidosis has meant unresponsiveness to
tuberculoprotein. However, as investigators have become cognizant of the
importance of using a battery of skin test reagents to evaluate cell-
mediated immunity, unreactivity to other environmental antigens such as
monilia, SK-SD, mumps, and trichophyton have been identified as well.
The incidence of anergy in sarcoid patients has varied from 30 to 70%,
depending on the number of antigens used and the disease activity of the
patient population studied (Broom and MacLaurin 1973, Crofton and
Douglas 1975, Mitchell and Scadding 1974, Scadding 1967, Siltzbach et al.
1974). In addition, many patients with sarcoidosis cannot be sensitized to a

"new" antigen such as dinitrochlorobenzene. The presence of anergy usually parallels the disease activity, with increased abnormalities noted in clinically symptomatic patients.

It should be pointed out with regard to anergy to tuberculoprotein that most patients with active sarcoidosis and myobacterial infections express positive tuberculin PPD skin tests. Thus, in patients with sarcoidosis, the appearance of a positive skin test, particularly in those patients being treated with corticosteroids, should make the clinician suspicious of active tuberculosis.

C. In Vitro Responses

Active disease is usually associated with a reduction in the number of circulating blood lymphocytes (Daniele and Rowlands 1976, Hedfors et al. 1974, Hoffbrand 1968, Ramachander et al. 1975, Sorensen et al. 1976). This lymphopenia represents an absolute reduction in the number of T cells. Furthermore, when one quantitates the T cell subsets, there is an increase in Fc-IgG (Tγ) receptor positive cells and a decrease in the Fc-IgM (Tμ) receptor positive population (Daniele and Rowlands 1976, Hedfors et al. 1974, Sorensen et al. 1976). The lymphopenia occurs in patients with acute and chronic active disease but not in patients with resolved disease. It should be noted that these changes in T-cell populations are not limited to patients with sarcoidosis.

Lymphocyte function per se has been extensively examined in patients with sarcoidosis. The vast majority of studies have documented abnormal proliferative responses to mitogens, environmental antigens, and allogenic stimuli in patients with active disease, but responses have been normal in patients in remission (Goldstein et al. 1978, Hirschorn et al. 1964, Kataria et al. 1973, Horsmanheimo 1974, Sharma et al. 1971, Siltzbach et al. 1971). Furthermore, lymphocytes from sarcoid patients fail to produce various lymphokines in response to mitogens and antigenic stimuli (Rocklin et al. 1972, Kataria et al. 1976, Tannenbaum et al. 1976). While most patients with sarcoidosis exhibit abnormal lymphocyte function in terms of lymphocyte proliferation and lymphokine production, it should be noted that some anergic patients have only a partial "defect" in their response (Rocklin et al. 1972, Tannenbaum et al. 1976). That is, both mitogen- and antigen-induced proliferation is comparable to that obtained for normal subjects, but lymphokine production is depressed. This dissociation between these two in vitro correlates of cell-mediated immunity has been observed in other diseases such as chronic mucocutaneous candidiasis and collagen-vascular diseases.

IX. Possible Explanations for Abnormalities
in Cell-Mediated Immunity in Sarcoid Patients

From the data accumulated thus far, no one single explanation would
account for the reduction in number and function of circulating T lymphocytes. However, several observations and hypotheses are worthwhile citing
here.

One of the most relevant observations concerns the issue of whether
the reduction of delayed-type skin test reactivity and in vitro lymphocyte
function reflect a deletion of the population of immunoreactive cells being
sampled, an intrinsic defect in their function, extrinsic factors modulating
their function, or a combination of these factors. With regard to the
deletion of immunoreactive cells, it is worth pointing out first that the
expression of skin reactivity requires adequate numbers of circulating
lymphocytes; usually a level greater than 1500 lymphocytes/mm^3 is
associated with normal skin reactivity. Therefore, an inadequate number
of peripheral lymphocytes in and of itself may be a sufficient explanation
for anergy. Lymphopenia per se, however, would not explain the abnormal
in vitro lymphocyte function because the cell numbers are adjusted to
compensate for reduced cell counts. The real question then is whether the
disease process has totally eliminated these cells or just made them
unavailable.

There is evidence to suggest that the latter possibility may be the
more reasonable one. First, when the disease resolves, the immunologic
abnormalities appear to be reversible. Second, sampling lymphocyte
function in other tissues (besides blood) containing lymphoid cells, such as
lymph nodes and bronchial lavage specimens of sarcoid patients, reveals
the presence of immunoreactive cells (Hunninghake et al. 1978a, 1978b,
1979, 1980). Lastly, studies in the animal models of granulomatous disease
indicate that there is an altered circulating pattern for T cells such that
these cells become sequestered in the central lymphoid organs and sites of
inflammation and do not recirculate in their usual fashion. Thus, it is
likely that one explanation for the apparent reduction in cell-mediated
immunity is that the immunoreactive cells are present in the granulomas
and not freely circulating in the blood, or present in the skin in sufficient
numbers to elicit a response, leading to a sampling error.

In addition to the above explanation, one must also consider whether
sarcoid lymphocytes available in the blood for study have an intrinsic defect
in their function, or whether their function is being modified by extrinsic
components such as regulatory cells or serum factors. It has not yet been
established that sarcoid lymphocytes are defective. However, there is
abundant evidence that suppressor cells and serum factors may contribute to

abnormal lymphocyte function. For example, there is an increased number of Tγ cells in the blood of sarcoid patients and increased monocyte suppressor activity in such patients (Goodwin et al. 1979, Katz and Fauci 1978).

The latter two observations provide circumstantial evidence that lymphocyte function is being down-regulated by T suppressor cells and monocytes in sarcoid patients with active disease. However, it has not been established whether the appearance of such regulatory cells is a primary factor or whether they develop secondarily as a result of the granulomatous response. Finally, it has been repeatedly shown that sera from sarcoid patients inhibit autologous lymphocyte function as well as cells from normal subjects (Belcher et al. 1974, Davies et al. 1980, Mangi et al. 1974). However, the nature of the inhibitory factor(s) present in these sera has not been clarified.

Taken together, the available evidence would suggest that the reduction in cell-mediated immunity in patients with sarcoidosis (and possibly patients with other granulomatous disease) is reversible, probably more apparent than real, and thus reflects a sampling error; the apparent reduction also may involve regulatory influences (cells and serum factors) that help modulate cell-mediated immunity. Further insight into the pathogenesis of this defect in cellular-immune function may come through the quantitating and making functional studies of lymphocyte subpopulations in granulomatous tissue, as well as through making clinical correlations and following the effects of treatment on these immunological parameters.

References

Belcher, R. W., Carney, J. F., and Nankervis, G. A. (1974). Effect of sera from patients with sarcoidosis on in vitro lymphocyte response. *Int. Arch. Allergy,* **46**:183.

Benacerraf, B. (1976). In *Role of Products of the Histocompatibility Gene Complex in Immune Responses.* Edited by D. H. Katz and B. Benacerraf. New York, Academic Press, p. 225.

Broom, B. C., and MacLaurin, B. P. (1973). Sarcoidosis: Correlation of delayed hypersensitivity, MLC reactivity and lymphocytotoxicity with disease activity. *Clin. Exp. Immunol.,* **15**:355–364.

Cantor, H., and Boyse, E. A. (1977). Lymphocytes as models for the study of mammalian cellular differentiation. *Immunol. Rev.,* **33**:105.

Cerottini, J. C., and Brunner, K. T. (1974). Cell-mediated cytotoxicity, allograft rejection and tumor immunity. *Adv. Immunol.,* **18**:67.

Chess, L., and Schlossman, S. F. (1977). Human lymphocyte subpopulations. *Adv. Immunol.,* **25**:213.

Crofton, J., and Douglas, A. (1975). *Respiratory Disease.* Oxford, Blackwell.

Daniele, R. P., and Rowlands, D. T., Jr. (1976). Lymphocyte subpopulations in sarcoidosis: Correlation with disease activity and duration. *Ann. Intern. Med.,* **85**:593–600.

Daniele, R. P., Dauber, J. H., and Rossman, M. D. (1980). Immunologic abnormalities in sarcoidosis. *Ann. Intern. Med.,* **92**:406.

David, J. R., and Rocklin, R. E. (1978). Lymphocyte mediators: The "lymphokines." In *Immunological Diseases.* Edited by M. Samter. Boston, Little, Brown, p. 307.

Davies, B. H., Jones, K. P., Evans, P., and Williams-Jones, W. (1980). Thymic lymphocyte responses in sarcoidosis: Effect of sera and levamisole. In *Proceedings of the 8th International Conference on Sarcoidosis and Other Granulomatous Disease.* Edited by W. J. Williams and B. H. Davies. London, Alpha Omega, pp. 477–484.

Faguet, G. B. (1978). Cellular immunity in sarcoidosis: Evidence for an intrinsic defect of effector cell function. *Am. Rev. Respir. Dis.,* **118**:89.

Geraint, J. D., Neville, E., and Walker, A. (1978). Immunology of sarcoidosis. *Am. J. Med.,* **59**:388.

Goldstein, R. A., Janicki, B. W., Mirro, J., and Foellmer, J. W. (1978). Cell-mediated immune responses in sarcoidosis. *Am. Rev. Respir. Dis.,* **117**:55–62.

Goodwin, J. S., DeHoratius, R., Israel, H., Peake, G. T., and Messner, R. (1979). Suppressor cell function in sarcoidosis. *Ann. Intern. Med.,* **90**:169–173.

Hedfors, E., Holm, G., and Petterson, E. (1974). Lymphocyte subpopulations in sarcoidosis. *Clin. Exp. Immunol.,* **17**:219–226.

Hirschorn, K., Schreibman, R. R., Bach, F. H., and Siltzbach, L. E. (1964). In vitro studies of lymphocytes from patients with sarcoidosis and lymphoproliferative diseases. *Lancet,* **2**:842–843.

Hoffbrand, B. I. (1968). Occurrence and significance of lymphopenia in sarcoidosis. *Am. Rev. Respir. Dis.,* **98**:107–110.

Horsmanheimo, M. (1974). Correlation of tuberculin-induced lymphocyte transformation with skin test reactivity and with clinical manifestations of sarcoidosis. *Cell. Immunol.,* **10**:329–337.

Hunninghake, G., Kelman, J., Weinberger, S., Young, R., Fulmer, J., and Crystal, R. G. (1978a). Lung lymphocyte subpopulations in sarcoidosis. *Clin. Res.,* **26**:448A.

Hunninghake, G. W., Kelman, J. A., Gadek, J. E., Elson, N. A., Fulmer, J. D., and Crystal, R. G. (1978b). Comparison of inflammatory and immune effector cell populations in lavage fluid and lung biopsies of patients with pulmonary fibrosis. *Am. Rev. Respir. Dis.,* **177**:68.

Hunninghake, G. W., Gadek, J. E., Kawanami, O., Ferrans, V. J., and Crystal, R. G. (1979). Inflammatory and immune processes in the human lung in health and disease: Evaluation by bronchoalveolar lavage. *Am. J. Pathol.,* **97**:149–206.

Hunninghake, G. W., Fulmer, J. D., Young, R. C., and Crystal, R. G. (1980). Comparison of lung and blood lymphocyte subpopulations in pulmonary sarcoidosis. In *Proceedings of the 8th International Conference on Sarcoidosis and Other Granulomatous Disease.* Edited by W. J. Williams and B. H. Davies. London, Alpha Omega, pp. 426–435.

Kataria, Y. P., Sagone, A. L., LoBuglio, A. F., and Bromberg, P. A. (1973). In vitro observations on sarcoid lymphocytes and their correlation with cutaneous anergy and clinical severity of disease. *Am. Rev. Respir. Dis.,* **108**:767–776.

Kataria, Y. P., LoBuglio, A. F., and Bromberg, P. A. (1976). Sarcoid lymphocytes spontaneous transformation and release of macrophage migration inhibition activity. *Am. Rev. Respir. Dis.,* **113**:315–323.

Katz, P., and Fauci, A. S. (1978). Inhibition of polyclonal B-cell activation by suppressor monocytes in patients with sarcoidosis. *Clin. Exp. Immunol.,* **32**:554–562.

Mangi, R. J., Dwyer, J. M., and Kantor, F. S. (1974). The effect of plasma upon lymphocyte responses in vitro: Demonstration of a humoral inhibitor in patients with sarcoidosis. *Clin. Exp. Immunol.,* **18**:519–528.

Mitchell, D. N., and Scadding, J. G. (1974). Sarcoidosis. *Am. Rev. Respir. Dis.,* **110**:774–802.

Moller, G., Ed. (1974). The immune response to infectious diseases. *Transplant. Rev.,* **19**:1.

Nelson, D. S. (1976). *Immunobiology of the Macrophage.* New York, Academic Press.

Ramachandar, K., Douglas, S. D., Siltzbach, L. E., and Taub, R. N. (1975). Peripheral blood lymphocyte subpopulations in sarcoidosis. *Cell. Immunol.,* **16**:422–426.

Rheinherz, E., and Schlossman, S. F. (1980). Regulation of the immune response: Inducer and suppressor T-lymphocyte subsets in human beings. *N. Engl. J. Med.,* **303**:370.

Rocklin, R. E., Sheffer, A. L., and David, J. R. (1972). *Sarcoidosis: A Clinical and in Vitro Immunologic Study.* New York, Academic Press, pp. 743–749.

Rose, N. R., and Friedman, H., Eds. (1980). *Manual of Clinical Immunology.* Washington, D.C., American Society of Microbiology.

Scadding, J. G. (1967). *Sarcoidosis.* London, Eyre and Spottiswoode.

Sharma, O. P., James, D. G., and Fox, R. A. (1971). A correlation of in vitro delayed type hypersensitivity and in vitro lymphocyte transformation in sarcoidosis. *Chest,* **60**:35–37.

Shearer, G., and Schmitt-Verhulst, A. (1977). A. Major histocompatibility complex restricted cell-mediated immunity. *Adv. Immunol.,* **25**:55.

Siltzbach, L. E., Glade, P. R., Hirshant, Y., Vieira, L. O. B. D., Celikoglu, I. S., and Hirschhorn, K. (1971). In vitro stimulation of peripheral lymphocytes in sarcoidosis. In *Fifth International Conference on Sarcoidosis.* Edited by L. Levinsky and F. Macholda. Prague, University Karlova, **217**:20.

Siltzbach, L. E., James, D. G., Neville, E., Turiaf, J., Battesti, J. P., Sharma, O. P., Hosada, Y., Mikami, R., and Odaka, M. (1974). Course and prognosis of sarcoidosis around the world. *Am. J. Med.,* **57**:847–852.

Sorenson, S. F., Hardt, F., and Veien, N. K. (1976). Estimation of lymphocyte subpopulation in the peripheral blood of patients with sarcoidosis. *Scand. J. Immunol.,* **5**:1117–1122.

Tannenbaum, H., Rocklin, R., Schur, P. H., and Sheffer, A. L. (1976). Immune function in sarcoidosis: Studies on delayed hypersensitivity, B and T lymphocytes, serum immunoglobulins and serum complement components. *Clin. Exp. Immunol.,* **26**:511–519.

Turk, J. L. (1975). Delayed hypersensitivity. In *Frontiers of Biology,* Vol. 4, 2nd ed. Amsterdam, North Holland.

8

Abnormalities of the Humoral Immune System in Sarcoidosis

RONALD P. DANIELE

University of Pennsylvania School of Medicine
Philadelphia, Pennsylvania

I. General

In contrast to the depression in cell-mediated immunity, which was described in the previous chapter, there is hyperreactivity of the humoral immune system in sarcoidosis. This is expressed mainly in two ways: an increased response to exogenous antigens and the development of auto-antibodies to host antigens.

Humoral immune responses are the end product of antigen interaction with bone-marrow-derived or bursal equivalent lymphocytes (B cells). Although antibody production is ultimately derived from B cells, it is well recognized that the response is controlled by a network of cell populations which include at least two subsets of thymus-derived lymphocytes (T cells) and phagocytic cells (Roitt 1981). The identity of these cell populations and their interactions were discussed in the previous chapter and will be reviewed briefly here.

The recognition phase of the immune response usually begins with antigen processing by the phagocyte (Fig. 1). This stage includes not only degradation of foreign substances but a poorly defined step which promotes optimal presentation of antigens to lymphocytes. Macrophage presentation

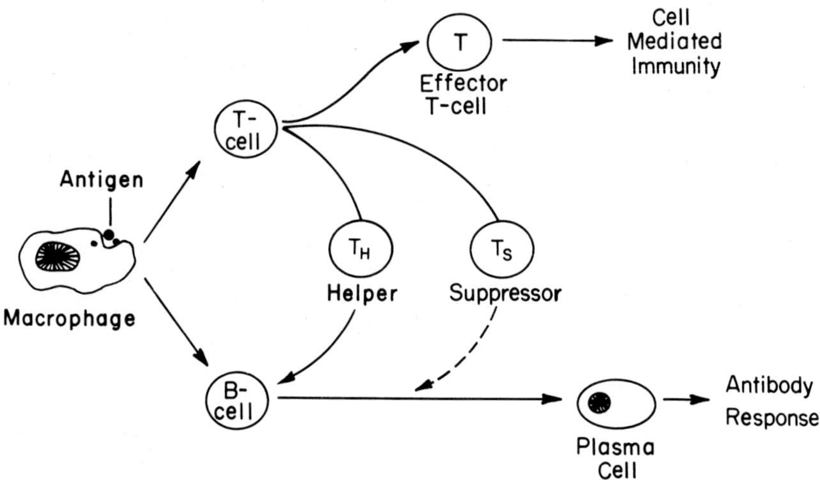

Figure 1   Diagram of the functional interrelations of subpopulations of lymphocytes and macrophages in cell-mediated and humoral immune responses.   (Modified from Daniele, Dauber, and Rossman, 1980.)

of antigens to cells within the lymphoid system results in predominantly a cellular or humoral immune response.   The type of response depends on a number of ill-defined factors including the size, route of entry, and physical and biological properties of the antigen.   Antigen recognition may lead to B-cell proliferation and differentiation into plasma cells, which actively synthesize and secrete antibodies to the inciting antigen.

The regulation of B-cell proliferation and differentiation involves at least two populations of T cells (Gershon 1974, Cantor and Boyse 1977a). One class of cooperative T cells, called helper T cells, is required for optimal antibody production to most antigens.*   The cooperation between B and T cells usually involves an antigen molecule which possesses two regions: a relatively large carrier determinant and a smaller one called a hapten which is coupled to the carrier.   Helper T cells distinguish the carrier region of the antigen and cooperate with B cells which recognize the hapten.   Helper T cells also require that antigen be physically presented to them by macrophages.   Once activated by antigen, helper T cells also require macrophages or dendritic cells to trigger specific B cells.   Although these three cell types are needed for B cell proliferation and differentiation,

---

*Certain large antigens that possess many repeating antigenic determinants may stimulate B cells without T-cell help.

the exact sequence and mechanism of interactions of these cells in vivo
have yet to be defined.

Another distinct subpopulation of T cells, called suppressor T cells,
inhibits or regulates the humoral response once it is initiated (Cantor and
Boyse 1977a). Less is known about the function of suppressor T cells.
For example, it is unclear whether they act upon macrophages, helper T
cells, B cells, or combinations of these cell populations. Nonetheless, the
balance between regulatory T cells (and macrophages) determines the outcome of antigenic recognition, which is ultimately expressed in the kind
(Ig class) and degree of the humoral response.

Until recently, T-cell subpopulations in man were only functionally
defined. Two advances have allowed more precise identification and
physical isolation of these subsets of T cells. First, it has been observed
that suppressor T cells have membrane receptors for the Fc portion of IgG
(Tγ), whereas helper T cells have receptors for IgM (Tμ) (Moretta et al.
1977). Indicator red cells (ox red blood cells) opsonized with IgG or IgM
bind the T-cell receptors and permit identification and separation of these
subpopulations of T cells in man.

More recently, these two functional subsets of T cells have been
identified with monoclonal antibodies directed to stable membrane
differentiation antigens (Reinherz and Schlossman 1980). This situation is
similar to what has been established in inbred strains of mice using thymus
cell differentiation antigens (e.g., Ly 1,2,3) (Cantor and Boyse 1977b). By
this approach, helper cells are identified by monoclonal antibodies directed
to T4 antigens on the cell membrane; suppressor T cells are recognized by
monoclonal antibodies to T8 antigens. Although it is not established
whether these two methods identify similar or identical T cells, their use
should aid greatly in understanding how these cell subpopulations act in
generating the immune response.

II. Abnormalities of Serum Immunoglobulins

One of the first recognized abnormalities of the humoral immune system
in sarcoidosis was an elevation in the serum levels of gammaglobulin
(above 3.5 g/100 ml). In a series involving 3676 patients from 11 cities
around the world, elevations in gamma globulin ranged between 23 and
96% of the patients, with the greatest levels in black populations in New
York and Los Angeles (James et al. 1976). Our experience in Philadelphia
involving 30 black patients revealed a prevalence of 50% (Daniele and
Rowlands 1976a). There is an increase in all immunoglobulin classes, but
IgG is the most consistently and persistently elevated (James et al. 1975,
Turner-Warwick 1978). Elevations in IgM have been associated with
erythema nodosum (Mustakallio et al. 1967).

Electrophoretic studies reveal a broad-based elevation in gamma globulins, indicating a polyclonal increase in immunoglobulins. That there is a humoral hyperresponsiveness to many antigens in patients with sarcoidosis is suggested by the frequency of specific serum antibodies. These include antibodies to mycobacterial (Chapman and Speight 1964) and mycoplasmal (Horsmanheimo et al. 1978) antigens; to a variety of viral antigens (Byrne et al. 1974) (e.g., herpes simplex, rubella, Epstein-Barr); and to isoagglutinins to small amounts of mismatched blood (Sands et al. 1955).

III. B-Cell Populations

With the evidence of hyperreactive humoral responses, it might be expected that the number of B cells would be increased. There is still controversy, however, over whether the proportion or absolute number of peripheral blood B cells is increased, decreased, or normal in patients with active sarcoidosis (Daniele and Rowlands 1976a, Hedfors et al. 1974, Fernandez et al. 1976). B cells are usually identified by the presence of surface immunoglobulin (SIg) or complement receptors (C3b) (Rowlands and Daniele 1975). Initially, we also found a discrepancy in the proportion of B cells identified by surface immunoglublin and complement receptors in patients with active disease (Daniele and Rowlands 1976a). However, the possibility was examined that the increase in cells exhibiting surface immunoglublulin was due to the binding of exogenous immunoglobulin to the surface of non-B cells (Daniele and Rowlands 1976a, Rossman et al. 1978). As indicated in Figure 2, when lymphocytes from sarcoid patients were cultured for 18 hr in the absence of autologous sera, the proportion of cells bearing (and synthesizing) surface immunoglobulin was significantly reduced by about 25%. Moreover, the proportion of cells detected by surface immunoglobulin after incubation was in good agreement with the proportion of cells identified by complement receptors. Thus, to accurately enumerate B cells in blood or other tissues, technical measures should be used that exclude cells that bind immunoglobulins to the lymphocyte membrane. These exogenous immunoglobulins may include autoantibodies to the lymphocytes (see below), labile immunoglobulin (Lobo et al. 1975), and immune complexes that bind the membrane Fc receptor. Although the proportion of cells expressing surface immunoglobulin may be normal, the absolute number of B cells in patients with active disease (acute and chronic) may be normal or reduced depending on the degree of lymphocytopenia (Daniele and Rowlands 1976a, Rossman et al. 1978).

Recently, an in vitro plaque-forming assay has been used to assess B-cell function in patients with sarcoidosis (Katz and Fauci 1978). Peripheral blood lymphocytes from sarcoid patients had low plaque-forming cell

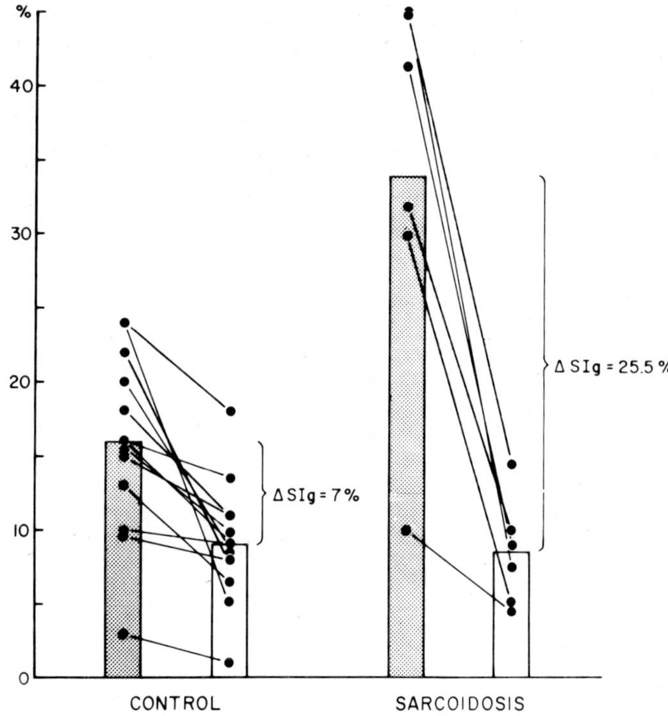

Figure 2 The percentage of peripheral blood lymphocytes bearing surface immunoglobulin (SIg) in control subjects and subjects with acute sarcoidosis. The height of the stippled bar represents the mean value before overnight culture. The height of the open bar represents the mean value after overnight culture in fetal calf serum; ΔSIg = the difference between the mean values. (Modified from Rossman, Dauber, and Daniele, 1978.)

responses compared to controls after activation by B-cell mitogens (pokeweed). Removal of adherent cells (monocytes) from the cell suspensions corrected the B-cell response. Unfortunately, these in vitro studies of B-cell function do not readily shed light on the regulatory mechanisms involved in the heightened B-cell activity found in vivo.

IV. Serum Autoantibodies

Another expression of humoral abnormalities in sarcoidosis is the appearance of autoantibodies directed at host antigens. These include antinuclear antibody (Veien et al. 1976) and rheumatoid factor (Oreskes and Siltzbach

1968).   Autoantibodies have not been consistently observed and do not appear to bear a relationship to the severity or clinical manifestations of the disease (Turner-Warwick 1978).   For example, although the prevalence of rheumatoid factor has been reported to be as high as 38% in patients with active sarcoidosis, it does not correlate with joint symptoms (Turner-Warwick 1978, Oreskes and Siltzbach 1969).

Autoantibodies to lymphocytes have also been observed in sarcoidosis (Daniele and Rowlands 1976b).   Using enriched (greater than 90%) T lymphocytes from a panel of normal donors with differing histocompatibility leukocyte antigen (HLA) phenotypes, autoantibodies to T cells were detected in the sera of about 50% of the patients with active disease.   The autoantibodies were cold reactive (at 4°C) and cytotoxic to about 30% of the enriched T cells.   By indirect immunofluorescent techniques, IgM was found to be the predominant immunoglobulin, but IgG was also detected to a lesser extent.

These findings have been confirmed and extended by Lobo and Suratt (1979) who found lymphocyte autoantibodies which were reactive to autologous lymphocytes in about 53% of the patients (range 21–83%). Moreover, these autoantibodies reacted with enriched populations of B lymphocytes as well as T cells.   The autolymphocytotoxins were also cold reactive, but only of the IgM class.   In these studies (Lobo and Suratt 1979) and our own (unpublished), there was no apparent correlation between lymphocyte autoantibodies and the stage of disease and degree of clinical activity.   The lack of a correlation between the presence of autolymphocytotoxins and clinical features of the disease differs from the findings in connective tissue disorders, such as systemic lupus erythematosus (SLE).   However, the presence of lymphocyte autoantibodies may provide clues in understanding the abnormalities in immunoregulation found in sarcoidosis.

V. Immune Complexes in Sarcoid Serum

Within the past 5 years, immune complexes have emerged as a prominent abnormality of sarcoidosis.   Table 1 summarizes the experience of four centers using different techniques to identify serum immune complexes (Hedfors and Norberg 1974, Gupta et al. 1977, Daniele et al. 1978, Mornex et al. 1979).   The prevalence of immune complexes in active disease (acute and chronic) varied between 23 and 70%.   The variability probably reflects the different techniques used to identify immune complexes.

The methods differ not only in their sensitivity but also in the information they provide (Theofilopoulos and Dixon 1979).   For example,

Table 1 Serum Immune Complexes in Sarcoidosis

Assay	Prevalence	Reference
Platelet aggregation	23%	Hedfors and Norberg (1974)
Raji cell and rheumatoid factor	51%[a]	Gupta et al. (1977)
Raji cell	39%	Daniele et al. (1978)
C1q binding	70%	Mornex et al. (1979)

[a]This value represents the percentage that was positive for one or both tests. For the Raji test alone, positive sera equaled 32%; for the monoclonal rheumatoid factor test, 40% were positive.

one of the first approaches to be used was the platelet aggregation test (Hedfors and Norberg 1974), which is based on the property of platelets to aggregate after IgG immune complexes interact with the Fc receptors on the platelet membrane. The method is sensitive but limited to IgG complexes and by the fact that other factors such as antiplatelet antibodies, myxoviruses, and certain enzymes will also induce platelet aggregation. Also, serum components such as rheumatoid factor and immune complexes containing complement may inhibit platelet aggregation.

The C1q assay detects large immune complexes (IgG and IgM) which must activate complement by the classic pathway. It is limited by the inability to distinguish nonspecifically aggregated Ig and other factors that will react with C1q, including double and single-stranded DNA, poly-ribonucleotides, and lipopolysaccharides (endotoxin).

Rheumatoid factor radioimmunoassays are highly sensitive. They detect relatively small complexes and are independent of complement-fixing properties of the complexes. The limitations of this test are that they detect only IgG complexes and may give positive results in the presence of high concentrations of monomeric IgG or of serum rheumatoid factor; the latter is an important consideration in view of the frequency of rheumatoid factor in sarcoid sera.

A recent advance in detecting serum immune complexes has been the use of Raji cells, a continuous line of human lymphoblastoid cells derived from a patient with Burkitt's lymphoma (Theofilopoulos and Dixon 1979). These cells lack detectable surface immunoglobulin but possess membrane receptors for components of complement (C1q, C3b, C3d, and C4b). An assay employing immunofluorescent or radiolabeled reagents can be used to identify complexes that bind the plasma membrane by the complement receptors. The technique is sensitive and reproducible and requires small volumes of serum. The limitations of the test are that it preferentially detects large complexes and that spurious results may occur from IgG lymphocyte autoantibodies.

It is generally agreed that no single test is ideal in having the sensitivity and specificity to detect immune complexes which vary in size, include all Ig classes, and may or may not fix complement. Thus, the use of more than one test has been recommended for optimal screening of immune complexes in patients' sera (WHO Scientific Group 1977). Based on the different techniques that have been reported (Table 1), it appears well established that immune complexes are a frequent abnormality in sarcoidosis.

Our experience involved the use of the Raji cell line and an indirect immunofluorescent assay (Daniele et al. 1978) (Fig. 3). Sera were examined in 44 patients with sarcoidosis who were separable into three distinct clinical groups: (1) acute disease (less than 1 yr), (2) chronic active disease (5 or more yr), and (3) resolved disease. As Table 2 indicates, about half the patients with acute disease had circulating immune complexes. Immune complexes were less frequent in patients with chronic disease, and absent in resolved disease. There was no apparent association between the presence of immune complexes and the stage of the disease or the presence of extrapulmonary lesions. Although it is unsettled whether there is such an association (Gupta et al. 1977), it is generally agreed that there is a high prevalence of immune complexes in patients with erythema nodosum and arthritis (James et al. 1975, Veien et al. 1976). It is unclear how immune complexes participate in the evolution of the disease. To establish a pathogenetic role for immune complexes in sera or biologic fluids, it is first necessary to demonstrate the deposition of immune complexes in involved tissues. It has been suggested that immune complexes are involved in the development of sarcoid granulomas. The presence of immunoglobulins

Table 2 Immune Complexes in Control Subjects and Patients with Sarcoidosis

| | Immune complexes | | Total |
| | Negative | Positive | number of |
Group	test	test	patients
Control subjects	12	0	12
Acute sarcoidosis	14	12	26
Chronic sarcoidosis	8	2	10
Resolved sarcoidosis	8	0	8

Source: Data from Daniele et al. (1978).

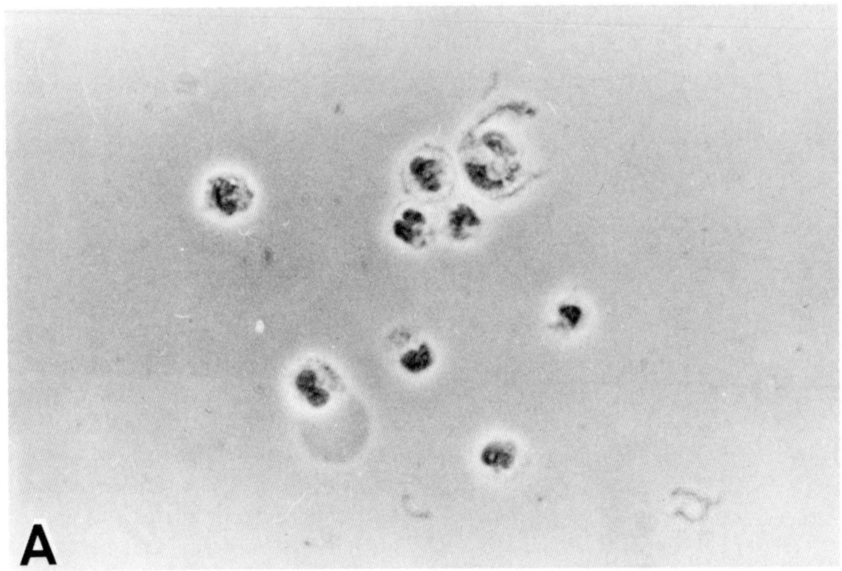

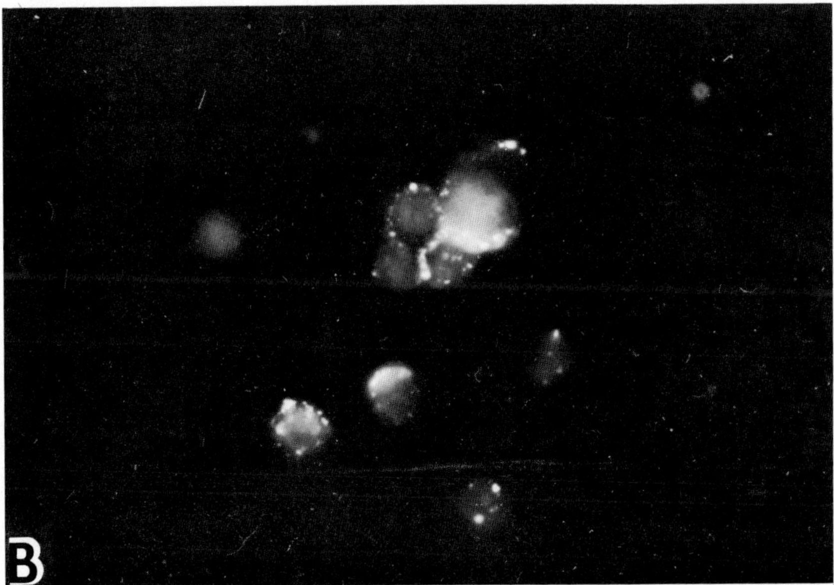

Figure 3 Immune complexes in sarcoid sera binding Raji cells. A. Phase contrast microscopy of Raji cells (original magnification X 400). B. Same preparation examined with fluorescent microscopy (original magnification X 400). (From Daniele, Dauber, and Rossman, 1980.)

and complement components in sarcoid granuloma provide some support for this idea (Ghose et al. 1974, Kataria et al. 1978).

Despite their presence, immune complexes usually do not lead to the renal and vascular lesions of other diseases in which immune complexes play a conspicuous role in pathogenesis (e.g., SLE). It is uncertain why certain immune complexes are injurious and others relatively benign. Factors that seem important are the size, the composition, and the capacity of immune complexes to resist host clearance. Relatively small immune complexes that persist in the circulation appear to be more pathogenic. Other important factors include their ability to fix complement and bind cell membranes and certain tissues (i.e., renal basement membrane). Which of these properties contributes to pathogenicity of the immune complexes in sarcoidosis remains unknown.

Because there is hyperreactivity of the humoral response, resulting in antibodies to both exogenous and endogenous antigens, it is likely that immune complexes are composed of extrinsic or intrinsic antigens or both. It is also possible that immune complexes contain antigenic determinants of the inciting agent(s) in sarcoidosis. The capacity of bulk Raji cell cultures to adsorb large concentrations of immune complexes on the cell membrane (Fig. 3) affords a promising approach to isolating and possibly identifying the specific etiologic agent(s) in this disease. Indeed, recent immunochemical techniques have succeeded in isolating and characterizing components of immune complexes in other situations (Theofilopoulos et al. 1978).

With the presence of circulating immune complexes, it might be expected that serum complement components would be depressed. However, in most reports, complement levels (C1q, CH50, and C3) are either normal or elevated (Buckley et al. 1966). One explanation for this finding is that complement consumption is exceeded by synthesis, as might occur in acute phase reactions. Support for this possibility comes from the fact that acute phase reactants, such as C-reactive protein, are elevated in the majority of patients with active sarcoidosis (Mornex et al. 1979).

Besides its possible role in the pathogenesis of the sarcoid lesions, immune complexes may also influence immune regulation. For example, immune complexes may alter the distribution and function of immune regulatory cells (T cells and macrophages). This possibility will be discussed below.

VI. Other Serum Factors

In addition to the recognized products of the immune system (e.g., auto-antibodies and immune complexes), it is important to place in some perspective the ill-defined serum and plasma factors that have been shown to influence both humoral and cell-mediated immunity in sarcoidosis.

As shown in Figure 4, our experience (unpublished) confirms that of others (Mangi et al. 1974) in that sera from sarcoid patients may inhibit the proliferative response of T cells to polyclonal mitogens. One explanation for this phenomenon is the presence of autoantibodies to T cells. However, some of the patients whose sera inhibited the proliferative response of their own and normal lymphocytes to T-cell mitogens lacked autoantibodies to T cells. Other inhibitory factors that might explain these findings include prostaglandins (Goodwin et al. 1979) and immune complexes (Zubler and Lambert 1977).

In a previous report (Daniele and Rowlands 1976b), serum factors were shown to inhibit the binding of sheep red blood cells to lymphocytes (E rosette), a test that identifies T cells. Initially, it was thought that this might be a sensitive assay for the identification of autoantibodies to T cells. However, after reexamining this phenomenon, we found that autoantibodies to T cells could not entirely explain the inhibition of E rosette formation. For example, certain patients' sera markedly inhibited E rosette formation by T cells but lacked lymphocyte autoantibodies (unpublished).

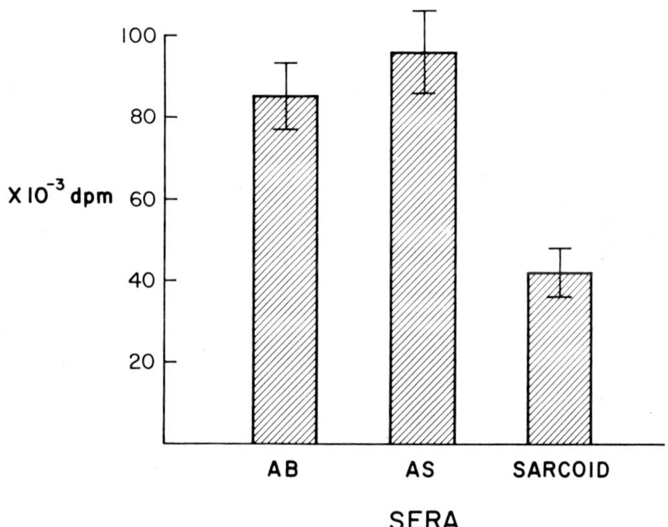

Figure 4 Effect of sarcoid sera on the proliferative response of normal human lymphocytes. DPM = disintegration per minute; AS = autologous serum; AB = pooled AB serum. Results are representative of eight experiments. The percent of inhibition ranged from 30 to 72% (unpublished results). Values equal mean ± SEM of an experiment performed in triplicate.

Recently, serum from sarcoid patients was also shown to suppress antibody responses as demonstrated by a plaque-forming assay (Izumi and Suginoshita 1980). Partial characterization of this factor showed that it was heat-stabile and not an immunoglobulin.

Although the identity and origin of these inhibitory mediators is unknown, they appear to act similarly to the regulatory factors which are liberated by and interact with the cells of the immune network.

VII. Possible Mechanisms of Humoral Abnormalities in Sarcoidosis

Table 3 summarizes the abnormalities of the humoral immune system in sarcoid. In general, there is a hyperreactivity of the B-cell system, which contrasts with the relative depression of the T-cell system. One explanation that may link these apparently discordant phenomena is that serum inhibitors or autoantibodies to T cells may be responsible for the functional alterations in the B cell system. As mentioned, B-cell proliferation and differentiation into immunoglobulin-secreting cells are modulated by the balance of helper and suppressor T cells. Thus, interference with suppressor T-cell and B-cell interaction might lead to exaggerated immunoglobulin responses. Conceivably, antibodies to suppressor T cells could account for the exaggerated response to antigens and elevations in serum immunoglobulins.

This possibility bears compelling similarities to certain collagen vascular diseases, such as systemic lupus erythematosus (SLE), in which there is B-cell

Table 3 Humoral (B-Cell) Abnormalities in Sarcoidosis

Polyclonal elevation of serum immunoglobulin

Exaggerated humoral response to certain antigens

High serum antibodies to
    Mycoplasma
    Virus (Epstein-Barr, rubella, parainfluenza, herpes simplex)

Autoantibodies to
    Rheumatoid factor
    Antinuclear antibody
    T cells

Circulating immune complexes

Decreased or normal number of B cells

Impaired B-cell function (blood)

hyperreactivity coupled with a depression in cell-mediated immunity. Recent studies have shown that in SLE there is a selective loss of T lymphocytes which is due to autoantibodies to suppressor T cells (Morimoto et al. 1980). The demonstration of antibodies to a fraction of T cells in sarcoidosis raises the possibility that a similar mechanism might exist. This possibility, however, remains to be examined.

There are several observations mentioned in Table 3 which apparently contradict the general pattern of humoral hyperresponsiveness. These include the normal or reduced numbers of circulating B cells and depressed B-cell function. The latter functional impairment can be completely or partially restored by removing adherent cells. Whether adherent cells (monocytes) are mediating the suppressive effect by secreting inhibitory molecules, such as prostaglandins, is not established. An alternative possibility involves an imbalance of regulatory T cells which has recently been demonstrated in the peripheral blood of sarcoid patients (Katz et al. 1978). For example, there is a relative increase in $T\gamma$ (suppressor) and a decrease in $T\mu$ (helper) lymphocytes.

But how does one then reconcile these facts with the hyperreactivity of the B-cell system? One explanation, which is receiving increasing support, is that the cells recovered from the blood of sarcoid patients do not validly reflect the immune inflammatory events occurring in this disease (Daniele et al. 1980, Crystal et al. 1981). Thus, to assess B-cell (and T-cell) function in sarcoid, it may be necessary to examine the antibody-generating plants or lymph nodes. In this context, the lung, which is involved in the majority of the cases of sarcoidosis, is also considered a semiautonomous lymphoid organ which generates both local humoral and cellular responses to inhaled antigens (Turner-Warwick 1978, Daniele 1980). In fact, when lung lymphocytes are recovered by lavage or surgical specimens from patients with sarcoid, there are more immunoglobulin-producing cells than in undiseased lungs (Lawrence et al. 1980, Hunninghake and Crystal 1981). These cells consist mainly of IgG and IgM classes (Hunninghake and Crystal 1981). Furthermore, there is a direct correlation between the number of bronchoalveolar T cells and the number of Ig-secreting cells (Hunninghake and Crystal 1981).

A recent preliminary observation, which bears on the finding of enhanced immunoglobulin production in the lung, is that increased numbers of helper T cells are recovered by bronchial lavage in sarcoid (Goldenheim et al. 1981, Hunninghake and Crystal 1982). The cells were identified by monoclonal antibodies directed to the specific membrane determinants of human helper T cells (OK4). Thus, in contrast to the blood, the ratio of helper to suppressor T cells is increased in the lung, favoring immunoglobulin production. Whether a similar situation exists in granulomatous lymph nodes is unknown.

It is unclear why there is an increased ratio of helper to suppressor T cells. One possibility is that serum inhibitors or lymphocyte autoantibodies are directed primarily at suppressor T cells and lead to such an imbalance. It should be emphasized, however, that it remains to be established whether cold-reactive autoantibodies to T cells in sarcoidosis play a significant role in vivo.

Another possibility to account for the immune imbalance is the presence of immune complexes. As shown in Figure 5, immune complexes

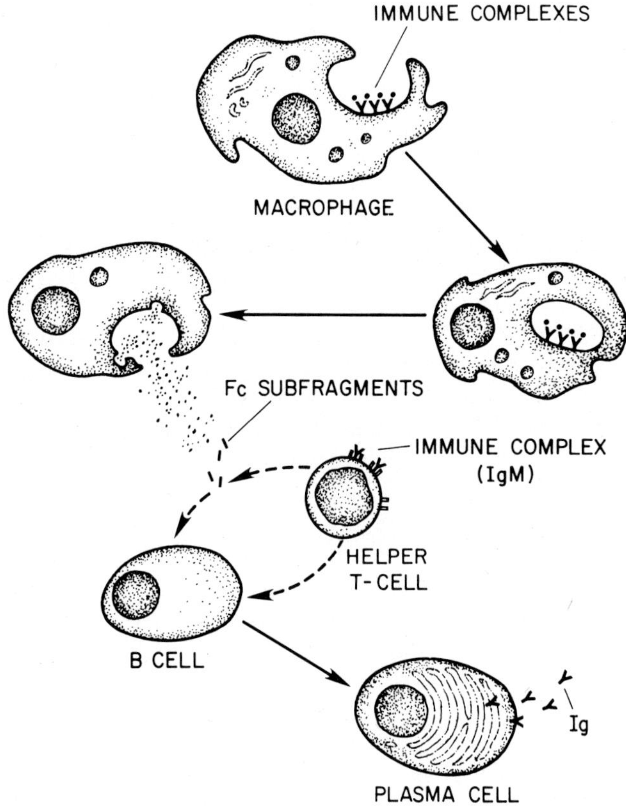

Figure 5 Mechanisms by which immune complexes may enhance B-cell function. Macrophages process immune complexes and release Fc subfragments which may stimulate helper T cells or B cells. IgM immune complexes may stimulate helper T cells. (Modified from Theofilopoulos and Dixon, 1980.)

may interact with several regulatory cell populations (Theofilopoulos and Dixon 1979, 1980). For example, macrophages may bind and process immune complexes, releasing Fc subfragments that stimulate helper T cells or B cells directly. Also, immune complexes containing IgM may react with the Fc receptor of Tμ or helper T cells causing the release of factors that facilitate proliferation and differentiation of B cells into plasma cells.

Clearly, these suggestions on the pathogenesis of humoral abnormalities are incomplete and largely speculative. They leave unanswered a number of important questions. For example, what are the origin and function of the suppressor monocytes and soluble inhibitors found in peripheral blood? Also, why is the ratio between helper and suppressor T cells in blood opposite to what is found in the lung? And finally, but of major importance, are these immunologic phenomena primary or secondary (epiphenomena) events which are involved in the granulomatous inflammation of sarcoidosis?

To answer these questions, it seems that efforts should be directed at the major foci of the inflammatory response, the lung and lymph nodes. Studies of the lymphocytes and accessory cells recovered from these sites may provide fresh insights into the pathogenesis of the disease and help clarify the nature of immune abnormalities.

References

Buckley, C. E., III, Nagaya, H., and Sieker, H. O. (1966). Altered immunologic activity in sarcoidosis. *Ann. Intern. Med.*, **64**:508–520.

Byrne, E. G., Evans, A. S., Fouts, D. W., and Israel, H. L. (1974). Serological hyperreactivity to Epstein-Barr virus and other viral antigens in sarcoidosis. In *Proceedings of the VIth International Conference on Sarcoidosis.* Edited by K. Iwai and Y. Hosoda. Baltimore, University Park Press, pp. 218–225.

Cantor, H., and Boyse, E. A. (1977a). Regulation of the immune response by T cell subclasses. *Contemp. Top. Immunobiol.*, **7**:47–67.

Cantor, H., and Boyse, E. A. (1977b). Regulation of cellular and humoral immune responses by T cell subclasses. *Cold Spring Harbor Symp. Quant. Biol.*, **41**:23–32.

Chapman, J. S., and Speight, M. (1964). Further studies of mycobacterial antibodies in the sera of sarcoidosis patients. *Acta Med. Scand., (Suppl.)*, **425**:61–67.

Crystal, R. G., Roberts, W. C., Hunninghake, G. W., Gadek, J. E., Fulmer, J. D., and Line, B. R. (1981). Pulmonary sarcoidosis: A disease characterized and perpetuated by activated lung T lymphocytes. *Ann. Intern. Med.*, **94**:73–94.

Daniele, R. P. (1980). Immune defenses of the lung. In *Pulmonary Diseases and Disorders.* Edited by A. P. Fishman. New York, McGraw-Hill, pp. 624–632.

Daniele, R. P., and Rowlands, D. T., Jr. (1976a). Lymphocyte subpopulations in sarcoidosis: Correlation with disease activity and duration. *Ann. Intern. Med.,* **85**:593–600.

Daniele, R. P., and Rowlands, D. T., Jr. (1976b). Antibodies to T cells in sarcoidosis. *Ann. NY Acad. Sci.,* **278**:88–110.

Daniele, R. P., McMillan, L. J., Dauber, J. H., and Rossman, M. D. (1978). Immune complexes in sarcoidosis. A correlation with activity and duration of disease. *Chest,* **74**:261–264.

Daniele, R. P., Dauber, J. H., and Rossman, M. D. (1980). Immunologic abnormalities in sarcoidosis. *Ann. Intern. Med.,* **92**:406–416.

Fernandez, B., Press, P., and Girard, J. P. (1976). Distribution and function of T and B cell subpopulations in sarcoidosis. *Ann. NY Acad. Sci.,* **278**:80–87.

Gershon, R. K. (1974). T cell control of antibody production. *Contemp. Top. Immunobiol.,* **3**:1–40.

Ghose, T., Landrigan, P., and Asif, A. (1974). Localization of immunoglobulin and complement in pulmonary sarcoid granulomas. *Chest,* **66**:264–268.

Goldenheim, P., Burton, R., Hurwitz, C., Kazemi, H., and Ginns, L. (1981). Identification of T cell subsets in sarcoidosis by monoclonal antisera and flow cytometry. *Am. Rev. Respir. Dis.,* (abstract), **123**(No. 4, Pt. 2): 58.

Goodwin, J. S., DeHoratius, R., Israel, H., Peake, G. T., and Messner, R. P. (1979). Suppressor cell function in sarcoidosis. *Ann. Intern. Med.,* **90**:169–173.

Gupta, R. C., Kueppers, F., DeRemee, R. A., Huston, K. A., and McDuffie, F. C. (1977). Pulmonary and extrapulmonary sarcoidosis in relation to circulating immune complexes. A quantification of immune complexes by two radioimmunoassays. *Am. Rev. Respir. Dis.,* **116**:261–266.

Hedfors, E., and Norberg, R. (1974). Evidence for circulating immune complexes in sarcoidosis. *Clin. Exp. Immunol.,* **16**:493–496.

Hedfors, E., Holm, G., and Petterson, D. (1974). Lymphocyte subpopulations in sarcoidosis. *Clin. Exp. Immunol.,* **17**:219–226.

Horsmanheimo, M., Jansson, E., Hannuksela, M., and Fudenberg, H. H. (1978). Studies in sarcoidosis: Intradermal mucoplasma test. *Am. Rev. Respir. Dis.,* **117**:975–979.

Hunninghake, G. W., and Crystal, R. G. (1981). Mechanisms of hypergammaglobulinemia in pulmonary sarcoidosis: Site of increased antibody production and role of T lymphocytes. *J. Clin. Invest.,* **67**:86–92.

Hunninghake, G. W., and Crystal, R. G. (1982). Pulmonary sarcoidosis, a disorder mediated by excessive helper T-lymphocyte activity at sites of disease activity. *N. Engl. J. Med.*, **305**:429–434.

Izumi, T., and Suginoshita, T. (1980). Plaque-forming cell response suppressive factor in sarcoidosis serum. In *Eighth International Conference on Sarcoidosis and Other Granulomatous Diseases.* Edited by W. J. Williams and B. H. Davies. Cardiff, Wales, Alpha Omega, pp. 449–458.

James, D. G., Neville, E., and Walker, A. (1975). Immunology of sarcoidosis. *Am. J. Med.*, **59**:388–394.

James, D. G., Neville, E., Siltzbach, L. E., Turiaf, J., Battesti, J. P., Sharma, O. P., Hosoda, Y., Mikami, R., Odaka, M., Villar, T. G., Djuric, B., Douglas, A. C., Middleton, W., Karlish, A., Blasi, A., Olivieri, D., and Press, P. (1976). A worldwide review of sarcoidosis. *Ann. NY Acad. Sci.* **278**:321–324.

Kataria, Y. P., Zafranas, A., and Sharma, H. M. (1978). Immunohistochemistry of human cutaneous sarcoidosis: A study of nine cases. *Hum. Pathol.*, **9**:517–522.

Katz, P., and Fauci, A. S. (1978). Inhibition of polyclonal B cell activation by suppressor monocytes in patients with sarcoidosis. *Clin. Exp. Immunol.*, **32**:554–562.

Katz, P., Haynes, B. F., and Fauci, A. S. (1978). Alteration of T lymphocyte subpopulations in sarcoidosis. *Clin. Immunol. Immunopathol.*, **10**:350–354.

Lawrence, E. C., Martin, R. R., Blaese, R. M., Teague, R. B., Awe, R. J., Wilson, R. K., Deaton, W. J., Bloom, K., Greenberg, S. D., and Stevens, P. M. (1980). Increased bronchoalveolar IgG-secreting cells in interstitial lung diseases. *N. Engl. J. Med.*, **302**:1186–1188.

Lobo, P. I., and Suratt, P. M. (1979). Studies on the autoantibody to lymphocytes in sarcoidosis. *J. Clin. Lab. Immunol.*, **1**:283–288.

Lobo, P. I., Westervelt, F. B., and Horwitz, D. A. (1975). Identification of two populations of immunoglobulin-bearing lymphocytes in man. *J. Immunol.*, **114**:116–119.

Mangi, R. J., Dwyer, J. M., and Kantor, F. S. (1974). The effect of plasma upon lymphocyte response in vitro. Demonstration of a humoral inhibitor in patients with sarcoidosis. *Clin. Exp. Immunol.*, **18**: 519–528.

Moretta, L., Webb, S. R., Grossi, C. E., Lydyard, P. M., and Cooper, M. D. (1977). Functional analysis of two human T cell subpopulations: Help and suppression of B cell responses by T cells bearing receptors for IgM or IgC. *J. Exp. Med.*, **146**:184–200.

Morimoto, C., Reinherz, E. L., Schlossman, S. F., Schur, P. H., Mills, J. A., and Steinberg, A. D. (1980). Alterations in immunoregulatory T cell subsets in active systemic lupus erythematosus. *J. Clin. Invest.*, **66**:1171–1174.

Mornex, J. F., Revillard, J. P., Vincent, C., Deteix, P., and Brune, J. (1979). Elevated serum β_2-microglobulin levels and C1q-binding immune complexes in sarcoidosis. *Biomedicine,* **31**:210–213.

Mustakallio, K. K., Vuopio, P., Videman, T., Venesmaa, P., and Putkonen, T. (1967). Immunoglobulins, haptoglobin and transferrin in sarcoidosis in relation to patients' Kveim reactivity and stage of the disease: An immuno-electrophoretic study. *Ann. Med. Intern. Fenniae,* **56**:19–21.

Oreskes, I., and Siltzbach, L. E. (1968). Changes in rheumatoid factor activity during the course of sarcoidosis. *Am. J. Med.,* **44**:60–67.

Reinherz, E. L., and Schlossman, S. F. (1980). Regulation of the immune response—Inducer and suppressor T lymphocyte subsets in human beings. *N. Engl. J. Med.,* **303**:370–373.

Roitt, I. M. (1981). *Essential Immunology,* 4th ed. Oxford, Blackwell.

Rossman, M. D., Dauber, J. H., and Daniele, R. P. (1978). Identification of activated T cells in sarcoidosis. *Am. Rev. Respir. Dis.,* **117**:713–720.

Rowlands, D. T., Jr., and Daniele, R. P. (1975). Surface receptors in the immune response. *N. Engl. J. Med.,* **293**:26–32.

Sands, J. H., Palmer, P. P., Mayock, R. L., and Creger, W. P. (1955). Evidence for serologic hyper-reactivity in sarcoidosis. *Am. J. Med.,* **19**:401–409.

Theofilopoulos, A. N., and Dixon, F. J. (1979). The biology and detection of immune complexes. *Adv. Immunol.,* **28**:89–220.

Theofilopoulos, A. N., and Dixon, F. J. (1980). Detection of immune complexes: Techniques and implications. *Hosp. Prac.,* **May**:107–121.

Theofilopoulos, A. N., Eisenberg, R. A., and Dixon, F. J. (1978). Isolation of circulating immune complexes using Raji cells: Separation of antigens from immune complexes and production of antiserum. *J. Clin. Invest.,* **61**:1570–1581.

Turner-Warwick, M. (1978). *Immunology of the Lung.* London, Edward Arnold, pp. 148–164.

Veien, N. K., Hardt, F., Bendixen, G., Ringsted, J., Brodthagen, H., Faber, V., Genner, J., Heckscher, T., Svejgaard, A., Sorensen, S. F., Wanstrup, J., and Wiik, A. (1976). Immunological studies in sarcoidosis: A comparison of disease activity and various immunological parameters. *Ann. NY Acad. Sci.,* **278**:47–51.

WHO Scientific Group (1977). The role of immune complexes in disease. Technical Series 606, Geneva, WHO, p. 5.

Zubler, R. H., and Lambert, P. H. (1977). Immune complexes in clinical investigation. In *Recent Advances in Clinical Immunology.* Edited by R. A. Thompson. New York, Churchill Livingstone, pp. 125–147.

Part Five

DIAGNOSTIC METHODS AND MEANS FOR FOLLOWING ACTIVITY OF SARCOIDOSIS

9

Bronchoalveolar Lavage in Sarcoidosis: An Approach for Assessing and Following Disease Activity

RONALD P. DANIELE, JAMES H. DAUBER,
and MILTON D. ROSSMAN

University of Pennsylvania School of Medicine
Philadelphia, Pennsylvania

I. Introduction

Although sarcoidosis can involve any organ, it has a striking predilection
for intrathoracic structures. In a large, worldwide study (James et al.
1976), close to 90% of cases had granulomas in lung, intrathoracic lymphoid
tissue, or both. It is also becoming appreciated that pulmonary involvement
may begin as diffuse mononuclear cell infiltration of alveolar septa and
airspaces (Rosen et al. 1978). These infiltrates may coalesce to form
discrete granulomas containing multinucleated giant cells. The inflammatory
process may proceed at variable rates in different parts of the lung. In
most cases, resolution occurs either spontaneously or with treatment, but
some cases culminate in fibrosis with destruction of the lung's gas exchanging
units.

This work was supported by the following grants from the National
Heart, Lung and Blood Institute: Young Investigator Award 1R23-HL-24500
(Dr. Rossman), Research Career Development Award 1K04-HL-00210
(Dr. Daniele), and grant R01-HL-23877.

Monitoring the activity of pulmonary inflammation in sarcoidosis by chest roentgenograms and pulmonary function tests is often unreliable. Because viable cells and soluble products from the lung can be recovered from the lung by lavage, this approach has been used to study the inflammatory events in sarcoidosis (Daniele et al. 1980, Crystal et al. 1981). In this chapter we will review the use of segmental bronchoalveolar lavage in sarcoidosis and indicate how it might be beneficial in evaluating patients with this disease.

II. Validity of Assessing Interstitial Lung Disease by Segmental Lavage

Several lines of evidence support the view that cells and soluble products recovered by segmental lavage may be used to assess the inflammatory activity in pulmonary parenchyma.

First, the types of cells obtained by *total* pulmonary lavage from experimental animals are similar to those recovered by segmental lavage from humans. For example, most cells recovered from several species (Gorenberg and Daniele 1976) and subhuman primates (Kazmierowski et al. 1976) are macrophages. The same is true for cells recovered from normal humans (Daniele et al. 1975, Daniele et al. 1979). Lymphocytes are also found in the lavage fluid from animals and man. That these cells are immunocompetent is demonstrated by their ability to proliferate when stimulated with mitogens and antigens and to synthesize antibodies in vitro (Daniele 1980). Thus, these cells can mount a local cellular or humoral immune response to antigens reaching the airways.

Second, using semiquantitative methods, it has been shown that the types and numbers of cells found in lavage fluid are similar to those found in the distal areas of the lung in several interstitital diseases, including idiopathic pulmonary fibrosis and sarcoidosis (Haslam et al. 1980, Hunninghake et al. 1981). Thus, the abnormalities in the distribution of cells recovered by bronchial lavage appear to reflect the cellularity found in the interstitium in each disease.

It should be emphasized, however, that correlations between the types and number of inflammatory cells recovered by lavage with those found in the interstitium are still preliminary. Uncertainties with respect to this approach involve (a) the need to quantify more precisely (e.g., by morphometric techniques) the number and type of inflammatory cells in the interstitium; (b) the contribution of the bronchi to cells found in lavage fluid (Rossman et al. 1981); and (c) sampling in interstitial diseases in which lesions are focal and nonrandomly distributed. Despite these reservations, it appears that types and numbers of cells recovered in lavage fluid of patients with sarcoidosis yield important information concerning the degree and progress of the parenchymal inflammatory response.

A. Methodological Considerations

Before discussing the results of lung lavage in sarcoidosis, it might be helpful to highlight some of the technical and procedural problems encountered in segmental bronchopulmonary lavage (Daniele and Dauber 1981). First we will discuss the bronchoscopic procedure itself and then review approaches to interpreting the results.

B. Lavage Procedure

Segmental lavage can be performed through a fiberoptic bronchoscopic or a balloon-tipped catheter. Since most lavages today are done with the bronchoscope, only this method will be addressed here.

Prior to bronchoscopy, subjects are premedicated with 0.4–0.6 mg atropine sulfate intramuscularly. Topical anesthesia of the nasal mucosa may be achieved with 2% viscous lidocaine and 4% lidocaine in isotonic saline (or other types of anesthetics with which the bronchoscopist is familiar). The bronchofiberscope is usually inserted transnasally and passed to the level of the hypopharynx. Topical anesthesia of the larynx is achieved by injecting 2% lidocaine through the aspiration channel. Anesthesia of the bronchial mucosa is achieved in the same way. The tip of the bronchoscope is advanced to a subsegmental middle or lower lobe bronchus. During insertion of the bronchoscope and final placement of the tip, it is usually more comfortable for the subject to be in a seated position. The tip of the bronchoscope is gently wedged into the bronchus.

Up to 300 ml of sterile isotonic saline is injected into the isolated subsegment in aliquots of 20–50 ml. Fluid may be injected at a rate of 5 ml/sec. Following each injection, fluid is recovered by aspiration and collected in a sterile 250-ml suction flask which is kept on ice. The flask is filled with 50 ml of Hanks' balanced salt solution (Grand Island Biological Company, Grand Island, NY) before collection of lavage fluid to provide nutritional support for the bronchoalveolar cells.

During the actual lavage procedure, the subject is in a recumbent position. This permits the use of lower aspiration pressures which appears to be important since viability of recovered cells is greater and contamination with columnar epithelial cells less when aspirating pressures are kept below minus 100 torr measured at the outlet of the trap. When such measures are employed, recovery of infused fluid usually exceeds 50% and viability of the aspirated cells is greater than 80%.

C. Complications of Bronchoalveolar Lavage

Fiberoptic bronchoscopy is a relatively safe procedure. The risks of
bronchoalveolar lavage derive primarily from insertion of the bronchoscope
(Gee and Fick 1980). Complications include reactions to the local
anesthesia (mainly tetracaine), injury to the laryngeal mucosa causing
laryngospasm, and hypoxemia during and after the procedure. The
hypoxemia associated with fiberoptic bronchoscopy may be exaggerated by
segmental lavage. Hypoxemia may also induce cardiac arrhythmias. In
about 10% of cases, there may be a transient fever with or without
infiltrates on chest roentgenogram. In most cases, this usually requires
only observation and symptomatic treatment. Rarely, a frank pneumonia
may develop.

To safeguard against these complications, all patients undergoing lavage
should have their vital signs and cardiac rhythm monitored throughout the
procedure and receive appropriate amounts of supplemental oxygen during
and after the procedure. Patients with severe pulmonary function impairment or unstable ischemic heart disease should be excluded from bronchoalveolar lavage studies.

D. Interpreting Lavage Data

Variation in the number of cells recovered results if the volume of fluid
instilled is not constant or if there is incomplete recovery of instilled fluid
for technical reasons (such as the subject coughing and expectorating lavage
fluid). To reduce variation from these causes, we have found it useful to
relate the cell yield to the volume of fluid recovered and express the result
as number of cells per volume (ml) of recovered lavage fluid.

Normalizing cell recovery by this method appears valid for several
reasons. First, as shown in Figure 1, the total number of cells correlates
well with the volume of lavage fluid recovered for healthy smoking and
nonsmoking subjects (Dauber et al. 1979, Daniele and Dauber 1981). A
similar relationship holds for patients with sarcoidosis ($r = 0.787$, $p <$
0.005). Second, the proportions of macrophages, lymphocytes, and neutrophils correlate poorly with the volume of lavage fluid recovered ($r < 0.4$ in
all cases). Third, the proportions of cells recovered from a single location
by repetitive lavage are similar (Weinberger et al. 1978). Finally, Davis
et al. (1978) found that when sequential boluses (60 ml) of lavage fluid
are introduced to the same site in the lung, the proportions of cells
(macrophages and lymphocytes) contained in the recovered fluid were
roughly comparable. Thus, a "small" lavage (120 ml) yields similar information about cell types as larger lavages (240 ml).

On the other hand, the concentration of soluble substances in lavage
fluid, such as protein, lipids, and carbohydrates, appears to depend on the

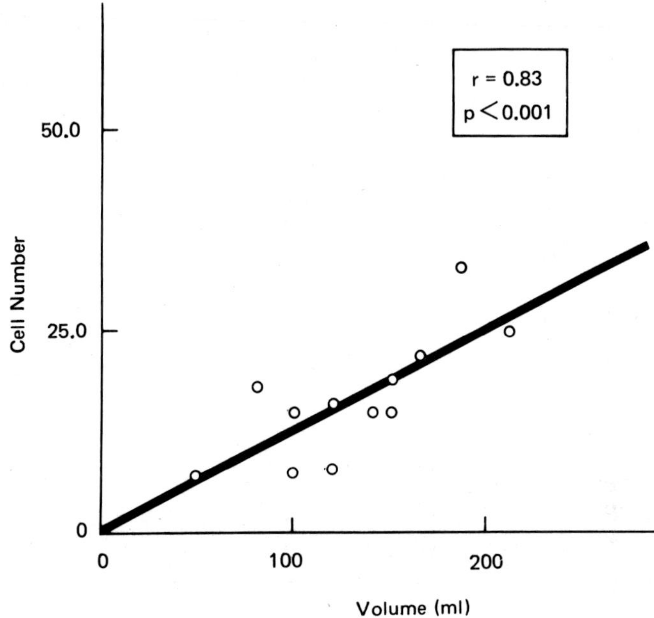

Figure 1 Correlation between number of cells recovered and volume of fluid aspirated for normal nonsmoking subjects. Similar results were obtained for asymptomatic smokers (data not shown). (From Daniele and Dauber [1981].)

volume of lavage fluid instilled (Davis et al. 1978). Thus, when results for soluble substances are reported, the volume of lavage fluid instilled and recovered should be equivalent and the values suitably standardized. Most investigators relate the concentration of a soluble substance, such as IgG, to the concentration of albumin in the lavage fluid (e.g., IgG:albumin ratio). Normalizing the concentration by relating it to the concentration of albumin also yields information on whether a given substance is actively or passively transported into the distal airways.

III. Results of Pulmonary Lavage in Sarcoidosis

In spite of variations in techniques and experimental approaches of lavage and study of bronchoalveolar cells, there is surprisingly good agreement in the results reported for sarcoidosis by investigators in the United States (Dauber et al. 1979, Hunninghake et al. 1979) and in Europe (Danel et al. 1979). In view of the unanimity of findings, we will present results which we have accumulated in the last 3 years to indicate the trends uncovered thus far. Since smoking affects the populations of bronchoalveolar cells (Daniele et al. 1979), results in smoking and nonsmoking patients with sarcoidosis must be compared with age-matched smoking and nonsmoking healthy subjects.

The cell recovery in nonsmoking sarcoidosis patients was increased compared to nonsmoking controls (Table 1). In contrast, no significant difference was noted when cell recovery from smoking patients with sarcoidosis was compared to smoking controls. It is noteworthy, however, that the yield of cells from nonsmoking and smoking patients with sarcoidosis was comparable. Also, recovery of lavage fluid and viability of the cells was similar in all groups (data not shown).

In nonsmoking patients with sarcoidosis there was a significant increase in the proportion of lung lymphocytes and a decrease in the proportion of macrophages compared to corresponding controls (Fig. 2). Similar results were obtained for smoking patients (not shown). The proportion of neutrophils in patients with sarcoidosis did not differ from that in controls and was comparable in nonsmoking and smoking patients with sarcoidosis (6 ± 2 vs. $2 \pm 0.3\%$, respectively).

Based on the cell recovery (Table 1) and distribution of bronchoalveolar cells (Fig. 2), lymphocyte yields in nonsmoking patients with sarcoidosis were markedly increased compared to controls. This also was

Table 1 Results of Lung Lavage Studies

	Normal (11 nonsmokers, 7 smokers)	Sarcoidosis (14 nonsmokers, 8 smokers)
Nonsmokers		
Cell yield	12.5 ± 1.4[a]	33 ± 5.9[b]
Macrophages	11 ± 1.3	23.2 ± 3.5[c]
Lymphocytes	1.1 ± 0.18	10.1 ± 3.6[b]
Smokers		
Cell yield	41.5 ± 5.7	30.3 ± 5.3[d]
Macrophages	38.6 ± 5.1	24 ± 3.9[c]
Lymphocytes	1.7 ± 0.33	5.6 ± 1.9[b]

[a]Values expressed at 10^4 cells/ml (mean $\pm$ SE).
[b]$p < 0.01$ (Students' t test).
[c]$p < 0.05$.
[d]$p > 0.05$ and not significant.

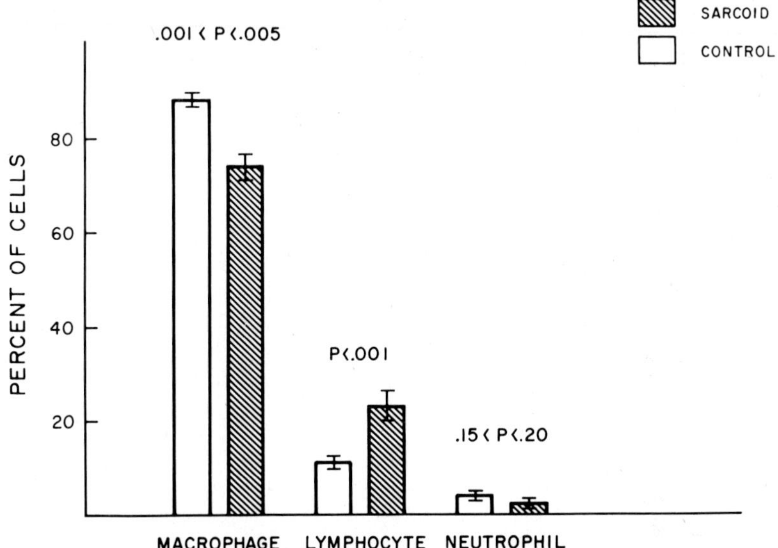

Figure 2 Results of differential cell counts of bronchoalveolar cells from nonsmoking patients with sarcoidosis and nonsmoking controls. Values are expressed as mean ± 1 SE percent of cells.

true for smoking patients with sarcoidosis (Table 1). Thus, increased numbers of lung lymphocytes are found in patients with active sarcoidosis, irrespective of the smoking history.

A. Lymphocyte Subpopulations in Lavage Fluid

In agreement with others (Hunninghake et al. 1979), we have found that the lymphocytosis in the bronchoalveolar airspaces of nonsmoking patients was due mainly to an increase of number of T cells (Dauber et al. 1979) (Fig. 3). On the other hand the proportion of B cells, determined by rosette formation with guinea pig red blood cells sensitized with antibody and complement (EAC rosettes), was normal. Similar results were found for patients with sarcoidosis who smoked (Fig. 3). Because of the increased recovery of total lymphocytes and the increased proportion of T cells in this population, the normalized recovery of T cells was increased four- to 10-fold.

The finding of increased numbers of T cells (and macrophages) in the lavage fluid of sarcoid patients lends credence to the hypothesis that the cells in the lavage fluid reflect the inflammatory events taking place in the

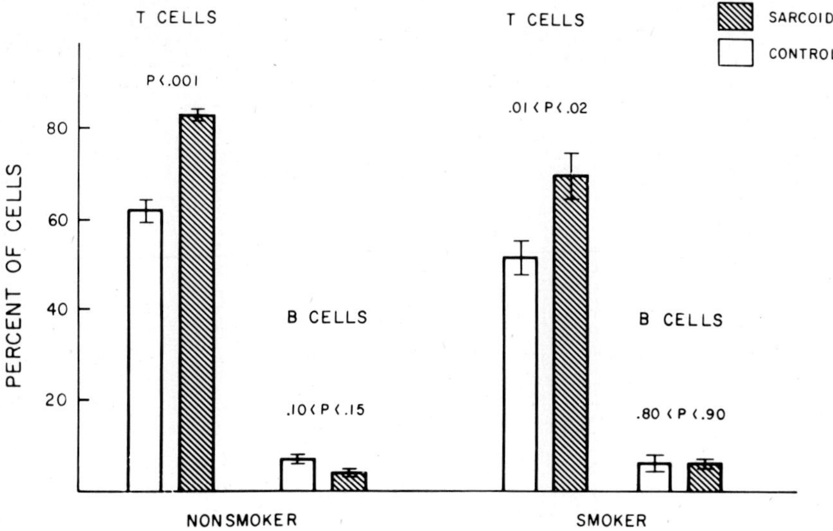

Figure 3 Subpopulations of bronchoalveolar lymphocytes in nonsmoking and smoking patients with sarcoidosis and corresponding controls. Values are expressed as mean ± 1 SE percent of total lymphocytes. [From Dauber, J. H., Rossman, M. D., and Daniele, R. P. (1979). Bronchoalveolar cell populations in acute sarcoidosis: Observations in smoking and non-smoking patients. *J. Lab. Clin. Med.*, **94**:862–871.]

lung parenchyma because this distribution of cell types is similar to what has been observed from lung biopsy specimens in patients with sarcoidosis (Hunninghake et al. 1981). Also, lymphocytes and macrophages are constituents of the interstitial infiltrates and granulomas of sarcoidosis.

Because granulomas are the hallmark of sarcoidosis, it has long been suspected that immunologic mechanisms play an important role in the pathogenesis of this disease. Additional support for an immunopathogenesis of sarcoidosis comes from the observation that increased numbers of activated T cells are recovered by lung lavage (Crystal et al. 1981, Dauber et al. 1979) (Fig. 4). Activated T cells in humans are identified by their ability to form stable rosettes with sheep erythrocytes at 37°C (Berger et al. 1976). These cells are increased in both smoking and nonsmoking patients with sarcoidosis, but in smoking patients, the increase is of borderline significance when compared to smoking controls (Dauber et al. 1979).

Lymphocytes that form stable rosettes at 37°C have an atypical structure by light and electron microscopy (Berger et al. 1976). Cells

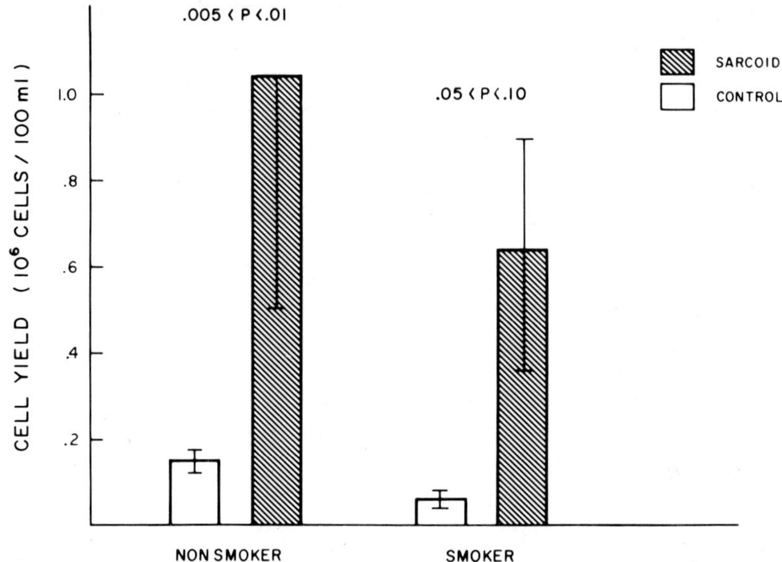

Figure 4 The yield of $37°$ E rosettes (activated T cells) in nonsmoking and smoking patients with sarcoidosis compared to corresponding controls. Values are expressed as the mean ± 1 SE number of cells per 100 ml of lavage fluid recovered. [From Dauber, J. H., Rossman, M. D., and Daniele, R. P. (1979). Bronchoalveolar cell populations in acute sarcoidosis: Observations in smoking and non-smoking patients. *J. Lab. Clin. Med.,* **94**:862–871.]

with similar morphological features are found in active lesions of sarcoidosis, particularly granulomas. Functionally, activated T cells appear to be stimulated from the resting state of the cell cycle (i.e., G_0) and committed to cell division (Rossman and Daniele, unpublished). This may explain why some lymphocytes recovered from blood and bronchoalveolar lavage divide spontaneously and release macrophage migration inhibition factor (Kataria et al. 1976) and chemotactic factors for monocytes (Hunninghake et al. 1980).

Other characteristics of activated T cells may be relevant to the pathogenesis of inflammatory lesions in sarcoidosis. For example, lymphocytes that are activated or stimulated by antigens or mitogens do not recirculate from blood to lymph but migrate preferentially to inflammatory foci. In addition, these cells possess enhanced effector functions, such as lymphokine production. Thus, the finding of increased numbers of T cells which form 37° rosettes in sarcoidosis raises the possibility that a population of activated lymphocytes plays an important role in the lungs' interstitial inflammatory response. Quantification of this cell population may also prove to be a sensitive measure of disease activity.

B. Comparison of Cell Populations in Lung and Blood

Comparison of lymphocyte populations in the lavage fluid and peripheral blood of patients with sarcoidosis reveals both similarities and differences (Daniele et al. 1980). As noted above, the number of lymphocytes and T cells is increased in lavage fluid, but in blood there usually is a lymphopenia due predominantly to a reduction in the number of T cells (Table 2) (Daniele and Rowlands 1976). In some cases the number of B cells in peripheral blood is normal, but in others it is reduced. In spite of the marked T-cell lymphopenia, the percentage and absolute number of activated T cells are increased (Rossman et al. 1978). There is a good correlation between the number of activated T cells in the lung and peripheral blood, which suggests that activated T cells in peripheral blood may be in transit to or derived from inflamed lung or other involved organs. Such a finding is not specific for sarcoidosis because activated T cells are also found in the peripheral blood of patients with acute lympho-

Table 2 Peripheral Blood Studies

	Sarcoidosis (n = 22)	Normal (n = 25)
Lymphocytes	1572 ± 110[a]	2179 ± 131[b]
T cells		
Number	925 ± 94	1504 ± 108[b]
Percent	58 ± 3.9	69 ± 1.9[c]
Activated T cells (37° rosettes)		
Number	126.0 ± 25.3	55.8 ± 7.8[b]
Percent	8.8 ± 1.6	2.7 ± 0.4[b]
B cells (EAC)		
Number	241 ± 47.5	304 ± 32 (NS)[d]
Percent	15.1 ± 2.7	14.5 ± 1.7 (NS)[d]

[a]Cells/mm^3 (mean $\pm$ SE).
[b]$p < 0.001$ (determined by Students' t test).
[c]$p < 0.01$.
[d]NS = not significant.

blastic leukemia (Borella and Sen 1975) and chronic hepatitis (Galili et al. 1975).

The differences in results of lymphocyte subpopulations in lung and blood underscore a point made earlier that future inquiries into the immune pathogenesis of sarcoidosis should be aimed at studying the immune cells present at the sites of active inflammation, particularly the lung.

C. IgG Levels in Lavage Fluid

As discussed in Chapter 8, serum IgG is consistently elevated in patients with sarcoidosis. Similarly, the concentration of IgG in lavage fluid appears to be elevated, as evidenced by an increased IgG:albumin ratio in patients compared to controls (Reynolds et al. 1977, Weinberger et al. 1978). The ratio of IgG:albumin in lavage fluid of patients with sarcoidosis exceeds that in their serum, suggesting that some of the IgG present in lavage fluid is secreted rather than passively transported into the distal airspaces. Support for this hypothesis comes from the recent observation that the number of cells recovered by lavage that secrete IgG and IgM in vitro is increased in patients with sarcoidosis compared to normals (Hunninghake and Crystal 1981).

D. Comparison of Bronchoalveolar Cells and Secretions in Interstitial Lung Diseases

The cells and proteins in bronchoalveolar lavage fluid from patients with other interstitial lung diseases have also been analyzed (Reynolds et al. 1977, Weinberger et al. 1978). The findings for hypersensitivity pneumonitis, idiopathic pulmonary fibrosis, and sarcoidosis are compared in Table 3. Although there are distinct patterns in the distribution and numbers of cell types, there is some overlap between diseases, particularly for sarcoidosis and hypersensitivity pneumonitis. In general the total number of cells recovered by lavage is increased in patients with these interstitial lung diseases compared to normal nonsmokers. There is a significant increase in the proportion and number of lymphocytes in lavage fluid in both sarcoidosis and hypersensitivity pneumonitis, but the proportion of lymphocytes is greater in the latter disease. In contrast, in idiopathic pulmonary fibrosis, the proportion of lymphocytes is usually normal (or slightly increased), but the proportion and number of neutrophils are markedly increased. Neutrophils may be normal or slightly increased in sarcoidosis and hypersensitivity pneumonitis, but they are substantially less in these diseases than in idiopathic pulmonary fibrosis.

IgG levels (IgG:albumin ratio) are elevated in all of these fibrotic diseases, but the greatest increase occurs in hypersensitivity pneumonitis.

Table 3 Bronchopulmonary Lavage: Cells and Secretions in Interstitial Lung Disease[a]

	Sarcoidosis	Hypersensitivity pneumonitis	Idiopathic fibrosis
Cell yield	↑	↑	↑
Alveolar macrophages[b]	↓	↓↓	↓
Lymphocytes[b]	↑	↑↑	N
Neutrophils[b]	N-↑	N-↑	↑↑
IgG:albumin	↑	↑	↑
IgM:albumin	A	+	A

[a]↑ = increase; ↓ = decrease; N = normal values; A = absent; + = present.
[b]Designations represent percentage changes.
Source: Daniele et al. (1980).

A unique feature of hypersensitivity pneumonitis is the finding of an elevated IgM:albumin ratio in lavage fluid; IgM is rarely detected in lavage fluid of normal subjects or patients with idiopathic pulmonary fibrosis.

A distinctive finding in the lavage fluid of patients with sarcoidosis is the spontaneous binding of lymphocytes to alveolar macrophages (macrophage-lymphocyte rosettes) (Yeager et al. 1977). The specificity and importance of the increased numbers of macrophage-lymphocyte rosettes are not established, but this finding lends support to the idea that the pathogenesis of the inflammation in sarcoidosis is related to interaction of macrophages with lymphocytes.

IV. Comparison of Lavage Results with Clinical Activity and Extent of Disease

There is general agreement that the number of lymphocytes recovered in bronchoalveolar lavage fluid correlates with disease activity in sarcoidosis. In patients who clearly have inactive disease, the proportion and number of lymphocytes recovered by lavage is normal (Crystal et al. 1981, Reynolds and Merrill 1979). In these patients, IgG levels (Reynolds and Merrill 1979) and the number of IgG-secreting cells (Hunninghake and Crystal 1981) in lavage fluid are also normal. The extent of pulmonary involvement may also correlate with the number of lymphocytes recovered in bronchoalveolar fluid. As shown in Figure 5, significantly greater numbers of lymphocytes were recovered from patients with stage II versus stage I disease (Rossman et al. 1982).

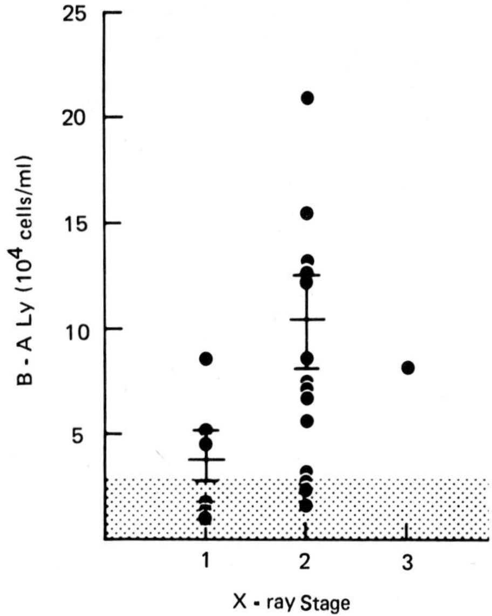

Figure 5 X-ray stage versus recovery of bronchoalveolar lymphocytes in 22 patients with newly diagnosed or active sarcoidosis. The hatched areas are the normal means ± 2 SD. Patients with stage II sarcoidosis had a greater lymphocytosis than did stage I patients (p < 0.02). (From Rossman et al. 1982).

Longitudinal studies correlating cells and secretions recovered in sequential lavages with progression or resolution of disease are more limited. Preliminary results, however, suggest that as disease resolves either spontaneously or as the result of steroid therapy, the number of lymphocytes recovered by bronchoalveolar lavage returns to normal (Crystal et al. 1981). These findings further support the notion that the degree of lymphocytosis in lavage fluid mirrors the intensity of the lung's inflammatory response in sarcoidosis.

V. Comparison of Lavage Results with Other Measures of Disease Activity

Additional support for the idea that the lymphocytosis in lavage fluid reflects the intensity of disease activity comes from correlative studies of cells in lavage fluid with gallium scanning and measurements of serum angiotensin enzyme activity.

The use of gallium scanning to evaluate inflammatory activity in sarcoidosis (and other interstitial lung diseases) will be discussed later (Chapter 12). It is noteworthy, however, that there is a good correlation between gallium uptake in the lung and the proportion of T lymphocytes recovered by bronchial lavage (Line et al. 1981). There is also good agreement between the level of gallium uptake in the lung and the degree of pulmonary inflammation as reflected in the cellularity of lung biopsy specimens (Niden et al. 1976).

Serum angiotensin-converting enzyme (ACE) activity is increased in many patients with active sarcoidosis (Lieberman 1975, Fanburg et al. 1976). In these patients it may also be useful in monitoring disease activity (DeRemee and Rohrbach 1980). Although this will be discussed in greater detail (Chapter 10), it is appropriate to mention here results of recent studies in which the number of lymphocytes recovered in broncho-alveolar lavage fluid was compared with the levels of serum angiotensin-converting enzyme (Stanislas-Leguern et al. 1979, Rossman et al. 1982). For patients with newly diagnosed disease, there was a good correlation between the number of lymphocytes recovered by lavage and the level of ACE in the serum (Fig. 6). In all cases in which ACE was elevated, the recovery of lymphocytes was increased (Rossman et al. 1982). On the other hand, 10 patients whose serum ACE values were normal had an increased recovery of lung lymphocytes. Thus, serum ACE may be normal

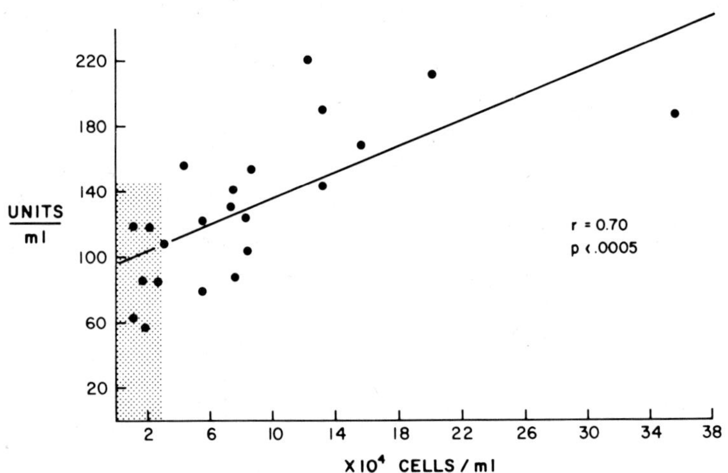

Figure 6 Recovery of bronchoalveolar lymphocytes versus serum-angiotensin-converting enzyme (SACE) activity. Bronchoalveolar lymphocytes are expressed as 10^4 cells/ml of lavage fluid recovered. SACE activity was measured by a radiochemical assay based on the release of tritiated hippuric acid from tritiated hippuryl glycylglycine (Rohatgi and Ryan 1980) and expressed as units/ml of serum. The hatched area is the normal mean ± 2 SD. The points represent the values found in 22 patients (smokers and nonsmokers) with newly diagnosed or active sarcoidosis. (From Rossman et al. 1982).

in patients with active disease. This finding suggests that the number of lymphocytes recovered by segmental lavage may be a more sensitive indicator of disease activity than serum ACE.

VI. Prospect

Besides determining the etiologic agent(s) in sarcoidosis, other major problems facing physicians who deal with this disease are finding reliable and precise methods for defining disease activity and developing effective forms of therapy. The quantification of cell types recovered by broncho-alveolar lavage appears to be one approach for measuring disease activity. Nonetheless, several questions about the use of this procedure remain to be answered. First, is it a sensitive measure of disease activity in all patients with sarcoidosis, *particularly* those with long-standing disease and fibrosis? Second, how can it be used most effectively in combination with less invasive measures of disease activity, such as serum angiotensin-converting enzyme activity or gallium scanning? And third, when and how often should bronchoalveolar lavage be repeated to define disease activity? Answers to these questions will provide a more rational basis for manage-ment of the disease, especially with respect to the need for and response to therapy.

References

Berger, B. M., Schuman, R. K., Daniele, R. P., and Nowell, P. C. (1976). E rosette formation at 37°C: A property of mitogen-stimulated human peripheral blood lymphocytes. *Cell. Immunol.,* **26**:105–113.

Borella, L., and Sen, L. (1975). E receptors on blasts from untreated acute lymphocytic leukemia (ALL): Comparison of temperature dependence of E rosettes formed by normal and leukemic lymphoid cells. *J. Immunol.,* **114**:187–190.

Crystal, R. G., Roberts, W. C., Hunninghake, G. W., Gadek, J. E., Fulmer, J. D., and Line, B. R. (1981). Pulmonary sarcoidosis: A disease characterized and perpetuated by activated lung T lymphocytes. *Ann. Intern. Med.,* **94**:73–94.

Danel, C., Arnoux, A., Marsac, J., Basset, F., and Chretien, J. (1979). Données cellulaires approtées par le lavage broncho-alveolaire (L.B.A.) au cours de diverses pathologies interstitielles. *INSERM,* **84**:489–498.

Daniele, R. P. (1980). Immune defenses of the lung. In *Pulmonary Diseases and Disorders.* Edited by A. P. Fishman. New York, McGraw-Hill, pp. 624–632.

Daniele, R. P., and Dauber, J. H. (1981). Collection and enrichment of human alveolar macrophages. In *Manual of Macrophage Methodology.* Edited by H. B. Herscowitz, H. T. Holden, J. A. Bellanti, and A. Ghaffar. New York, Marcel Dekker, pp. 23–30.

Daniele, R. P., Altose, M. D., and Rowlands, D. T., Jr. (1975). Immuno-competent cells from the lower respiratory tract of normal human lungs. *J. Clin. Invest.,* **56**:986–995.

Daniele, R. P., Dauber, J. H., and Rossman, M. D. (1979). Lymphocyte populations in the bronchoalveolar air spaces: Recent observations in asymptomatic smokers and non-smokers. *INSERM,* **84**:193–210.

Daniele, R. P., Dauber, J. H., and Rossman, M. D. (1980). Immunologic abnormalities in sarcoidosis. *Ann. Intern. Med.,* **92**:406–416.

Daniele, R. P., and Rowlands, D. T., Jr. (1976). Lymphocyte subpopulations in sarcoidosis: Correlation with disease activity and duration. *Ann. Intern. Med.,* **85**:593–600.

Dauber, J. H., Rossman, M. D., and Daniele, R. P. (1979). Broncho-alveolar cell populations in acute sarcoidosis: Observations in smoking and non-smoking patients. *J. Lab. Clin. Med.,* **94**:862–871.

Davis, G. S., Low, R. B., and Visco, G. (1978). Comparative analysis of sequential samples in human pulmonary lavage. *Am. Rev. Respir. Dis.,* **117**:327 (abstr.).

DeRemee, R. A., and Rohrbach, M. S. (1980). Serum angiotensin-converting enzyme activity in evaluating the clinical course of sarcoidosis. *Ann. Intern. Med.,* **92**:361–365.

Fanburg, B. L., Schoenberger, M. D., Bachus, B., and Snider, G. L. (1976). Elevated serum angiotensin I converting enzyme in sarcoidosis. *Am. Rev. Respir. Dis.,* **114**:525–528.

Galili, U., Eliakim, M., Slavin, S., and Schlesinger, M. (1975). Lymphocyte subpopulations in chronic active hepatitis: Increase in lymphocytes forming stable E rosettes. *Clin. Immunol. Immunopathol.,* **4**:538–544.

Gee, J. B. L., and Fick, R. B., Jr. (1980). Bronchoalveolar lavage (editorial). *Thorax,* **35**:1–8.

Gorenberg, D. J., and Daniele, R. P. (1976). Characterization of immuno-competent cells recovered from the respiratory tract and tracheo-bronchial lymph nodes of normal guinea pigs. *Am. Rev. Respir. Dis.,* **114**:1099–1105.

Haslam, P. L., Turton, C. W. G., Heard, B., Lukoszek, A., Collins, J. V., Salsbury, A. J., and Turner-Warwick, M. (1980). Bronchoalveolar lavage in pulmonary fibrosis: Comparison of cells obtained with lung biopsy and clinical features. *Thorax,* **35**:9–18.

Hunninghake, G. W., and Crystal, R. G. (1981). Mechanisms of hyper-gammaglobulinemia in pulmonary sarcoidosis. Site of increased antibody production and role of T lymphocytes. *J. Clin. Invest.,* **67**:86–92.

Hunninghake, G. W., Fulmer, J. D., Young, R. C., Jr., Gadek, J. E., and Crystal, R. G. (1979). Localization of the immune response in sarcoidosis. *Am. Rev. Respir. Dis.,* **120**:49–57.

Hunninghake, G. W., Gadek, J. E., Young, R. C., Jr., Kawanami, O., Ferrans, V. J., and Crystal, R. G. (1980). Maintenance of granuloma formation in pulmonary sarcoidosis by T lymphocytes within the lung. *N. Engl. J. Med.,* **302**:594–598.

Hunninghake, G. W., Kawanami, O., Ferrans, V. J., Young, R. C., Jr., Roberts, W. C., and Crystal, R. G. (1981). Characterization of the inflammatory and immune effector cells in the lung parenchyma of patients with interstitial lung disease. *Am. Rev. Respir. Dis.,* **123**: 407–412.

James, D. G., Neville, E., Siltzbach, L. E., Turiaf, J., Battesti, J. P., Sharma, O. P., Hosoda, Y., Mikami, R., Odaka, M., Villar, T. G., Djuric, B., Douglas, A. C., Middleton, W., Karlish, A., Blasi, A., Olivieri, D., and Press, P. (1976). A worldwide review of sarcoidosis. *Ann. N.Y. Acad. Sci.,* **278**:321–324.

Kataria, Y. P., LoBuglio, A. F., and Bromberg, P. A. (1976). Sarcoid lymphocytes: Spontaneous transformation and release of macrophage migration inhibition activity. *Am. Rev. Respir. Dis.,* **113**:315–323.

Kazmierowski, J. A., Fauci, A. S., and Reynolds, H. Y. (1976). Characterization of lymphocytes in bronchial lavage fluid from monkeys. *J. Immunol.,* **116**:615–618.

Lieberman, J. (1975). Elevation of serum angiotensin-converting enzyme (ACE) level in sarcoidosis. *Am. J. Med.,* **59**:365–372.

Line, B. R., Hunninghake, G. W., Keogh, B. A., Jones, A. E., Johnston, G. S., and Crystal, R. G. (1981). Gallium-67 scanning to stage the alveolitis of sarcoidosis: Correlation with clincal studies, pulmonary function studies, and bronchoalveolar lavage. *Am. Rev. Respir. Dis.,* **123**:440–446.

Niden, A. H., Mishkin, F. S., and Khurana, M. L. (1976). [67]Gallium citrate lung scans in interstitial lung disease. *Chest,* **69**:266–268.

Reynolds, H. Y., Fulmer, J. D., Kazmierowski, J. A., Roberts, W. C., Frank, M. M., and Crystal, R. G. (1977). Analysis of cellular and protein content of broncho-alveolar lavage fluid from patients with idiopathic pulmonary fibrosis and chronic hypersensitivity pneumonitis. *J. Clin. Invest.,* **59**:165–175.

Reynolds, H. Y., and Merrill, W. W. (1979). Analysis of bronchoalveolar lavage in normal humans and patients with diffuse interstitial lung diseases. *INSERM,* **84**:227–250.

Rohatgi, P. K., and Ryan, J. W. (1980). Simple radioassay for measuring serum activity of angiotensin-converting enzyme in sarcoidosis. *Chest,* **78**:69–76.

Rosen, Y., Athanassiades, T. J., Moon, S., and Lyons, H. A. (1978). Non-granulomatous interstitial pneumonitis in sarcoidosis: Relationship to the development of epithelioid granulomas. *Chest,* **74**:122–125.

Rossman, M. D., Dauber, J. H., and Daniele, R. P. (1978). Identification of activated T cells in sarcoidosis. *Am. Rev. Respir. Dis.,* **117**:713–720.

Rossman, M. D., Dauber, J. H., Cardillo, M. E., and Daniele, R. P. (1982). Pulmonary sarcoidosis: Correlation of serum angiotensin-converting enzyme with blood and bronchoalveolar lymphocytes. *Am. Rev. Respir. Dis.,* **125**:366–369.

Rossman, M. D., Daniele, R. P., and Dauber, J. H. (1981). Nodular endobronchial sarcoidosis: A study comparing blood and lung lymphocytes. *Chest,* **79**:427–431.

Stanislas-Leguern, G., Marsac, J., Arnoux, A., and Lecossier, D. (1979). Serum angiotensin-converting enzyme and bronchoalveolar lavage in sarcoidosis. *Lancet,* **1**:723.

Weinberger, S. E., Kelman, J. A., Elson, N. A., Young, R. C., Jr., Reynolds, H. Y., and Fulmer, J. D. (1978). Bronchoalveolar lavage in interstitial lung disease. *Ann. Intern. Med.,* **89**:459–466.

Yeager, H., Jr., Williams, M. C., Beekman, J. F., Bayly, T. C., Beaman, B. L., and Hawley, R. J. (1977). Sarcoidosis: Analysis of cells obtained by bronchial lavage. *Am. Rev. Respir. Dis.,* **116**:951–955.

10

Serum Angiotensin 1-Converting Enzyme in the Diagnosis and Determination of Activity of Sarcoidosis

BARRY L. FANBURG

New England Medical Center Hospital
Tufts University School of Medicine
Boston, Massachusetts

I. General

The finding of an elevation of angiotensin 1-converting enzyme in serum of patients with sarcoidosis was first reported by Lieberman in 1974 (Lieberman 1974). Subsequently, this observation was confirmed by a large number of other laboratories (Table 1). The percentage of patients with sarcoidosis with levels of angiotensin 1-converting enzyme greater than 2 standard deviations above the control mean as measured by these laboratories varies from 34 to 88%. Hence, the sensitivity of this testing procedure for sarcoidosis is variable, and there is obviously a high incidence of false negative results.

The reason for the large variability in sensitivity is unclear since most laboratories doing this assay have used a similar synthetic substrate, hippuryl-l-histidyl-l-leucine, despite the differences in physical techniques for the assay, such as spectrophotometry (Cushman and Cheung 1971a), fluorimetry (Friedland and Silverstein 1976a), or radioisotope counting (Rohrbach and DeRemee 1979). Although there is a potential problem that the assay may measure peptidases other than angiotensin 1-converting enzyme, this does not seem to be the case for serum under the conditions

Table 1 Serum Angiotensin 1-Converting Enzyme in Sarcoidosis

Reference	No. of subjects tested		Serum level (nmol/min/ml ± SD)	Percent elevated > 2 SD
Lieberman (1975)	Sarcoid	17	13.67 ± 2.26[a]	88.2
	Control	172	7.6 ± 2.0[a]	
Lieberman (1976)	Sarcoid	64	15.76 ± 7.4[a]	83
	Control	172	7.6 ± 2.0[a]	
Silverstein et al. (1976a)	Sarcoid	58	48.3 ± 4.8 (SEM)	43
	Control	63	28.6 ± 0.94 (SEM)	
Fanburg et al. (1976)	Sarcoid	56	52.7 ± 24.4	48
	Control	84	28.2 ± 11.3	
Studdy et al. (1978)	Sarcoid	90	55 ± 23	43–48
	Control	80	34 ± 9	
Rohrback and DeRemee (1979)	Sarcoid	42	71.9 ± 19.2	79
	Control	60	40.2 ± 8.6	
Khoury et al. (1979)	Sarcoid	26	35.5 ± 10.7	81
	Control	18	17.4 ± 4.6	
Rømer (1979)	Sarcoid	85	38.4 ± 14.4	41
	Control	116	24.4 ± 6.2	
Gupta et al. (1979)	Sarcoid	80	46.2 ± 20.6 (untreated)	67 (untreated)
			38.1 ± 23.1 (treated)	
	Control	55	26.8 ± 4.8	

[a]Values should be multiplied by a factor of 3 due to incorrect calculation in the report.

of the assay (Fanburg et al. 1976, Oparil et al. 1976). Part of the variability in sensitivity of the test could be related to the variable criteria used in establishing a diagnosis of sarcoidosis, but this seems unlikely since criteria were stringent in most studies.

II. Elevation of Angiotensin 1-Converting Enzyme in Other Diseases

With the exception of some diseases unlikely to be clinically confused with sarcoidosis, such as Gaucher's disease (Lieberman and Beutler 1976, Silverstein and Friedland 1977), leprosy (Lieberman and Rea 1977), occasional cases of miliary tuberculosis (Thomas et al. 1979), idiopathic respiratory distress syndrome of the newborn infant (Mattioli et al. 1975), and primary biliary cirrhosis (Studdy et al. 1978), an elevated serum level of angiotensin 1-converting enzyme appears to be relatively specific for sarcoidosis. An exception may occur for patients with silicosis and asbetosis. Gröhagen-Riska and associates (1980) reported that 7 of 22 patients with silicosis and three of 18 with asbestosis had elevated levels of serum angiotensin 1-converting enzyme. Yotsumoto and associates (1980) reported elevations in patients with silicosis and liver cirrhosis. Also, other occasional isolated exceptions have been reported (Abboy et al. 1980). The enzyme has been found to be within normal limits in sera of a large number of patients with other diseases that may cause diagnostic confusion with sarcoidosis. These include tuberculosis, lymphoma, pulmonary neoplasm, inflammatory bowel disease, granulomatous hepatitis (Lieberman 1975, 1976, Silverstein et al. 1976a, Fanburg et al. 1976, Studdy et al. 1978) and beryllium disease (Sprince et al. 1980).

III. Source of Angiotensin 1-Converting Enzyme

Two questions have arisen repeatedly concerning the elevated angiotensin 1-converting enzyme in sera of patients with sarcoidosis: (a) What is the source of this increased enzyme? and (b) Do levels of angiotensin 1-converting enzyme in serum reflect the "activity" of sarcoidosis? Answers to these questions require some background information about the biology and biochemistry of angiotensin 1-converting enzyme.

The site of production of serum angiotensin 1-converting enzyme in normal individuals is not currently known. This enzyme, which catalyzes the conversion of angiotensin 1 to vasoactive angiotensin 2 and inactivates bradykinin by its dipeptidyl hydrolase activity, is known to be located on, or in, several cells of the body. The primary location appears to be the endothelial cell, where the enzyme is present on the plasma membrane, an advantageous site for direct contact with substrates in the plasma (Smith and Ryan 1973, Ryan et al. 1975, Caldwell et al. 1976). The large amount of the enzyme in lung is probably due to the large surface area of the pulmonary vasculature. The enzyme is also present to a lesser extent in pulmonary macrophages (Friedland et al. 1977) and appears to be associated with fibroblasts (Rubin and Dobbs 1979, Weinberg et al. 1982). It has been localized on epithelial cells of the proximal tubule of the kidney (Ward et al. 1977) and on brush borders of gut epithelium (Wigger and Stalcup 1978, Ward et al. 1980). Although found in high concentrations in testes and epididymous (Cushman and Cheung 1971b), the cellular localization in these organs has not been established. There has been no clear demonstration that any of these cells are able to secrete the enzyme actively under physiologic conditions. Also, concentration of the enzyme is low in the liver (Cushman and Cheung 1971b), and this organ has not been demonstrated to be a source of its production.

It is possible that the epithelioid cell, or some variant of this cell, is the source of the elevated serum angiotensin 1-converting enzyme in sarcoidosis. Lymph nodes from patients with sarcoidosis have high levels of the enzyme (Silverstein et al. 1976a, 1976b, 1977, 1979) and show immunohistochemical positively for the enzyme (Pertschuk et al. 1980). Cultured cells from lymph nodes of patients with sarcoidosis have been reported to release increased amounts of the enzyme into culture medium as compared to normal lymph nodes (Okabe et al. 1980). It may be that the source of the elevated enzyme in sera of patients with sarcoidosis differs from that of normal subjects. However, no qualitative differences have so far been demonstrated between the enzyme in normal serum and that in serum of patients with sarcoidosis (Friedland and Silverstein 1976a). No studies have been done to exclude the possibility that elevated levels of serum angiotensin 1-converting enzyme in sarcoidosis may represent a decrease in degradation of the enzyme. There is no information about the turnover of serum angiotensin 1-converting enzyme.

Some attempts have been made to evaluate levels of angiotensin 1-converting enzyme from sources other than the serum in patients with sarcoidosis. The enzyme has been assessed in materials from bronchial lavage, and it has been found to be elevated in bronchoalveolar macrophages (Hinman et al. 1979) but not in noncellular material from the lavage. The elevation in macrophages may be relevant to that in serum in sarcoidosis if a "macrophage-like" cell is the source of the elevated enzyme. However, it is curious that there is no elevation in bronchoalveolar lavage noncellular material if secretion of enzyme by the macrophage is playing a role in its elevation in serum. Hence, the source of elevated enzyme in serum in sarcoidosis remains uncertain. In normal individuals, the concentration of angiotensin 1-converting enzyme is elevated relative to albumin in noncellular lavage material as compared to that of serum (Lanzillo and Fanburg 1979). This finding suggests a selective secretory mechanism by some cell in the airways, but its relevance to sarcoidosis is currently unknown.

If elevated angiotensin 1-converting enzyme of patients with sarcoidosis does represent overproduction by a cell such as the epithelioid cell, it raises an interesting question regarding the mechanism that triggers the production of this protein. If derepression of a gene is the mechanism, the associated elevation of lysozyme (Pasquel et al. 1973, Zorn et al. 1980) would suggest that more than one genetic site has been affected. A more logical assessment of the related molecular chemistry will await clearer data on the source of enzyme in the serum in sarcoidosis. Furthermore, why the elevation of the enzyme in serum occurs in some patients, but not in others, needs clarification. If the epithelioid cell is the source of the elevated serum enzyme in patients with sarcoidosis, it may be that all patients with sarcoidosis have elevated enzyme levels in lymph nodes, but only some have a sufficiently high rate of production, release, or impaired clearance to result in an elevated level in the serum. This concept is supported by the data of Pertschuk et al. (1980).

IV. Relation of Elevated Level of Enzyme to "Activity" of Disease

Granted that antiotensin 1-converting enzyme is elevated in a large number of patients with sarcoidosis, does its elevation reflect the "activity" of the disease? This is a very difficult question to answer since we do not have a precise definition of activity of sarcoidosis with which to make comparisons. In a general way, activity is usually considered to represent (a) rapid development or progression of respiratory or other symptoms; (b) recent appearance or rapid progression of radiological findings; (c) histological presence of granulomas; and (d) rapid progression of physiologic changes. Inflammatory cellular changes in bronchoalveolar lavage and positivity of gallium scans are under investigation as other indicators of activity of sarcoidosis and are discussed in another section of this chapter. An indirect measurement of activity is related to response to steroids. For correlation of activity with serum levels of angiotensin 1-converting enzyme, the general approaches have been to assess levels of the serum enzyme as other indicators of the disease worsen or improve, or to evaluate the influence of steroid therapy on levels of the serum enzyme. The results from these studies have been somewhat variable and there is still a need to accumulate more data from large populations of patients studied prospectively.

Two studies in which attempts have been made to assess serum angiotensin 1-converting enzyme levels longitudinally in relation to changes in clinical status of patients with sarcoidosis are those of DeRemee and Rohrbach (1980) and Ueda and associates (1980). Both studies concluded that angiotensin 1-converting enzyme levels closely parallel and occasionally antedate changes in clinical status of patients either undergoing spontaneous remission or being treated with prednisone. In the study by DeRemee and Rohrbach (1980), eight spontaneous remissions were correlated with decreasing levels of serum angiotensin 1-converting enzyme; 13 of 18 patients treated with glucocorticosteroids had a statistically significant correlation between indices of clinical improvement and serum angiotensin 1-converting enzyme levels. More recently, Yotsumoto (in press) reported that the serum angiotensin 1-converting enzyme level decreased more rapidly in corticosteroid-treated patients than in those with spontaneous remissions and attributed the decrease both to a suppressive effect of corticosteroids on angiotensin 1-converting enzyme produced by inflammatory cells and to a possible direct depressor effect of corticosteroids on serum angiotensin 1-converting enzyme levels.

In addition to the longitudinal studies noted above, several investigators have attempted to correlate serum levels of angiotensin 1-converting enzyme with the use of steroids for treatment. Silverstein and associates (1976b) reported that serum levels of angiotensin 1-converting enzyme decreased in 15 of the 16 patients who were placed on prednisone. Grönhagen-Riska et al. (1980) found decreases following steroid therapy in serum enzyme in 11 patients with elevated levels of enzyme. Studdy et al. (1978) found significantly lower levels of serum angiotensin 1-converting enzyme in patients with sarcoidosis who were taking steroids than in those who were not. Fanburg et al. (1976) also reported lower levels of the serum enzyme in patients taking steroids than in those not taking them, but a statistically significant difference was not established. A similar result was noted for treated and untreated patients by Gupta et al. (1979). Hence, although there are reasonably valid indications that steroids cause both remission of sarcoidosis and lowering of levels of serum angiotensin 1-converting enzyme, the evidence is not conclusive that the two end results are coupled to one another or that steroids invariably lower serum angiotensin 1-converting enzyme in sarcoidosis in remission.

There does not appear to be a close correlation between the stages of sarcoidosis and serum angiotensin 1-converting enzyme (Fanburg et al. 1976, Studdy et al. 1978, Gupta et al. 1979, DeRemee and Rohrbach 1980). Possible conclusions concerning this finding are that (a) stages of disease do not reflect quantitation of granulomatous tissue, or (b) stages of disease do reflect quantitation of granulomatous tissue, but the quantity of tissue affected does not correlate with levels of enzyme in the serum. Until better methods for quantifying granulomatous tissue are found, it may be impossible to resolve this question.

V. Conclusion

In conclusion, it currently appears that serum angiotensin 1-converting enzyme has some value, albeit an imperfect one, in diagnosing and following the course of sarcoidosis. Development of methods for achieving better sensitivity with the test, without sacrificing specificity, are desirable. Measurements of absolute amounts of enzyme, as opposed to enzymatic activity, may be helpful in this respect. Furthermore, additional studies of large population groups to access the relationship of enzymatic activity to the "activity" of the disease would be useful. Information is also needed about the possible role of this enzyme in the pathogenesis of sarcoidosis.

References

Abboy, R., Kanada, D., and Shama, D. P. (1980). Serum angiotensin converting enzyme in sarcoidosis. In *Sarcoidosis and Other Granulomatous Diseases.* Edited by W. J. Williams and B. H. Davies. Cardiff, Wales, Alpha Omega, pp. 273–276.

Caldwell, P. R. B., Seegal, B. C., Hsu, K. G., Das, M., and Soffer, R. L. (1976). Angiotensin-converting enzyme: Vascular endothelial localization. *Science,* **191**:1050–1051.

Cushman, D. W., and Cheung, H. S. (1971a). Spectrophotometric assay and properties of the angiotensin-converting enzyme of rabbit lung. *Biochem. Pharmacol.,* **20**:1637–1648.

Cushman, D. W., and Cheung, H. S. (1971b). Concentrations of angiotensin converting enzyme in tissues of the rat. *Biochim. Biophys. Acta,* **250**:261–265.

DeRemee, R. A., and Rohrbach, M. S. (1980). Serum angiotensin-converting enzyme activity in evaluating the clinical course of sarcoidosis. *Ann. Intern. Med.,* **92**:361–365.

Fanburg, B. L., Schoenberger, M. D., Bachus, B., and Snider, G. L. (1976). *Am. Rev. Respir. Dis.,* **114**:525–528.

Friedland, J., and Silverstein, E. (1976b). Similarity in some properties of serum angiotensin converting enzyme from sarcoidosis in patients and normal subjects. *Biochem. Med.,* **15**:178–185.

Friedland, J., and Silverstein, E. (1976a). A sensitive fluorimetric assay for angiotensin converting enzyme. *Am. J. Clin. Pathol.,* **66**:416–424.

Friedland, J., Setton, C., and Silverstein, E. (1977). Angiotensin converting enzyme: Induction by steroids in rabbit alveolar macrophages in culture. *Science,* **197**:64–65.

Grönhagen-Riska, C., Selroos, O., Fröseth, B., Fynrquist, F., Hellström, P. E., Kurppa, K., and Wägar, G. (1980). Increased serum angiotensin converting enzyme (ACE) in sarcoidosis, silicosis and asbestosis. In *Sarcoidosis and Other Granulomatous Diseases.* Edited by W. J. Williams and B. H. Davies. Cardiff, Wales, Alpha Omega, pp. 266–272.

Gupta, R. G., Oparil, S., and Szidon, J. P. (1979). Clinical significance of serum angiotensin-converting enzyme levels in sarcoidosis. *J. Lab. Clin. Med.,* **93**:940–949.

Hinman, L. M., Stevens, C., Matthey, R. A., and Gee, J. B. L. (1979). Angiotensin convertase activities in human alveolar macrophages: Effects of cigarette smoking and sarcoidosis. *Science,* **205**:202–203.

Khoury, F., Teasdale, P. R., Smith, L., Jones, O. G., and Carter, J. R. (1979). Angiotensin-converting enzyme in sarcoidosis: A British study. *Br. J. Dis. Chest,* **73**:382–388.

Lanzillo, J. J., and Fanburg, B. L. (1979). Angiotensin-converting enzyme in bronchoalveolar lining fluid (letter). *Lancet,* **1**:1199.

Lieberman, J. (1974). A new confirmatory test for sarcoidosis. Serum angiotensin converting enzyme: Effect of steroids and chronic lung disease. Annual Meeting of American Thoracic Society/American Lung Association, Cincinnati, Ohio.

Lieberman, J. (1975). Elevation of serum angiotensin-converting-enzyme (ACE) level in sarcoidosis. *Am. J. Med.,* **59**:365–372.

Lieberman, J. (1976). The specificity and nature of serum-angiotensin converting enzyme (serum ACE) elevations in sarcoidosis. *Ann. N.Y. Acad. Sci.,* **278**:498–513.

Lieberman, J., and Beutler, E. (1976). Elevation of serum angiotensin-converting enzyme in Gaucher's disease. *N. Engl. J. Med.,* **294**: 1442–1444.

Lieberman, J., and Rea, T. H. (1977). Serum angiotensin-converting enzyme in leprosy and coccidioidomycosis. *Ann. Intern. Med.,* **87**:422–425.

Mattiolli, A., Zakheim, R. M., Mullis, K., and Molteni, A. (1975). Angiotensin-1-converting enzyme activity in idiopathic respiratory distress syndrome of the newborn infant and in experimental alveolar hypoxia in mice. *J. Pediatr.,* **87**:97–101.

Okabe, T., Suzuki, A., Ishikawa, H., Yotsumoto, H., Ohsawa, N. (1981). Cells originating from sarcoid granulomas in vitro. *Am. Rev. Respir. Dis.,* **124**:608–612.

Oparil, S., Low, J., and Koerner, T. J. (1976). Altered angiotensin 1 conversion in pulmonary disease. *Clin. Sci. Mol. Med.,* **51**:537–543.

Pascual, R. S., Gee, J. B. L., and Finch, S. C. (1973). Usefulness of serum lysozyme measurement in diagnosis and evaluation of sarcoidosis. *N. Engl. J. Med.,* **289**:1074–1076.

Pertschuk, L. P., Silverstein, E., and Friedland, J. (1980). Immunologic diagnosis of sarcoidosis, detection of angiotensin-converting enzyme in sarcoid granulomas. *Am. J. Clin. Pathol.,* **75**:350–354.

Rohrbach, M. S., and DeRemee, R. A. (1979). Serum angiotensin converting enzyme activity in sarcoidosis as measured by a simple radiochemical assay. *Am. Rev. Respir. Dis.,* **119**:761–767.

Rømer, F. K. (1979). Angiotensin-converting enzyme in sarcoidosis. *Acta Med. Scand.,* **206**:27–30.

Rubin, D. B., and Dobbs, L. G. (1979). Angiotensin converting enzyme activity in fibroblasts and endothelial cells. *J. Cell Biol.,* **83**:98a.

Ryan, J. W., Ryan, U. S., Schultz, D. R., Whitaker, C., Chung, A., and Dorer, F. E. (1975). Subcellular localization of pulmonary angiotensin-converting enzyme (kininase II). *Biochemistry,* **146**: 497–499.

Silverstein, E., and Friedland, J. (1977). Elevated serum and spleen angiotensin converting enzyme and serum lysozyme in Gaucher's disease. *Clin. Chim. Acta,* **74**:21–25.

Silverstein, E., Friedland, J., Lyons, H. A., and Gourin, A. (1976a). Elevation of angiotensin converting enzyme in granulomatous lymph nodes and serum in sarcoidosis: Clinical and possible pathogenic significance. *Ann. N.Y. Acad. Sci.,* **278**:498–513.

Silverstein, E., Friedland, J., Lyons, H. A., and Gourin, A. (1976b). Markedly elevated angiotensin converting enzyme in lymph nodes containing non-necrotizing granulomas in sarcoidosis. *Proc. Natl. Acad. Sci. U.S.A.,* **73**:2137–2141.

Silverstein, E., Friedland, J., and Ackerman, T. (1977). Elevation of granulomatous lymph-node and serum lysozyme in sarcoidosis and correlation with angiotensin-converting enzyme. *Am. J. Clin. Pathol.,* **68**:219–224.

Silverstein, E., Pertschuk, L. P., and Friedland, J. (1979). Immunofluorescent localization of angiotensin converting enzyme in epithelioid and giant cells of sarcoidosis granulomas. *Proc. Natl. Acad. Sci. U.S.A.,* **76**:6646–6648.

Sprince, N. L., Kazemi, H., and Fanburg, B. L. (1980). Serum angiotensin 1 converting enzyme in chronic beryllium disease. In *Sarcoidosis and Other Granulomatous Diseases.* Edited by W. J. Williams and B. H. Davies. Cardiff, Wales, Alpha Omega, pp. 287–290.

Smith, U., and Ryan, J. W. (1973). Electron microscopy of endothelial and epithelial components of the lungs: Correlations of structure and function. *Fed. Proc.*, **32**:1957–1966.

Studdy, P., Bird, R., James, D. G., and Sherlock, S. (1978). Serum angiotensin-converting enzyme (SACE) in sarcoidosis and other granulomatous disorders. *Lancet*, **2**:1332–1334.

Thomas, A. V., Ansari, A., Khurana, M., and Niden, A. H. (1979). Elevated serum angiotensin converting enzyme in miliary tuberculosis (abstract). *Am. Rev. Respir. Dis.*, **119**:86.

Ueda, E., Kawabe, T., Tachibana, T., and Kokubu, T. (1980). Serum angiotensin-converting enzyme activity as an indicator of prognosis in sarcoidosis. *Am. Rev. Respir. Dis.*, **121**:667–671.

Ward, P. E., Schultz, W., Reynolds, R. E., and Erdös, E. G. (1977). Metabolism of kinins and angiotensins in the isolated glomerulus and brush border of rat kidney. *Lab. Invest.*, **36**:559–606.

Ward, P. E., Sheridan, M. A., Hammon, K. J., and Erdös, E. G. (1980). Angiotensin 1 converting enzyme (kininase II) of the brush border of human and swine intestine. *Biochem. Pharmacol.*, **29**:1525–1529.

Weinberg, K. S., Douglas, W. H. J., MacNamee, D. R., Lanzillo, J. J., and Fanburg, B. L. (1982). Angiotensin-1-converting enzyme localization on cultured fibroblasts by immunofluorescence. *In Vitro*, **18**: 400–406.

Wigger, H. J., and Stalcup, S. A. (1978). Distribution and development of angiotensin converting enzyme in the fetal and newborn rabbit, an immunofluorescence study. *Lab. Invest.*, **38**:581–585.

Yotsumoto, H., Mikami, R., Yokoyama, H., and Hosoda, Y. (1980). Interassay variance of SACE and the change of ACE activity during corticosteroid therapy. In *Sarcoidosis and Other Granulomatous Diseases*. Edited by W. J. Williams and B. H. Davies. Cardiff, Wales, Alpha Omega, pp. 276–282.

Yotsumoto, H. (in press). Longitudinal observations of serum angiotensin converting enzyme activity in sarcoidosis with and without treatment. *Chest*.

Zorn, S. K., Stevens, C. A., Schachter, E. N., and Gee, J. B. L. (1980). The angiotensin converting enzyme in pulmonary sarcoidosis and the relative diagnostic value of serum lysozyme. *Lung*, **157**:87–94.

11

Diagnostic Value of the Kveim Reaction

HAROLD L. ISRAEL

Jefferson Medical College
Thomas Jefferson University
Philadelphia, Pennsylvania

I. Introduction

Opposing views regarding the diagnostic value of the Kveim reaction have
been summarized by Siltzbach (1974) and Israel (1974a). A review of 17
studies of the diagnostic value of the Kveim test published since that time
indicates that the issue must still be considered unsettled. Although some
reports show the test to be sensitive and specific, others demonstrate the
reaction to be insensitive and nonspecific (Table 1). If poor results are
attributed to the use of unreliable test materials, it must be recognized
that these materials are employed by investigators only because better
ones are not available.

Siltzbach (1969) enumerated the following drawbacks to the Kveim
test: the 4–6 weeks necessary for maturation of the nodule, the need for
biopsy, the insufficient number of reliable test materials, the problems in
histological interpretation, and the ignorance of the active principle in sarcoidal
tissue that evokes the reaction. Another drawback pointed out later
(Karlish 1971) was the need to defer corticosteroid treatment until the test
was completed. Two decades later, none of these drawbacks has been

Table 1 Clinical Trials of Kveim Tests (1972–1980)

| Test materials | Percentage positive | | Country | Reference |
	Sarcoidosis	Controls		
CSL	65	17	U.S.	Israel (1974b)
Yugoslavia	88	0	Yugoslavia	Behrend et al. (1974)
CSL	68	20	Australia	Hurley and Sullivan (1974)
Edinburgh	74	0	U.K., U.S.	Douglas et al. (1976)
K12	58	1	U.K.	Bradstreet et al. (1976)
Various	48	26	U.K., Japan	Williams et al. (1976)
Dutch	35	25	Netherlands	Kooy et al. (1976)
Edinburgh	69	1	Worldwide	Middleton and Douglas (1980)
CRL	67	0	U.S.	Kataria et al. (1980)
Swiss	44	4	Japan	Hongo et al. (1980)
K19	73	1	U.K.	Bradstreet et al. (1980)
Turiaf	74	1	France	Turiaf et al. (1980)
Polish	61	22	Poland	Zych and Szymanska (1980)
Swedish	73	3	Sweden	Nillson et al. (1978)
Various	66	–	U.K.	Mitchell et al. (1976)
CSL, Danish	40	–	Denmark	Veien et al. (1979)
K19	45	–	U.K.	Mitchell et al. (1980)

eliminated, and the clinical importance of the Kveim test has diminished with the development of newer diagnostic tools such as transbronchial biopsy through the fiberoptic bronchoscope, measurement of serum angiotensin 1-converting enzyme (ACE) levels, bronchoalveolar lavage, and gallium scanning.

II. History

Williams and Nickerson (1935) first reported that use of a saline suspension of a ground cutaneous sarcoid lesion produced a cutaneous papule in a test subject within 24 hr, and that this papule disappeared in 8–21 days. These reactions were noted in four patients with sarcoidosis (in retrospect two had Crohn's disease) and were not present in control subjects. Kveim (1941) first reported the use of a similar preparation and the delayed development of a small indurated papule that on microscopic study showed granulomas similar to those of the natural disease. Nelson (1949) was the first person in the United States to describe the use of the Kveim reaction, obtaining a positive test in 11 of 15 patients with cutaneous sarcoidosis, but he regarded the reaction as having prognostic rather than diagnostic value.

Siltzbach et al. (1954) reported that 86% of 58 patients having proven sarcoidosis with various types of involvement gave positive tests and urged its application as a specific test for the disease. Siltzbach (1969) reported the first large-scale trial on 750 subjects, 165 of whom had proven sarcoidosis. Positive tests were obtained in 94% of those with stage I and stage II sarcoidosis, and 73% of those with stage III and normal roentgenograms, frequencies not approached by subsequent investigators. Worldwide trials were instituted employing Siltzbach's test materials, and in 1966 results were reported in 763 patients with sarcoidosis; positive tests were obtained in only 52% of these individuals (Siltzbach 1967).

Hurley and Bartholomeucz (1967) reported that the Commonwealth Serum Laboratories (CSL) in Australia had produced a Kveim test material that gave concordant results in 121 of 125 simultaneous tests with Chase-Siltzbach test materials. The CSL test materials were regarded as validated by this comparison and were distributed widely to investigators during the next few years. No further large-scale studies with Chase-Siltzbach materials were subsequently carried out, and the next international trials employed CSL materials and were reported by Hurley and Bartholomeucz (1971) to give positive tests in 59% of 510 proven cases of sarcoidosis and 1.7% of 722 patients not suffering from sarcoidosis. However, Israel and Goldstein (1971) reported that false positive reactions had been encountered in a variety of other diseases, notably tuberculous lymphadenitis and lymphoma. Subsequent reports described positive reactions in Crohn's disease (Karlish 1970) as well as in normal subjects (Izumi et al. 1974). It became obvious that CSL materials were no longer reliable, either as a result of unexpected deterioration or of a flaw in the original trials.

Although subsequent publications by Siltzbach (1974) and Middleton and Douglas (1980) indicate that some preparations maintain sensitivity and specificity, the unexpected deterioration of what had been validated as a reliable test material cast a damper on the use of the Kveim test. Kveim test material is available in only a few locations. In the United Kingdom it is available through the Colindale Laboratories of London, and a commercial preparation is manufactured in Switzerland. It has not been approved for use in the United States and no major pharmaceutical manufacturers have prepared it for large-scale distribution. Although enthusiastic reports regarding its diagnostic value continue to be presented at sarcoidosis conferences, the number of papers on the Kveim reaction has dwindled in the past few years. Cumulative *Index Medicus* citations for the years 1979–1980 include only six papers on the Kveim test compared to the 32 papers on angiotensin 1-converting enzyme studies in sarcoidosis.

III. Nature of the Kveim Reaction

The effective principle in the Kveim material is particulate and is located intracellularly. It is insoluble in water and resistant to alcohol, chloroform, and radiation (Siltzbach and Taub 1978). Efforts to produce a soluble granuloma-inducing factor have invariably been unsuccessful (Middleton and Douglas 1980). Whether the particulate factor represents part of the cell membrane or is phagocytosed material has not been determined. The reaction is difficult to classify immunologically, falling into none of the conventional types I to IV immunological reactions. As a result, textbooks of immunology devote little attention to this reaction. A similar torpid granulomatous response has been encountered in leprosy and zirconium hypersensitivity dermatitis. The active principle in the lepromin test which evokes the Mitsuda reaction is derived from crude suspensions of lepromatous tissue. It is interesting that the purified bacillary antigen produces an early reaction, but not the delayed granulomatous reaction (Kooij and Gerritsen 1958). The granulomatous dermatitis that occurs in some users of zirconium-containing deodorants has been shown (Shelley and Hurley 1958) to be a hypersensitivity phenomenon. Patients who develop granulomatous inflammation from zirconium salts show a Kveim-like reaction to injection of these compounds.

IV. Kveim Test Materials

Investigators have reported induction of Kveim reactions in sarcoidosis patients with the use of a variety of test materials (Israel 1974a), but undoubtedly the most potent test materials are those prepared from sarcoidal spleens or lymph nodes. Curiously, there is little correlation between the intensity of granulomatous involvement of the tissue extracted and its granuloma-inducing potency. Fibrotic tissues or those obtained from patients after corticosteroid therapy may yield more potent Kveim test material than tissues from early cases with extensive granuloma formation (Shelley and Hurley 1958). Most reports (Douglas et al. 1976, Kataria et al. 1980) indicate that Kveim test materials remain intact at room temperature or in refrigerators for 5 years or more, but reports by Nelson and Schwimmer (1956) and Hurley et al. (1975) indicate a loss of sensitivity and specificity during storage. A Colindale K19 antigen that gave positive results in 73%

of patients with sarcoidosis from 1973 to 1977 (Bradstreet et al. 1980) showed positivity in only 43% of patients tested in 1977–1978 (Veien et al. 1979), suggesting a possible loss in sensitivity of the stored material.

Meijer et al. (1975) obtained different results with different preparations from the same spleen, indicating that new batches may not be equivalent to older ones. Ripe et al. (1974) prepared a membrane fraction of sarcoid lymph nodes that gave large and more frequent reactions than the whole antigen. Although the supernatants alone gave no reactions, when the supernatants were coupled with Sephadex particles, positive reactions were obtained in five of 15 patients. However, the Sephadex alone produced positive reactions in two of the 15 patients.

Whether the later batches of CSL antigen lost their specificity or lacked it initially is open to question. Several studies (Hurley and Bartholomeucz 1967, Izumi et al. 1974) reported excellent specificity with lots 002 and 003. However, Williams et al. (1976) found many reactions in Crohn's disease with these batches, and Hurley et al. (1975) in a retest observed false positive reactions with the early batches as well. It is clear that the change was not due to introduction of foreign material in the preparation, as was suggested at the time, since the reactions evoked by the CSL antigen were epithelioid ones and not foreign body reactions. Perhaps the failure to detect false positive reactions in the early batches was due to the fact that no one expected them and, hence, did not test enough controls with tuberculous lymphadenitis, Crohn's disease, and lymphoma to discover the nonspecificity of the test material.

Although proponents of the Kveim test continue to insist that "good" test materials remain stable and specific, there appears to be no practical way of ensuring that later batches remain reliable. The need for close surveillance of test materials has been emphasized since the discovery of variability in the CSL preparation (Siltzbach 1974), but there is presently no agency that monitors and reports on Kveim test materials. Thus, it will be noted from Table 1 that since 1972 there have been no reports on testing with Chase-Siltzbach test material except for two small studies (Nillson et al. 1978, Teirstein et al. 1976) which actually indicate a much lower yield (60–66%) than had been observed in earlier studies. To obviate this problem, it has been our practice to use two different test materials in each case, considering that antigens are stable so long as concordance is observed in the majority of cases.

V. Histological Interpretation

Pathologists without special experience in interpreting Kveim reactions frequently differ in their interpretation, varying not only as to whether granulomatous inflammation is present but also as to whether the granulomas are of foreign body origin. A controlled comparison of interpretation by two expert British pathologists (Williams et al. 1976) has been reported, but unfortunately tests were done with five different test materials that resulted in positive reactions in only 47% of sarcoidosis patients and in 27% of patients with Crohn's disease, tuberculosis, and collagen disorders. The two observers concurred on positive readings in 75% of cases, were in partial agreement in 23%, and were in complete disagreement only in 2%. A study comparing the interpretation of 66 slides by five Japanese pathologists was also based on tests made with a variety of antigens. Agreement among the five readers was obtained in 21 slides, among four readers in 20 slides, and among three readers in 11 slides (Iwai et al. 1974).

No controlled trial of histological interpretation with large numbers of tests employing Siltzbach, Edinburgh, or other apparently stable antigens has been published. The variability of the reaction in rigidly controlled studies, however, is demonstrated in a study that matched tests using two British preparations and the Siltzbach suspension (Nillson et al. 1978). Although positive tests were obtained in 66% of patients with sarcoidosis there was considerable discrepancy in matched tests. Thus, in the 12 patients who had positive reactions, concordance of the two tests occurred in only seven of the pairs. The most recent report of matched tests was by Veien et al. (1979) employing Danish and CSL test materials. Their behavior was consistent, but positive tests were obtained in only 40% of sarcoidosis patients, suggesting extreme conservatism in reading.

VI. Clinical Correlates of the Kveim Reaction

All investigators have noted that the frequency of positive Kveim tests is highest in patients with erythema nodosum, cutaneous sarcoidosis, and stage I roentgenograms. This has been interpreted by most observers to be a reflection of "early" sarcoidosis, but our own studies (Israel and Goldstein 1971, Israel and Washburne 1980) show a significant relationship to the presence of lymphadenopathy but not to duration of disease. We have been especially impressed by the frequency of negative tests in patients found to have transient hilar adenopathy due to sarcoidosis. Aside from this phenomenon the Kveim reaction provides no particularly prognostic information; some patients with chronic indolent sarcoidosis remain Kveim-positive for decades.

The lower frequency of Kveim reaction in patients without mediastinal or hilar adenopathy is shown in several recent studies. In a study done in Philadelphia (Table 2) Kveim tests were positive in 91 of 113 patients with adenopathy, and in four of 16 patients with stage III or stage 0 disease (Israel and Washburne 1980). Middleton and Douglas (1980), in

Table 2 Kveim Tests (1974–1976)

Hilar/mediastinal adenopathy	Black		White	
	Tested	Positive	Tested	Positive
Present	55	51[a,b]	58	50[a,b]
Absent	5	1[b]	11	3[b]
Subacute	45	40[a]	58	38[a]
Chronic	15	12	11	5
Total	60	52[a]	69	43[a]

[a]Significant difference between black and white patients.
[b]Significant difference between patients with and without adenopathy.
Source: Israel and Washburne (1980).

an international study, reported 507 positive tests among 677 patients with stage I–II roentgenograms and 129 positive tests among 236 patients with stages 0 and III roentgenograms. Bradstreet et al. (1980) reported positive tests in 75% of 1774 patients with stage I–II disease and in only 29% of patients with stage 0 and III roentgenograms.

In our experience (Table 2) the Kveim test is significantly more often positive in black patients (81%) than in whites (62%). Thus, the Kveim test is unusually positive in obvious cases of sarcoidosis, easily identified by characteristic roentgenographic and cutaneous changes. A specific test for sarcoidosis would be most helpful in atypical cases, and it is in such patients without the telltale lymphadenopathy and cutaneous lesions that the Kveim test is very often negative. This conclusion is supported by the results of a recent analysis of Kveim tests performed at Johns Hopkins Hospital (Harber et al. 1981). The odds of positivity were found to be 10 times greater in a young black female with a stage I x-ray than in a white male over 30 with ocular sarcoidosis and a stage 0 x-ray.

VII. In Vitro Kveim Reactions

A series of papers a decade ago reported that circulating white cells from patients with sarcoidosis exhibited inhibition of leukocyte and macrophage migration on exposure to Kveim antigens, offering promise that an in vitro Kveim test could be devised (Becker et al. 1972, Hardt and Wanstrup 1969, Williams et al. 1972). Subsequent studies (Hardt et al. 1976, Horsmanheimo et al. 1978) failed to confirm these observations, and these investigators have concluded as a consequence that the Kveim reaction is not a lymphocyte-mediated process. Whether for this reason, or because of the impossibility of isolating a soluble antigen, it appears at present that the Kveim phenomenon cannot be duplicated in vitro.

VIII. Comparison of Kveim Test and Transbronchial Biopsy

Mitchell in a recent study of the diagnostic yield of transbronchial biopsy through the fiberoptic bronchoscope (1980), compared these results with Kveim tests in 29 patients investigated by both procedures (Table 3). Transbronchial biopsy provided a diagnosis in 24 of 29 patients, while an unequivocally positive Kveim test was obtained in only 13 patients. From this study, carried out in the Brompton Hospital with a long experience with the Kveim test and employing the widely distributed Colindale K19 test antigen, it appears that the Kveim test has a low sensitivity for sarcoidosis.

Teirstein et al. (1976) reported Kveim tests in 25 patients with sarcoidosis who had had fiberoptic bronchoscopy. Twenty of the 25 had granulomas demonstrable by transbronchial biopsy. Seven of the Kveim tests were incomplete, while three tests were invalidated by the need for high-dose corticosteroid therapy. Of the 15 tests completed, only nine were positive. Three patients had both positive biopsy and Kveim test, six had positive biopsy only, and three had a positive Kveim test only.

Table 3 Comparison of Results of Transbronchial Biopsy or Biopsy of Bronchial Mucosa, or Both, and Results of Kveim Tests in 29 Patients Investigated by Both Procedures[a]

| | Biopsy | | |
Kveim test	Positive[b]	Negative	Total
Positive	11	2	13
Equivocal	3	1	4
Negative	10	2	12
Total	24	5	29

[a]Transbronchial lung biopsy and Kveim test were carried out in 21 patients; biopsy of bronchial mucosa and Kveim test were carried out in eight patients.
[b]Epithelioid and giant-cell granulomas were present.
Source: Mitchell et al. (1980).

Bronchoscopy thus provided not only a more rapid result but a higher yield, uninfluenced by lack of patient compliance in returning for reading or by an urgent need for corticosteroid therapy. The only disadvantages to bronchoscopic biopsy are the need for hospitalization and the hazards of the procedure, which appear to be minimal in experienced hands.

IX. Comparison of Kveim Test and Serum Angiotensin-Converting Enzyme Assays

No matched trials have been reported, although Siltzbach et al. (1980) noted in a recent study of 139 patients that Kveim tests were positive in 79% of patients with sarcoidosis while only 56% had elevated angiotensin 1-converting enzyme (ACE) levels. We have compared these tests simultaneously in 40 patients with active sarcoidosis. Kveim tests were positive in 70% of patients, and ACE elevations were noted with an equal frequency. However, as Table 4 shows, only 43% of patients were positive to both tests, and 55% were positive only to one test. Only a single patient had a negative Kveim test and a normal serum ACE level.

It appears that the Kveim reaction and the enzyme elevations are different parameters of the disease. Concurrence of the two tests represents strong evidence for the diagnosis of sarcoidosis, but unfortunately such concurrence was obtained in less than half of our patients with active sarcoidosis. On the other hand, a normal serum ACE level and failure to react to a reliable Kveim test material indicate that the likelihood of sarcoidosis is small. This time-consuming method for determining that other investigations are necessary may be useful in patients who are completely well, but is unjustifiable in patients who are ill.

Table 4 Kveim Tests and ACE Levels in Active Sarcoidosis

No. of patients	Kveim test[a]	ACE level[b]
17	Positive	Elevated
11	Positive	Normal[b]
11	Negative	Elevated
1	Negative	Normal[b]

[a]Duplicate tests employing Swiss, Edinburgh 2H, and Kataria test materials.
[b]Normal mean ± 2 SD. Men 16–36 units, women 12–30 units.

X. Conclusion

None of the drawbacks to the Kveim test enumerated 20 years ago has been eliminated, and more productive and more convenient diagnostic tools have been developed. Were the Kveim reaction a truly reliable test for demonstrating the presence or absence of sarcoidosis, its use would still be desirable. As it is, the unavailability of Kveim test material in the United States has not proven to be a significant handicap in the diagnosis and management of patients suspected of having sarcoidosis.

References

Becker, F. W., Krull, P., Deicher, H., and Kalden, J. R. (1972). Leukocyte migration test in sarcoidosis. *Lancet,* **1**:120–123.

Behrend, H., Djuric, B., and Aleksic, N. (1974). Experience with our Kveim antigen. In *Proceedings of the Sixth International Conference on Sarcoidosis.* Edited by K. Iwai and Y. Hosoda. Tokyo, University of Tokyo Press, pp. 60–67.

Bradstreet, C. M. P., Dighero, M. W., and Mitchell, D. N. (1976). The Kveim test: Analysis of results of tests using Colindale (K12) material. *Ann. N.Y. Acad. Sci.,* **278**:681–686.

Bradstreet, C. M. P., Dighero, M. W., and Mitchell, D. N. (1980). The Kveim test: Analysis of results of tests using K19 materials. In *Sarcoidosis and Other Granulomatous Diseases.* Edited by W. J. Williams and B. H. Davies. Cardiff, Wales, Alpha Omega, pp. 674–677.

Douglas, A. C., Wallace, A., Clark, J., Stephens, J. H., Smith, I. E., and Allan, N. C. (1976). The Edinburgh spleen: Source of a validated Kveim-Siltzbach test material. *Ann. N.Y. Acad. Sci.,* **278**:671–679.

Harber, P., Terry, P., and Johns, C. (1981). Predictors of positive Kveim test results. *Am. Rev. Respir. Dis.,* **123**:52.

Hardt, F., and Wanstrup, J. (1969). Sarcoidosis—An in vitro Kveim reaction based on the leukocyte migration test. *Acta Pathol. Microbiol. Scand.,* **76**:493–494.

Hardt, F., Veien, N., Bendixen, G., Brodthagen, H., Faber, V., Genner, J., Hecksher, T., Ringsted, J., Sorensen, S. F., Wanstrup, J., and Wiik, A. (1976). Immunologic studies in sarcoidosis: A comparison of in vivo and in vitro Kveim tests. *Ann. N.Y. Acad. Sci.,* **278**:711–716.

Hedfors, E. (1980). Sarcoidosis. In *Clinical Immunology.* Edited by C. W. Parker. Philadelphia, Saunders, pp. 556–582.

Hongo, O., Fukushiro, R., Hosoda, Y., Odaka, M., Izumi, T., Iwai, K., Matsui, M., Hiraga, Y., Ito, Y., Yoneda, R., Osada, H., Tachibana, T., Shigematsu, N., Horikawa, M., and Fruie, T. (1980). Analysis of results of the Kveim tests using Swiss Kveim antigen. In *Sarcoidosis and Other Granulomatous Diseases.* Edited by W. J. Williams and B. H. Davies. Cardiff, Wales, Alpha Omega, pp. 668–669.

Horsmanheimo, M., Horsmanheimo, A., Fudenberg, H., and Siltzbach, L. E. (1978). Leukocyte migration test (LMAT) in sarcoidosis using Kveim test material. *Br. J. Dermatol.,* **79**:263–270.

Hurley, T. H., Sullivan, J. R., and Hurley, J. V. (1975). Reaction to Kveim test material in sarcoidosis and other diseases. *Lancet,* 1:494–496.

Hurley, T. H., and Bartholomeucz, C. (1967). The Kveim test. Results obtained in sarcoid and non-sarcoid patients with simultaneous use of Australian (CSL) and American (Chase-Siltzbach type I, USA) Kveim suspensions. In *Proceedings of the Fourth International Conference on Sarcoidosis.* Paris, Masson, pp. 194–200.

Hurley, T. H., and Sullivan, J. R. (1974). Results obtained with Australian Kveim test material, 1966–1972. In *Proceedings of the Sixth International Conference on Sarcoidosis.* Edited by K. Iwai and Y. Hosoda. Tokyo, University of Tokyo Press, pp. 73–76.

Hurley, T. H., and Bartholomeucz, C. (1971). An international Siltzbach-Kveim test study using an Australian (CSL) test material, 1966–1969. In *Proceedings of the Fifth International Conference on Sarcoidosis.* Prague, Univ. Charles Press, pp. 343–348.

Israel, H. L., and Goldstein, R. A. (1971). Relation of Kveim antigen test to lymphadenopathy. Study of sarcoidosis and other diseases. *N. Engl. J. Med.,* **284**:345–349.

Israel, H. L., and Washburne, J. D. (1980). Characteristics of sarcoidosis in black and white patients. Analysis of 162 recent cases. In *Sarcoidosis and Other Granulomatous Diseases.* Edited by W. J. Williams and B. H. Davies. Cardiff, Wales, Alpha Omega, pp. 497–507.

Israel, H. L. (1974a). The Kveim test is not a specific test for sarcoidosis. In *Controversy in Internal Medicine.* Edited by F. J. Ingelfinger. Philadelphia, Saunders, pp. 339–348.

Israel, H. L. (1974b). Observations on the mechanism and specificity of the Kveim reaction. In *Proceedings of the Sixth International Conference on Sarcoidosis.* Edited by K. Iwai and Y. Hosoda. Tokyo, University of Tokyo Press, pp. 60–67.

Iwai, K., Fukushiro, R., Kobata, Y., Izumi, T., Hirako, T., Hongo, O., and Odaka, M. (1974). Kveim reaction–Disagreement in results and tentative criteria. In *Proceedings of the Sixth International Conference on Sarcoidosis.* Edited by K. Iwai and Y. Hosoda. Tokyo, University of Tokyo Press, pp. 57–59.

Izumi, T., Kobara, Y., Morioka, S., Sato, A., and Tsuji, S. (1974). False positive reaction in the Kveim test using the CSL material. In *Proceedings of the Sixth International Conference on Sarcoidosis.* Edited by K. Iwai and Y. Hosoda. Tokyo, University of Tokyo Press, pp. 77–78.

Karlish, A. M. (1970). Kveim test in Crohn's disease. *Lancet,* 2:977–978.

Karlish, A. J. (1971). The effect of steroids on the development of the Kveim reaction. In *Proceedings of the Fifth International Conference on Sarcoidosis.* Edited by L. Levinsky and F. Macholda. Prague, Univ. Charles Press, pp. 367–370.

Kataria, Y. P., Sharma, O. M., Israel, H. L., and Rogers, M. (1980). Kveim antigen CR-1: Its sensitivity and specificity in sarcoidosis, a cooperative study. In *Sarcoidosis and Other Granulomatous Diseases.* Edited by W. J. Williams and B. H. Davies. Cardiff, Wales, Alpha Omega, pp. 660–667.

Kooij, R. J., and Gerritsen, T. (1958). On the nature of the Mitsuda and the Kveim reaction. *Dermatologica,* 116:1–27.

Kooy, R., Ruitenberg, E. J., Sirks, J. L., Stam, J., and Meyer, S. (1976). Experience with a Dutch Kveim suspension in men and guinea pigs. *Ann. N.Y. Acad. Sci.,* 278:717–721.

Kveim, A. (1941). En ny og Spesifik Kutan-Reakjon Ved Boecks Sarcoid. *Nord. Med.,* 9:1969–1972. (Preliminary report on new and specific cutaneous reaction in Boecks sarcoid).

Meijer, S., Stam, J., and Sirks, J. L. (1975). Reaction to Kveim test material in sarcoidosis. *Lancet,* 1:808.

Middleton, W. G., and Douglas, A. C. (1980). Further experience with Edinburgh prepared Kveim-Siltzbach test suspension. In *Sarcoidosis and Other Granulomatous Diseases.* Edited by W. J. Williams and B. H. Davies. Cardiff, Wales, Alpha Omega, pp. 655–659.

Mitchell, D. M., Mitchell, D. N., Collins, J. V., and Emerson, C. J. (1980). Transbronchial lung biopsy through fibreoptic bronchoscope in diagnosis of sarcoidosis. *Br. Med. J.,* 1:679–680.

Mitchell, D. N., Sutherland, K., Bradstreet, C. M. P., and Dighero, M. W. (1976). Validation and standardization of Kveim test suspensions prepared from 2 human spleens. *J. Clin. Pathol.,* 29:203–210.

Nelson, C. T. (1949). Kveim reaction in sarcoidosis. *Arch. Dermatol. (Suppl.),* 60:377–389.

Nelson, C. T., and Schwimmer, B. (1956). The specificity of the Kveim reaction. *J. Invest. Dermatol.,* 6:57–60.

Nillson, B. S., Hanngren, A., Lins, R. E., Ripe, E., Ivemark, B., Askergren, J., and Suudblad, R. (1978). Acute phase of sarcoidosis with splenomegaly and hypercalcemia. *Scand. J. Respir. Dis.,* 59:199–209.

Ripe, E., Hanngren, A., Izumi, T., Nilsson, B. S., and Unge, G. (1974). On the active principle in the Kveim antigen. In *Proceedings of the Sixth International Conference on Sarcoidosis.* Edited by K. Iwai and Y. Hosoda. Tokyo, University of Tokyo Press, pp. 51–53.

Shelley, W. B., and Hurley, H. J. (1958). The allergic origin of zirconium deodorant granulomas. *Br. J. Dermatol.,* **70**:75–101.

Siltzbach, L. E. (1974). Surveillance of Kveim test results. In *Proceedings of the Sixth International Conference on Sarcoidosis.* Edited by K. Iwai and Y. Hosoda. Tokyo, University of Tokyo Press, pp. 77–78.

Siltzbach, L. E., and Taub, R. N. (1978). Sarcoidosis. In *Immunologic Diseases,* 3rd ed. Edited by M. Samter. Boston, Little Brown, pp. 548–569.

Siltzbach, L. E., Ehrlich, J. C., and Nickerson, O. O. (1954). Kveim reaction in sarcoidosis. *Am. J. Med.,* **16**:790–803.

Siltzbach, L. E. (1967). An international Kveim test study in sarcoidosis. In *Proceedings of the Fourth International Conference on Sarcoidosis.* Paris, Masson, pp. 201–213.

Siltzbach, L. E. (1969). The Kveim test in sarcoidosis. *JAMA,* **178**: 476–482.

Siltzbach, L. E. (1974). The Kveim test is a reliable means of diagnosing sarcoidosis. In *Controversy in Internal Medicine.* Edited by F. J. Ingelfinger. Philadelphia, Saunders, pp. 349–358.

Siltzbach, L. E., Krakoff, L., Dorph, D., and Teirstein, A. S. (1980). Elevated levels of serum angiotensin-converting enzyme (kininase II) and lysozome levels in sarcoidosis. In *Sarcoidosis and Other Granulomatous Diseases.* Edited by W. J. Williams and B. H. Davies. Cardiff, Wales, Alpha Omega, pp. 298–302.

Teirstein, A. S., Chuang, M., Miller, A., and Siltzbach, L. E. (1976). Flexible-bronchoscope biopsy of lung and bronchial wall in intrathoracic sarcoidosis. *Ann. N.Y. Acad. Sci.,* **278**:522–526.

Turiaf, J., Basset, F., Menault, M., and Jeanjean, X. (1980). The Kveim test: A personal experiment using an allergen obtained from a sarcoid spleen. In *Sarcoidosis and Other Granulomatous Diseases.* Edited by W. J. Williams and B. H. Davies. Cardiff, Wales, Alpha Omega, p. 678.

Veien, N. K., Stahl, D., Genner, J., and Hou-Jensen, K. (1979). Kveim test in sarcoidosis. A report of a Danish Kveim material. *Dan. Med. Bull.,* **26**:6–9.

Williams, W. J., Seal, R. E. M., and Davies, K. J. (1976). International Kveim histology trial. *Ann. N.Y. Acad. Sci.,* **278**:607–699.

Williams, R. H., and Nickerson, D. A. (1935). Skin reactions in sarcoidosis. *Proc. Exp. Biol. Med.,* **33**:403–405.

Williams, W. J., Bioli, E., Jones, D. J., and Dighero, M. W. (1972). The Kmif (Kveim induced macrophage migration inhibition factor) test in sarcoidosis. *J. Clin. Pathol.,* **25**:951–954.
Zych, D., and Szymanska, D. (1980). Evaluation of the diagnostic value of six various Kveim-Siltzbach test suspensions in sarcoidosis. In *Sarcoidosis and Other Granulomatous Diseases.* Edited by W. J. Williams and B. H. Davies. Cardiff, Wales, Alpha Omega, pp. 682–686.

12

Gallium-67 Scanning as an Indicator of the Activity of Sarcoidosis

BRUCE R. LINE,* GARY W. HUNNINGHAKE,†
BRENDAN A. KEOGH, and RONALD G. CRYSTAL

National Institutes of Health
Bethesda, Maryland

I. Introduction

Pulmonary sarcoidosis is a chronic disorder characterized by inflammation
of the alveolar structures ("alveolitis"), interstitial noncaseating granulomata,
changes in the alveolar epithelial, endothelial, and mesenchymal cells, and,
in some individuals, interstitial fibrosis (Scadding 1967, Spencer 1977,
Crofton and Douglas 1975, Mitchell et al. 1977, Rosen et al. 1978,
Crystal et al. 1981a). Although the classic hallmark of sarcoidosis is the
granuloma, it is now recognized that the alveolitis precedes and modulates
the formation of the granulomata as well as the other derangements of the
lung that are characteristic of this disease (Weinberger et al. 1978, Keogh
and Crystal 1980, Hunninghake et al. 1979a, 1976b, 1980a, 1980b,
1980d, 1981d, Hunninghake and Crystal 1981a, Carrington et al. 1976,
Takahashi 1970, Teilum 1964, Judd et al. 1975, Crystal et al. 1981a,b).
Thus, it is now understood that the alveolitis of sarcoidosis is responsible

---

Present Affiliation
        *Albany Medical Center Hospital, Albany, New York
        †University of Iowa Hospitals and Clinics, Iowa City, Iowa

for the loss of functioning alveolar-capillary units suffered by these patients. In this context, it is critical that the clinician caring for patients with sarcoidosis have a means to evaluate the alveolitis of the disease.

It is the purpose of this chapter to describe one technique, thoracic gallium-67 scanning, that, in combination with bronchoalveolar lavage, accomplishes this goal. To demonstrate this, we will first describe how gallium-67 scans are performed and interpreted. Then, to explain why the gallium-67 scan is useful in evaluating the alveolitis of sarcoidosis, we will detail the current concepts of the pathogenesis of this disease, particularly as related to the character of the alveolitis. With this as a background, we will return to a discussion of the gallium-67 scan to assess its validity as a means to quantify the intensity of the alveolitis of sarcoidosis and its use in staging patients with this disease and making decisions about therapy.

II. Performing and Interpreting Gallium-67 Scans in Sarcoidosis

Gallium-67 is a cyclotron-produced radionuclide with a half-life of 78 hr. After the intravenous injection of 50 μCi/kg ^{67}Ga citrate, most of the isotope is bound to serum proteins; 10–20% of the administered dose is removed from the body unchanged through the kidneys and gastrointestinal tract (Nelson et al. 1972). Images of the distribution of gallium-67 are usually obtained 48–72 hr after tracer administration to allow the non-specific body background activity to fall to low levels (Larson et al. 1973). Because a significant quantity of gallium-67 is eliminated from the body through the gastrointestinal tract, patients are often given laxatives during this 2- to 3-day period to lower radiation exposure and to keep colonic activity from interfering with scan interpretation.

Images of the distribution of gallium-67 in the thorax and abdomen may be produced by large-field-of-view scintilation cameras which collect gallium-67 gamma emmissions from a region comparable in size to that of a standard chest roentgenogram. Alternatively, both anterior and posterior images of the tracer distribution may be produced using a dual probe rectilinear scanner which passes slowly over the head, chest, and abdomen. We prefer rectilinear scans over gamma camera images because the scanner records tracer activity in both thorax and abdomen at distance and information density settings that are easily standardized; these factors are critically important in staging and following patients with sarcoidosis.

A. Scan Evaluation

In normal individuals, rectilinear scans show physiologic gallium-67 uptake in the liver, spleen, and skeletal structures (spine, ribs, and pelvis) (Fig. 1).

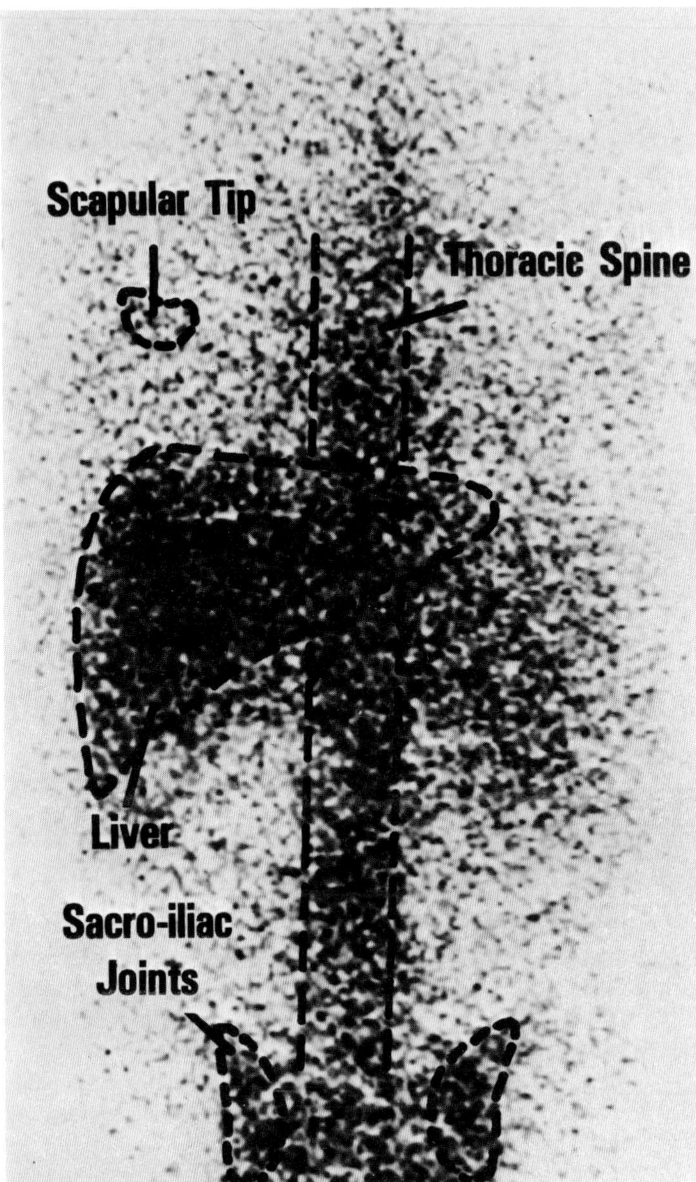

Figure 1 Example of normal posterior rectilinear scan of the thorax and abdomen. There is normal physiologic uptake of gallium-67 uptake in skeletal tissues (scapular tips, spine, pelvis, sarcoiliac joints), liver, and spleen. The pulmonary uptake is comparable to background as determined from the abdominal activity below the kidneys.

The image region over the lungs is usually just slightly above the non-specific body background due to rib uptake.

The intensity of gallium-67 uptake by the lungs of patients is difficult to evaluate quantitatively because patient body morphology, imaging technique, and observer subjectivity all affect the accuracy to which estimates can be made. To reduce these sources of variation, we use only posterior gallium-67 scans to evaluate sarcoidosis. This view is less influenced by differences in patient size, sex, and body habitus than anterior scans (Line et al. 1978, 1981).

We further reduce observer subjectivity by calculating an index (the "^{67}Ga index"), a semiquantitative estimate of the degree of gallium-67 uptake by the lung. This index is generated by combining estimates of the relative lung area and the relative uptake intensity of each abnormal region of thoracic gallium-67 localization (Line et al. 1981) (Fig. 2). The uptake area is estimated as a percentage of the total lung area to adjust for differences in image size between patient studies. The uptake intensity* is individually graded on a scale of 0 to 4 to minimize the effects of body background and the quantity of administered tracer. Intensity grade 0 (body background), is determined from lower abdominal uptake in areas free of colonic tracer activity. Intensity grade 4 is determined from the most intense body uptake; this is usually the liver but may be a region of the lung itself. The ^{67}Ga index is then computed by multiplying the uptake area by the intensity grade for each region with increased gallium-67 uptake, and by summing these products to obtain the total index value.

To illustrate computation of the ^{67}Ga index, three main regions of gallium-67 uptake are outlined in the lung of a 42-year-old man with active pulmonary sarcoidosis (Fig. 2). The uptake in the right upper lung includes 20% of the lung image area with a grade 2 intensity, equivalent to 20% × 2 or 40 ^{67}Ga index units. The two localizations of grade 1 intensity in the mid and lower lung zones involve a total of 50% of the lung image area (30% + 20%), and account for 50% × 1 or 50 ^{67}Ga index units. Thus, the combined ^{67}Ga index for this patient study would be 40 plus 50 units or 90 ^{67}Ga index units. Although the highest possible ^{67}Ga index is 400 units (i.e., assuming 100% of the lung involved with an intensity of 4+; 100 × 4 = 400 units), normal individuals show ^{67}Ga indices of 50 or less index units with no regions of uptake having greater than a grade 1 intensity (Fig. 1). In this context, gallium-67 scans of the lung parenchyma are considered positive if they are found to have an uptake of more than 50 ^{67}Ga index units.

---

*The intensity of gallium-67 uptake in each region of the scan is the function of the tracer concentration in that region and the depth of the lung.

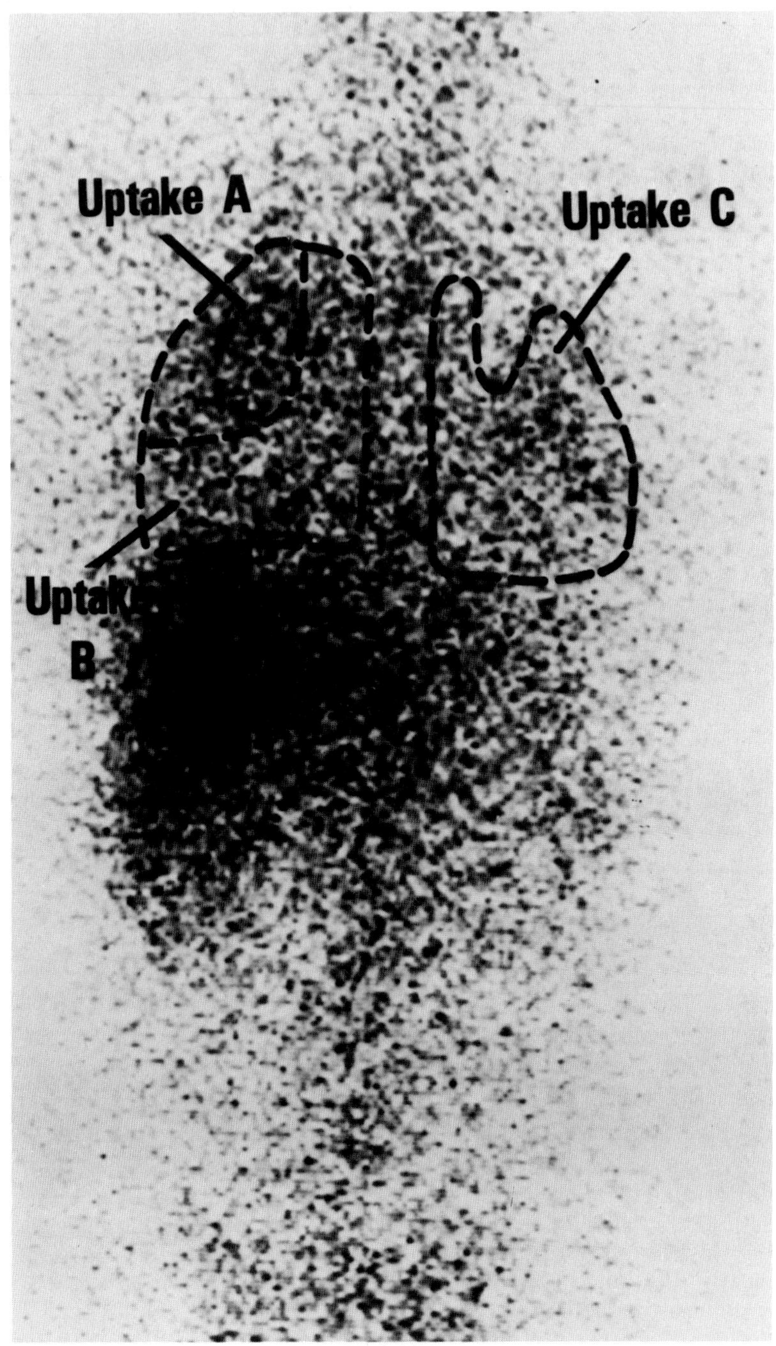

Figure 2 Example of ^{67}Ga index computation in a 42-year-old man with pulmonary sarcoidosis. Three regions show uptake greater than the background area. Region A (intensity = 2, area = 20%, index = 40 units), region B (intensity = 1, area = 20%, index = 20 units), and region C (intensity = 1, area = 30%, index = 30 units) are summed to give a total ^{67}Ga index of 90 units.

B. Gallium-67 Scans in Patients with Sarcoidosis

Although normal individuals show little gallium-67 uptake in pulmonary parenchyma (Larson et al. 1973), two-thirds of patients with sarcoidosis demonstrate significant pulmonary uptake ($>$50 ^{67}Ga index units) (Line et al. 1981, Crystal et al. 1981b) (Figs. 3 and 4). The gallium-67 may be distributed throughout the lung, but often it occurs in more localized non-segmental regions. Gallium-67 scans with ^{67}Ga index values greater than 150 often show diffuse patterns of uptake primarily in the mid and lower lung fields. Forty-five percent of patients show index values greater than or equal to 100, while 13% show values greater than or equal to 200 index units. In general, however, the pattern of uptake on the scan is highly variable in distribution, intensity, and extent of lung involvement.

During the course of the disease, the pattern may change rapidly in character, with different regions of the lung being involved with varying intensity patterns. For example, over a 2-year interval of follow-up, a patient showed intense nodal and central lung uptake (Fig. 5), which spontaneously resolved and then subsequently recurred in a pattern involving the lung parenchyma in the right upper and mid lung zones.

In addition to the gallium-67 uptake in the lung parenchyma, more than two-thirds of the patients with sarcoidosis show abnormal uptake either in extrathoracic tissues or in intrathoracic hilar and paratracheal nodes (Line et al. 1981). Localizations are commonly observed in the parotid glands and nasopharynx (Fig. 6a); they may be found in the cervical, suprascapular, axillary, paraaortic, inguinal, and femoral lymph nodes (Fig. 6b); in the spleen (Fig. 6c); and in bone marrow (Fig. 6d). Rarely, we have observed extrathoracic gallium-67 uptake without coexisting abnormal accumulations of tracer within the thorax.

C. Use of Thoracic Gallium-67 Scans in Sarcoidosis

Two uses have been suggested for thoracic gallium-67 scans in sarcoidosis: (a) to establish the diagnosis; and (b) to help quantify the alveolitis of the parenchymal disease.

Figure 3 Examples of posterior rectilinear gallium-67 scans in pulmonary sarcoidosis. (A) Diffuse pulmonary uptake involving mid and lower lung regions in a 27-year-old woman; ^{67}Ga index = 90 units. (B) Bilateral hilar lymph node and diffuse right lower lobe uptake in a 34-year-old woman; ^{67}Ga index = 40 units. (C) Diffuse moderate-intensity pulmonary uptake with prominent uptake in hilar region and in parotid glands in a 27-year-old man; ^{67}Ga index = 180 units. (D) Diffuse high-intensity ^{67}Ga uptake in a 35-year-old man; ^{67}Ga index = 340 units.

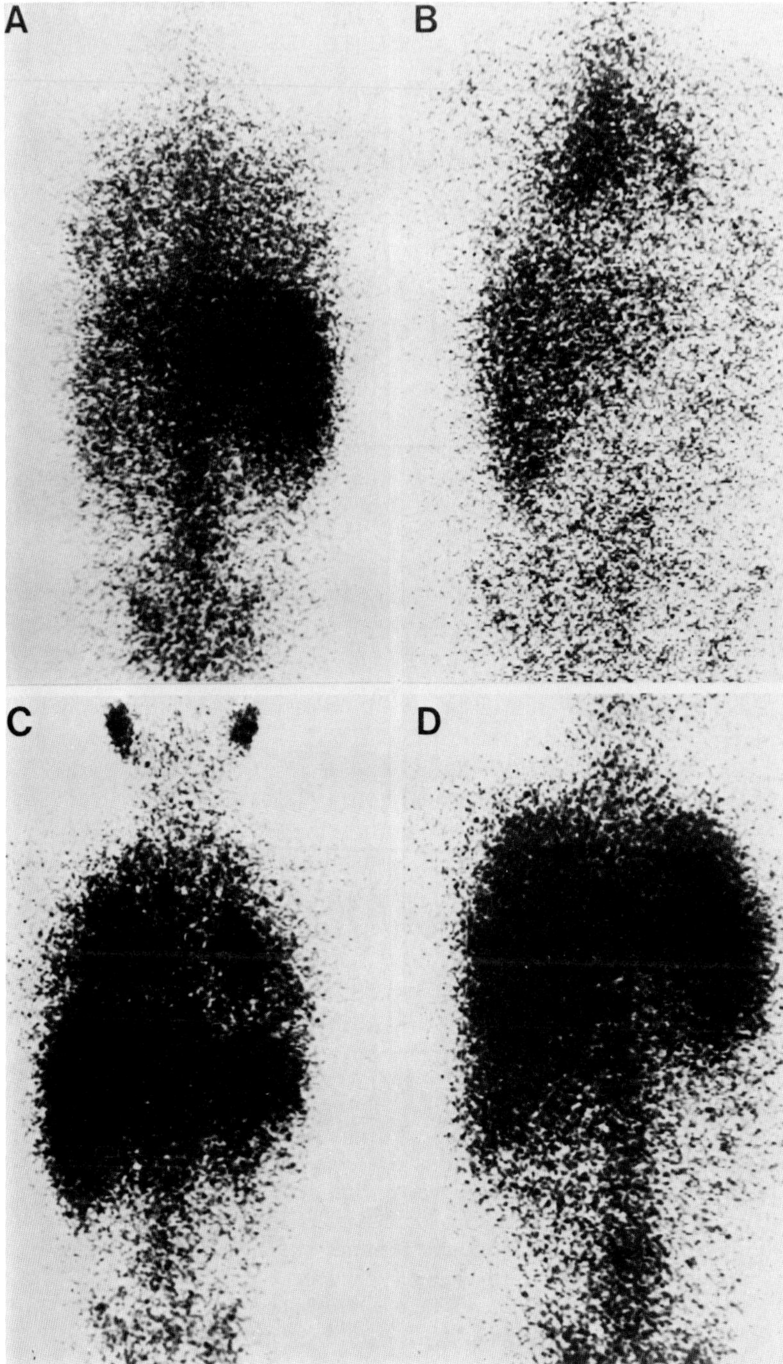
A
B
C
D

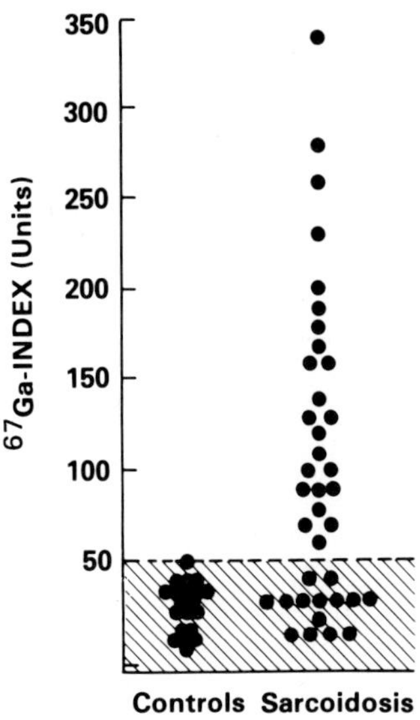

Figure 4 Distribution of ^{67}Ga indices in control patients and in patients with sarcoidosis. Nineteen scans in control subjects show ^{67}Ga index values below 50 ^{67}Ga index units. Sixty-three percent of 38 patients with sarcoidosis show a ^{67}Ga index greater than or equal to 50 ^{67}Ga index units; 45% had a ^{67}Ga index greater than or equal to 100 units and 13% had values greater than or equal to 200 units.

While the gallium-67 scan is positive in most patients with sarcoidosis, it certainly is not specific for this disease. To date, a variety of acute and chronic lung disorders have been described with positive gallium-67 scans (Crystal et al. 1981a, Keogh and Crystal 1981) (Table 1).

It has been suggested that the diagnostic specificity of gallium-67 scanning can be improved by requiring both a positive gallium-67 scan and an elevated serum angiotensin converting enzyme to make the diagnosis (Nosal et al. 1979). However, it is now recognized that, like gallium-67 scans, serum-angiotensin-converting enzyme can be elevated in a variety of disorders, and thus is not specific for sarcoidosis (Crystal et al. 1981b,

---

Figure 5 Serial posterior gallium-67 scans over a 1-year interval in a 24-year-old woman with sarcoidosis. (A) Prominent hilar node and proximal lower lobe uptake are apparent, as is diffuse low-intensity distal parenchymal uptake. (B) Two months later there is spontaneous, nearly complete resolution of mediastinal uptake, but persistent diffuse parenchymal involvement. (C) Nine months after the initial scan there is intense right upper lung and moderate bilateral mid lung zone uptake as well as parotid and splenic involvement. (D) Eleven months after the initial scan the pattern is similar to that at 9 months, but with involvement of lower lung zones as well.

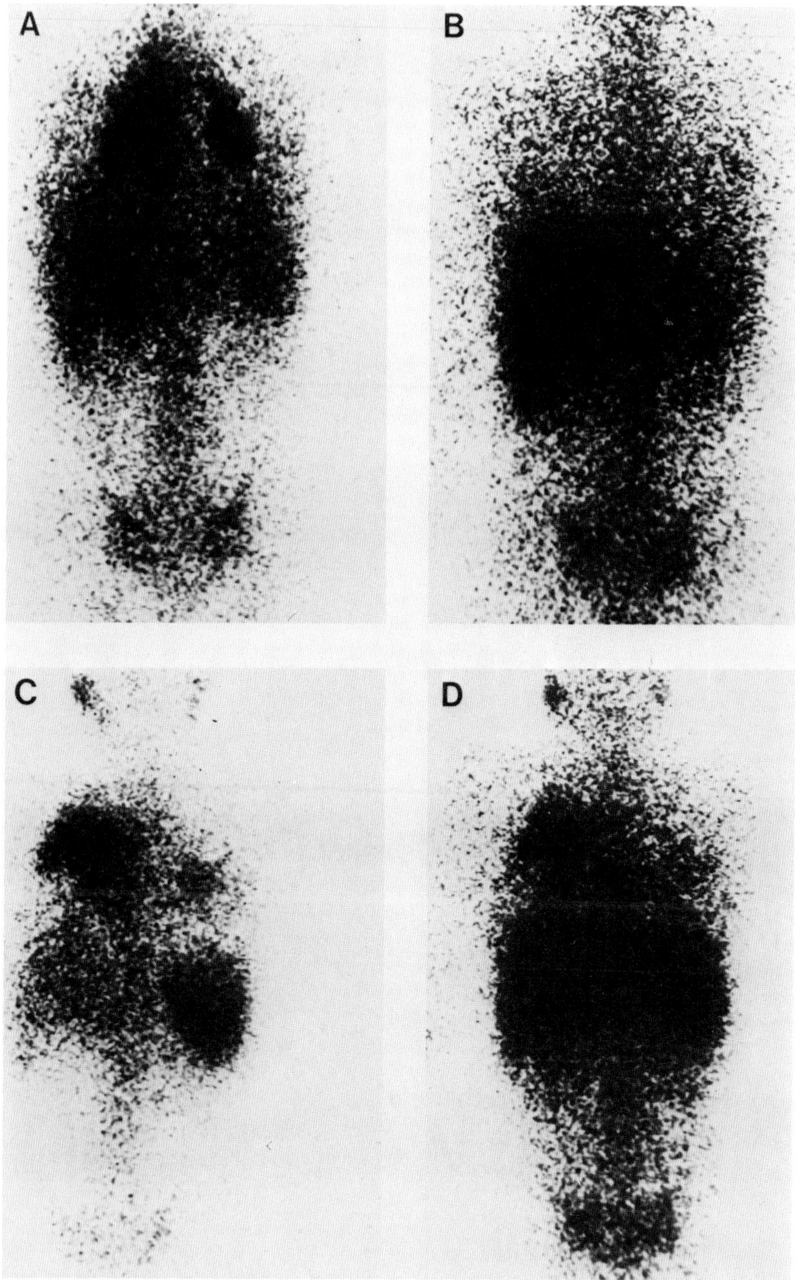

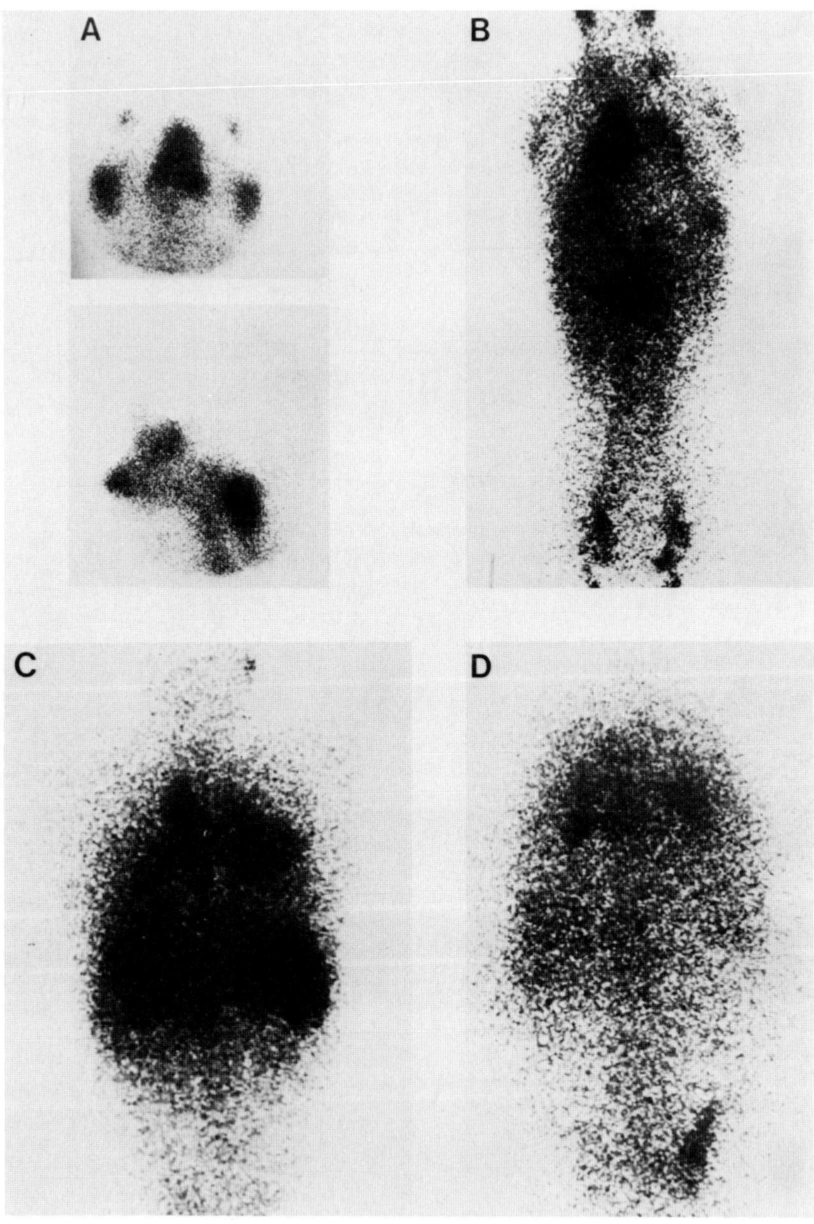

Figure 6 Extrathoracic localization of gallium-67 in sarcoidosis. (A) Nasopharyngeal and parotid gland uptake of gallium-67 in a 24-year-old man with sarcoidosis. Clinical evidence of involvement of the nasopharynx

Table 1 Lung Diseases Demonstrating Positive Thoracic Gallium-67 Scans

Interstitial disorders
  Sarcoidosis (Line et al. 1981, Crystal et al. 1981)
  Silicosis (Dige-Peterson et al. 1972, Higashi et al. 1972, Siemsen et al. 1974)
  Asbestosis (Siemsen et al. 1974)
  Radiation pneumonitis (Kinoshita et al. 1974, Siemsen et al. 1976)
  Bleomycin toxicity (Richman et al. 1975)
  Systemic lupus erythematosus (Niden et al. 1976, Teates and Hunter 1975)
  Cyclophosphamide toxicity (MacMahon and Bekerman 1978)
  Idiopathic pulmonary fibrosis (Line et al. 1978)
  Histiocytosis-X (Javaheri et al. 1979)
  Wegener's granulomatosis (Alpert 1980)
  Coal-workers' pneumoconiosis (Barkman et al. 1980)

Infectious disorders
  Bacterial pneumonitis (Bell et al. 1971)
  Bacterial abscess (Bell et al. 1971)
  Tuberculosis (Siemsen et al. 1976)
  Filariasis (Van der Schoot et al. 1972)
  Aspergillosis (Fogh et al. 1974)
  Pneumocystis carinii (Levenson et al. 1976)
  Blastomycosis (Rose and Varkey 1978)
  Cytomegalovirsus (Hamed et al. 1976)

Neoplastic disorders
  Primary malignancies (Thesingh et al. 1978)
  Metastatic malignancies (Teates et al. 1978)

Figure 6 (Continued)
was present, but the parotid glands were clinically normal. (B) Thoracic and extrathoracic gallium-67 localization in a 29-year-old woman with systemic sarcoidosis. Gallium uptake is present in cervical, supraclavicular, axillary, hilar, para tracheal, and para aortic lymph nodes, and in pulmonary parenchyma at the lung bases. (C) Right paratracheal, diffuse pulmonary parenchymal, and splenic gallium-67 uptake in a 29-year-old woman with sarcoidosis. Mild left parotid uptake is barely evident. (D) Extrathoracic uptake in the left posterior iliac crest, and diffuse pulmonary parenchymal uptake with mediastinal and bilateral hilar involvement in a 63-year-old man with sarcoidosis.

Lieberman et al. 1979). Thus, in our experience, the gallium-67 scan is a useful adjunct to the diagnosis of sarcoidosis, but does not make the diagnosis. To diagnose sarcoidosis we rely on characteristic clinical, roentgenographic, physiologic, bronchoalveolar lavage (see Table 2 and Crystal et al. 1981b for discussion of the characteristic findings), and gallium-67 scanning to strongly suggest the diagnosis. We then confirm the diagnosis of sarcoidosis by the characteristic morphology in lung parenchyma obtained by open biopsy or (more commonly) by trans-bronchial biopsy (often performed at the same time as lavage).

The major use of gallium-67 scanning in pulmonary sarcoidosis is as a method to quantify the alveolitis of the disease. However, to understand the validity and use of the gallium-67 in this regard, it is first necessary to understand the pathogenesis of the disease.

III. Pathogenesis of Pulmonary Sarcoidosis

Since the alveolitis of sarcoidosis precedes granuloma formation and other derangements of the alveolar structures, an understanding of the pathogenesis of this disease was not possible until a methodology was developed to investigate the alveolitis of patients with active disease. The methodology that permitted this was the adaptation of the fiberoptic bronchoscope to sample the epithelial fluid of the lower respiratory tract of the human, thus enabling investigators to obtain large numbers of the inflammatory and immune effector cells present in the alveolar structures (Reynolds and Newball 1974, Reynolds et al. 1977, Hunninghake et al. 1979a). When the first sarcoidosis patients were studied with this approach (Yeager et al. 1977, Weinberger et al. 1978, Hunninghake et al. 1979b), the results were striking: It became immediately apparent that pulmonary sarcoidosis was not a disease of nonspecific depression of cellular immunity as had been thought, but rather was associated with an intense cellular immune response in the alveolar structures.

In this context, the current concept of the pathogenesis of pulmonary sarcoidosis is that two effector cell types, the lung T lymphocyte and the alveolar macrophage, together modulate the characteristic derangements of this disorder (Fig. 7) (Crystal et al. 1981b, Hunninghake et al. 1980a, Hunninghake and Crystal 1981b). A recognition of the importance of both cell types is critical not only to understanding the pathogenesis of the disease, but also to understanding why gallium-67 scanning is so useful in staging these patients.

Table 2 Bronchoalveolar Lavage Evaluation of the Inflammatory and Immune Effector Cells Present in the Alveolar Structures of Patients with Pulmonary Sarcoidosis[a]

Cell	Normal	Inactive pulmonary sarcoidosis	Active pulmonary sarcoidosis
Lymphocytes	<10%	↑	↑↑
T lymphocytes	65–80%[b]	↑	↑↑
T_γ	5–10%[b]	↑	↑↑
$T_{37°}$[c]	5–12%[b]	↑	↑↑
$T_{lymphokine}$[c]	Not detected	±↑	↑↑
T_{helper}(TH)	35–55%[d]	–	↑↑
$T_{suppressor}$(Ts)	18–32%[d]	↑	↓
TH/Ts	1.8–1	↓	↑↑
B lymphocytes	4–10%[b]	–	–
IgG secreting	0.1–0.4%[e]	↑	↑↑
IgM secreting	0.1–0.2%[e]	±↑	±↑
IgA secreting	0.2–0.4%[e]	–	–
Alveolar macrophages	>90%[f]	↓	↓↓
Interleukin-l	Not detected	±↑	↑↑
Fibronectin	Basal level	±	↑
Fibroblast growth factor	Not detected	±	↑↑
Antigen presentation	Basal level	↑	↑
Polymorphonuclear leukocytes	<1%	–	–
Neutrophils	<1%	–	–
Eosinophils	<1%	–	–
Basophils	<1%	–	–

[a]See Hunninghake et al. 1979a, 1979b, 1980a, 1980b, 1980c, 1980d, 1981a, 1981e, Hunninghake and Crystal, 1981b).
[b]Percentage of total lymphocytes recovered.
[c]T_γ = T lymphocytes with Fc receptors for IgG; $T_{37°}$ = T lymphocytes that bind sheep red blood cells at 37°C; T lymphokine = T lymphocytes that produce mediators such as monocyte chemotactic factor.
[d]Percentage of total T lymphocytes recovered.
[e]Percentage of total B lymphocytes recovered.
[f]Percentage of total cells recovered.
Arrows indicate change in distribution of cells compared to normals; ↓ = decreased; – = no change; ±↑ = mildly increased; ↑ = increased; ↑↑ = markedly increased.

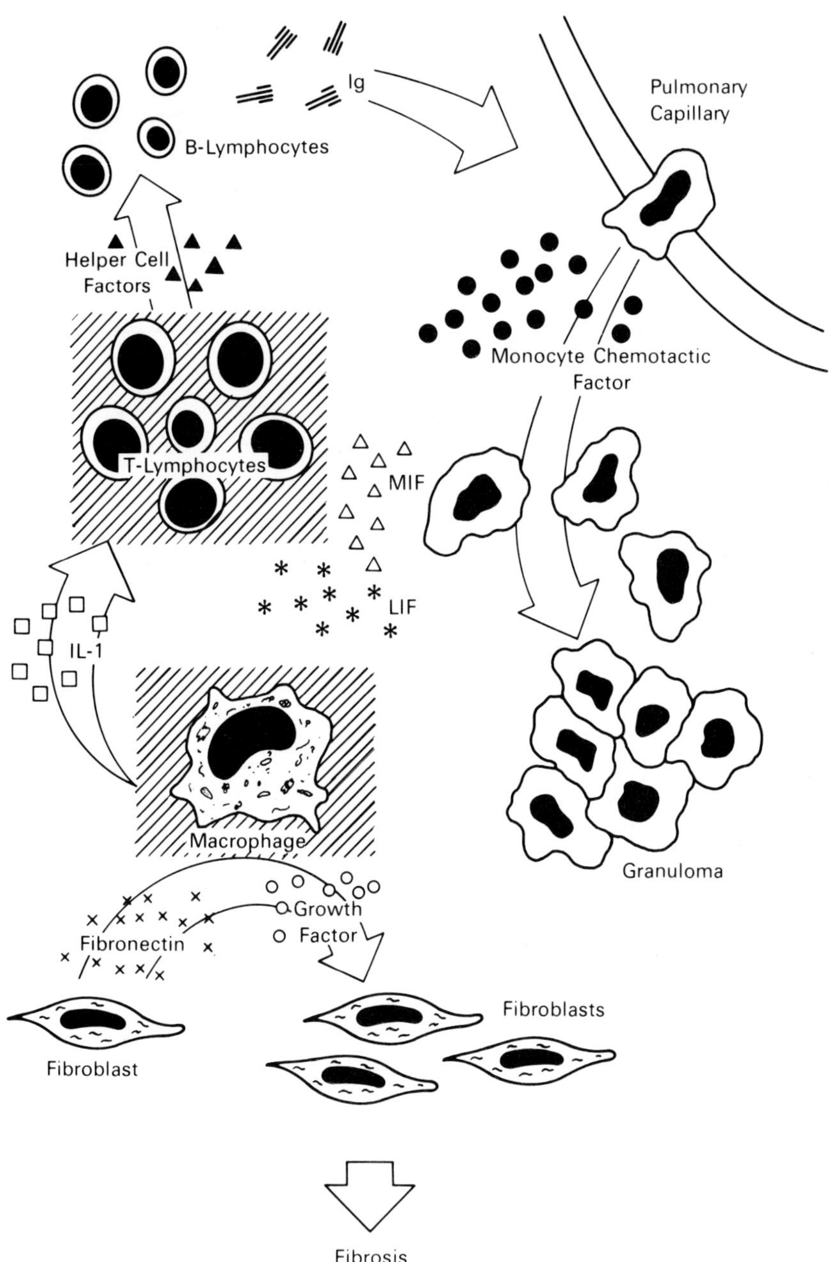

Figure 7 Current concepts of the pathogenesis of pulmonary sarcoidosis. T lymphocytes in the sarcoid lung are activated for unknown reasons, possibly by stimuli from macrophages such as interleukin-l (IL-l). As a result of their activation, the lung T lymphocytes release monocyte chemotactic factor, attracting blood monocytes to lung. Monocytes are

A. Role of Lung T Lymphocytes

As determined by analysis of bronchoalveolar lavage fluid, the effector cells present in the alveolar structures of normal nonsmokers consist of >90% alveolar macrophages, <10% lymphocytes, and <1% polymorphonuclear leukocytes (Table 2) (Hunninghake et al. 1979a). "Normal" cigarette smokers have similar lavage findings, but in contrast to nonsmokers, 3–5% of the lung effectors are neutrophils. Of the lymphocytes present in the normal alveolar structures, 65–80% are T lymphocytes, 4–10% are B lymphocytes, and the remainder are null cells. In terms of the total inflammatory and immune effector cells present in the lower respiratory tract, up to 8% are T cells while <1% are B cells. This is true for nonsmokers and cigarette smokers (Hunninghake et al. 1979a, 1980d).

In marked contrast to normals, patients with active pulmonary sarcoidosis are characterized by a major increase in the proportions of lymphocytes in the lower respiratory tract (Weinberger et al. 1978, Hunninghake et al. 1979b, Crystal et al. 1981b, Danel et al. 1979, Yeager et al. 1977, Rossman et al. 1979, Dauber et al. 1979, Daniele et al. 1980). In fact, patients with clinical criteria associated with "active" disease (e.g., fever, weight loss, erythema nodosum, and progressive deterioration of lung function) have nearly sixfold the normal proportion of lung lymphocytes (Weinberger et al. 1978, Crystal et al. 1981b).

When the number of T lymphocytes in the lungs of patients with sarcoidosis is expressed as a proportion of the total inflammatory and immune effector cells present, it becomes apparent that this disease is characterized not only by an increase in the proportion of lung lymphocytes, but also by a shift in the effector cell populations toward an intense T lymphocyte alveolitis (Table 2). Whereas in normal individuals T lymphocytes account for 8% or less of all inflammatory and immune effector cells within the alveolar structures, in an unselected series of

---

Figure 7 (Continued)
precursors of macrophages, epithelioid cells, and multinucleated giant cells, which comprise granuloma. Other T-lymphocyte factors such as migration inhibitory factor (MIF) and leukocyte inhibitory factor (LIF) likely contribute to granuloma formation. Activated sarcoid lung T lymphocytes also produce helper cell factors which stimulate normal B lymphocytes in a polyclonal fashion to differentiate into immunoglobulin-secreting cells, which produce antibodies to a wide variety of antigens. Besides producing interleukin-1, alveolar macrophages from patients with active sarcoidosis also produce fibronectin, a glycoprotein that acts as a chemoattractant for fibroblasts, and a growth factor that stimulates fibroblast replication. Together, these factors recruit and expand the number of fibroblasts in the interstitium, resulting in fibrosis.

patients with untreated sarcoidosis, T lymphocytes represent 31 ± 8% of the effector cells present (Crystal et al. 1981b). Furthermore, given that biopsies of patients with sarcoidosis show 5–20 times more effector cells within alveolar structures than normal (Mitchell and Scadding 1974, Mitchell et al. 1977, Carrington et al. 1976, Boros 1978, Rosen et al. 1978, Takahasi 1970), it is apparent that the shift toward T lymphocytes observed by bronchoalveolar lavage actually reflects a vast increase in the absolute numbers of T lymphocytes in the lungs of these patients. This marked increase in lung T lymphocytes in active pulmonary sarcoidosis is unaffected by cigarette smoking: The only difference between a smoking sarcoid patient and a nonsmoking sarcoid patient is that the former has neutrophils in the alveolar structures while the latter does not.*

In patients with active pulmonary sarcoidosis, many of the lung T lymphocytes appear to be activated as defined by a number of criteria, including (a) spontaneous incorporation of increased amounts of tritiated thymidine (Hunninghake et al. 1980a), (b) rosetting with sheep red blood cells at 37°C (Hunninghake et al. 1979b, 1980a, 1980d, 1981d, Crystal et al. 1981b, (c) activating normal B lymphocytes to differentiate into immunoglobulin-secreting cells (Hunninghake and Crystal 1981c), and (d) releasing large amounts of monocyte chemotactic factor, macrophage migration inhibitory factor, and leukocyte inhibitory factor, mediators that are important for granuloma formation (Hunninghake et al. 1979b, 1980a, 1980b, Crystal et al. 1981b). The lung T lymphocyte population of patients with active disease is also characterized by an increased proportion of helper T lymphocytes and a decreased proportion of suppressor T lymphocytes (Hunninghake and Crystal 1981). These observations are important because helper T lymphocyte populations are critical to the production of various mediators such as "helper factors" that stimulate B lymphocytes to secrete immunoglobulin. Compared to sarcoid patients with active disease, those with inactive disease have smaller numbers of T lymphocytes in their lavage fluid and these T lymphocytes appear to be less activated. In addition, their ratio of lung helper T lymphocytes to lung suppressor T lymphocytes is similar to that found in normal individuals.

B. Role of B lymphocytes

Because of the increased numbers of T cells in lavage fluid, the relative proportions of B lymphocytes are decreased in patients with active disease (Table 2). The absolute number of these cells in the alveolar structures is

---

*There are some data suggesting that nonsmoking patients with late stages of sarcoidosis may have neutrophils in the alveolar structures, thus explaining some of the destructive aspects of the late-stage disease (Roth et al. 1981).

likely increased, however, because the total number of lung inflammatory and immune effector cells is markedly increased in these patients (Hunninghake et al. 1980a, Crystal et al. 1981b). In addition, the relative proportions of lung B cells that are spontaneously secreting IgG are markedly increased in sarcoidosis (Hunninghake and Crystal 1981c). This is in contrast to the blood of the same patients in which the proportions of B lymphocytes that are spontaneously secreting immunoglobulin are normal. Since lung, but not blood B cells, are producing large amounts of immunoglobulins in pulmonary sarcoidosis, it is reasonable to hypothesize that the elevated levels of immunoglobulin found in lung lavage fluid and in serum of these patients are produced by lung B lymphocytes that diffuse from lung to blood.

One interesting aspect of the hypergammaglobulinemia of sarcoidosis is that it appears to be polyclonal in nature, i.e., it is comprised of antibodies to a wide variety of antigens, including self-antigens (Gupta et al. 1977, Oresbes and Siltzbach 1968, Hedfors and Norberg 1974, Hirshaut et al. 1970, Daniele et al. 1978, Daniele and Rowlands 1976). Although it is possible that this increased production of immunoglobulins results from a continual abnormal response of these patients to multiple antigens, recent studies have demonstrated that an important stimulus for antibody formation in these patients is the presence of activated T cells in the alveolar structures. In this regard, highly purified lung T cells (but not blood T cells) from patients with active pulmonary sarcoidosis are capable of stimulating normal B cells in vitro (without added antigens or mitogens) to differentiate into immunoglobulin-secreting cells (Hunninghake and Crystal 1981c).

There are two in vitro correlates of this observation: (a) There is a direct correlation between the number of T lymphocytes and the number of immunoglobulin-secreting cells in bronchoalveolar lavage fluid from these patients; and (b) as discussed above, antibody production in patients with sarcoidosis is localized to sites of disease since polyclonal activation of B cells results in the secretion of antibodies with specificities toward multiple antigens. These observations explain, at least in part, the presence of high titers of antibodies to a wide variety of antigens, including self-antigens, in these patients.

While it is clear that lung B lymphocytes are actively producing immunoglobulins in sarcoidosis, the relevance of this phenomenon to the pathogenesis of the disease is not known. Although current concepts suggest it is an epiphenomenon unrelated to the morphological derangements characteristic of this disease, there are no data to exclude the possibility that at least a portion of the antibodies present in these patients are directed at an antigen that initiated the underlying process. In this context, there are animal data to suggest that antigen-specific antibodies can trigger granuloma formation (Spector and Heesom 1969).

C. Role of Alveolar Macrophages

Although the relative proportions of alveolar macrophages are decreased in lavage fluid of patients with active sarcoidosis, the absolute number of macrophages in the lower respiratory tract is markedly increased (Table 2) (Hunninghake et al. 1980a, Crystal et al. 1981b). Several lines of evidence suggest significant numbers of these macrophages are activated; including (a) macrophages from patients with active disease spontaneously releasing interleukin-l (also called lymphocyte-activating factor), a monokine that activates T lymphocytes (Hunninghake et al. 1981c), (b) macrophages from patients with sarcoidosis secrete large amounts of fibronectin, a large (220,000 dalton), adhesive glycoprotein that modulates fibroblast attachment to the extracellular matrix and serves as a chemoattractant for fibroblasts (Rennard et al. 1981a), (c) macrophages from these individuals release a growth factor that stimulates lung fibroblasts to replicate (Bitterman et al. 1981a, 1981b), and (d) alveolar macrophages from sarcoid patients "present" antigen to autologous T lymphocytes in an enhanced manner, i.e., alveolar macrophages from sarcoid patients respond to antigens much more actively than do macrophages from normals (Venet et al. in press).

All of these macrophage functions have relevance to the pathogenesis of sarcoidosis. For example, the production of interleukin-l may be important in expanding the numbers of activated T lymphocytes within the lung; since the T lymphocyte is responsible for attracting monocytes to the lung, this provides a mechanism whereby the macrophage indirectly modulates granuloma formation. Since fibronectin is a chemoattractant for fibroblasts, its release by sarcoid alveolar macrophages helps explain the increased number of fibroblasts at sites of disease activity. In addition, release of a growth factor for fibroblasts by alveolar macrophages also expands the number of fibroblasts once they have been recruited to the milieu of the macrophage. Finally, while enhanced antigen presentation by the alveolar macrophage may be an epiphenomenon, it is also possible that it is central to pathogenesis of the disease, i.e., independent of the etiology of sarcoidosis, an enhanced response of the macrophage to any antigen it encounters may provide one mechanism that keeps lung T lymphocytes activated in these patients.

D. How The Alveolar Structures Are Deranged in Sarcoidosis

In the context of recognizing that the alveolitis precedes the derangements of the alveolar structures that characterize sarcoidosis, and with the insight that the alveolitis is comprised of T lymphocytes and alveolar macrophages that are activated in a characteristic fashion, it is possible to understand how the alveolar structures are deranged in this disorder. Although the states of activation of lung T lymphocytes and alveolar macrophages are undoubtly linked in this disease, it appears that the activated T lymphocytes are primarily responsible for granuloma formation and that the activated macrophages are primarily responsible for the interstitial fibrosis.

The ability of lung T cells to attract monocytes (the precursors of macrophages, epitheloid cells, and multinucleated giant cells, i.e., the building blocks of granulomata) to the alveolar structures is critical to the pathogenesis of the granulomata of sarcoidosis. Activated lung T cells not only secrete monocyte chemotactic factor which attracts monocytes to sites of granuloma formation, but also secrete a variety of other lymphokines, including macrophage migration inhibitory factor and leukocyte inhibitory factor, which are likely important in modulating granuloma formation (Hunninghake et al. 1980a, 1980b, Crystal et al. 1981b). Just by their bulk alone, the granulomata are associated with at least some degree of alteration of epithelial, endothelial, and mesenchymal cells that comprise the normal alveolar structures. Although it is unclear whether it is the granulomata alone, or the combination of alveolitis and granuloma which mediate these cellular alterations, it is clear that in some cases the granulomata significantly contribute to the eventual end stage of alveolar-capillary units.

Although it had been thought that the interstitial fibrosis of sarcoidosis was due to an activation of fibroblasts such that each cell produced more collagen, current concepts of the fibrosis of this disease suggest that the increased amounts of collagen found in the alveolar structures result from increased numbers of collagen-producing cells, with each producing normal amounts of collagen. In the context of sarcoidosis, the macrophage clearly plays a central role: By secreting fibronectin it attracts fibroblasts and by secreting a growth factor it expands the numbers of fibroblasts (Rennard et al. 1981a, Bitterman et al. 1981b). Thus, fibroblasts are increased in number in the areas of active disease. Since collagen is a major secretory product of these cells, the result is an increase in the amount of collagen in the local milieu, i.e., fibrosis. Thus, by virtue of their ability to recruit and increase the number of fibroblasts, the alveolar macrophage plays a significant role in mediating the fibrosis of sarcoidosis.

IV. Staging Patients with Pulmonary Sarcoidosis: Evaluation of Lung T Lymphocytes and Alveolar Macrophages

Since activated lung T lymphocytes and alveolar macrophages are the critical determinants of parenchymal injury in sarcoidosis, it is important that the clinician have methods available that can be used to repetitively evaluate the intensity of the alveolitis and distinguish this from the extent of derangement to the alveolar structures (i.e., granulomata, changes in parenchymal cells, and fibrosis). Since the primary determinant of lung parenchymal injury in sarcoidosis is the intensity of the inflammatory and immune effector processes within the alveolar structures, a rational approach to staging these patients necessitates distinguishing between the present status of the alveolitis and the derangements to the alveolar structures that have resulted from alveolitis that has been present in the past. It is important to recognize, however, that the clinical, roentgenographic, and physiologic criteria that have been traditionally used to stage patients with sarcoidosis are neither specific for, nor sensitive to, the alveolitis of sarcoidosis (Crystal et al. 1981a,b, Keogh and Crystal 1980, 1981). Rather, these criteria primarily evaluate the extent of parenchymal derangement.

A. Staging by Roentenographic Criteria

Although the classic roentgengraphic methods of staging sarcoidosis have been useful from an epidemiologic point of view, it is now apparent that the chest film cannot be used to gauge disease activity. The insensitivity of the chest film in detecting the alveolitis of sarcoidosis is best exemplified by x-ray stage I (i.e., hilar adenopathy with normal parenchyma); biopsy data have demonstrated that all of these individuals have varying degrees of alveolitis (Rosen et al. 1978, Rosen et al. 1977, Young et al. 1968, Huang et al. 1979). Furthermore, the extent of chest roentgenogram abnormality clearly bears little relationship to the alveolitis; for example, there is no correlation between x-ray stage and the activity of disease as quantified by bronchoalveolar lavage or by gallium-67 scans (Fig. 8). In our experience, it is not uncommon to find normal gallium-67 uptake in regions of stable pulmonary infiltrates in serial roentgenograms. At the other extreme, patients with normal or minimally abnormal chest roent-genograms may have intense, diffuse gallium-67 uptake in the lung. In addition, we have yet to find a patient with purely nodal uptake of gallium-67; this is consistent with the biopsy evidence that patients with stage I roentgenograms (nodal disease only) all have parenchymal sarcoidosis as well. For example, a patient with nodal disease (Fig. 3b) also has uptake above background in the right lower lung. These findings are con-sistent with the observations of others that gallium-67 scanning is probably more sensitive to the alveolitis of sarcoidosis than is the chest film (Siemsen et al. 1976).

B. Staging by Physiologic Criteria

Although functional testing is more sensitive to pulmonary sarcoidosis than the chest film, pulmonary function tests can be normal in the presence of

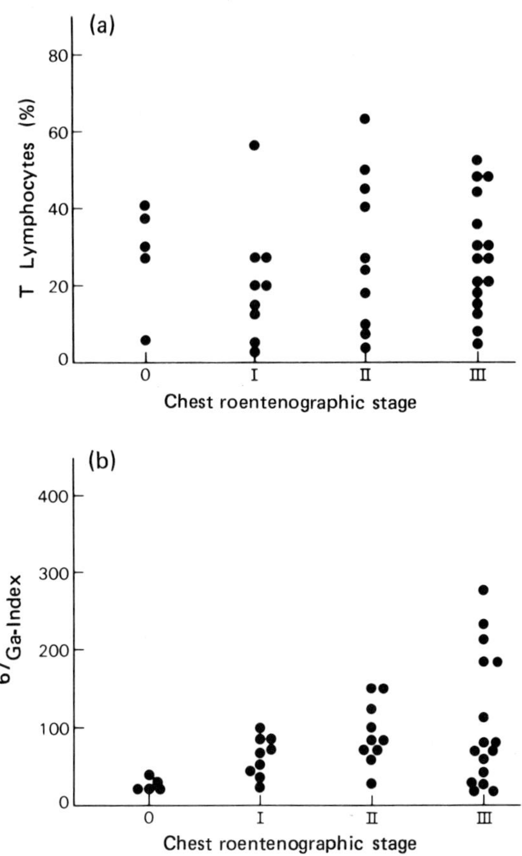

Figure 8 Evaluation of the ability of the chest roentgenogram to estimate the activity of the alveolitis of pulmonary sarcoidosis. (a) Comparison of the percentage of cells recovered by bronchoalveolar lavage that are T lymphocytes to the x-ray stage. (b) Comparison of the gallium-67 index to x-ray stage. The x-ray classification includes: stage 0 = normal, stage I = hilar adenopathy only; stage II = hilar adenopathy and parenchymal involvement; stage III = parenchymal involvement only. Evidence of active alveolitis can be found in all x-ray stages. Although the most intense gallium-67 scans are often found in the more advanced x-ray stage, positive gallium-67 scans (i.e., ^{67}Ga index values > 50) can be present when there is no evidence of parenchymal disease by x-ray (e.g., stage I).

an alveolitis. The most complete analysis of function-structure relationships in sarcoidosis has been carried out by Juang and colleagues (1979), who compared various physiologic tests with open lung biopsy findings in 81 individuals. While lung function tests generally correlated with the overall severity of the morphological findings, functional tests could not distinguish between alveolitis, granulomata, and fibrosis. A similar conclusion can be drawn from our series: There is little relationship between the degree of alveolitis as measured by bronchoalveolar lavage or gallium-67 scanning and the extent of functional impairment (Figs. 9 and 10).

The physiologic findings associated with sarcoidosis, i.e., reduced lung volume, reduced carbon monoxide diffusing capacity, and hypoxia that worsens with exercise, show little relationship to the proportion of T lymphocytes assessed by bronchoalveolar lavage or to the degree of gallium-67 uptake. Although it seems reasonable that the pulmonary function tests that assess the integrity of the alveolar structures would be sensitive to the accumulation of inflammatory and immune effector cells, the available data suggest that the lung function tests are not specific for the extent of parenchymal inflammation. The reasons for this likely reflect the fact that physiologic tests are more sensitive to structural derangement (e.g., granulomata and fibrosis) than to alveolitis.

C. Staging by Clinical Criteria

The intensity of the alveolitis of sarcoidosis and gallium-67 scanning as assessed by bronchoalveolar lavage is not related to patient age, sex, duration of symptoms, smoking history or current smoking status (Line et al. 1981). In addition, although various clinical criteria are often suggested as indicating "active" sarcoidosis (e.g., weight loss, malaise, weakness, fever, cough, progressive dyspnea on exertion, and anergy), it is now recognized that such criteria are insensitive to, and not specific for, the alveolitis, and are likely influenced by the extent of lung derangement (e.g., fibrosis) as well as by disease in organs other than lung (Crystal et al. 1981b).

D. Staging by Blood Test Criteria

Various blood studies have been proposed as monitors of disease activity including sedimentation rate, serum calcium, the presence of immune complexes, elevations of serum lysozyme, and, most recently, elevations of serum-angiotensin-converting enzyme (Crystal et al. 1981b). Although angiotensin-converting enzyme is probably the best of those blood tests suggested, there is little evidence that any changes in the blood necessarily reflect changes in the density and activation of effector cells within the alveolar structures. In this context, attempts to correlate serum-angiotensin-converting enzyme to the status of sarcoid alveolitis as reflected in the numbers lung T lymphocytes have shown little correlation (Schoenberger

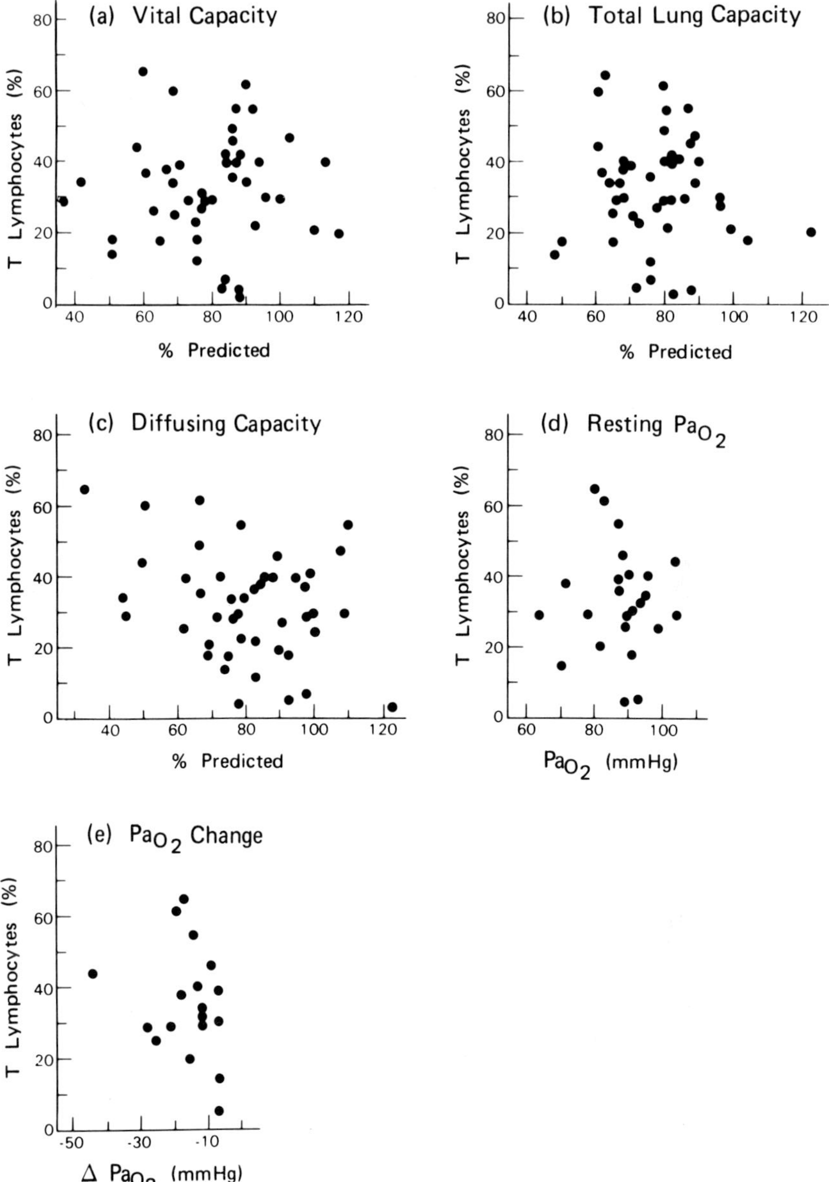

Figure 9 Evaluation of the sensitivity and specificity of lung function tests as monitors of the intensity of the alveolitis of pulmonary sarcoidosis. The intensity of the alveolitis was quantified by bronchoalveolar lavage. The proportion of lung effector cells that are T lymphocytes are compared to (a) vital capacity (percent predicted); (b) total lung capacity (percent predicted); (c) diffusing capacity (single breath, percentage predicted value based on alveolar volume and hemoglobin); (d) resting arterial oxygen tension (mmHg); and (e) change in arterial oxygen tension with exercise $[Pa_{O_2} \text{ (exercise)} - Pa_{O_2} \text{ (rest)}]$.

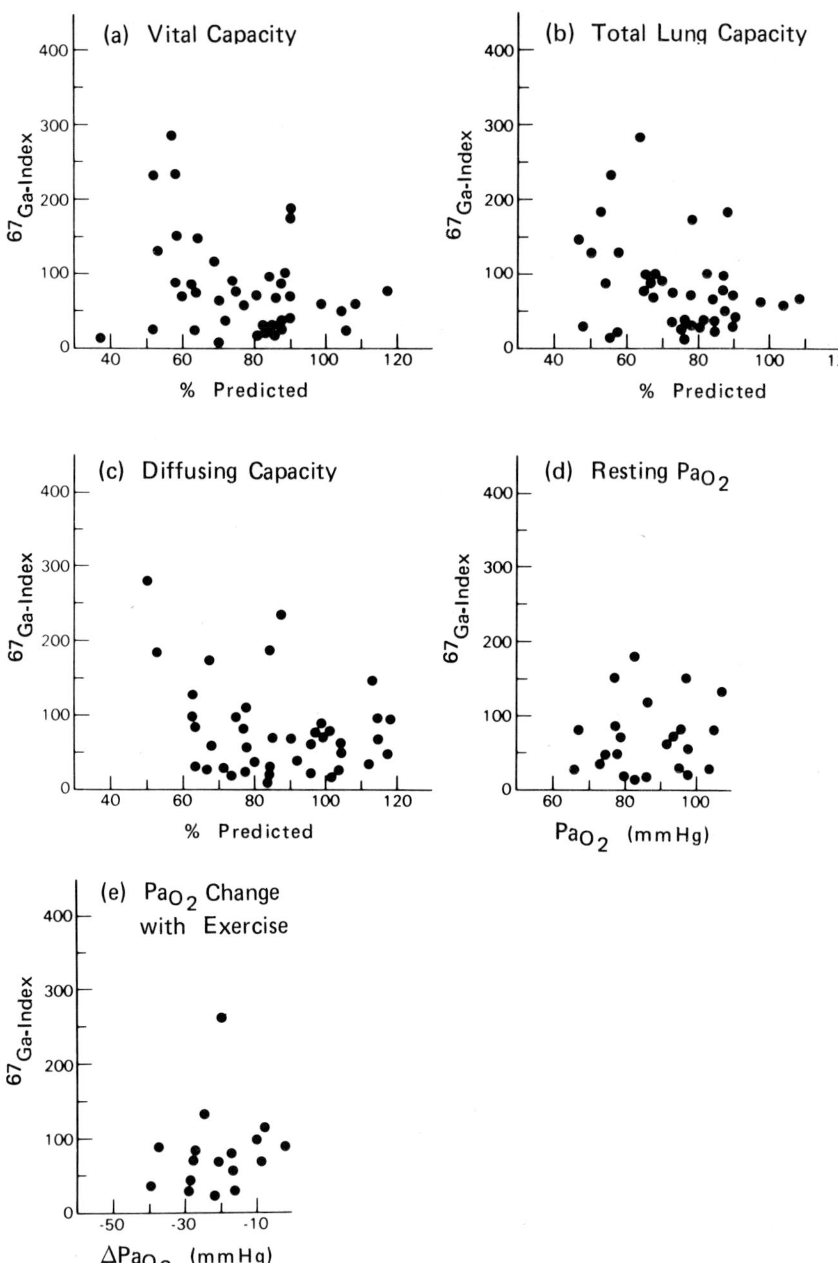

Figure 10 Evaluation of the sensitivity and specificity of lung function tests as monitors of the intensity of the alveolitis of pulmonary sarcoidosis. The intensity of the alveolitis was quantified by gallium-67 scanning. The ^{67}Ga index for each patient is compared to (a) vital capacity (percentage predicted); (b) total lung capacity (percentage predicted); (c) diffusing

et al. 1981a, 1981b). In addition, both false positives (i.e., high serum-angiotensin-converting enzyme with a normal proportion of lung T cells) and false negatives (i.e., normal serum-angiotensin-converting enzyme in the presence of a marked T cell alveolitis) are observed.

E. Staging by Bronchoalveolar Lavage and Gallium-67 Scanning Criteria

The optimal monitor of the alveolitis of sarcoidosis would indicate the number of activated alveolar macrophages and T lymphocytes per unit region of lung, i.e., the density of the effector cells that determine derangement to the alveolar structures. Neither bronchoalveolar lavage nor gallium-67 does exactly that, but each comes close, and both methods are far superior to any clinical, roentgenographic, or physiologic methods available (Crystal et al. 1981b, Keogh and Crystal 1980). In addition, since bronchoalveolar lavage most reflects the intensity of the T lymphocyte alveolitis and gallium-67 scanning the intensity of the activated alveolar macrophage, the combination of bronchoalveolar lavage and gallium-67 scanning gives the broadest overview of the alveolitis of sarcoidosis currently available.

F. Use of Bronchoalveolar Lavage in Staging Sarcoidosis

Bronchoalveolar lavage is particularly useful for quantifying the T-lymphocyte component of the alveolitis. In normal lung, T lymphocytes represent $<8\%$ of all effector cells present (Hunninghake et al. 1979a). In contrast, lavage of untreated patients with sarcoidosis demonstrates that T lymphocytes represent up to 65% of all inflammatory and immune effector cells present (Crystal et al. 1981b). In addition, comparison of the histological estimate of the intensity of the alveolitis (i.e., relative number of effector cells per unit paranchyma) to the proportion of T lymphocytes recovered by lavage has shown that the proportion of lavage T lymphocytes is an excellent predictor of the presence of high- or low-intensity alveolitis in lung biopsies from these patients (Fig. 11) (Crystal et al. 1981b, Hunninghake et al. 1980a).

   To demonstrate this, biopsy specimens were divided histologically into groups characterized by either high- or low-intensity alveolitis by grading the number of mononuclear cells within the alveolar structures. These groups were then compared to the findings of bronchoalveolar lavage in

---

Figure 10 (Continued)
capacity (single breath, percentage predicted value based on alveolar volume and hemoglobin); (d) resting arterial oxygen tension (mmHg); and (e) change in arterial oxygen tension with exercise [Pa_{O_2} (exercise) $-$ Pa_{O_2} (rest)].

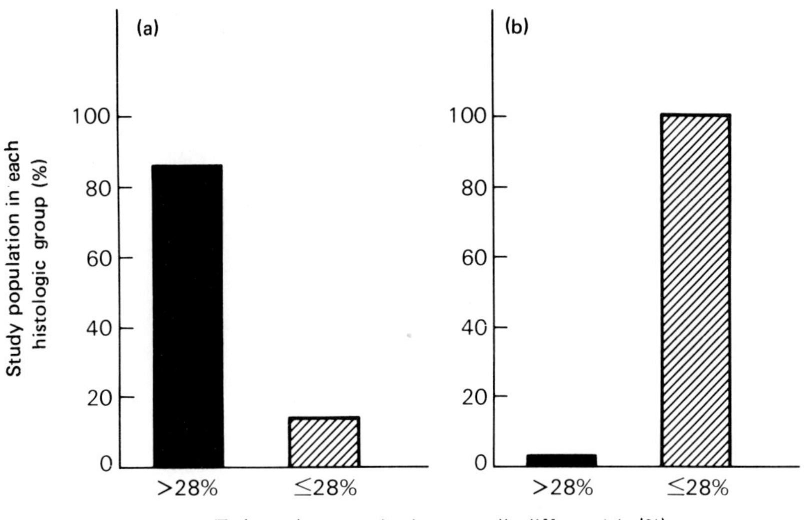

Figure 11 Assessment of disease activity in pulmonary sarcoidosis by quantification of lung T lymphocytes by bronchoalveolar lavage compared to the assessment of disease activity by open lung biopsy. Patients were divided by biopsy criteria into (a) a high-intensity alveolitis group and (b) a low-intensity alveolitis group. The two biopsy groups were then characterized by the proportion of lavage inflammatory and immune effector cells that were T lymphocytes. (i.e., patients in whom >28% of all cells recovered by lavage were T lymphocytes, and patients in whom ≤28% of all cells recovered by lavage were T lymphocytes). Most patients with high-intensity alveolitis by histological criteria had >28% T lympho-cytes in the lavage cell differential. In contrast, most patients with low-intensity alveolitis by histological criteria had ≤28% T lymphocytes in the lavage cell differential.

which the same patients were grouped by the proportion of T lymphocytes recovered. Nearly all patients with high-intensity alveolitis by histological criteria had more than 28% T lymphocytes as a proportion of their total lavage inflammatory and immune effector cells, whereas all patients with low-intensity alveolitis by biopsy had ≤28% T lymphocytes (Fig. 11). Furthermore, evaluation of the function of the T-lymphocyte populations recovered by lavage of patients with sarcoid has shown that for all individuals in whom >28% of the effector cells present were T lympho-cytes, those T-cell populations (a) had a ratio of helper-to-suppressor cells greater than normal, (b) were secreting monocyte chemotactic factor, and

(c) were capable of polyclonally activating normal B cells to produce immunoglobulin (Hunninghake and Crystal 1981a).

Thus, the empiric observation has been made that a shift in lavage cell populations toward relatively more T lymphocytes (i.e., >28% of effector cells), generally signifies (a) a marked increase in intensity of the alveolitis per unit lung parenchyma, and (b) activation of the lung T-lymphocyte populations. In this context, bronchoalveolar lavage is an extremely useful method by which to quantify the alveolitis of sarcoidosis.

G. Use of Gallium-67 Scanning in Staging Sarcoidosis

It has been known for some time that gallium-67 localizes in inflammatory foci, and thoracic gallium scanning is now an established method by which to evaluate the alveolitis of a variety of chronic interstitial lung disorders (Kanno 1971, Dige-Peterson 1972, Crystal et al. 1981b, Line et al. 1978, 1981). However, until recently, the mechanism causing patients with active sarcoidosis to have positive thoracic gallium-67 scans was not known.

Although it has been suggested that "capillary leak" secondary to inflammation may be responsible for positive gallium-67 scans (Ito et al. 1971), the fact that patients with noninflammatory pulmonary capillary leak disorders (e.g., cardiac-induced pulmonary edema) have negative gallium scans suggests serum leak is not the mechanism. A much more tenable hypothesis is that the effector cell populations in the alveolar structures are responsible, likely by the activated effector cells taking up the gallium-67. However, since normal individuals have alveolar macro-phage and T, B, and null lymphocytes in their alveolar structures, the fact that they have negative gallium-67 scans suggests either that these cells are not responsible for the gallium-67 uptake in active sarcoidosis or that they are not present in sufficient numbers and/or states of activation in normals to result in a positive scan.

To evaluate this concept, comparisons were made between the ^{67}Ga index and the percentage of various inflammatory and immune effector cells recovered by bronchoalveolar lavage in our series of patients with sarcoidosis. In this analysis, highly significant correlations were observed between the amount of gallium-67 taken up by the lung parenchyma and the proportions of lavage cells that were T lymphocytes (Fig. 12) (Line et al. 1981). However, while such an analysis strongly suggests that T lymphocytes are responsible for the positive gallium-67 scans in sarcoidosis, it is also possible that this observation reflects a secondary effect, i.e., that while T lymphocytes are involved, it is another cell type that is taking up gallium-67 and also modulating the numbers and/or state of activation of the T-cell populations (Crystal et al. 1981, Line et al. 1981).

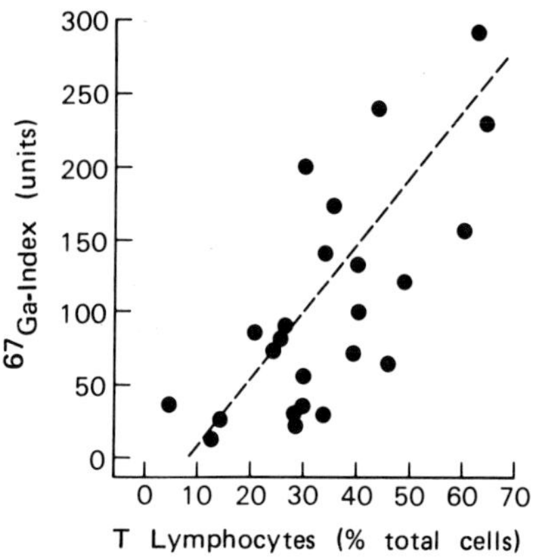

Figure 12 Comparison of the ^{67}Ga index with the differential percentage of bronchoalveolar lavage cells that are T lymphocytes. Highly significant correlations between the ^{67}Ga index and the percentage of T lymphocytes are noted (p = 0.0001, r = 0.71).

To test this hypothesis, Hunninghake and colleagues (1981b) lavaged patients with sarcoidosis who had just had gallium-67 scans, recovered the effector cells from the lower respiratory tract, and separated the various cell types to determine which cells contained the gallium-67 (Hunninghake et al. 1981b). The results were striking: Greater than 95% of the gallium-67 was associated with the alveolar macrophages (Table 3). To evaluate this observation further, alveolar macrophages obtained from normal individuals and patients with active pulmonary sarcoidosis were exposed to gallium-67 in vitro. Interestingly, only the macrophages from the sarcoid patients took up gallium-67, confirming the in vivo observations and explaining why normal individuals have negative gallium-67 scans even though they have large numbers of macrophages in their alveolar structures, that is, a positive gallium-67 scan in sarcoidosis indicates large numbers of activated alveolar macrophages.

Table 3 Distribution of ^{67}Ga in Fluid and Cells Recovered by Bronchoalveolar Lavage of Patients with Sarcoidosis[a]

	Distribution of ^{67}Ga in bronchoalveolar lavage fluid and cells			
Condition	Fluid	Cells	Macrophages	T lymphocytes
Sarcoidosis	<1%	>99%	>95%	<5%

[a]See Hunninghake et al. 1981c for details; data obtained from 10 patients with sarcoidosis who underwent bronchoalveolar lavage 72 hr following injection with ^{67}Ga-citrate.

This finding gives further support to the concept of a strong link between the two major activated cell types in the sarcoid lung, the alveolar macrophage and the T lymphocyte, i.e., while the ^{67}Ga index correlates with the proportion of T cells in the lower respiratory tract, it is the activated alveolar macrophages that primarily are responsible for gallium-67 uptake. In addition, this observation is consistent with the concept that alveolar macrophages play a role in modulating the shift in effector cell populations in the sarcoid lung toward more T lymphocytes (Hunninghake et al. 1981c).

H. Combined Lavage and Gallium-67 Scan Criteria in Staging Sarcoidosis

Using the concepts elucidated above, Keogh and colleagues (1981) have established criteria for "high-intensity alveolitis" and "low-intensity alveolitis" based on lavage and gallium-67 scans. Empirically, the criteria for high-intensity alveolitis were established as a positive gallium-67 scan (i.e., a ^{67}Ga index >50 units) and the percentage of lavage T lymphocytes as greater than 3.5 times the highest proportions found in normals (i.e., normals ≤8%; high-intensity alveolitis >28%). The criteria for low-intensity alveolitis include all other patients, that is, a normal gallium-67 scan and/or lavage T cells ≤28%. When used prospectively to follow patients with untreated sarcoidosis, the validity of such criteria were striking. Of those with untreated high-intensity alveolitis, 63% deteriorated in at least one lung functional parameter over a 6-month period. In contrast, of those with untreated low-intensity alveolitis, 8% deteriorated over the same period.

It has long been recognized that the status of patients with pulmonary sarcoidosis can change spontaneously. This is clearly observed when patients are followed with lavage and gallium-67 scanning. Individuals with high-intensity alveolitis can spontaneously revert to low-intensity and vice versa. In our experience, the reversion from high- to low-intensity alveolitis is much more common than from low to high, consistent with the well-known clinical fact those with stable disease usually do not deteriorate.

I. Therapy Decisions in Sarcoidosis

When deciding on therapy, screening studies that directly assess the intensity of the sarcoid alveolitis are clearly preferable to those that are either nonspecific for pulmonary disease or are confounded by the presence of irreversible structural and functional changes. Thus, it is understandable that conventional monitors of disease severity (e.g., chest roentgenograms and pulmonary function tests) might not be sensitive to the efficacy of corticosteroids even if they were to ameliorate an active sarcoid alveolitis.

Since patients with sarcoidosis at high risk to deteriorate (high-intensity alveolitis) exhibit characteristic alterations in their cell populations obtained by bronchoalveolar lavage and in their ^{67}Ga index values which distinguish them from patients with quiescent disease (low-intensity alveolitis), the use of these techniques should allow patients with high-intensity alveolitis to be identified so that irreversible functional derangements of the alveolar structures can be avoided with prompt and appropriate therapy. All available evidence suggests that the prospective use of ^{67}Ga scanning and bronchoalveolar lavage in the staging of patients with sarcoidosis will provide a rational approach to the use of corticosteroids that has not been previously available.

References

Alpert, L. (1980). Pulmonary uptake of gallium-67 in Wegener's granulomatosis. *Clin. Nucl. Med.,* **5**:53–56.

Barkman, H. W., Kawner, R. E., Rom, W. N., and Welch, D. M. (1980). Gallium-67 citrate imaging in coal workers pneumoconiosis (CWP). *Am. Rev. Respir. Dis.,* **121**:221.

Bell, E. G., O'Mara, R. E., Henry, C. A., Subramanian, G., McAfee, J. G., and Brown, L. C. (1971). Non-neoplastic localization of ^{67}Ga citrate. *J. Nucl. Med.,* **12**:338–339.

Bitterman, P., and Crystal, R. (1981a). Pulmonary alveolar macrophages (AM) secrete a growth factor (GF) causing human lung fibroblasts to replicate. *Am. Rev. Respir. Dis.,* **123**:50.

Bitterman, P., Hunninghake, G., Keogh, B., Rossi, G., Line, B., and Crystal, R. G. (1981b). Evidence for locus regulating immune processes causing familiar pulmonary fibrosis. *Clin. Res.,* **49**:314A.

Boros, O. L. (1978). Granulomatous inflammations. *Prog. Allergy,* **24**:183–267.

Carrington, C. B., Gaensler, E. A., Milaus, J. P., Schacter, A. W., Burke, G. W., and Goff, A. M. (1976). Structure and function in sarcoidosis. *Ann. N.Y. Acad. Sci.,* **278**:265–282.

Crofton, J., and Douglas, A. (1975). *Respiratory Disease.* Oxford, England, Blackwell Scientific Publications.

Crystal, R. G., Roberts, W. C., Hunninghake, G. W., Gadek, J. E., Fulmer, J. D., and Line, B. R. (1980). Pulmonary sarcoidosis: A disease characterized and perpetuated by activated lung T-lymphocytes. *Ann. Intern. Med.,* **94**:73–94.

Crystal, R. G., Gadek, J. E., Ferrans, V. J., Fulmer, J. D., Line, B. R., and Hunninghake, G. W. (1981a). Interstitial lung disease: Current concepts of pathogenesis, staging, and therapy. *Am. J. Med.,* **70**: 542–568.

Crystal, R. G., Roberts, W. C., Hunninghake, G. W., Gadek, J. E., Fulmer, J. D., and Line, B. R. (1981b). Pulmonary sarcoidosis: A disease characterized and perpetuated by activated lung T-lymphocytes. *Ann. Intern. Med.*, **94**:73–94.

Danel, C., Arnoux, A., Marsac, J., Basset, F., and Chreitien, J. (1979). Cellular data from bronchoalveolar lavages in various interstitial lung diseases. *Bull. Europ. Physiopathol. Respir.*, **15**:42–43.

Daniele, R. P., and Rowlands, D. T. (1976). Antibodies to T-cells in sarcoidosis. *Proc. N.Y. Acad. Sci.*, **278**:88–100.

Daniele, R. P., McMillan, L. J., Dauber, J. H., and Rossman, M. D. (1978). Immune complexes in sarcoidosis: A correlation with activity and duration of disease. *Chest,* **74**:261–264.

Daniele, R. P., Dauber, J. H., and Rossman, M. D. (1980). Immunologic abnormalities in sarcoidosis. *Ann. Inter. Med.*, **92**:406–416.

Dauber, J. H., Rossman, M. D., and Daniele, R. P. (1979). Bronchoalveolar cell populations in acute sarcoidosis: Observations in smoking and non-smoking patients. *J. Lab. Clin. Med.*, **94**:862–871.

Dige-Peterson, H., Heckscher, T., and Hertz, M. (1972). ^{67}Ga-scintigraphy in non-malignant lung diseases. *Scand. J. Respir. Dis.*, **53**:314–319.

Fogh, J., Bettelsen, S., and Schmidt, A. (1974). Diagnostic value of ^{67}Ga-scintigraphy in chest surgery. *Thorax,* **29**:26–31.

Gupta, R. C., Kueppers, F., DeRemee, R. A., Huston, K. A., and McDuffie, P. C. (1977). Pulmonary and extrapulmonary sarcoidosis in relation to circulating immune complexes: A quantification of immune complexes by two radioimmunoassays. *Am. Rev. Respir. Dis.*, **116**:261–266.

Hamed, I. A., Wenzel, J. E., Leonard, J. C., Altschuler, G. P., and Pederson, J. A. (1979). Pulmonary cytomegalovirus infection: Detection by Gallium 67 imaging in the transplant patient. *Arch. Intern. Med.*, **139**:286–288.

Hedfors, E., and Norberg, R. (1974). Evidence for circulating immune complexes in sarcoidosis. *Clin. Exp. Immunol.*, **16**:493–496.

Higasi, T., Nakayama, Y., Murata, A., Nakamura, K., Skugiyama, M., Kawaguchi, T., and Susuki, S. (1972). Clinical evaluation of ^{67}Ga-citrate scanning. *J. Nucl. Med.*, **13**:196–201.

Hirshaut, Y., Slade, P. B. D., Vierira, L. D., Ainbender, E., Dvorak, B., and Siltzbach, L. E. (1970). Sarcoidosis, another disease associated with serological evidence for herpes-like virus infection. *N. Engl. J. Med.*, **283**:502–504.

Huang, C. T., Heurich, A. E., Rosen, Y., Moon, H. A., and Lyons, H. A. (1979). Pulmonary sarcoidosis: Roentenographic, functional, and pathologic correlations. *Respiration,* **37**:337–345.

Hunninghake, G. W., and Crystal, R. G. (1981a). Pulmonary sarcoidosis:
   A disorder mediated by excess helper T-lymphocyte activity at sites
   of disease activity. *N. Engl. J. Med.*, **305**:420–434.
Hunninghake, G. W., and Crystal, R. G. (1981b). Inflammatory and
   immune mechanisms in chronic diseases of the lung parenchyma. In
   *Proceedings of the 6th Irwin Strasburger Memorial Seminar on
   Immunology.* Edited by G. W. Siskind (in press).
Hunninghake, G. W., and Crystal, R. G. (1981c). Mechanisms of hyper-
   gammaglobulinemia in sarcoidosis: Site of increased antibody
   production and role of T-lymphocytes. *J. Clin. Invest.*, **67**:86–92.
Hunninghake, G. W., Gadek, J. E., Kawanami, O., Ferrans, V. J., and
   Crystal, R. G. (1979a). Inflammatory and immune processes in the
   human lung in health and disease: Evaluation by bronchoalveolar
   lavage. *Am. J. Pathol.*, **97**:149–206.
Hunninghake, G. W., Fulmer, J. D., Young, R. C., Gadek, J. E., and
   Crystal, R. G. (1979b). Localization of the immune response in
   sarcoidosis. *Am. Rev. Respir. Dis.*, **120**:49–57.
Hunninghake, G. W., Keogh, B. A., Line, B. R., Gadek, J. E., Kawanami,
   O., Ferrans, V. J., and Crystal, R. G. (1980a). Pulmonary sarcoidosis:
   Pathogenesis and therapy. In *Basic and Clinical Aspects of Granulo-
   matous Diseases.* Edited by D. Boros and T. Yoshida. New York,
   Elsevier, pp. 274–290.
Hunninghake, G. W., Gadek, J. E., Young, R. C., Jr., Kawanami, O.,
   Ferrans, V. J., and Crystal, R. G. (1980b). Maintenance of granu-
   loma formation in pulmonary sarcoidosis by T-lymphocytes within
   the lung. *N. Engl. J. Med.*, **302**:594–598.
Hunninghake, G. W., Gadek, J. E., Szapiel, S. V., Strumpf, I. J., Kawanami,
   O., Ferrans, V. J., Keogh, B. A., and Crystal, R. G. (1980c). The
   human alveolar macrophage. In *Methods in Cell Biology.*
   Edited by C. C. Harris, B. F. Trump, and G. D. Stoner. New York,
   Academic Press, pp. 94–112.
Hunninghake, G. W., Fulmer, J. D., Young, R. C., and Crystal, R. G.
   (1980d). Comparison of lung and blood lymphocyte subpopulations
   in pulmonary sarcoidosis. In *Proceedings of the 8th International
   Conference on Sarcoidosis and Other Granulomatous Disease.*
   Edited by W. J. Williams and B. H. Davies. London, Alpha Omega,
   pp. 426–435.
Hunninghake, G. W., Keogh, B. A., Line, B. R., and Crystal, R. G. (1981a).
   Short course intravenous Solu-Medrol: A new approach to the therapy
   of pulmonary sarcoid. *Am. Rev. Respir. Dis.*, **123**:99.
Hunninghake, G. W., Line, B. R., Szapiel, S. V., and Crystal, R. G.
   (1981b). Activation of inflammatory cells increases the localization
   of gallium-67 at sites of disease. *Clin. Res.*, **49**:171A.

Hunninghake, G. W., Broska, P., Haber, R., Keogh, B., Line, B., and Crystal, R. G. (1981c). Correlation of lung T-cell and macrophage function with disease activity in pulmonary sarcoid. *Clin. Res.*, **49**:550A.

Hunninghake, G. W., Kawanami, O., Ferrans, V. J., Young, R. C., Jr., Roberts, W. C., and Crystal, R. G. (1981d). Characterization of the inflammatory and immune effector cells in the lung parenchyma of patients with interstitial lung disease. *Am. Rev. Respir. Dis.*, **123**: 407–412.

Ito, Y., Okunyama, S., Awano, T., Takahashi, K., Sato, T., and Kanno, I. (1971). Diagnostic evaluation of ^{67}Ga scanning of lung cancer and other diseases. *Radiology*, **101**:355–362.

Javaheri, S., Levine, B. W., McKusick, K. A. (1979). Serial ^{67}Ga scanning in pulmonary eosinophic granuloma. *Thorax*, **34**:822–823.

Judd, P. A., Finnegan, P., and Curran, R. C. (1975). Pulmonary sarcoidosis: A clinicopathologic study. *J. Pathol.*, **115**:191–198.

Kanno, I. (1971). Diagnostic evaluation of ^{67}Ga scanning of lung cancer and other diseases. *Radiology*, **101**:355–362.

Keogh, B. A., and Crystal, R. G. (1980). Pulmonary function testing in interstitial pulmonary disease: What does it tell us? *Chest*, **78**:856–865.

Keogh, B. A., and Crystal, R. G. (1981). Chronic interstitial lung disease. In *Current Pulmonology*. Edited by D. H. Simmons. New York, Wiley, pp. 237–340.

Keogh, B., Hunninghake, G., Line, B., Price, D., Young, R., and Crystal, R. (1981). Alveolitis parameters as prediators of the natural history of pulmonary sarcoidosis. *Clin. Res.*, **49**:447A.

Kinoshita, F., Ushito, T., Maekawa, A., Ariwa, R., and Kubo, A. (1974). Scintiscanning of pulmonary diseases with Gallium-67 citrate. *J. Nucl. Med.*, **15**:227–233.

Larson, S. U., Milder, M. S., and Johnson, G. S. (1973). Interpretation of the ^{67}Ga photoscan. *J. Nucl. Med.*, **14**:208–214.

Levenson, S. M., Warren, R. D., Richman, S. D., Johnston, G. S., and Chalsner, B. A. (1976). Abnormal pulmonary gallium accumulation in *P. carinii* pneumonia. *Radiology*, **119**:395–398.

Lieberman, J., Nosal, A., Schlessner, L. A., and Sastre-Foker, A. (1979). Serum angiotensin-converting enzyme for diagnosis and therapeutic evaluation of sarcoidosis. *Am. Rev. Respir. Dis.*, **120**:329–335.

Line, B. R., Fulmer, J. D., Reynolds, H. Y., Roberts, W. C., Jones, A. E., Harris, E. K., and Crystal, R. G. (1978). Gallium-67 citrate scanning in the staging of idiopathic pulmonary fibrosis: Correlation with physiology, morphology and bronchoalveolar lavage. *Am. Rev. Respir. Dis.*, **118**:355–365.

Line, B. R., Hunninghake, G. W., Keogh, B. A., Jones, A. E., Johnston, G. S., and Crystal, R. G. (1981). Gallium-67 scanning to stage the alveolitis of sarcoidosis: Correlation with clinical studies, pulmonary function studies and bronchoalveolar lavage. *Am. Rev. Respir. Dis.*, **123**:440–446.

MacMahon, H., and Bekerman, C. (1978). The diagnostic significance of gallium lung uptake in patients with normal chest radiograph. *Radiology*, **127**:189–193.

Mitchell, D. N., and Scadding, J. G. (1974). Sarcoidosis. *Am. Rev. Respir. Dis.*, **110**:774–802.

Mitchell, D. N., Scadding, J. G., Heard, B. E., and Hinson, K. F. W. (1977). Sarcoidosis: Histopathological definition and clinical diagnosis. *J. Clin. Pathol.*, **30**:395–408.

Nelson, B., Hayes, R. L., Edwards, C. L., Kniseley, R. M., and Andrews, G. A. (1972). Distribution of gallium in human tissues after intravenous administration. *J. Nucl. Med.*, **13**:92–100.

Niden, A. H., Mishkin, F. S., and Kuurhana, M. L. (1976). Gallium-67 citrate lung scans in interstitial lung disease. *Chest*, **69**:266–268.

Nosal, A., Schleissner, L. A., Mishkin, F. S., Lieberman, J. (1979). Angiotensin-1-converting enzyme and gallium scan in noninvasive evaluation in sarcoidosis. *Ann. Intern. Med.*, **90**:328–331.

Oresbes, I., and Siltzbach, L. E. (1968). Changes in rheumatoid factor activity during the course of sarcoidosis. *Am. J. Med.*, **44**:6067.

Rennard, S., and Crystal, R. (1981). Fibronectin in human broncho-pulmonary lavage fluid: Elevation of patients with interstitial lung disease. *J. Clin. Invest.*, **69**:113–122.

Rennard, S. I., Hunninghake, G. W., Bitterman, P. B., and Crystal, R. G. (1981). Production of fibronectin by the human alveolar macrophage: A mechanism for the recruitment of fibroblasts to sites of tissue injury in the interstitial lung diseases. *Proc. Natl. Acad. Sci. U.S.A.* (in press).

Reynolds, H. Y., and Newball, H. H. (1974). Analysis of proteins and respiratory cells obtained from human lungs by bronchial lavage. *J. Lab. Clin. Med.*, **84**:559–573.

Reynolds, H. Y., Fulmer, J. D., Kazmierowski, J. A., Roberts, W. C., Frank, M. M., and Crystal, R. G. (1977). Analysis of bronchoalveolar lavage fluid from patients with idiopathic pulmonary fibrosis and chronic hypersensitivity pneumonitis. *J. Clin. Invest.*, **59**:165–175.

Richman, S. D., Levenson, S. M., Bunn, P. A., Flinn, G. S., Johnson, G. S., and Devita, V. T. (1975). ^{67}Ga accumulation in pulmonary lesions associated with bleomycin toxicity. *Cancer*, **36**:1966–1972.

Rose, H. D., and Varkey, B. (1978). Micronazole treatment of relapsed pulmonary blastomycosis. *Amer. Rev. Respir. Dis.*, **118**:403–408.

Rosen, Y., Amorosa, J. K., Mason, S., Cohen, J., and Lyons, H. A. (1977). Occurrence of lung granulomas in patients with stage I sarcoidosis. *Am. J. Roentgenol.,* **129**:1083-1985.

Rosen, Y., Athanassiades, T. J., Moon, S., and Lyons, H. A. (1978). Nongranulomatous interstitial pneumonitis in sarcoidosis: Relationship to the development of epithelioid granulomas. *Chest,* **74**:122-125.

Rossman, M. D., Daniele, R. P., and Dauber, J. H. (1979). Broncho-alveolar lymphocytes in sarcoidosis. *Am. Rev. Respir. Dis.,* **119**:795.

Roth, C., Huchon, G. J., Arnoux, A., Stanislas-LeGruen, G., Marsac, J. H., and Chretien, J. (1981). Bronchoalveolar cells in advanced pulmonary sarcoidosis. *Am. Rev. Respir. Dis.,* **121**:9-12.

Scadding, J. G., and Hinson, K. F. W. (1967). Diffuse fibrosing alveolitis (diffuse interstitial fibrosis of the lungs): Correlation of history at biopsy with prognosis. *Thorax,* **22**:291.

Schoenberger, C. I., Line, B. R., Keogh, B. A., Hunninghake, G. W., Crystal, R. G. (1982). Lung inflammation in sarcoidosis: Comparison of serum angiotensin converting enzyme levels with bronchoalveolar lavage and gallium-67 scanning assessment of the T-lymphocyte alveolitis. *Thorax,* **37**:19-25.

Schoenberger, C., Rosenberg, D., and Crystal, R. (1981b). Angiotensin-converting enzyme (ACE) in bronchoalveolar lavage fluid: Correlation with diagnosis and serum ACE. *Am. Rev. Respir. Dis.,* **123**:99.

Siemsen, J. K., Sargent, E. N., Grebe, S. F., Windsor, D. W., Wentz, D., and Jacobson, G. (1974). Pulmonary concentration of ^{67}Ga in pneumoconiosis. *Radiology,* **113**:765.

Siemsen, J. K., Grebe, S. F., Sargent, E. N., and Wentz, D. (1976). Gallium-67 scintigraphy of pulmonary diseases as a complement to radiography. *Radiology,* **118**:371-375.

Spector, W. G., and Heesom, N. (1969). The production of granulomata by antigen-antibody complexes. *J. Pathol.,* **98**:31-39.

Spencer, H. (1977). *Pathology of the Lung.* New York, Pergammon.

Takahashi, M. (1970). Histopathology of sarcoidosis and its immunological basis. *Acta Pathol.,* **20**:171-182.

Teates, C. D., and Hunter, J. G. (1975). Gallium scanning as a screening test for inflammatory lesions. *Radiology,* **116**:383-387.

Teates, C. D., Bray, S. T., and Williamson, B. R. (1978). Tumor detection with ^{67}Ga-citrate: A literature survey (1979-1978). *Clin. Nucl. Med.,* **3**:453-455.

Thesingh, C. W., Driessen, O. M., Daems, W. T. (1978). Accumulation and localization of gallium-67 in various types of primary lung carcinoma. *J. Nucl. Med.,* **19**:28-30.

Teilum, G. (1964). Morphogenesis and development of sarcoid lesions: Similarities to the group of collagenesis. *Acta Med. Scand.,* **425**:14-18.

Van der Schoot, J. B., Groen, A. S., and De Jong, J. (1972). Gallium-67 scintigraphy in lung diseases. *Thorax,* **27**:543–546.

Venet, A. R., Hunninghake, G. W., Clretien, J., and Crystal, R. G. (1982). Macrophage T-cell interactions in sarcoid: Antigen presentation by alveolar macrophage. In *Proceedings of the 9th International Conference on Sarcoidosis and Other Granulomatous Disorders.* Paris. In press.

Weinberger, S. E., Kelman, J. A., Elson, N. A., Young, R. C., Jr., Reynolds, H. Y., Fulmer, J. D., and Crystal, R. G. (1978). Bronchoalveolar lavage in interstitial lung disease. *Ann. Intern. Med.,* **89**: 459–466.

Yeager, J., Williams, M. D., Beekman, J. F., Bayly, T. C., Beaman, B. L., and Hawley, R. J. (1977). Sarcoidosis: Analysis of cells obtained by bronchial lavage. *Am. Rev. Respir. Dis.,* **116**:951–955.

Young, R. L., Lordon, R. E., Krumholz, R. A., Harkleoad, L. E., Branam, G. E., and Weg, J. G. (1968). Pulmonary sarcoidosis. I. Pathophysiologic correlations. *Am. Rev. Respir. Dis.,* **97**:997–1008.

13

Fiberoptic Bronchoscopy in the Diagnosis of Sarcoidosis

ALVIN S. TEIRSTEIN

The Mount Sinai Medical Center
New York, New York

I. General

Despite the lengthy, intensive search for an in vitro diagnostic test, the definitive diagnosis of sarcoidosis still requires demonstration of noncaseating epithelioid granulomas in specimens obtained from organ biopsy, or, according to some investigations, a positive Kveim-Siltzbach test. Since sarcoidosis is a systemic disease involving almost every body tissue, a variety of biopsy sites are available for diagnosis. These include lacrimal glands and conjunctiva, oronasal mucosa, peripheral lymph nodes, skin, liver, and spleen, and even gastrointestinal and rectal mucosae. Because intrathoracic manifestations of sarcoidosis play a preeminent role in the clinical presentation and course of the disease, most attention has focused on the lung, mediastinum, and scalene fat pad as particularly rewarding loci for biopsy proof of sarcoidosis.

To qualify as a favorable site for biopsy, the tissue must offer the following advantages: (a) high frequency of true positive biopsies (sensitivity), (b) low frequency of false positive biopsies (selectivity), (c) minimal morbidity, (d) minimal expense, and (e) simplicity.

Many biopsy procedures are employed infrequently because they fail to fulfill one or more of the foregoing criteria. For example, liver biopsy is quite sensitive, detecting granulomas in as many as 95% of patients with sarcoidosis. However, liver granulomas indistinguishable from those in sarcoidosis occur in a variety of diseases. Therefore, liver biopsy is unselective and is a poor diagnostic procedure in sarcoidosis. Open lung biopsy, on the other hand, is quite sensitive and selective, but the expense and morbidity of this procedure, and the availability of numerous less traumatic procedures, make open lung biopsy an infrequently employed diagnostic procedure in sarcoidosis.

Bronchoscopic biopsy in the diagnosis of sarcoidosis was first reported by Benedict in 1941 using the rigid bronchoscope (Benedict and Castleman 1941). Its importance in the diagnosis of the more chronic stages of sarcoidosis was emphasized by several subsequent investigators (Olsen 1946, Jacob 1949, Friedman et al. 1963). Rigid bronchoscopy limits visualization and biopsy to the major bronchi and a minority of the smaller airways, primarily in the middle and lower lobes and lingula. In addition, the rigid instrument is poorly tolerated by the awake patient, and often requires general anesthesia. With the introduction of the flexible forceps by Hennessy (1968), and finally the fiberoptic bronchoscope by Ikeda (1968), the major failings of the rigid bronchoscope were overcome.

Ikeda stressed the relative comfort of the patient, the greater range of visibility, and the increased diagnostic yield offered by the flexible bronchoscope when compared with the rigid instrument and emphasized the unique utility of the new instrument in the study of patients with suspected lung cancer (Ikeda 1970). Subsequently, a rapid succession of reports emphasized the value of the flexible bronchoscope for obtaining forceps biopsy of the lung in patients with diffuse, interstitial lung diseases (Levin et al. 1974, Joyner et al. 1975, Teirstein et al. 1975). In addition to a significant high diagnostic yield in a variety of infections, metastatic carcinoma, and interstitial pneumonitis, flexible fiberoptic bronchoscopy was found to be particularly fruitful for obtaining lung tissue showing noncaseating epithelioid granulomas in patients with sarcoidosis.

At the present time, flexible, fiberoptic bronchoscopy with forceps biopsy of the lung and bronchial wall is the invasive procedure that best fulfills the criteria for biopsy in the diagnosis of sarcoidosis. This is the first procedure that should be performed, if tissue biopsy is desired, when the Kveim-Siltzbach test is negative or unavailable, and when the patient does not demonstrate an easily biopsied dermal lesion, conjunctival gland, or superficial lymph node.

II. Materials and Methods

The most commonly used instrument in the United States is the Olympus Flexible Bronchofiberscope Type BF-5B2. This instrument has an outer diameter of 5.7 mm with an inner 2-mm channel through which secretions may be aspirated and a flexible brush or biopsy forceps introduced. By means of a remote control lever, the tip of the fiberscope may be moved through an arc of 160° (130° anterior and 30° posterior flexion). A teaching or lecture head allows an instructor and student to share the view of the tracheobronchial tree. With the brilliant illuminating systems available, excellent 35-mm endoscopic photography or 8-mm cinematography is possible.

A. Materials

For local anesthesia, the following materials are recommended:

20 cc 2% lidocaine solution

Topical anesthetic ointment

Hand nebulizer

Emesis basin

Gauze pads

Disposable 10-cc syringe

For collection of specimens, the following equipment is required:

Suction apparatus

Suction trap collecting bottles

Polyethylene connecting tubes

Glass slides, cytologic fixative

1-cm squares of filter paper

10% formalin specimen jar

Sterile gloves

10-cc nonbacteriostatic saline

Disposable 10-cc syringe

Ancillary supplies required are:

10 cc 1:100,000 epinephrine

Disposable 10-cc syringe

Cold sterilization of the fiberscope is accomplished by thorough washing with soap and water including the passage of a cleansing brush through the aspiration channel, followed by immersion in 2% PVP-I solution (Betadine). This can be readily effected by immersing the instrument for 30 min in a ¾-in. diameter polyethylene tube with a corked distal end. This allows the control head of the fiberscope to remain out of the sterilizing solution. The solution is sucked into the aspiration channel with a disposable 10-cc syringe. After sterilization, the solution is washed out with saline and the instrument is dried with 10% isopropyl alcohol.

B. Collection of Specimens

Secretions are obtained via suction applied to a trap-collecting bottle connected to the 2-mm aspiration channel of the bronchoscope. The secretions are suitable for bacteriologic and cytologic analyses.

Brushings are obtained with a bronchial brush attached to a flexible cable and introduced through the aspiration channel of the fiberscope. For cytology, the brush is applied directly to glass slides which are immediately sprayed with a standard cytologic fixative. Alternatively, the brush may be immersed in a test tube containing sterile saline. With either method, the specimen must be delivered promptly to the cytology laboratory for processing. Several unfixed specimen slides are submitted to the bacteriology laboratory for Gram's, acid-fast, and special stains for fungi and *Pneumocystis carinii*.

With the 2-mm biopsy forceps introduced through the aspiration channel, multiple biopsies may be obtained via fluoroscopic control. The specimens are placed on 1-cm square pieces of filter paper which are immediately immersed in 10% formaldehyde. Where indicated, "touch prints" are made before immersion, or tissue may be placed in sterile saline for bacteriologic studies.

C. Methods

Careful explanation of the procedure is imperative to allay patient anxiety and ensure maximum cooperation. As premedication, we prefer 60 mg of codeine, 100 mg of sodium phenobarbital, and 0.4 mg of atropine injected subcutaneously 30 min before bronchoscopy. The patient may be seated in an otolaryngology examining chair or may be recumbent on a variety of examining tables. Since fluoroscopy is essential to bronchofiberoscopy, our studies are performed with the patient recumbent on the fluoroscopy table.

Either the oral or nasal route may be used, with or without prior insertion of an endotracheal tube. The nasal and oral pharynges are sprayed with approximately 5 cc of 2% lidocaine. Silicone is applied to the distal lens of the bronchoscope to prevent fogging, and lidocaine jelly or ointment is applied to the sides of the distal 3 in. of the bronchoscope. The instrument is then introduced. The vocal cords are observed for motion, and 1 cc of 2% lidocaine solution is introduced through the bronchoscopic channel directly onto the vocal cords. After approximately 30 sec, the instrument is passed through the vocal cords into the upper trachea. This often causes a brief period of stridor which is always promptly overcome with the introduction of 1 cc of 2% lidocaine solution. The bronchoscope is then passed into the desired lung and to the areas of the bronchial tree under study. Additional 1-cc doses of lidocaine are introduced as required to control coughing. This is usually necessary when entering a new division of the bronchial tree, particularly in the less dependent upper lobes and anterior segments. Aspiration of secretions, brushing of lesions, and biopsies are then carried out as previously described. When indicated, a polyethylene tube is passed through the bronchoscopic channel into a specific segment under study and 10 cc of iodinized contrast media is introduced for bronchography.

Since open-lung biopsy yields nearly 100% positive diagnoses in sarcoidosis, failure to attain this ideal frequency of positive diagnoses by fiberoptic bronchoscopy has raised the issue of adequacy of sampling. Although biopsy of the bronchial wall without parenchymal lung tissue often demonstrates granulomas supporting the diagnosis, lung specimens with identifiable alveoli are more likely to be diagnostic. Attempts have been made to establish the desired minimum number of biopsies that will give the highest frequency of positive diagnoses in sarcoidosis. Fechner et al. (1977) proposed that in any given patient, the diagnosis of diffuse, interstitial lung disease is established by the first two or three broncho-scopic biopsy specimens or not at all. On the other hand, Roethe et al. (1980) recommend ten bronchoscopic biopsies to obtain the diagnosis in at least 95% of patients with sarcoidosis. In a well-structured statistical study, Gilman and Wang (1980) established that a diagnostic yield of 90% is achieved in patients with sarcoidosis with four biopsies, and that the cost and time of additional biopsies is not justified by the minimal increase in diagnoses. Koerner's report in 1975, in which the diagnosis of sarcoidosis was established in 91% of patients by flexible bronchoscopy, was followed by several additional studies confirming his findings (Koerner et al. 1975, Koontz et al. 1976, Levin et al. 1974, Whitcomb et al. 1978).

An updated review of the use of fiberoptic bronchoscopy in sar-coidosis allows one to assess the role of the fiberscope in the diagnostic schema for sarcoidosis. From February 1973 to February 1981, 114 patients with sarcoidosis underwent fiberoptic bronchoscopy at The Mount Sinai Medical Center in New York. The results of these procedures are listed in Table 1. Eighty-one percent of patients had a positive diagnosis

Table 1　Results of Fiberoptic Bronchoscopy in 114 Patients with Sarcoidosis

X-ray stage	No. of patients	Biopsy positive
I	21	13 (62%)
II	36	31 (86%)
III	57	48 (82%)
Total	114	92 (81%)

for sarcoidosis by bronchoscopic biopsy. When subdivided according to the radiographic stage of sarcoidosis, bronchoscopic biopsy was positive in 62% of patients with stage I, 86% with stage II, and 82% with stage III sarcoidosis. The higher percentage of positive biopsies in patients with stages II and III sarcoidosis is expected since these patients with radiographic evidence of parenchymal disease have more intense infiltration of the lungs than patients with stage I disease. It is noteworthy that even in this latter group of patients with clear lung fields, most have demonstrable pulmonary granulomas by forceps biopsy of the lung. This confirms previous open lung biopsy studies and pulmonary function data which have demonstrated sarcoid involvement of the lungs and the restrictive type of pulmonary function alterations in patients with stage I sarcoidosis (Miller et al. 1980, Rosen et al. 1977).

The proportion of patients in each of the three radiographic stages undergoing fiberoptic bronchoscopy was unusually heavily weighted in favor of patients in the more advanced stages of sarcoidosis. Thus, 93 of the 114 (81%) had stages II and III disease, and only 21 (19%) had stage I. This disproportion stands in marked contrast to the radiographic grouping of the usual population encountered with sarcoidosis; for example, at the Mount Sinai Medical Center in New York, Siltzbach reported the radiographic grouping of patients to be 43% in stage I, 35% in stage II, and 14% in stage III (Siltzbach 1967). Eight percent had normal chest radiographs (Renz et al. 1972). These percentages are similar to the distribution by radiographic stages at several other large centers around the world (Siltzbach et al. 1974).

This disparity in the distribution of patients undergoing diagnostic bronchoscopy and the total sarcoidosis population is readily explained by a knowledge of the sequence of the diagnostic procedure. At The Mount Sinai Medical Center, for example, the diagnosis is established by the intracutaneous Kveim-Siltzbach test in the overwhelming majority of patients with suspected sarcoidosis. With this highly specific test,

Siltzbach has reported 92% positive diagnoses in 311 patients with sarcoidosis (Siltzbach 1961a). However, the frequency of positive Kveim test reactions tends to decrease with chronicity of the disease (Siltzbach 1961b). Thus, one of the major reasons for performance of flexible bronchoscopy was a negative Kveim-Siltzbach test. Since most patients with radiographic stage I sarcoidosis had a positive Kveim-Siltzbach test, relatively few in this early radiographic stage underwent diagnostic bronchoscopy. However, a larger proportion of patients with stages II and III sarcoidosis had a negative Kveim-Siltzbach test and required fiberoptic bronchoscopy for diagnosis. Fiberoptic bronchoscopy was also performed in some patients with severe dyspnea who were deemed too ill to wait the 4 weeks required for maturation of the Kveim-Siltzbach papule. Finally, patients exhibiting diffuse pulmonary infiltrations with no discernible lymphadenopathy often presented a diagnostic challenge, since similar radiographic patterns are encountered in a host of interstitial pulmonary diseases as well as in sarcoidosis. Fiberoptic bronchoscopy was performed in this group as an integral part of the study of patients with unknown diffuse interstitial lung disease, many of whom had negative Kveim-Siltzbach tests.

It is apparent that the Kveim-Siltzbach test and fiberoptic bronchoscopy are complementary studies in the diagnosis of sarcoidosis, with the Kveim-Siltzbach test yielding a higher percentage of positive diagnoses in radiographic stage I sarcoidosis, and fiberoptic bronchoscopy being more rewarding in stages II and III. In our experience the diagnosis of sarcoidosis was established by Kveim-Siltzbach tests and/or lung biopsy via the flexible fiberoptic bronchoscope in 92% of patients, most of whom were in the more chronic stages of the disease. In the remaining nine patients, the diagnosis was obtained by scalene lymph node biopsy in eight and open lung biopsy in one.

The ascendancy of flexible fiberoptic bronchoscopic biopsy in the diagnosis of sarcoidosis was emphasized by a study of 209 medical centers around the world reported at the VIII International Conference on Sarcoidosis (Teirstein et al. 1980). Each investigator was asked to submit the favored sequence of diagnostic procedures performed at his center. The respondents were divided into 106 who had valid Kveim-Siltzbach antigen, and 103 who did not. The responses in order of preference are tabulated in Table 2. It is apparent that in centers with valid Kveim-Siltzbach antigen the intracutaneous test was the preferred diagnostic procedure performed in stage I sarcoidosis, followed by flexible bronchoscopic lung biopsy. In stages II and III sarcoidosis, the order was reversed. Where no Kveim-Siltzbach antigen was available, bronchoscopic biopsy was clearly the primary diagnostic procedure, with either scalene lymph node biopsy or mediastinoscopy the second choice.

Table 2 Mean Rank of Diagnostic Procedures[a]

	Kveim antigen	Fiberoptic bronchoscopy	Scalene node biopsy	Mediastinoscopy	Liver biopsy
Stage I					
Kveim (106)	2.22	2.45	2.62	2.88	3.43
No Kveim (103)		1.58	2.29	2.24	3.15
Stages II and III					
Kveim (106)	2.39	2.07	2.78	2.97	3.44
No Kveim (103)		1.35	2.39	2.33	3.07

[a]From the VIII International Conference on Sarcoidosis; 106 responders with
Kveim, 103 without Kveim.
Obtained by assigning value of 1 through 5 according to order of preference and
computing average value. The more preferred procedure has the lower mean
rank.
Source: Teirstein, Siltzbach, and Dorph (1980).

The pathologist must exercise great caution in basing the diagnosis of
sarcoidosis on the analysis of 2-mm biopsy specimens obtained at fiberoptic
bronchoscopy. The demonstration of noncaseating epithelioid granulomas is
not necessarily diagnostic of sarcoidosis. Mycobacterial and fungal diseases
may manifest the same histology on small biopsy specimens. Special
stains for acid-fast bacilli and fungi must be performed. Failure to
demonstrate these organisms, while important, does not guarantee that an
infectious agent is absent.

We have seen two patients in whom bronchoscopic biopsies showed
"noncaseating epithelioid granulomas consistent with sarcoidosis" and negative
stains for acid-fast bacilli. In both patients the Kveim-Siltzbach test was
negative and cultures obtained at bronchoscopy eventually grew tubercle
bacilli. In a third patient, the specimen obtained at bronchoscopy was
reported to show "caseating epithelioid granulomas consistent with tuberculosis." However, in this patient, the clinical course did not improve with
antituberculosis therapy, and a subsequent Kveim-Siltzbach test was positive.
Open lung biopsy confirmed the diagnosis of sarcoidosis.

Fiberoptic bronchoscopy is not without risk. Credle et al. (1974)
reported morbidity and mortality related to drugs used in premedication,
insertion of the flexible instrument, and lung biopsy and brushing.
Hypoxemia, hemorrhage, arrhythmias, and pneumothorax have all been
reported with varying frequency (Elguindi et al. 1979, Kleinholz and Fussel
1973, Luck et al. 1978, Palmer and Wirts 1957, Pereira et al. 1978, Rentz
et al. 1972; Teirstein et al. 1976, 1977, Zavala 1976). In our group,

among 114 patients undergoing flexible bronchoscopy for the diagnosis of sarcoidosis, pneumothorax occurred in two, neither of whom required intubation of the hemithorax. Three additional patients had brisk hemorrhage. In two, approximately 200 cm^3 of blood were expectorated, and hemoptysis of approximately 100 cm^3 occurred in a third patient. No morbidity due to preanesthesia or the passage of the bronchoscope was encountered. There were no deaths.

III. Summary

1. Flexible fiberoptic bronchoscopy with forceps biopsy of the lung yields a high frequency of diagnosis in patients with all radiographic stages of sarcoidosis.

2. The frequency of positive diagnosis is greater than 80% in patients with radiographic-visible parenchymal infiltrations (stages II and III).

3. The risks of bronchoscopic biopsy in sarcoidosis are minimal and confined to approximately 2% with small pneumothoracies and 3% with hemorrhages of from 100 to 200 cm^3.

4. Flexible fiberoptic bronchoscopy with forceps biopsy of the lung is the preferred initial invasive diagnostic procedure when the Kveim-Siltzbach test is negative or unavailable and there is no readily biopsied conjunctival, lymph node, or skin lesion available.

References

Benedict, E. H., and Castelman, B. (1941). Sarcoidosis with bronchial involvement. *N. Engl. J. Med.*, **224**:186–189.

Credle, W. F., Smiddy, J. F., and Elliott, R. C. (1974). Complications of fiberoptic bronchoscopy. *Am. Rev. Resp. Dis.*, **109**:67–71.

Elguindi, A. S., Harrison, G. N., Abdulla, A. M., Chaudhary, B. A., Vallner, J. J., Kolbeck, R. C., Speir, W. A., Jr. (1979). *Cardiac Rhythm Disturbances During Fiberoptic Bronchoscopy: A Prospective Study.* St. Louis, C. V. Mosby, pp. 557–561.

Fechner, R. E., Greenberg, S. D., Wilson, R. K., and Stevens, P. M. (1977). Evaluation of transbronchial biopsy of the lung. *Am. J. Clin. Pathol.*, **68**:17–20.

Friedman, O. H., Blaugrund, S. M., and Siltzbach, L. E. (1963). Biopsy of the bronchial wall as an aid in diagnosis of sarcoidosis. *JAMA*, **183**:120–124.

Gilman, M. J., and Wang, K. P. (1980). Transbronchial lung biopsy in sarcoidosis. *Am. Rev. Resp. Dis.*, **122**:721–724.

Hennessy, J. J. (1968). Bronchial brushing and transbronchial forceps
    biopsy in the diagnosis of pulmonary lesions. *Dis. Chest,* **53**:377–389.
Ikeda, S. (1968). Flexible bronchofiberscope. *Keio J. Med.,* **17**:1.
Ikeda, S. (1970). Flexible bronchofiberscope. *Ann. Otol. Rhinol.
    Laryngol.,* **79**:916–919.
Jacob, E. (1949). Sarcoidosis lesions revealed by bronchoscopy. *Acta
    Clin. Belg.,* **4**:301–310.
Joyner, L. R., and Scheinhorn, D. J. (1975). Transbronchial forceps lung
    biopsy through the fiberoptic bronchoscope. *Chest,* **67**:532–535.
Kleinholz, E. J., and Fussel, J. (1973). Arterial blood gas studies during
    fiberoptic bronchoscopy. *Am. Rev. Respir. Dis.,* **108**:1014.
Koerner, S. K., Sakowity, A. J., Appelman, R. I., Becker, N. H., and
    Shoenbaum, S. W. (1975). Transbronchial lung biopsy for the
    diagnosis of sarcoidosis. *N. Engl. J. Med.,* **293**:268–270.
Koontz, C. H., Joyner, L. R., and Nelson, R. A. (1976). Transbronchial
    lung biopsy via the fiberoptic bronchoscope in sarcoidosis. *Ann.
    Intern. Med.,* **85**:64–66.
Levin, D. C., Wicks, A. B., and Ellis, J. H., Jr. (1974). Transbronchial
    lung biopsy via the fiberoptic bronchoscope. *Am. Rev. Respir. Dis.,*
    110:4.
Luck, J. C., Messeder, O. H., Rubenstein, M. J., Morrissey, W. L., and
    Engel, T. R. (1978). Arrhythmias from fiberoptic bronchoscopy.
    Chest, **74**:2.
Miller, A., Einstein, K., Thornton, J., Teirstein, A. S., and Siltzbach, L. E.
    (1980). Physiologic classification and staging of intrathoracic
    sarcoidosis. Eighth International Conference on Sarcoidosis and Other
    Granulomatous Diseases, pp. 331–336.
Olsen, H. M. (1946). Boeck's sarcoid: Report of case in which diagnosis
    was made by bronchoscopic exam and biopsy. *Ann. Otol.,* **53**:629–
    637.
Palmer, E. D., and Wirts, W. C. (1957). Survey of gastroscopic and
    esophagoscopic accidents. *JAMA,* **164**:2012.
Pereira, W., Jr., Kovnat, D. M., and Snider, G. L. (1978). A prospective
    cooperative study of complications following flexible fiberoptic
    bronchoscopy. *Chest,* **73**:813–816.
Renz, L. E., Smiddy, J. F., Rauscher, C. R., Kerby, G. R., and Ruth, W.
    E. (1972). Bronchoscopy in respiratory failure. *JAMA,* **219**:619.
Roethe, R. A., Fuller, P. B., Byrd, R. B., and Hafermann, D. R. (1980).
    Transbronchial lung biopsy in sarcoidosis. *Chest,* **77**:400–402.
Rosen, Y., Amorosa, J. K., Moon, S., Cohen, J., and Lyons, H. A. (1977).
    Occurrence of lung granulomas in patients with stage I sarcoidosis.
    Am. J. Radiol., **129**:1083–1085.

Siltzbach, L. E. (1961a). Current status of the Nickerson-Kveim reaction. *Am. Rev. Respir. Dis.* (Suppl.), **84**:89–93.

Siltzbach, L. E. (1961b). The Kveim test in sarcoidosis: A study in 750 patients. *JAMA,* **178**:476–482.

Siltzbach, L. E. (1967). Clinical features and management. *Med. Clin. North Am.,* **57**:483–502.

Siltzbach, L. E., James, D. G., Neville, E., Turiaf, J., Battesti, J. P., Sharma, O. P., Hosoda, Y., Mikami, R., and Odaka, M. (1974). Course and prognosis of sarcoidosis around the world. *Am. J. Med.,* **57**:847–852.

Teirstein, A. S., Chuang, M. T., and Miller, A. (1975). Application of the flexible bronchoscope. *Mount Sinai J. Med.,* **42**:81–94.

Teirstein, A. S., Chuang, M. T., Miller, A., and Siltzbach, L. E. (1976). Flexible bronchoscope biopsy of lung and bronchial wall in intrathoracic sarcoidosis. VII International Conference on Sarcoidosis and Other Granulomatous Disorders. *Ann. N.Y. Acad. Sci.,* **278**:522–527.

Teirstein, A. S., Chuang, M. T., Choy, A. R., and Miller, A. (1977). Fiberoptic bronchoscopy in the diagnosis of sarcoidosis. *Mount Sinai J. Med.,* **44**:740–743.

Teirstein, A. S., Siltzbach, L. E., and Dorph, D. (1980). Report of international questionnaire regarding diagnostic procedures in sarcoidosis: The impact of fiberoptic bronchoscopy. *Eighth International Conference on Sarcoidosis and Other Granulomatous Diseases.* Cardiff, Wales, Alpha Omega, pp. 233–237.

Whitcomb, M. E., Domby, W. R., Hewley, P. C., and Kataria, Y. P. (1978). The role of fiberoptic bronchoscopy in the diagnosis of sarcoidosis. *Chest,* **74**:205–208.

Zavala, E. C. (1976). Pulmonary hemorrhage in fiberoptic transbronchial biopsy. *Chest,* **70**:584–588.

14

Biopsy of Tissues Other Than the Lung in the Diagnosis of Sarcoidosis

D. GERAINT JAMES

Royal Northern Hospital and St. Thomas' Hospital
London, England
and University of Miami School of Medicine
Miami, Florida

I. Introduction

This chapter is concerned with the histologic confirmation of the diagnosis of sarcoidosis by biopsy of tissues other than the lung. The differential diagnosis of pulmonary infiltration, uveitis, or erythema nodosum is often so wide that histologic confirmation becomes necessary. Moreover, patients troubled by their disease in later years are frequently those in whom clinical diagnosis was not supported by histologic confirmation initially, and so treatment was delayed until it was too late to be effective.

II. Historical Background

A retrospective comparison of 11 intensively investigated series comprising 3676 patients with sarcoidosis was reported to the Seventh International Conference on Sarcoidosis in New York City (James et al. 1976). They were observed and followed in London, New York, Paris, Los Angeles, Tokyo, Lisbon, Novi Sad, Edinburgh, Reading, Geneva, and Naples. The results of this 11-city survey show the most popular methods for obtaining a histologic diagnosis of sarcoidosis during the quarter-century between

1950 and 1975. The methods varied in different centers, depending on local interests (Table 1). For instance, it can be seen that aspiration liver biopsy was popular in London, whereas bronchoscopy was a routine procedure in Paris. Most centers did lymph node biopsies, and this reflected the popular techniques of scalene node biopsy and mediastinoscopy during those years. Histologic support was obtained by lymph node biopsy in about one-half the cases, and histologic confirmation in the other half was divided among biopsies of skin, liver, bronchus, and a variety of other tissues.

The Kveim-Siltzbach skin test also had popular support in this world survey (Table 2). It was positive in about four-fifths of patients. It was found to be a reliable, safe, and simple outpatient technique for delineating multisystem sarcoidosis from the numerous other causes of systemic and local nonspecific sarcoid tissue reactions.

The patients in these series were of differing ethnic groups and from different climates and environments. Nevertheless, there was an extraordinary parallelism of the clinical findings and of the techniques used in those days.

Table 1 Number of Patients and Patterns of Histologic Confirmation of Sarcoidosis in a Worldwide Survey

Center	Bronchus	Lymph node	Skin	Liver biopsy	Other tissues	Total histologic confirmation
London	0	100	82	76	42	300
New York	0	89	31	12	33	165
Paris	243	49	16	12	44	364
Los Angeles	2	53	19	38	32	144
Tokyo	0	118	19	9	10	156
Reading	45	46	33	9	78	211
Lisbon	16	36	18	9	7	86
Edinburgh	0	109	16	10	29	164
Novi Sad	15	115	8	15	17	170
Naples	7	212	1	0	1	221
Geneva	1	33	4	19	24	81
Total number	284	960	237	198	317	2062
Total percent	14	47	12	10	17	100

Source: James et al. (1976a).

Table 2 Histologic Confirmation of Sarcoidosis by Kveim-Siltzbach Tests, Using Different Test Materials from Around the World

Center	No. done	Positive	
		No.	Percent
London	466	384	82
New York	311	285	92
Paris	261	202	77
Los Angeles	50	36	72
Tokyo	141	76	54
Reading	408	331	81
Lisbon	55	43	78
Edinburgh	222	141	64
Novi Sad	205	167	81
Naples	27	15	56
Geneva	43	36	84
Total	2189	1714	78

Source: James et al. (1976a).

III. Present Procedures

Within a few years, techniques for obtaining histology have changed, mainly as a result of the popularity of fiberoptic bronchoscopy. Nonetheless, a wide variety of techniques is available to suit the interests of all disciplines.

A. Fiberoptic Bronchoscopy

Flexible forceps biopsy is commendable because it yields both bronchial and lung tissue and appears to be more specific for sarcoidosis than are other biopsies, such as lymph node and liver. This procedure will be discussed in another section of the book.

B. Skin

Original observations on sarcoidosis were made by dermatologists. Tenneson (1892) did a skin biopsy of a patient with lupus pernio and provided the essential histologic description of "predominance of epithelioid cells and a variety of giant cells" in the skin lesions. Hutchinson

(1877, 1898) had already described the skin lesions accurately but did not have much luck with skin biopsy. His patient, Mrs. Mortimer, was 64 years old when she developed lupus pernio. He presented her to a meeting of the Dermatological Society of London in 1895, when the concensus of opinion favored the diagnosis of sarcoma, and urged skin biopsy for histologic proof. Hutchinson suggested this course of action to Mrs. Mortimer with the result that he did not see her again for 2 years. Nowadays it is, of course, the first tissue to be biopsied if there is skin involvement.

The dermatologist has virtually no difficulty, for skin biopsy is a simple procedure. His only dilemma is to decide whether the sarcoid granuloma confronting him is the multisystem disorder sarcoidosis or a local nonspecific sarcoid tissue reaction. There are pointers to their differentiation (Table 3).

C. Lymph Node Biopsy

Lymph node biopsy has been universally favored over the years as a means for confirming the diagnosis of sarcoidosis. Its popularity is evident in the

Table 3 Differences Between the Multisystem Disorder, Sarcoidosis, and a Nonspecific Local Sarcoid Tissue Reaction

Feature	Multisystem sarcoidosis	Local sarcoid-tissue reaction
No. of systems involved	Several	Usually one
Age group	20–50 yr	Any
Chest radiograph	Abnormal in 87%	Normal
Slit lamp examination of eyes	Abnormal in 15%	Normal
Tuberculin skin test	Negative in 66%	Variable
Kveim-Siltzbach skin test	Positive in 78%	Always negative
Serum angiotensin 1-converting enzyme	Elevated in 60%	Normal
Calcium metabolism	Abnormal in 20%	Normal
Response to corticosteroids	Good	Variable
Other treatments	Indomethacin Oxyphenbutazone Chloroquine P-aminobenzoate Methotrexate	Depends on cause Anti-infective Immunosuppressives

world series (Table 1) because lymph node biopsy was positive in 960 (47%) patients—as popular as all other techniques put together. Any accessible lymph node is acceptable, but a right scalene lymph node biopsy is the most popular. The mediastinal lymph node chain ascends on the right side. Right paratracheal lymphadenopathy is very frequent, and this leads to the high incidence of positive right scalene node biopsies. Variations in the technique led to mediastinoscopy and to mediastinotomy, but fiberoptic bronchoscopy has now overshadowed all these techniques.

D. Aspiration Liver Biopsy

This procedure remains a popular and simple technique for obtaining evidence of hepatic granulomas. It is important that serial sections are made through the block; if this is done, hepatic granulomas are found in two-thirds or more of patients with sarcoidosis. Identical granulomas may be found in tuberculosis, brucellosis, schistosomiasis, and in certain liver diseases, so the onus shifts back to the clinician to relate the clinical information to the histologic evidence obtained.

In two independent surveys the most common cause of epithelioid granulomas found on liver biopsy were sarcoidosis and underlying liver disorders, including primary biliary cirrhosis (Neville et al. 1975, Klatskin 1976). Ova are readily recognizable in schistosomiasis when one is alert to the possibility. Acid-fast bacilli are demonstrable in only one-tenth of patients with tuberculosis, so the differentiation of sarcoidosis and tuberculosis is made on other grounds. The Kveim-Siltzbach test is of added value in diagnosis since it is positive in about 70% of patients with sarcoidosis but is consistently negative in patients with hepatic granulomas from other causes (Table 4) (Neville et al. 1975, Klatskin 1976).

Scheuer (1980) subdivides hepatic granulomas obtained by biopsy into four groups:

1. The cause of the granuloma is seen in tissue sections, for example, ova of *Schistosoma* or tubercle bacilli.

2. Granulomas adjacent to bile ducts suggest primary biliary cirrhosis.

3. Clusters of fibrosing granulomas in portal tracts suggest sarcoidosis.

4. The cause in unknown. (About 10% remain in this category.)

The granuloma in sarcoidosis is large, well organized, and usually near portal tracts. There may be multinucleate giant cells and other inclusions. Central necrosis is minimal and the reticulin network is well preserved. Clusters of basophilic epithelioid cells and a thin peripheral ring of lymphocytes surround the lesion. Healing is by sclerosis. The granuloma is converted into an acellular mass of hyaline material with a fibrous capsule. Since the hepatic lesions are focal and fibrosis is restricted to

Table 4 A Comparison of Hepatic Granulomas Investigated at Yale (Klatskin)[a] and London (James)[b]

Hepatic granulomas	Yale		London	
	No.	Percent	No.	Percent
Total	565	100	138	100
Causes				
Sarcoidosis	217		75	
Liver disease	174	85	41	88
Tuberculosis	70		3	
Schistosomiasis	19		1	
Undiagnosed	37	7	14	10
Positive Kveim test	389	69	100	72

[a]Klatskin (1979).
[b]Neville et al. (1975).

healing lesions, sarcoidosis does not produce the diffuse fibrosis and nodular regeneration of cirrhosis (Sherlock 1981).

E. Aspiration of the Spleen

Selroos (1976) has pioneered fine-needle aspiration biopsy of the spleen. The aspiration device consists of a 0.7–0.8 mm needle on a 10–20 ml disposable syringe with a Luer adaptor. The needle is inserted into the tenth intercostal space, 3–4 cm dorsal to the midaxillary line. Selroos finds that even local anesthesia in his hardy Finn patients is unnecessary. The patient holds his breath in midexpiration. The aspirated material is spread on glass slides, air-dried, and stained with May-Grunwald-Giemsa stain. His only contraindications to the procedure are an overt hemorrhagic diathesis or a platelet count below $100,000/mm^3$. Selroos aspirates the spleen even when it is not enlarged. He now has experience with this technique in over 600 patients (personal communication) and regards it as his first choice for obtaining diagnostic histology. It is a simple, safe bedside technique in his hands, and he stresses its attraction of providing histologic confirmation of sarcoidosis within 1 hr.

F. Peritoneoscopy

Many gastroenterologists favor peritoneoscopy because it provides the twin advantages of visualizing the viscera together with an easy means for obtaining histology. Tachibana (1976) studied 65 sarcoidosis patients with asymptomatic hepatic lesions by peritoneoscopy, and he was able to obtain biopsies of liver granulomas in 51 of these patients by direct vision. In 6 of these 51 patients he also noted nodules on the surface of the spleen. Biopsies of these splenic nodules revealed characteristic sarcoid granulomas. This technique not only visualizes the granulomatous nodules on the surface of the liver and spleen and allows direct-vision biopsy, but also has provided elegant color photographs as a permanent record of these abnormalities.

G. Muscle Biopsy

The small submitted biopsy for sarcoid granulomas may become evident only on multiple serial sections. Scadding (1967) reviewed the historical background of this procedure, and there is very little new information on it. This means that it is not a popular method for making the histologic diagnosis. Muscle involvement occurs as frequently as that of any other tissues in both acute and chronic forms of the disorder. What is important for the future is that those who do muscle biopsies should endeavor to correlate myositis and other types of muscle involvement with the clinical picture elsewhere and to make sure that they are dealing with multisystem sarcoidosis and not a local sarcoid tissue reaction in muscle. They should also determine whether the muscle granulomas are a feature of acute or chronic sarcoidosis.

H. Minor Salivary Gland Biopsy

Biopsy of the minor salivary glands is a simple outpatient technique. The lower lip is everted and a chalazion clamp is applied at random. Local anesthesia is injected into a mental foramen; an incision 4–6 mm long and 1–2 mm deep is made, and one or two minor salivary glands are excised. The incision is closed with silk or plain gut sutures. Noncaseating granulomas wee obtained in 58% of patients with sarcoidosis in one series of 75 patients (Nessan and Jacoway 1979). Granulomas were obtained in one of three patients with a normal chest radiograph and in three-fifths of patients with hilar adenopathy or pulmonary involvement by chest roentgenogram.

I. Conjunctiva

I have reviewed a personal series of 818 patients with histologically confirmed multisystem sarcoidosis and, in particular, 224 patients with ocular sarcoidosis to determine the value of conjunctival biopsy (Figure 1). The most frequent lesions are anterior uveitis in 66%, posterior uveitis in 14%, and conjunctival involvement in 19% (James et al. 1976b). Con-

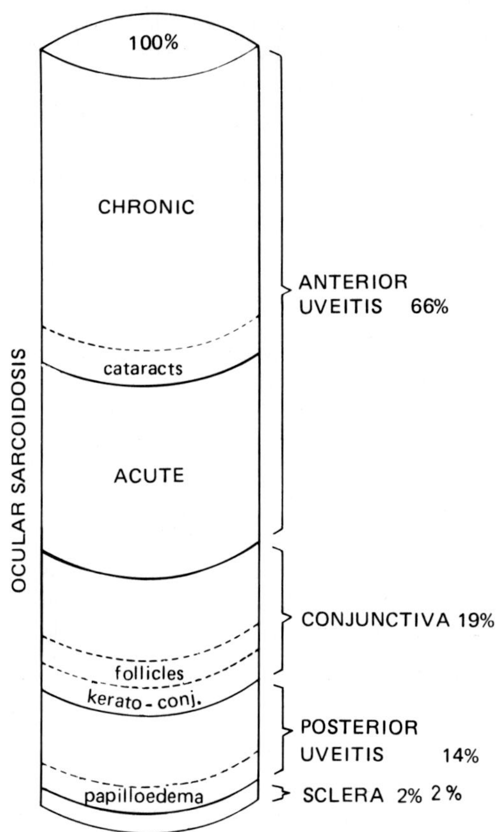

Figure 1 Distribution of ocular involvement in 224 patients with sarcoidosis of the eye.

junctival follicles were evident in only nine patients, and granulomas were readily obtained on biopsy of these follicles. Phlyctenular or nonspecific conjunctivitis occurred in another 28 patients, and granulomas were obtained particularly from obvious phlyctenules. However, blind biopsy of the normal conjunctiva was unrewarding and is rarely helpful. This is unfortunate because this approach comprised the vast majority of patients with anterior or posterior uveitis. Biopsy of the lacrimal gland is valuable in the small group of black patients with florid sarcoid lesions including enlarged lacrimals. In the great majority of patients with uveitis we are obliged to turn to other organ systems for histology.

Having painted this gloomy British picture of the place of conjunctival biopsy in the assessment of sarcoidosis, I shall redress the balance by quoting the much rosier experience in one part of Finland. Anni Karma

Table 5 The Differential Diagnosis of Sarcoid Granulomas of the Upper Respiratory Tract

Features	Sarcoidosis of the upper respiratory tract	Leprosy	Tuberculosis	Wegener's granulomatosis	Extrinsic allergic alveolitis
Female:male	3:1	1:1	1:1	1:2	1:2
Age at onset (yr)	20–30	Any	Any	25–55	20–50
Race	Any	Tropical	Asian	Any	Any
Clinical involvements					
Nasal skin	Yes	Yes	Yes	No	—
Skin elsewhere	Yes	Yes	No	Yes	—
Intrathoracic	Always	±	Always	Frequent	Yes
Iritis	Yes	Yes	No	Yes	—
Neuropathy	No	Yes	No	No	—
Renal failure	No	No	No	Yes	—
Skin tests					
Tuberculin	Negative	±	Positive	±	Negative
Kveim-Siltzbach	Positive	Negative	Negative	—	Negative
Histology	Sarcoid	Sarcoid	Sarcoid	Granulomatous angiitis	Granulomas encompassing foreign body
SACE[a]	Elevated	Normal	Normal	Normal	Normal
Microbiology	Negative	Mycobacteria	Mycobacteria	Negative	Negative
Treatment	Steroids, chloroquine	Dapsone, transfer factor	Rifampicin, isoniazid	Steroids, azathioprine, cyclophosphamide	Steroids

[a]SACE = serum angiotensin-converting enzyme.

(1979) analyzed a series of 79 patients with ocular sarcoidosis and obtained histologic evidence of conjunctival granulomas in 37, an incidence of 17% of 218 patients examined. A pitfall that cannot be overemphasized is that conjunctival biopsy may produce nonspecific foreign body giant cell granulomas, and these must not be misconstrued as the granulomas of sarcoidosis.

J. Upper Respiratory Tract

Our series of 818 patients with sarcoidosis includes 53 patients (6%) with sarcoidosis of the upper respiratory tract. We obtained histologic evidence of sarcoidosis from several sites of the upper respiratory tract, often from more than one. These sites included nasal mucosa in 36 patients, laryngeal and pharyngeal mucosa in 8, sinuses in 8, and parotid gland in 10 patients. Sarcoidosis of the upper respiratory tract occurs three times more frequently in women than men and usually presents in the third and fourth decades of life. It is commonly associated with lupus pernio. The natural history of sarcoidosis of the upper respiratory tract is often indolent (Neville et al. 1976).

When granulomas are found on biopsy of the upper respiratory tract, it is important to decide whether they represent multisystem sarcoidosis or are due to tuberculosis, Wegener's granulomatosis, or leprosy (Table 5). Villar (1976) widens the differential diagnosis still further by including extrinsic allergic alveolitis due to inhaled particles. He and his group have found granulomas in the nasal mucosa so frequently that they have substituted nasal biopsy for lung biopsy in the diagnosis of inhalational interstitial pulmonary disease.

K. The Heart

Myocardial sarcoidosis is difficult to recognize clinically. Its recognition does not pose a great problem if a patient with florid multisystem sarcoidosis develops bundle branch block, arrhythmias, congestive cardiac failure, pericarditis, or clinical evidence of cardiomyopathy. However, sudden death due to myocardial sarcoidosis may occur in an otherwise healthy asymptomatic individual. Between these two extremes lie patterns of involvement, including cardiomyopathy, in which endocardial biopsy may be indicated. This technique is easily performed by those accustomed to cardiac catheterization. It can be done at the same time as catheterization of the left or right side of the heart. It is recommended by Japanese workers as an aid to the diagnosis of myocardial sarcoidosis when serial changes show worsening of the ECG or vectorcardiography reveal disturbances of conduction (Numao et al. 1980).

References

Hutchinson, J. (1877). *Illustrations of Clinical Surgery.* London, Churchill, p. 42.

Hutchinson, J. (1898). Case of Mortimer's malady. *Arch. Surg.,* **9**: 307–315.

James, D. G., Neville, E., Siltzbach, L. E., Turiaf, J., and Battesti, J. P. (1976a). A worldwide review of sarcoidosis. *Ann. N.Y. Acad. Sci.,* **278**:321–334.

James, D. G., Neville, E., and Langley, D. A. (1976b). Ocular sarcoidosis. *Trans. Ophthalmol. Soc. U.K.,* **96**:133–139.

Karma, A. (1979). Ophthalmic changes in sarcoidosis. *Acta Ophthalmol.* (Suppl.), 141.

Klatskin, G. (1976). Hepatic granulomata: Problems in interpretation. *Ann. N.Y. Acad. Sci.,* **278**:427–432.

Nessan, V. J., and Jacoway, J. R. (1979). Biopsy of minor salivary glands in the diagnosis of sarcoidosis. *N. Engl. J. Med.,* **301**:922–924.

Neville, E., Piyasena, K. H. G., and James, D. G. (1975). Granulomas of the liver. *Postgrad. Med. J.,* **51**:361–365.

Neville, E., Mills, R. G. S., and James, D. G. (1976). Sarcoidosis of the upper respiratory tract and its relation to lupus pernio. *Ann. N.Y. Acad. Sci.,* **278**:416–425.

Numao, Y., Sekiguchi, M., Fruie, T., Matsui, Y., Izumi, T., and Mikami, R. (1980). A study of cardiac involvement in 963 cases of sarcoidosis by ECG and endomyocardial biopsy. In *Eighth International Conference on Sarcoidosis.* Edited by W. J. Williams and B. H. Davies. Cardiff, Wales, Alpha Omega.

Scadding, J. G. (1967). *Sarcoidosis.* London, Eyre and Spottiswoode.

Scheuer, P. J. (1980). *Liver Biopsy Interpretation,* 3rd ed. London, Bailliere, Tindall.

Selroos, O. (1976). Fine-needle aspiration biopsy of the spleen in diagnosis of sarcoidosis. *Ann. N.Y. Acad. Sci.,* **278**:517–521.

Sherlock, S. (1981). *Diseases of the Liver and Biliary System,* 6th ed. Oxford, Blackwell, and Chicago, Year Book Publishing.

Tachibana, T. (1976). Peritoneoscopy of sarcoid hepatosplenomegaly. *Ann. N.Y. Acad. Sci.,* **278**:520.

Tenneson, M. (1892). Lupus pernio. *Bull. Soc. Franc. Dermatol. Syph.,* **3**:417.

Villar, T. (1976). Nasal granulomas. *Ann. N.Y. Acad. Sci.,* **278**:426.

Part Six

DECISION ANALYSIS AND THERAPY

15

A Decision Analytic View of the Diagnosis of Sarcoidosis

JONATHAN E. GOTTLIEB, BARRY L. FANBURG,
and STEPHEN G. PAUKER

New England Medical Center Hospital
Tufts University School of Medicine
Boston, Massachusetts

I. Summary

Although sarcoidosis has long been recognized as a distinct clinical entity, establishing its presence in an individual patient is often fraught with uncertainty, and universally accepted criteria for the institution of therapy are lacking. Recently, physicians have begun to apply the techniques of decision analysis to complex clinical problems in which uncertainty predominates. This discipline allows the clinician to specify explicitly the assumptions underlying diagnostic and therapeutic decisions and to combine information from a variety of sources in a logical and consistent manner. In this chapter we shall perform a set of clinical decision analyses on a subset of the diagnostic challenges which this disease presents. We shall

Supported in part by training grant T15LM07027 from the Computers in Medicine Program, grant 1P01LM03374 from the National Library of Medicine, and grant 1P41RR01096 from the Division of Research Resources, National Institutes of Health. Dr. Pauker is the recipient of Research Career Development Award 1K04GM00349 from the National Institute of General Medical Sciences, Bethesda, Maryland.

primarily concern ourselves with the issue of establishing the diagnosis of sarcoidosis, that is, with the interpretation of diagnostic results that are not pathognomonic. The purpose of this chapter is not to analyze all, or even most, diagnostic and therapeutic dilemmas in this complex disease, but rather to awaken the reader's interest in this new approach to clinical decision making.

II. Introduction

Despite decades of investigation, physicians continue to debate about the diagnosis and treatment of sarcoidosis, in large part due to the lack of an established etiology and to the absence of a "gold standard" for diagnosis. Most authorities include several clinical, radiological, and histologic features in their diagnostic criteria since other disease processes can simulate sarcoidosis in many ways. Certainly, all three features may occasionally suggest sarcoidosis in patients later proven to have other diseases. For these reasons, several authors have proposed that rigorous efforts be made to exclude alternative diagnoses and that patients felt to be suffering from sarcoidosis be constantly subject to review and further testing.

Although universally recognized, the uncertainties surrounding the diagnosis of sarcoidosis have not generally been expressed in explicit terms. Underlying these uncertainties is the nature of the disease: Sarcoidosis is associated with a high likelihood of spontaneous resolution and only modest disability (James 1979). Since no etiologic agent has been established, the diagnosis is largely inferred from a constellation of clinical findings (Mitchell and Scadding 1974).

We shall first examine some of those inferences in analytic terms. The interpretation of any clinical finding depends on two classes of information: the likelihood of each possible diagnosis before (or prior to) knowledge of the finding, and the relative likelihoods of that finding occurring in each possible diagnosis. These two information streams can then to combined in a formal, explicit, and consistent manner (Gorry et al. 1978, Schwartz et al. 1981). First, let us consider the issue of clinical presentation or *prior probability*.

III. Toward a Confident Diagnosis of "Nil" Disease

Since most patients with sarcoidosis follow a benign course, one might consider the diagnosis of sarcoidosis in these patients as the establishment of the presence of a self-limited or "nil" disease. By using the term "nil" disease, we do not mean to imply that establishing the diagnosis is unimportant; rather, its importance often lies in excluding the presence of other more serious and more potentially treatable disorders. In this context, there is an analogy between findings that argue for the diagnosis of sarcoidosis and so-called normal findings (Gorry et al. 1978) that argue for the absence of serious disease. Of course, this rather limited view applies only to those patients without indications for therapy. In patients with progressive pulmonary impairment or major organ system involvement, sarcoidosis can occasionally be a serious, life-threatening disease.

Since the diagnosis of sarcoidosis is often not established with certainty, we can view the diagnostic process as changing the likelihood of the presence of sarcoidosis and the other diseases which often fall within its differential diagnostic spectrum. The strength of one's belief (Schafer 1976) in the presence of any disease can be expressed as a probability. In a patient with many characteristic features of sarcoidosis and no atypical ones (for example, a young woman with bilaterally symmetrical hilar adenopathy and erythema nodosum), the clinician may feel that the diagnosis is nearly 100% certain, that is, sarcoidosis would have a probability very near 1.00. In a patient with a more ambiguous picture (for example, cough and diffuse pulmonary infiltrates but no hilar adenopathy), the probability of sarcoidosis would be far lower since many other disorders could produce a similar picture.

Of course, the clinician's willingness to "make a diagnosis" of sarcoidosis depends not only on the likelihood of the disease but also on the consequences of that classification. If making the diagnosis results in either the termination of the diagnostic workup or the institution of potentially harmful therapy (such as administering steroids to a patient who could have tuberculosis), then the consequences of those actions must be reflected in the certainty required to label the patient as suffering from sarcoidosis. For example, if there were a small but real chance that the patient had lymphoma, the clinician might be unwilling to diagnose sarcoidosis based on hilar adenopathy alone. On the other hand, if the alternative diagnostic possibility were berylliosis, the physician might very well comfortably diagnose sarcoidosis and terminate further testing.

The difference in these two examples lies in the consequences of the erroneous diagnosis of sarcoidosis: In one case, the patient's prognosis could be severely compromised, whereas in the other case there would be little effect on the patient's course. The basis of this distinction lies in the contrasting natures of the diseases under consideration. Sarcoidosis is usually a rather mild process compared to alternatives such as lymphoma, tuberculosis and other infections. Since it has a high likelihood of spontaneous resolution and little morbidity, sarcoidosis can be thought of as a nil disease *in comparison to some of the alternative diagnoses.* A confident diagnosis of sarcoidosis is then the confident conclusion that other serious and treatable diseases are absent.

In considering the differential diagnosis of a granulomatous tissue reaction, Lofgren (1964) portrayed the universe of granulomatous diseases as broadly divided into two subsets: those of known origin (e.g., tuberculosis and berylliosis) and those of unknown origin (e.g., sarcoidosis). Although that view may still be useful, we propose that the universe of disorders that arise in the differential diagnosis of sarcoidosis be divided into the subsets nil disease and "more serious or treatable disease," as shown in Figure 1.

IV. Variations in Prior Probabilities

Let us consider three alternative case histories:

> *Patient A:* A 27-year-old woman with malaise, diffuse arthralgias, and a painful rash, typical of erythema nodosum, on her shins. Bilateral symmetrical hilar adenopathy is present on chest x-ray.

> *Patient B:* A 37-year-old man complaining of fever, night sweats, and cough, and with cervical adenopathy on physical examination. A left upper lobe infiltrate and bilateral hilar adenopathy are present on chest x-ray. A 5U PPD skin test results in 8 mm of induration at 48 hr.

> *Patient C:* A 57-year-old man who smoked heavily all his adult life presents with fever, weight loss, dyspnea, and cough of 6 months' duration. A reticulonodular infiltrate in the left upper lobe and bilateral hilar adenopathy are seen on chest x-ray.

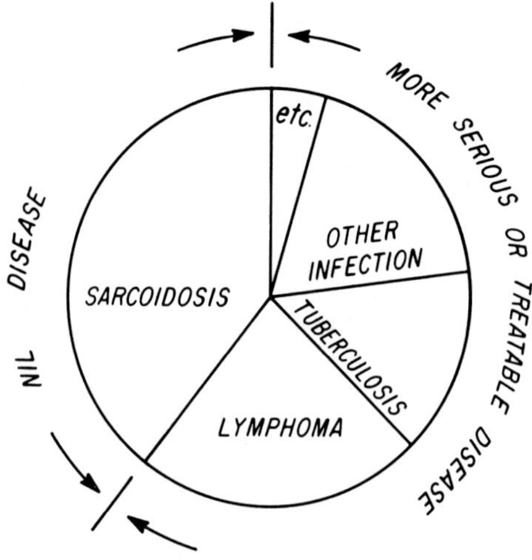

Figure 1 Differential diagnosis of sarcoidosis. Among the diseases that must be considered, sarcoidosis is often (fairly) benign while malignancies and infections are often more serious and require prompt treatment.

Although each patient may have sarcoidosis, the probability of that diagnosis varies markedly: Patient A presents a classic picture of acute sarcoidosis; patient B has findings very suggestive of tuberculosis; patient C quite likely has a malignancy. For illustrative purposes, assume that the major diagnostic considerations in each patient are sarcoidosis, an infectious disease (e.g., tuberculosis) and a malignant disease (e.g., lymphoma or lung cancer). Further assume that the clinicians caring for these patients estimated the likelihoods of the various diagnoses to be as shown in Table 1. Using these case histories as starting points, we shall examine the impact of a variety of diagnostic tests on the diagnostic spectra. In each case, we shall assume that the test results are suggestive of or consistent with the presence of sarcoidosis. We shall also examine each test result in a fourth situation, as a screening procedure in a clinically well Irish male. The prevalence of sarcoidosis in such patients is no more than 40 in 100,000 (Levinsky et al. 1976) and will thereby provide some measure of test performance when the prior probability of sarcoidosis is very low.

As stated above, the prior probability of a disease is the likelihood of that disease before the test under consideration is performed. In practice, this is often an estimate based on the physician's knowledge and experience. It is far better to supply these estimates quantitatively, as shown in Table 1, than with terms such as "high likelihood," "remote possibility," "moderate suspicion," and the like. If nonquantitative terms are used, there is inherent ambiguity: One physician may regard "high probability" to mean "greater than 95%" while another may regard it to signify "anything over 50%." Although quantitative probability estimation is not without its own errors (Tversky and Kahneman 1974), the advantage of using a common language and the ability to combine probability estimates by well-defined rules (see below) far outweigh the disadvantages and the small amount of retraining required.

Table 1 Prior Probabilities for Three Illustrative Cases

Presentation	Probability of:		
	Sarcoidosis	Infection	Malignancy
Case A: Young woman with rash and hilar adenopathy	99%	0.5%	0.5%
Case B: Young man with fever and pulmonary infiltrate	25%	70%	5%
Case C: Heavy smoker with weight loss, cough, and reticulonodular infiltrate	10%	2%	88%

Of course, the introduction of quantitation may appear to introduce greater precision that actually exists. Quantitative estimates can reflect the same degree of imprecision as can qualititative ones, except that the imprecision must be explicitly stated. One can estimate, for example, that a probability falls somewhere between 50 and 100% and can then perform calculations to determine the impact of this uncertainty on the diagnostic picture.

In some settings, usually when screening entire populations, the prior probability of disease may be known with precision. For example, the prevalence of sarcoidosis in Irish males is based on careful epidemiologic survey. More commonly, in dealing with individual patients, the prior probability cannot be precisely specified because the wealth of clinical information known about the patient may make him somewhat different from "typical" patients reported in the literature. In such cases, the literature can serve as an anchor point to, or initial approximation of the prior probability, but that estimate must be adjusted, based on the specifics of the case, by the clinician's experienced clinical judgment.

V. Interpreting a Test Result

Diagnostic tests are performed to determine whether a disease is present in a particular patient. Since a perfect test for sarcoidosis (i.e., one without false positive or false negative results) does not exist, even after performing diagnostic procedures the clinician will not be able to establish the presence or absence of this entity with certainty. Thus, the results of any diagnostic test must be interpreted probabilistically. In other words, the test will, if it provides any diagnostic information, modify the likelihood of some or all of the diagnoses under consideration. Again, these revised likelihoods are best expressed as probabilities. Since such estimates are made after knowledge of the test result, they are called *posterior probabilities,* although the terms "revised likelihood" and "predictive value" are sometimes used.

In fact, most published series report these probabilities directly. For example, in one group of asymptomatic patients with bilateral hilar adenopathy (Winterbauer et al. 1973), all patients (i.e., 100%) were ultimately found to have sarcoidosis. The experienced clinician will surely recognize that this study cannot be readily extrapolated to all patients in his practice with hilar adenopathy. Some unusual selection or referral pattern must have generated these perfect results. Certainly, some individuals from a larger universe of patients would ultimately be shown not to have sarcoidosis.

The issue of selection is precisely why the physician cannot directly use the posterior probabilities reported in the literature. Such reports are

only relevant if the particular patient being seen by the clinician shares
all the characteristics of patients in the reported series. Unfortunately, as
explained above, patients vary markedly in their clinical presentations, and
as we shall demonstrate below, those variations must have major impacts
on test interpretation.

The clinical meaning of any diagnostic results must be based on two
distinct kinds of information: the likelihood of disease before the test is
performed and the relative likelihoods of the observed result in each
diagnosis being considered. We shall first describe the characteristics of
some clinical tests commonly used in evaluating patients suspected of having
sarcoidosis and then shall introduce a procedure (i.e., Bayes rule) for
integrating the two streams of information.

VI. Characteristics of a Test

The information that a diagnostic test provides can be summarized by the
relative likelihoods of occurrence of each potential finding in patients
known either to have or not to have the disease under consideration. In
this section we shall assume that the results of the test are reported in a
binary manner—either positive or negative. In a later section, we shall
consider tests that are reported quantitatively. To report the probability
of a specific result in patients either known to have or known to be free
of a specific disease, one must have an independent gold standard for
determining the patients' true state. Since patients with disease are considered separately from those without disease, the prior probability of
disease in the study population is generally not important—as long as the
population includes enough patients from each group. Since the diagnostic
information that a test provides must be based on or "conditioned on"
the gold standard diagnosis, these measures of test performance are called
conditional probabilities.

The most commonly used conditional probabilities are sensitivity
and specificity. Sensitivity is defined as the probability of a positive
result in patients known (by the external gold standard) to have the
disease; it is sometimes called the true positive rate. The likelihood of a
negative result in patients with disease is the false negative rate. Specificity
is the probability of a negative result in patients known not to have the
disease; it is sometimes termed the true negative rate. The complement of
specificity is the false positive rate, the likelihood of a positive result in
patients without the disease. These interrelationships are summarized in a
two-by-two table (Table 2).

Unfortunately, sensitivity and specificity alone cannot be used for
test interpretation; they are defined in patients known to have or to be
free of the disease. The clinician does not know in which group his

Table 2 Characteristics of a Diagnostic Test in a Typical Study
(A Two-by-Two Table)

| | | Test result | | |
		Positive	Negative	Total
Gold standard	Disease present	a	b	a + b
	Disease absent	c	d	c + d
	Total	a + c	b + d	a + b + c + d

Prior probability = (a + b)/(a + b + c + d).
Sensitivity = a/(a + b).
False negative rate = b/(a + b).
Specificity = d/(c + d).
False positive rate = c/(c + d).
Posterior probability after positive result = a/(a + c).
Posterior probability after negative result = b/(b + d).

patient belongs; his task is to deduce the likelihood of disease based on
the clinical presentation and the test result. If the test were perfectly
sensitive, all diseased patients would have a positive test, and a negative
result would exclude the disease. Of course, this does not necessarily
imply that all patients having a positive result have the disease because
false positive results could also occur unless the test were also perfectly
specific. Contrariwise, if the test were perfectly specific, then all
patients without disease would have a negative test, and a positive result
would assure the presence of disease. Of course, unless the test were also
perfectly sensitive, this would not imply that all patients with negative
test results were free of the disease bacause false negative results might
occur.

 If both false negative and false positive results might occur, then
intuitive estimates about the likelihood of disease would be difficult and
surprisingly inaccurate. In such settings, formal methods of combining
prior and conditional probabilities should be used (Bayes 1763).

 In later sections of this chapter, we shall consider the interpretation
of a variety of diagnostic procedures that can alter the likelihood of
sarcoidosis. Although each test might yield either a result suggestive of
sarcoidosis or one suggestive of some other disease, in the examples
developed below we shall usually consider positive test results, that is,
results suggestive of sarcoidosis. As examples, we shall initially deal with

four diagnostic procedures: conjunctival biopsy, the Kveim test, liver biopsy, and transbronchial biopsy of the lung. The sensitivity and specificity (of a result suggestive of sarcoidosis) in the first three tests is quite independent of the patient's clinical presentation. The conditional probabilities of a lung biopsy showing noncaseating granulomata depends on whether pulmonary involvement is present and therefore will vary with clinical presentation. The conditional probabilities of these tests are summarized in Table 3.

Before introducing Bayesian reasoning in detail, we must consider several problems that plague its application to the diagnosis of sarcoidosis. First, the specification of conditional probabilities requires an independent gold standard of diagnosis, and in sarcoidosis no such standard exists. Of course, this situation is not unique in medicine: Many diseases are inferred from a constellation of clinical findings rather than based on an absolute diagnostic standard. For example, the diagnosis of acute nontransmural myocardial infarction cannot, in life, be established with certainty. All available tests are known to have both false positive and false negative results. One often relies on the overall clinical picture (as it meets some preestablished criteria) and on the test of time. In defining the presence of sarcoidosis, one must rely on the combination of clinicoradiological and histologic findings and on the evolution of disease.

Second, as mentioned above, one must pay particular attention to the "disease not present state" when considering sarcoidosis. If the

Table 3 Conditional Probabilities of Diagnostic Tests for Sarcoidosis

Test	Sensitivity	Specificity
Conjunctival biopsy	0.15	0.99
Kveim test	0.90	0.85
Liver biopsy	0.75	0.60
Lung biopsy		
Without overt pulmonary disease (case A and screening)	0.20[a]	0.99
With overt pulmonary disease (cases B and C)	0.85	0.96[b]

[a]This number lies somewhere between that of case A and screening and is given as an example.
[b]This number is a weighted average. The conditional probability of non-caseating granulomata on lung biopsy is 0.05 in infection and 0.01 in malignancy.
The numbers used are for illustrative purposes and may vary depending on the source of information.

patient is symptomatic (having, for example, cough, fever, dyspnea, or an abnormal chest x-ray), some abnormal condition is usually present. The distinction is not, therefore, between sarcoidosis and "no disease," but between sarcoidosis and some other disease. Furthermore, the alternative diagnoses under consideration are frequently more serious and/or more treatable than is sarcoidosis itself.

VII. Clinical Application of Bayes Rule

With these considerations in mind, we may now approach the problem faced by the clinician: Given a particular clinical presentation and a particular test result, what is the posterior (that is, the revised) likelihood of sarcoidosis? The technique for combining data from these two diagnostic sources is called Bayes rule and can be visualized as follows: imagine a room (A) filled with patients whose clinical presentation is similar to the patient under consideration so that the proportion of patients with each diagnosis corresponds to the distribution of prior probabilities in this patient. Of course, the diagnosis of each individual in the room is not known, only the aggregate totals. Next assume that a diagnostic test is performed and those patients with a positive result are directed into a second room (B), leaving those the negative results behind. What then is the probability that an individual in room B has sarcoidosis? Our best estimate of that probability is the proportion of patients in room B who have sarcoidosis, that is, the ratio of the number of patients with a positive test *and* sarcoidosis to the number of patients with positive test results. Although this relation can be expressed as a formula,* we have found two other calculational approaches, one diagrammatic and one tabular, to be more clinically useful.

In Figure 2, we interpret a conjunctival biopsy in case A, the young woman with rash and hilar adenopathy. Consider a cohort of 100,000 women just like this patient in whom the prior probability of sarcoidosis is 0.99 (Table 1). Thus, 99,000 of these women would, in fact, have sarcoidosis and 1000 would not. Conjunctival biopsy has 15% sensitivity (Crick et al. 1961) and near perfect specificity (Fong and Israel 1979) (see Table 3). Thus, of the 99,000 women with sarcoidosis, 14,850 would have truly positive biopsies, whereas of the 1000 women without sarcoidosis, 10 would have falsely positive biopsy results. Thus, a total of 14,860

---

*If P_d is the prior probability of disease, sens is the sensitivity, and spec is the specificity, then the posterior probability equals

$$(P_d \times \text{sens})/\{(P_d \times \text{sens}) + [(1 - P_d) \times (1 - \text{spec})]\}$$

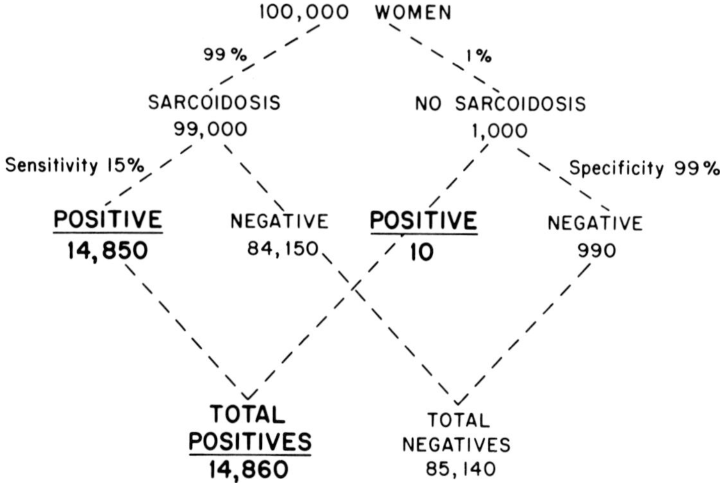

Figure 2   Interpretation of a conjunctival biopsy in case A.   Consider a cohort of 100,000 women in whom the prevalence of sarcoidosis is 99%. With a sensitivity of 15% and a specificity of 99%, conjunctival biopsy will be positive in 14,860 women of which 14,850 (99.93%) will actually have the disease.   Of the 85,140 women with negative biopsies, 84,150 (98.83%) will nevertheless have sarcoidosis.

biopsies would be positive, and the posterior probability of sarcoidosis after a positive conjunctival biopsy would be 14,850/14,860 or 0.9993.   The positive result changed our diagnostic impressions only very slightly because we were already quite sure that sarcoidosis was present.   The situation would be similar if a negative result were obtained.   We would expect 85,140 negative conjunctival biopsies of which 84,150 would come from women with sarcoidosis.   Thus, the revised probability would be 84,150/ 85,140 or 0.9884—minimally different from the prior probability.

It would seem, then, that conjunctival biopsy has little impact on the diagnosis.   That conclusion is valid, however, only when the prior probability of sarcoidosis is high.   In contrast, let us apply the same diagnostic test to case C, the heavy smoker with weight loss and cough.   In this case, the prior probability of sarcoidosis is only 10% (Table 1).   We shall use this case as an opportunity to introduce the tabular method of test interpretation.   In Table 4, we shall first interpret a positive result and then a negative one.

As can be seen in the upper portion of Table 4, we first list each diagnosis under active consideration—sarcoidosis, infection, and malignancy.

Table 4 Interpretation of a Conjunctival Biopsy in Case C

Diagnosis	A Prior probability	B Conditional probability of a positive result	C Product	D Revised probability
Sarcoidosis	0.10	0.15	150	150/240 = 0.625
Infection	0.02	0.01	2	2/240 = 0.008
Malignancy	0.88	0.01	88	88/240 = 0.367
			240	

Diagnosis	A Prior probability	B Conditional probability of a negative result	C Product	D Revised probability
Sarcoidosis	0.10	0.85	850	850/9760 = 0.087
Infection	0.02	0.99	198	198/9760 = 0.020
Malignancy	0.88	0.99	8712	8712/9760 = 0.893
			9760	

In column A we next record the prior probabilities in any consistent scale.
Here we have chosen to use percentages. In column B we then list the
conditional probabilities of the observed test result, in this example a
positive result. In sarcoidosis, the conditional probability is the sensitivity,
while that in infection and malignancy is the false positive rate. Next, in
column C, we record the separate pairwise products of the entries in
columns A and B. Finally, the revised or posterior probabilities (column
D) are calculated by dividing each entry in column C by the sum of
column C. Thus, we see that the probability of sarcoidosis in case C
has increased from 10% to 63% on the basis of a positive conjunctival
biopsy. Certainly the implications of such a shift on management would
be important to consider.

On the other hand, the lower half of Table 4 details the interpretation of a negative conjunctival biopsy. That result would have very little
diagnostic impact, lowering the probability of sarcoidosis from 10% to 9%

while increasing the probability of malignancy by a like amount. Thus, a single diagnostic test—the conjunctival biopsy—can transmit very different amounts of clinical information, depending on the specific characteristics of the patient to whom the test is applied.

VIII. The Interpretation of Positive Biopsy Results

Since this monograph is directed at the diagnosis of sarcoidosis, let us now turn our attention to positive test results—results that increase the likelihood of sarcoidosis. We shall consider four clinical settings (cases A, B, C, and "screening Irishmen") and four diagnostic tests, as detailed in Tables 1 and 3. The results of these 16 Bayesian analyses are summarized in Table 5. In general, the higher the prior probability, the higher the posterior probability. A minor exception occurs in the application of transbronchial lung biopsy to cases B and C, both of whom have interstitial infiltrates on chest x-ray. The prior probability of sarcoidosis is 2.5 times as likely in case B (25% versus 10%), but the posterior probability of sarcoidosis is slightly higher in case C (90% versus 86%). This apparent discrepancy occurs because the finding of noncaseating granulomata on biopsy is far more likely in infections than in malignancies, and because infection is the most likely diagnosis in case B but is a quite unexpected possibility in case C.

These 19 examples should have convinced the reader not only of the importance of explicit, Bayesian test interpretation but also of the relative simplicity of each individual calculation. Quite obviously, the major effect is that of the prior probability of disease. We have therefore calculated the impact of a positive result in each of these four diagnostic tests on

Table 5 Posterior Probabilities of Sarcoidosis After Various Positive Test Results

		Posterior probability after positive			
Setting	Prior probability	Conjunctival biopsy	Kveim test	Liver biopsy	Transbronchial biopsy
Case A	0.99	0.999	0.998	0.995	0.997
Case B	0.25	0.833	0.667	0.385	0.857
Case C	0.10	0.625	0.400	0.172	0.897
Screening	0.0004	0.006	0.002	0.001	0.008

all possible prior probabilities of disease, that is, with the prior probability ranging from zero to unity.

These analyses are summarized in Figure 3. The prior probability of sarcoidosis is displayed on the horizontal axis; the posterior probability is displayed on the vertical axis. Each test is depicted by a single line on the graph. Although the sensitivity and specificity of lung biopsy vary with pulmonary involvement, the diagnostic implications are essentially identical—the increase in sensitivity is just offset by the decrease in specificity. In general, more information is provided by invasive tests with the exception of liver biopsy.

From this figure one can gain an overall appreciation of the impact of positive test results on the likelihood of sarcoidosis. Specifically, different tests are to be preferred in different clinical settings. Similar calculations can be performed for negative test results; in that case both conjunctival biopsy and lung biopsy in the absence of overt pulmonary disease provide the least information while the Kveim test provides the most. With this realization, the clinician may be able to select more effectively among alternative diagnostic procedures.

IX. Beyond Sensitivity and Specificity

Up to this point we have considered tests that are reported as either positive or negative. The usefulness of such diagnostic procedures depends on three separate factors: first, the clinical setting (i.e., the prior probabilities);

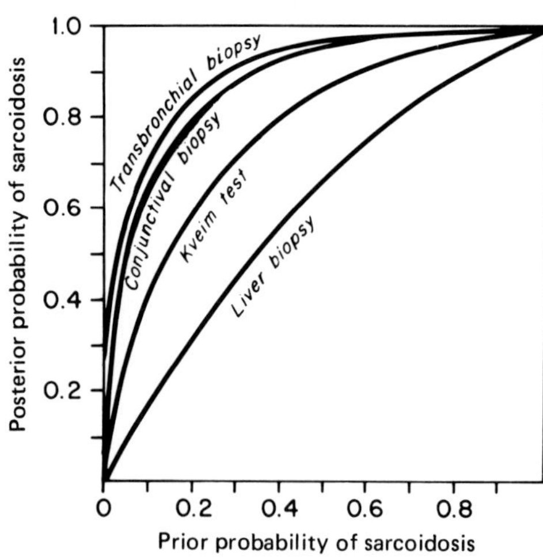

Figure 3 Relation of prior and posterior probabilities of sarcoidosis for four diagnostic tests. The horizontal axis shows the prior probability. Each line corresponds to a positive result on a single diagnostic test. The vertical axis depicts the resulting posterior, or revised, probability based on the application of Bayes rule.

second, the conditional probabilities; and third, the assumed criterion of positivity. Certainly, when reporting histologic or radiological test results, pathologists and radiologists may vary considerably in the strictness of their interpretations, that is, in whether they choose to label a particular biopsy or x-ray as positive. Even if the pathologist or radiologist foregoes classifying the material presented to him, the clinician will superimpose his own interpretation on the radiological or histologic description. If the test is interpreted using strict criteria for sarcoidosis, the false positive rate will be relatively low (that is, the specificity will be high)—at the expense of a lowered sensitivity. On the other hand, if the test in interpreted using lax criteria, sensitivity will be enchanced—at the expense of diminished specificity.

Clearly, the classification of the complex results of a diagnostic procedure as simply positive or negative is, in some sense, "information destructive;" all positives are grouped together and the relative strength of positivity is not distinguished. Of course, such an approach has definite advantages. With a well-established criterion for labeling results, it becomes possible to study test performance in patients whose diagnoses have been established by some external standard and thereby to measure sensitivity and specificity. These two conditional probabilities, then, are not innate measures of test performance: They measure the performance of the test under a particular criterion of classification. If that criterion were to change, so would sensitivity and specificity.

In this section we shall consider more directly the innate performance of diagnostic tests and shall consider how one might establish an appropriate criterion for classification. We shall demonstrate how Bayesian reasoning can be applied to a particular test result without superimposing a classification scheme that discards relevant clinical information. To clarify our consideration of test results, we shall move from histologic and radiological procedures which are often reported in ambiguous, qualitative terms (such as, "consistent with," "highly suggestive of," "cannot be excluded") to an enzymatic assay that is customarily reported quantitatively. In terms of the diagnosis of sarcoidosis, we shall consider as an example the serum level of angiotensin 1-converting enzyme.

Commonly, results are reported as abnormal when they fall more than two standard deviations beyond the mean of the control population. This criterion guarantees that the specificity will be 97.5% (in a one-tailed test where only abnormally high values are called positive); 2.5% of a normal population will lie in the upper tail. Unfortunately, this method has at least three serious flaws.

First, it ignores the distribution of test results in patients with sarcoidosis. If that distribution were narrow and widely separated from the distribution of results in patients without sarcoidosis, then a more strict criterion (a higher cutoff value) might be used. If the distribution of results in patients with sarcoidosis had major overlap with the normal distribution, a more lax criterion (a lower cutoff value) might be chosen to avoid a very low sensitivity. These considerations will be explained in more detail later.

Second, the "two standard deviations criterion" ignores the prior probability of sarcoidosis in the population to be screened or in the patient to be examined. If the prevalence were low, a relatively strict criterion might be applied to avoid a large number of false positive results. In other words, if the prior probability were low, the test would be applied to a large number of individuals without sarcoidosis, and the effect of the false positive rate would be greatly magnified. Conversely, if the prior probability of sarcoidosis were high, a relatively lax criterion might be preferable.

Third, the "two standard deviations criterion" ignores the relative costs of different classification errors. A type I error would classify a patient without sarcoidosis as actually having the disease. Since such patients are usually suffering from another disease, often one that is more serious or more treatable, such errors may delay necessary diagnosis and treatment. A type II error would fail to make the diagnosis of sarcoidosis and would thereby subject patients to unnecessary and perhaps risky diagnostic procedures or therapies.

Of course, even if more rational methods are used to establish the definition of a positive test result, the physician must be wary of bias introduced by the spectrum of patients included in the control group (Ransohoff and Feinstein 1978). When the performance of a test is first reported, the control group is often comprised of randomly selected members of a disease-free population. Such individuals would be quite dissimilar from patients with sarcoidosis and would be unlikely to show elevated test results. Thus, the initially reported specificity is quite high. As the test is used clinically, however, it is often applied to patients with diseases similar to sarcoidosis (e.g., granulomatous diseases, pulmonary diseases, or lymphoproliferative diseases), and, depending on the test, these patients could be more likely to have elevated results despite the absence of sarcoidosis. Furthermore, when a test is initially developed in the laboratory, its sensitivity is often reported on patients with classic or advanced disease; false negatives may be uncommon. In clinical use, however, the test is often applied to confusing cases that may involve unusual or minimal forms of the disease. In such patients, sensitivity might well be lower.

These relations are summarized in Figure 4. Each panel shows the distribution of test results in patients with (right-hand distribution) and without (left-hand distribution) sarcoidosis. For any criterion or cutoff

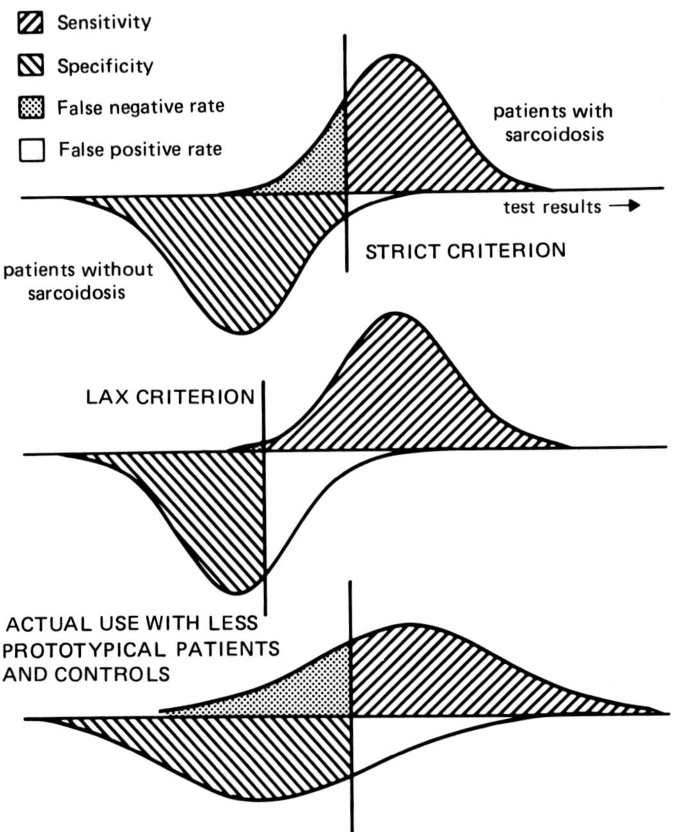

Figure 4 Distributions of test results in patients with and without sarcoidosis. The upper distribution corresponds to patients with sarcoidosis while the lower (inverted) distribution corresponds to patients free of that disease. The vertical line represents the cutoff criterion for definition of a positive result. The sensitivity, specificity, false positive rate, and false negative rate correspond to various shaded areas. The top panel shows a strict criterion; the middle panel shows a lax criterion; the bottom panel shows a strict criterion applied to less typical patients.

value (depicted by a vertical line) the test sensitivity corresponds to the right diagonally hatched area and the test specificity corresponds to the left diagonally hatched area. The top panel depicts a relatively strict criterion while the middle panel shows the effect of making the criterion more lax. In the bottom panel, the criterion of positivity is unchanged but the effect of changing patient populations is shown, with patients free of sarcoidosis becoming more abnormal and with patients suffering from sarcoidosis becoming less classic.

X. The Bayesian Interpretation of Quantitative Results

Let us now turn to the interpretation of a diagnostic test that is reported quantitatively, and let us ignore the issue of classification. We shall deal directly with the reported value, that is, the serum level of angiotensin 1-converting enzyme (ACE). We shall assume that the distributions of test results in patients with sarcoidosis and those without sarcoidosis are both Gaussian (i.e., bell-shaped), and that their respective means and standard deviations are known. Combining a variety of studies on ACE (for purposes of illustration), we shall take the mean plus or minus the standard deviation to be 49 ± 15 units/ml in sarcoidosis and 28 ± 9 units/ml in patients without sarcoidosis. These two distributions are displayed in Figure 5. With these values one can calculate the sensitivity and specificity for the ACE assay for various cutoff criteria (Table 6). The

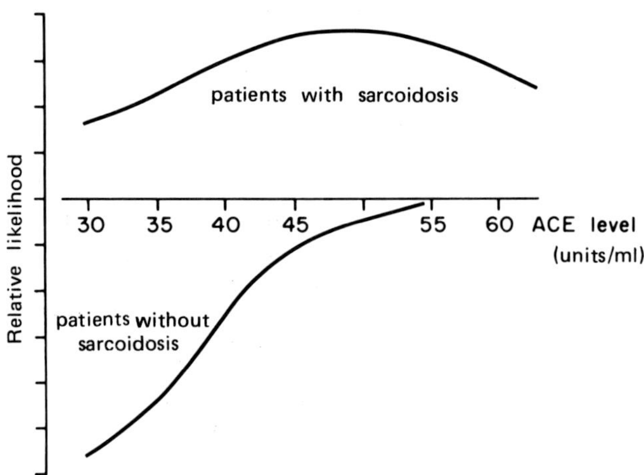

Figure 5 Distributions of serum levels of angiotensin 1-converting enzyme in patients with and without sarcoidosis. The formJat is analagous to that in Figure 4. The upper distribution shows patients with sarcoidosis while the lower (inverted) distribution corresponds to patients free of that disease. The distribution of patients with sarcoidosis is somewhat flatter since the standard deviation of that distribution is larger.

Table 6 Effect of Classification Criterion on Meaning of Results of Angiotensin 1-Converting Enzyme (ACE)

	ACE level (units/ml)						
	30	35	40	45	50	55	60
Sensitivity	0.898	0.824	0.726	0.606	0.482	0.345	0.233
Specificity	0.587	0.782	0.908	0.971	0.993	0.999	0.9998
If positive (above cutoff)							
Likelihood ratio	2.17	3.80	7.89	20.9	68.9	345	1164
Posterior probability if observed in:							
Case A (Prior = 0.99)	0.995	0.997	0.999	1.00	1.00	1.00	1.00
Case B (Prior = 0.25)	0.420	0.558	0.725	0.874	0.958	0.991	0.997
Case C (Prior = 0.10)	0.195	0.296	0.467	0.699	0.884	0.976	0.992
Screening (Prior = 0.0004)	0.001	0.002	0.003	0.008	0.027	0.121	0.318
If negative (below cutoff)							
Likelihood ratio	5.75	4.44	3.31	2.46	1.92	1.53	1.30
Posterior probability if observed in:							
Case A (Prior = 0.99)	0.945	0.957	0.968	0.976	0.981	0.984	0.987
Case B (Prior = 0.25)	0.055	0.070	0.091	0.119	0.148	0.179	0.204

Table 6 (Continued)

	\multicolumn{7}{c}{ACE level (units/ml)}						
	30	35	40	45	50	55	60
Case C (Prior = 0.10)	0.019	0.024	0.032	0.043	0.055	0.068	0.079
Screening (Prior = 0.0004)	0.0001	0.0001	0.0001	0.0002	0.0002	0.0003	0.0003

same approach can be taken if one uses other means and standard deviations for control and diseased groups; only the sensitivities and specificities would differ.

Having determined how the sensitivity and specificity of the angiotensin 1-converting enzyme assay vary with the criterion for classification, we can now utilize Bayes rule to determine the posterior probability of sarcoidosis in each for the four prototypical situations we have been using (i.e., cases A, B, and C, and screening). The results of these 56 applications of Bayes rule are displayed in Table 6. The upper half of the table shows the implications of a positive ACE level, that is, one above the cutoff criterion; the lower portion of the table displays the posterior probabilities for a negative ACE test at each cutoff level. Obviously, a positive test increases the probability of sarcoidosis whereas a negative test result lowers the likelihood. The two rows labeled "likelihood ratio" provide measures of the information content of the ACE test at each cutoff level. The likelihood ratio for a positive result is defined as sensitivity/(false negative rate). A likelihood ratio of 1 implies that the result carries no diagnostic information, that is, the posterior probability will equal the prior probability. The higher the likelihood ratio, the more information that the result carries. Thus, the more strict (i.e., the higher) the cutoff criterion, the more information that a positive result implies, but the less information a negative result conveys. Conversely, the more lax the criterion is, the greater is the information provided by a negative result, but the less by a positive result.

Of course, any such classification scheme is information-destructive, that is, it neglects the distance of the observed result from the criterion. If the cutoff criterion is an ACE level of 45 units/ml (roughly 2 SD above the mean of the distribution of results in patients without sarcoidosis), a level of 46 and a level of 60 would not be distinguished. To take full account of all the information provided by a specific observed level, the physician should use the conditional probability of that result (and not of all results above an arbitrary cutoff) in patients with and without sarcoidosis. Referring to Figure 5, we can see that these two conditional probabilities correspond to the relative *heights* of the two distributions at any given ACE level, rather than to the *areas* in the two tails.

The ratio between the height of the distribution of ACE results in patients with sarcoidosis and that in patients without sarcoidosis is called the "likelihood quotient" and is displayed in Table 7. A likelihood quotient of 1 implies that the result does not change the probability of sarcoidosis; quotients above unity imply that the likelihood of sarcoidosis is increased by the ACE result, while quotients below 1 imply that the probability is decreased. An ACE level above 38 units/ml will increase the likelihood of sarcoidosis while a level below 38 units/ml will decrease it.

In Table 7 we have also provided the results of 28 applications of Bayes rule corresponding to our four clinical situations and seven different ACE levels. It is interesting to compare this conclusion to the "two

Table 7 Interpretation of Angiotensin 1-Converting Enzyme (ACE) Level (Using All Information)

	Observed ACE level (units/ml)						
	30	35	40	45	50	55	60
Likelihood quotient	0.276	0.529	1.21	3.45	11.9	55.2	262
Posterior probability if observed in:							
Case A (Prior = 0.99)	0.965	0.981	0.992	0.997	0.999	1.00	1.00
Case B (Prior = 0.25)	0.084	0.150	0.288	0.535	0.799	0.948	0.987
Case C (Prior = 0.10)	0.030	0.055	0.119	0.277	0.570	0.860	0.967
Screening (Prior = 0.0004)	0.0001	0.0002	0.0005	0.001	0.005	0.022	0.095

standard deviation criterion" of 45. By that criterion, an ACE level of 40 would be negative and lower the likelihood of sarcoidosis in case C, for example, from 10% to 4% (Table 6, bottom). In stark contrast, the proper interpretation of that ACE level would actually increase the likelihood of sarcoidosis from 10% to 12% (Table 7), a threefold difference.

XI. Choosing a Cutoff Criterion

Although comparing the conditional probability of the observed value clearly provides more accurate information, it is time-consuming and physicians will likely continue to use cutoff criteria when interpreting a quantitative diagnostic test, labeling any given result as positive or negative. In that case, can one provide any rational basis for selecting the criterion used to define a positive result? Obviously, the answer is yes, and the technique utilizes another method of displaying some of the data in Table 6. Clearly, both sensitivity and specificity vary with the cutoff criterion; in fact, they vary inversely with one another. A strict criterion increases specificity and decreases sensitivity; a lax criterion increases sensitivity at the expense of decreased specificity. As shown in Figure 6, we can plot the true positive rate against the false positive rate for various cutoffs, obtaining a receiver operating characteristic (or ROC) curve (McNeil et al. 1975). The more convex that curve, that is, the more it approaches the upper left corner of the graph, the better is the diagnostic test that it describes. Moving the cutoff criterion to the right in Figure 5 (making it more strict) corresponds

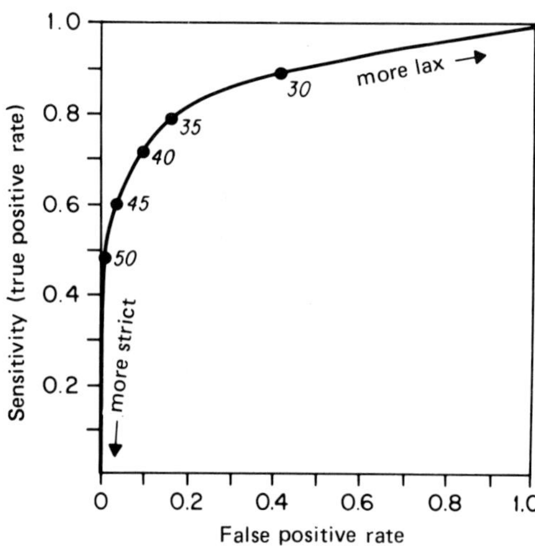

Figure 6 Receiver operator characteristic curve for serum levels of angiotensin 1-converting enzyme. The horizontal axis is the false positive rate (1 minus the specificity); the vertical axis is the true positive rate (sensitivity). The numbers along the curve correspond to the cutoff criterion (in units/ml) for each definition of sensitivity and specificity.

to moving along the ROC curve to the left; making the cutoff criterion more lax (moving to the left in Figure 5) corresponds to moving along the ROC curve to the right.

Given an ROC display, one can select the optimal cutoff on the basis of three additional facts: the prevalence of sarcoidosis in the population being tested, the cost of type I errors (i.e., diagnosing sarcoidosis in a patient with another disease), and the cost of type II errors (i.e., failing to diagnose sarcoidosis in a patient who actually has the disease). Note the use of the term "population" It makes no sense to establish a cutoff criterion when dealing with an individual patient. In that setting it would be far more rational to utilize all the information that the ACE assay can provide. Criteria for test interpretation are only rational if the test is going to be applied to many patients. Since we have not yet developed an approach to measuring costs, risks, and benefits, we shall not actually define the optimal cutoff for ACE determinations. Such cutoffs will clearly vary from setting to setting, depending on the prevalence of sarcoidosis and what diagnostic and therapeutic procedures will ensue after test interpretation.

Let us assume that the costs have been measured and labeled as $C_{error\ I}$ and $C_{error\ II}$. Also assume that the population prevalence of sarcoidosis is P_s. It can be shown that the optimal operating point on the ROC curve is the point where the slope of the curve (that is, the slope of a straight line tangent to the curve) is $(1 - P_s)(C_{error\ I})/(P_s)(C_{error\ II})$. The astute reader will deduce that the operating point should move toward the upper right end of the ROC curve when prevalence is high and the cost of type I errors is low. Contrariwise, the optimal operating point should move toward the lower left when prevalence is low and the cost of type II errors is low. In most clinical situations, the cost of type I errors will exceed the cost of type II errors. Thus, one should tend to operate toward the lower end of the ROC curve (i.e., with a strict criterion) unless the population prevalence of sarcoidosis is very high.

XII. Choosing to Terminate the Diagnostic Evaluation

In the final section of this chapter, let us return to the issues with which we began. Assuming that the patient has no evidence of major organ involvement or progressive pulmonary dysfunction (which would be indications for corticosteroid therapy), the major management dilemma that faces the physician is when to make the diagnosis of sarcoidosis—to label the patient as having this relatively benign disease—and thereby to terminate the current phase of diagnostic evaluation.

As mentioned above, this decision can beget several consequences. If the patient actually has sarcoidosis and the diagnosis is made, that is, the label is applied, then the patient escapes the risk, cost, and inconvenience of further diagnostic testing or even unnecessary therapy for some other disease (because diagnostic procedures are imperfect and therapy might be instituted based on erroneously positive test results). Such a patient suffers no harm in carrying the diagnosis since we have assumed, in this example, that a major organ is not threatened; hence, corticosteroid therapy would not be begun. On the other hand, if the patient actually was suffering from another disease, applying the sarcoidosis label would delay establishing the correct diagnosis and would delay the administration of specific therapy for what may be a life-threatening, yet treatable, disease.

In this section we shall approach this choice analytically, that is, in a given patient should the clinician make the presumptive diagnosis of sarcoidosis or should he proceed with further diagnostic evaluation? We shall utilize the principles of clinical decision analysis to consider this dilemma in an explicit and logical manner. This formal approach to medical decision making consists of five distinct steps: (a) structuring the problem, (b) assigning probabilities to various chance events, (c) assigning utilities or relative values to various potential outcomes, (d) calculating the optimal strategy, and (e) examining all assumptions through sensitivity analysis to determine under what specific circumstances the optimal choice would be different. In this section we cannot develop the logical basis for these tools; we shall simply apply them to the problem at hand and refer the interested reader to other sources (Raiffa 1968, Weinstein 1980) for more information on these techniques.

The notation we shall use for structuring this choice is the decision tree in Figure 7. The square decision node at the left denotes the choice— to diagnose sarcoidosis (upper branch) or to continue the diagnostic evaluation (lower branch). Even if the patient is diagnosed as having sarcoidosis, the patient may actually have some other disorder, since none of the current diagnostic tests for sarcoidosis is perfect. Although the differential diagnosis of sarcoidosis may comprise a lengthy list, we will limit our analysis to the two alternate possibilities that are of greatest clinical concern: infection and malignancy. In this analysis we shall not distinguish further among the infections and malignancies in the differential diagnosis of sarcoidosis. Both of these entities are serious and may improve if specific therapy is administered, but the patient may suffer irreparable harm if diagnosis and therapy are delayed.

The likelihood that the patient actually has each entity can be represented, as shown by the round chance node labeled A, as a probability. Since we assume that these three diagnoses are exhaustive and mutually exclusive (the patient actually has one and only one of them), we only need specify the probability of infection (P_i) and the probability of

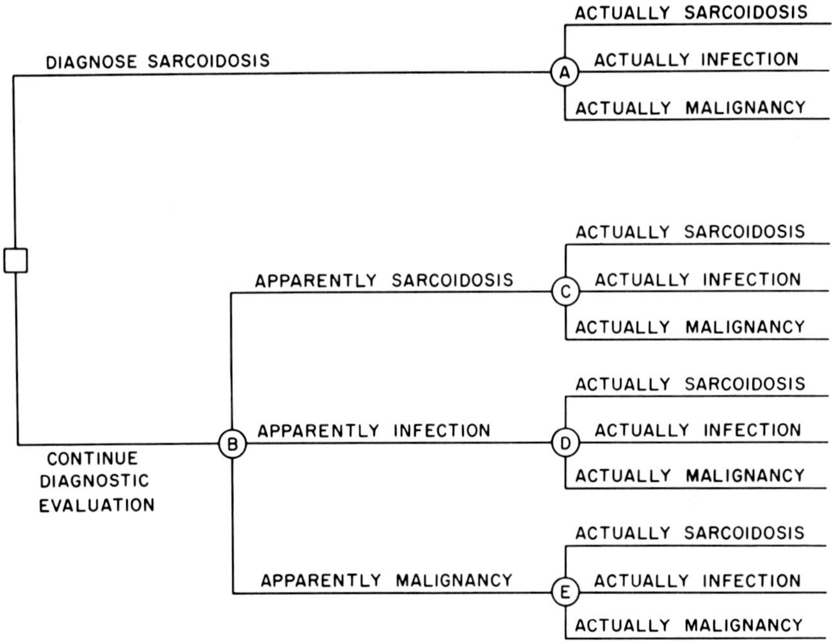

Figure 7 Decision tree for analysis of whether or not to continue diagnostic workup in a patient who may have sarcoidosis. The decision is denoted by the square node. The five circular nodes (A–E) denote chance events that can be described in terms of probabilities.

malignancy (P_m). The probability of sarcoidosis is then ($1 - P_i - P_m$). Next consider the lower branch of the square decision node. If further testing is performed, the patient will eventually be classified as having one of these entities (chance node B with branches "apparently sarcoid," "apparently infection," and "apparently malignancy"). In each case (nodes C, D, and E) the patient's actual diagnosis may be different, labeled "actually sarcoid," "actually infection," and "actually malignancy."

Let us assume that the diagnostic workup is imperfect and that the conditional probabilities of each diagnosis are as described in Table 8. Although not derived from experimental data, such conditional probabilities might be obtained from transbronchial biopsy, for example, where the probability of obtaining noncaseating granulomata in known sarcoidosis might be 0.80, and where such granulomata might also be seen in 5% of infections (including tuberculosis) and in 1% of malignancies producing a clinical picture of sarcoidosis. From these data we can calculate the yield

Table 8 Conditional Probabilities for Further Diagnostic Evaluation

	Apparent diagnosis after evaluation		
	Sarcoidosis	Infection	Malignancy
Actual diagnosis			
Sarcoidosis	0.80	0.15	0.05
Infection	0.05	0.90	0.05
Malignancy	0.01	0.01	0.98

of the proposed diagnostic evaluation. The diagnosis "apparently sarcoid" can arise in three different ways: from patients who actually have sarcoidosis (with probability 0.8), from patients with infections and falsely negative workup (with probability 0.05) and from patients with malignancy (probability 0.01). Since the prior probabilities are $(1 - P_i - P_m)$, P_i, and P_m, respectively, the probability of the "apparently sarcoid" branch of node B is $0.8 (1 - P_i - P_m) + 0.05 P_i + 0.01 P_m$. By like calculation, the probability of "apparently infection" is $0.15 (1 - P_i - P_m) + 0.9 P_i + 0.01 P_m$, and that of "apparently malignancy" is $0.05 (1 - P_i - P_m) + 0.05 P_i + 0.98 P_m$.

The branch probabilities for nodes C, D, and E can be calculated by Bayes rule given the prior probabilities and the information in Table 8. For example, the probability of infection given the "apparent" diagnosis of sarcoidosis (middle branch of node C) is calculated as the ratio of the probability of the workup's showing "apparently sarcoidosis" while the patient actually has sarcoidosis ($0.05 P_i$) to the probability of "apparently sarcoidosis" calculated above, or $0.05 P_i/(0.05 P_i + 0.01 P_m + 0.8 (1 - P_i - P_m))$.

Having specified the structure and probabilities, let us now turn to the issue of outcomes. Since this book is concerned with sarcoidosis, we shall not focus on the details of prognosis if the patient actually has infection or malignancy. Rather, we shall measure the relative value or utility of each outcome state (there are 12 outcomes depicted in Fig. 7) in terms of the chances of a good result. As shown in Table 9, our utility scale will run from 0 (death) to 100 (a good result). We assume that sarcoidosis and infection will both yield good results if properly treated, where proper treatment for sarcoidosis in this patient is no therapy. We assume that the best possible outcome in properly treated malignancy is 70 and that untreated infection and malignancy have utilities of 50 and 20, respectively. Thus, we assume that malignancy, even if properly diagnosed and treated, will yield an outcome only 70% as good as that of properly

Table 9 Utilities of Potential Outcomes

| | Utility | |
Outcome	Ignoring cost of workup	Including cost of workup
Sarcoidosis		
Untreated	100	100-C
Treated as infection	95	95-C
Treated as malignancy	90	90-C
Infection		
Properly treated	100	100-C
Undiagnosed and untreated	50	50-C
Undiagnosed and treated as malignancy	45	45-C
Malignancy		
Properly treated	70	70-C
Undiagnosed and untreated	20	20-C
Undiagnosed and treated as infection	18	18-C

treated sarcoidosis or infection. In addition, malignancy and infection will have significantly diminished utility if diagnosis and therapy are delayed. We further assume that unnecessary anti-infective or antineoplastic therapy will exact some toll, ranging from 2 to 10 units depending on the setting. Finally, we shall assign a cost C to the diagnostic workup.

Next we must calculate the average or expected utility for each strategy. This expected utility is found by "averaging out" at each chance node, that is, by calculating a weighted average of utilities, where the weights are determined by the likelihood of each outcome's occurring. For the strategy "diagnose sarcoidosis" the expected utility is found by summing the branchwise products of utility and probability at node A. Thus we have $100 (1 - P_i - P_m) + 50 P_i + 20 P_m$. The calculation for "continue diagnostic evaluation" is done in two stages. First, calculate the expected utility of nodes C, D, and E. Then calculate the expected utility of node B using the expected utilities just calculated and multiplying each by the proper branch probability for each branch of node B. After simplification, we have the expected utility of "diagnose sarcoid" (EU_{DX}) equals $100 - 50 P_i - 80 P_m$, and the expected utility of "continue diagnostic evaluation" (EU_{EVAL}) equals $98.75 - 4 P_i - 29.77 P_m - C$. For any combination of P_i, P_m, and C, we can calculate EU_{DX} and EU_{EVAL} and determine which is greater.

The preferred strategy is the one with the higher expected utility. For example, if the probability of infection is 70% and the probability of malignancy is 5% (case B), the probability of sarcoidosis is 25% and EU_{DX} is 61 while EU_{EVAL} is $94.46 - C$. Thus, the workup should continue unless C, the cost or risk of evaluation, exceeds 33.46 on the utility scale. Since it is very unlikely that the risk of a poor outcome as a consequence of diagnostic workup even approaches this level, it is clear that diagnostic evaluation should continue.

Although one might tabulate these results for all possible values of these three variables, the results of this analysis can be better grasped diagrammatically. Consider Figure 8. The probability of infection is depicted along the horizontal axis, and the probability of malignancy is depicted along the vertical axis. Since the sum of these probabilities cannot exceed 1, the legally defined points in the figure lie in the right triangle

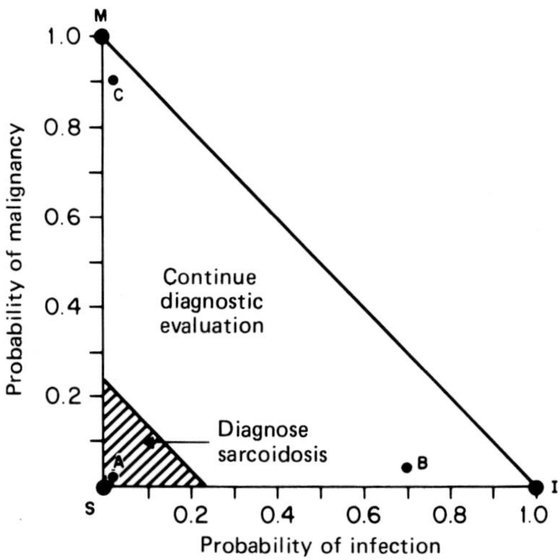

Figure 8 Sensitivity analysis of the prior probabilities of infection and malignancy. Each patient can be summarized by the probability of infection (horizontal axis) and the probability of malignancy (vertical axis); *a* denotes a unique point. If the point lies in the shaded area, sarcoidosis should be diagnosed and the workup terminated. Points A, B, and C correspond to the patients described in Table 1. Points I, M, and S correspond to patients known to have infection, malignancy, and sarcoidosis, respectively.

below the 45° line. Each point in that triangle corresponds to a unique set of prior probabilities, where the probability of sarcoidosis equals $(1 - P_i - P_m)$. Thus, a patient known to have sarcoidosis would be depicted by point S, one known to have infection would be depicted by point I, and one known to have malignancy would fall at point M. We can then divide the triangle into two regions, depending on whether the optimum strategy is to "diagnose sarcoid" (shaded area) or to "continue diagnostic evaluation" (unshaded area).

First, of course, we must specify a value for C, the cost of continued diagnostic testing. For illustrative purposes, let us choose a rather high value (10 units), assuming that the diagnostic procedure is dangerous and fraught with complications. Setting $EU_{DX} = EU_{EVAL}$ and solving for P_m in terms of P_i, we find that a straight line running almost at 45° separates the two regions. Any point falling in the shaded region would correspond to a patient who would be better served by diagnosing sarcoidosis and terminating the evaluation; any point falling above the threshold line (Pauker and Kassirer 1975, 1980) would correspond to a patient who should continue down the diagnostic pathway. On this same figure, points A, B, and C correspond to the patients presented in Table 1. We can see that diagnostic evaluation could be terminated and the diagnosis of sarcoidosis can be made in the young woman with hilar adenopathy, but diagnostic workup should continue in the patients suspected of probably having infection or malignancy. Of course, our assumed value of 10 for the cost of evaluation may be far too high.

In Figure 9, we have plotted (on a different scale) a family of threshold lines for various values of C. It is worth noting that even if C were 0, there would be a small region wherein the workup should be terminated. This occurs because we assumed that the workup is imperfect; thus, patients very likely actually to have sarcoidosis might be subjected to unnecessary therapies.

Obviously, the position of the threshold lines in Figures 8 and 9 depends critically on the assumptions we made about the accuracy of diagnostic evaluation and the relative utilities (risks and benefits) of the various possible treatments of patients with each diagnosis. If we had assumed that diagnostic evaluation were less accurate or if the risk of inappropriate therapy were higher, then each "diagnose sarcoid" region would be increased in size by shifting the corresponding threshold line upward and to the right. Conversely, the greater the benefit of appropriate treatment of malignancy, the more each line would be shifted away from point M, increasing the region above the line and making its slope somewhat flatter.

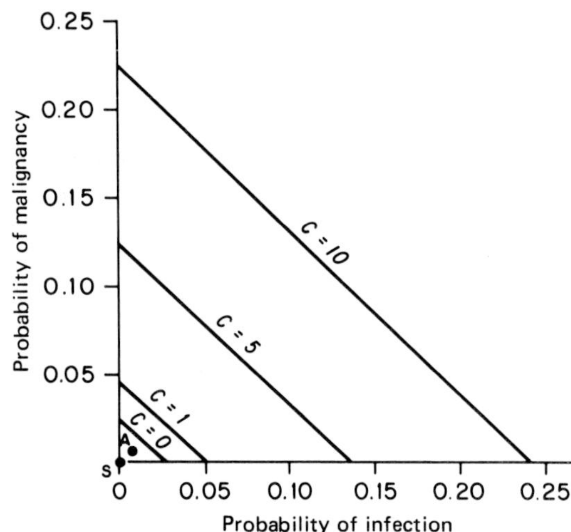

Figure 9 Effect of the cost of diagnostic evaluation on the threshold for diagnosing sarcoidosis. The format is identical to that in Figure 8, except for the expansion of the vertical and horizontal scales. Each threshold line corresponds to a specific assumed "cost" of the diagnostic evaluation. The line C = 10 corresponds to Figure 8. For each cost, diagnostic evaluation should be terminated if the point corresponding to a particular patient falls below the corresponding threshold line.

XIII. Conclusion

This analysis has been predicated on many assumptions, assumptions that some readers may not accept. However, our deliberately provocative assumptions have been explicitly stated so that they might be examined, criticized, and changed. Indeed, the major advantage of this approach is its explicit nature. We do not argue that our conclusions are correct and immutable. Rather, they are trial balloons, if you will, a first pass at bringing rationality to an uncertain area in medicine. We invite the interested reader to alter any assumptions and recalculate the probabilities and expected utilities to determine the impact of those changes on the optimal choice.

Finally, the purpose of this chapter was not to provide final answers, not to close off further discussion of these interesting and important dilemmas. Rather, our purpose was to introduce the concepts to the reader and to provide a language and technology for discussing many vital issues in the diagnosis of sarcoidosis.

References

Bayes, T. (1763). An essay toward solving a problem in the doctrine of chance. *Phil. Trans. R. Soc. Lond.*, **53**:370–375.

Crick, R. P., Hoyle, C., and Smellie, H. (1961). The eyes in sarcoidosis. *Br. J. Ophthalmol.*, **45**:461–481.

Fong, K. F., and Israel, C. W. (1979). Conjunctival biopsy in the diagnosis of sarcoidosis. *South. Med. J.*, **72**:124–126.

Gorry, G. A., Pauker, S. G., Schwartz, W. B. (1978). The diagnostic importance of the normal finding. *N. Engl. J. Med.*, **298**:486–489.

James, D. G. (1979). Sarcoidosis. In *Cecils' Textbook of Medicine*. Edited by P. B. Beeson, W. McDermott, and J. B. Wyngaarden. Philadelphia, Saunders, pp. 209–216.

Levinsky, L., Cumminsky, J., Rømer, R. K., Wurm, K., Buss, J., Dorken, H., Steinbruck, P., Zaumseil, P., Jaroszewicz, W., Mandi, L., Szegedy, G., Centea, A., Burilkov, T., Blasi, A., Olivieri, D., Mariani, B., Bisetti, A., Goldman, S., Djuric, B., Lazarous, P., and Celokoglu, S. I. (1976). Sarcoidosis in Europe: A cooperative study. Proceedings of the VIIth International Conference on Sarcoidosis and Other Granulomatous Disorders. *Ann. N.Y. Acad. Sci.*, **278**:335–346.

Lofgren, S. (1964). Concepts of sarcoidosis. *Acta Med. Scand. (Suppl. 425)*, **176**:3–6.

McNeil, B. J., Keeler, E., Adelstein, S. J. (1975). Primer on certain elements of medical decision making. *N. Engl. J. Med.*, **293**:211–215.

Mitchell, D. N., and Scadding, J. G. (1974). Sarcoidosis. *Am. Rev. Respir. Dis.*, **110**:774–802.

Pauker, S. G., Kassirer, J. P. (1975). Therapeutic decision making: A cost-benefit analysis. *N. Engl. J. Med.*, **293**:229–234.

Pauker, S. G., and Kassirer, J. P. (1980). The threshold approach to clinical decision making. *N. Engl. J. Med.*, **302**:1109–1117.

Raiffa, H. (1968). *Decision Analysis*. Reading, Mass., Addison Wesley.

Ransohoff, D. F., and Feinstein, A. R. (1978). Problems of spectrum and bias in evaluating the efficacy of diagnostic tests. *N. Engl. J. Med.*, **299**:926–930.

Schwartz, W. B., Wolfe, H. J., and Pauker, S. G. (1981). Pathology and probabilities—a new approach to biopsy interpretation. *N. Engl. J. Med.*, **305**:917–923.

Shafer, G. (1976). *A Mathematical Theory of Evidence*. Princeton, N.J., Princeton University Press.

Tversky, A., and Kahneman, D. (1974). Judgment under uncertainty: Heuristics and biases. *Science*, **185**:1124–1131.

Weinstein, M. C., Fineberg, H. V. (1980). *Clinical Decision Analysis*. Philadelphia, W. B. Saunders.

Winterbauer, R. H., Belic, N., and Moores, K. D. (1973). A clinical
interpretation of bilateral hilar adenopathy. *Ann. Intern. Med.*,
78:65–71.

16

Treatment of Sarcoidosis

BARRY L. FANBURG

New England Medical Center Hospital
Tufts University School of Medicine
Boston, Massachusetts

I. General

As seen in the previous chapter on decision analysis, the consideration of
treatment of sarcoidosis should be preceded by a correct diagnosis of
sarcoidosis. Therapy may be counterproductive with an incorrect diagnosis.
Hence, a major effort must be directed toward establishing the diagnosis
before any consideration of therapy for the disease.

Once a diagnosis is established, options regarding therapy are limited
and include: (a) no therapy, assuming that sarcoidosis may be a "nil"
disease that has a high likelihood of spontaneous complete or incomplete
resolution without impairment of organ function, and (b) treatment with
corticosteroids, probably the most effective and least toxic of the known
therapies for the granulomatous component of the disease (Turiaf et al.
1976). Alternative forms of therapy exist, but there is no evidence for
increased efficacy compared to corticosteroids. The rationale for making
one of the above decisions usually rests as much on individual experience
as on critically derived data.

Studies concerning therapy for sarcoidosis are difficult to interpret
because the presentation and course of the disease are so variable. First,

the disease has a limited course in a large proportion of patients. Why this is so in some individuals and not in others is not known. Sarcoidosis is usually a generalized disease, although some manifestations may not be obvious. The probability of a spontaneous resolution is often recognized by the physician experienced with this disease. For example, the so-called stage 0 disease (the asymptomatic patient with bilateral symmetrical hilar lymphadenopathy seen on chest x-ray) is recognized to have a 70–80% probability of spontaneous resolution (Israel 1974). On the other hand, when there are chest x-ray findings compatible with fibrosis (e.g., honey-combing or retraction), there is virtually no likelihood of spontaneous resolution and perhaps little chance of more than partial resolution with corticosteroid therapy. Similarly, the incidence of spontaneous complete remission decreases with any evidence of overt pulmonary parenchymal disease (Siltzbach 1967). Any partial resolution with therapy probably is due to an effect on granulomas, since pulmonary parenchymal infiltrates will generally respond to corticosteroids (Johns et al. 1976) and fibrosis is irreversible. Pulmonary fibrosis in sarcoidosis has the added feature of at times being quite extensive and stable without causing functional impairment.

A second difficulty with a decision concerning therapy is that corticosteroid therapy for sarcoidosis is generally recognized not to be curative, even when there is an initial response to steroids (Hoyle et al. 1967, Johns et al. 1974). In one series of 152 patients treated with corticosteroids in which there was a high percentage of satisfactory clinical responses, 78% of the patients relapsed when therapy was stopped (Johns et al. 1974). A rational interpretation of this observation is that the stimulus for granuloma formation (whatever that may be) persists and the process is only temporarily abated with corticosteroid therapy. Therefore, in any decision regarding therapy, it must be kept in mind that the therapy is unlikely to be curative, but may be effective until spontaneous resolution occurs.

It might be inferred that therapy has little benefit for the patient who is going to have a limited course of sarcoidosis and a spontaneous resolution since this patient is not going to have any residue of the sarcoidosis process. In a controlled study of 37 patients with hilar lymphadenopathy, control and treated groups did not differ significantly either at the end of a 3-month period of treatment with steroids or at 5.2 years after completion of therapy (Israel et al. 1973). Hence, in this case the risks associated with several weeks to months of therapy probably outweigh the benefits, unless for some reason there is unusual discomfort such as that associated with arthritis or severe airway symptoms such as cough or wheezing (Mitchell and Scadding 1974).

A greater dilemma exists with patients who have prolonged manifesta-tions of sarcoidosis leading to severe functional impairment of various organs in some individuals and to minimal impairment in others. Unfortunately, at the time of the initial diagnosis, we may not be able to separate progressive disease from that which will spontaneously resolve or will have few sequelae. Perhaps methods that define "activity" of sarcoidosis, as discussed elsewhere in the book, will eventually be helpful in solving this problem. With progression of fibrosis and organ functional impairment, the life span may be decreased and the case fatality rate may be as high as 10% (Siltzbach 1967, Mayock et al. 1963, Fanburg and Nash 1974). Hence, we are faced with a decision regarding therapy with a medication that has potential side effects and a risk/benefit ratio that is only vaguely understood.

II. Therapy with Corticosteroids

Figure 1 shows a possible therapeutic approach to sarcoidosis. Sarcoidosis might be considered a potentially self-limited disease, not requiring treatment unless function of a vital organ is impaired. Examples of this situation are asymptomatic patients with bilateral symmetrical hilar

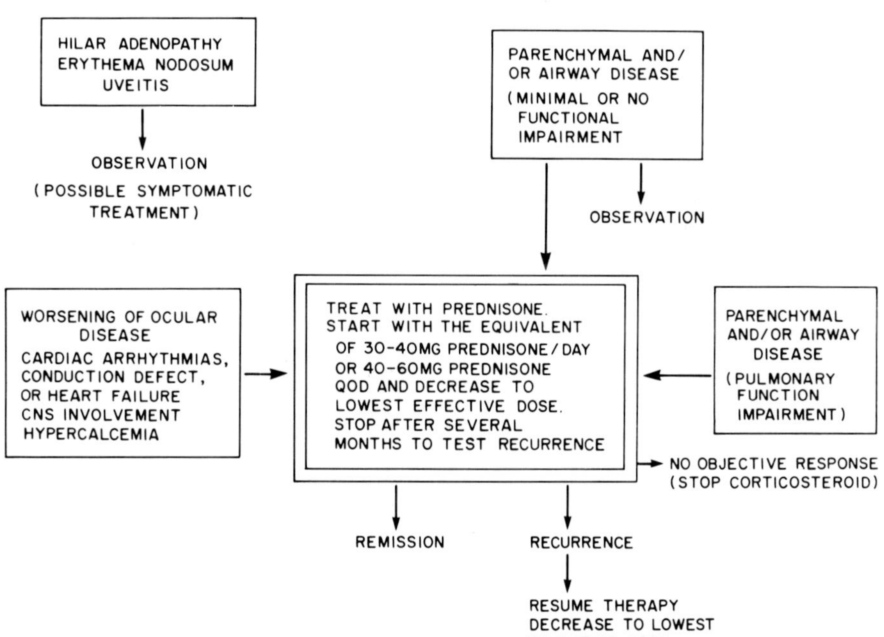

Figure 1   Therapeutic approaches to sarcoidosis.

lymphadenopathy and/or minimal interstitial pulmonary disease as evidenced only by chest x-ray. With our current state of knowledge and available therapy, this approach seems to be reasonable, assuming that the patient will be followed periodically until resolution or stability of the disease is assured.

Decisions regarding therapy for patients who have significant functional impairment of vital organs are at some times quite easy; at other times they are very difficult. Therapy (although recognized to have potential side effects) seems clearly justified in cases with cardiac, central nervous system, ocular, or significant pulmonary impairment or metabolic derangement (i.e., hypercalcemia) that may lead to organ impairment. A committee of the Medical Section of the National Tuberculosis and Respiratory Disease Association in 1971 described the following indications for therapy of sarcoidosis: (a) progressive pulmonary impairment or respiratory symptoms, (b) progressive impairment of visual acuity, (c) myocardial sarcoidosis with electrocardiographic evidence of conduction defects, (d) central nervous system sarcoidosis, (e) disfiguring cutaneous lesions, and (e) persistent hypercalcemia or hypercalciuria with renal insufficiency. In these cases, it is readily recognized that the potential benefit probably outweighs the risks associated with therapy (Friedman et al. 1976, Delaney 1977, Winnacher et al. 1968, Turner 1977, Maddrey 1970). Nevertheless, it should be kept in mind that even vital organ dysfunction may not be responsive to corticosteroids if the dysfunction is due to scarring.

A more difficult decision regarding therapy involves the patient in whom organ impairment is detected by pulmonary function testing. Here we may be faced with a large incidence of some functional impairment, perhaps artifactually thought to be discordant with other organ functional impairment, simply because attention has been directed toward the lung and other organs have not been sufficiently tested by sensitive methods to assure their absence of marginal impairment. Hence, we may not wish to start therapy, based only on moderate pulmonary functional impairment that might not be of any consequence. Because no clear data are available, this decision often becomes a judgmental one. Certainly, a case for institution of corticosteroids can usually be made when patients have pulmonary symptoms or show marked pulmonary functional impairment (Turief et al. 1976). Other parameters to be followed such as the cellularity of bronchial lavages, which is discussed in another section of this book, are currently being considered in the assessment of whether a patient should receive therapy. Here, too, more longitudinal data are needed to assess the likelihood of spontaneous resolution despite evidence of activity of disease by these other parameters.

Assuming we have made the decision to treat—and that decision currently means the use of a corticosteroid—we must select the dose and frequency of therapy. There does not appear to be a clear preference of the type of corticosteroid that would be superiorly suited for therapy, and doses and schedules have been derived from those known by experience to work. The most commonly used treatment is oral prednisone. One rational approach is to start with 30–40 mg of prednisone daily, a dose known to be usually effective (Johns et al. 1976). Some parameter or parameters should be selected for ascertaining effectiveness of this therapy, and once an improvement is achieved the dose should be tapered to the lowest effective dose. At times this can be as low as 5-10 mg of prednisone per day.

The parameter to determine effectiveness should be one that reflects activity of disease and is often not agreed upon. It could mean clinical improvement, functional improvement, chest x-ray clearing, the lowering of serum angiotensin 1-converting enzyme, changes in cellularity of bronchial lavages, or alterations in gallium scanning. Data regarding these various indications of activity of disease are discussed in other portions of the book. These parameters are not universally agreed upon as useful measurements of activity of disease. However, some parameter of disease should change with therapy to justify its continuation. Generally, if a response is going to occur, it will do so within several (perhaps 4-8) weeks. When there is no evidence of a response after several weeks, it seems logical to conclude that the disease has progressed to a fibrotic stage and to discontinue therapy so as to avoid the long-term side effects of corticosteroids (a high cost/benefit ratio). When steroids are effective and the dose is being tapered, it is worthwhile trying an alternate day schedule.

Some experience has been gained with the use of an alternate day schedule of corticosteroids from the start of therapy (MacGregor et al. 1969, Harter et al. 1963). Usually patients are begun at a somewhat higher dose of alternate day therapy, in the order of 40-60 mg of prednisone (Sheagren et al. 1973, Block and Light 1973). The apparent ineffectiveness of aerosolized steroid as a therapy for sarcoidosis is discussed in Chapter 3 by Dr. Henry Williams.

It should be emphasized that the decision regarding steroid therapy in sarcoidosis is usually predicated on the likelihood of the need for long-term therapy for several months to years. One should always attempt to achieve the lowest "effective" dose of steroid therapy. Tuberculosis is no longer a common complication in patients treated with corticosteroids (Israel 1974), probably because of more accurate initial diagnoses. Therefore, routine antituberculosis therapy in patients with sarcoidosis receiving corticosteroids appears unnecessary unless the tuberculin skin test is positive.

III. Alternatives to Steroid Therapy

A few medications other than corticosteroids, including chloroquine
(Siltzbach 1967, Morse et al. 1961, Brodthagen 1968, Siltzbach and
Teirstein 1964) and methotrexate (Lacher 1968, Israel 1970) are at least
partly effective in the treatment of sarcoidosis. Oxyphenbutazone (Sharma
1972), allopurinol (Rosof 1976), and levamisole (Rosenthal et al. 1976)
also have been proposed as treatments for sarcoidosis. Chloroquine and
methotrexate may be more effective against cutaneous than against
pulmonary sarcoidosis (Siltzbach 1967, Veirn 1977).

There is no substantive evidence that the above medications are
more effective than corticosteroids or might produce further improvement
beyond that gained with corticosteroids. As with corticosteroids, these
drugs are not curative. Because of the potential toxicity of chloroquine
and methotrexate (Siltzbach 1967, Veirn 1977, Hughes et al. 1971), they
should be withheld unless corticosteroids are contraindicated.

References

Block, A. J., and Light, R. W. (1973). Alternate day steroid therapy in
    diffuse pulmonary sarcoidosis. *Chest,* **63**:494–504.
Brodthagen, H. (1968). Chloroquine in pulmonary sarcoidosis. *Lancet,*
    1:1157.
Delaney, P. (1977). Neurologic manifestations in sarcoidosis: Review of the
    literature, with a report of 23 cases. *Ann. Intern. Med.,* **87**:336–345.
Fanburg, B. L., and Nash, G. (1974). Case records of the Massachusetts
    general hospital: Sarcoidosis with cor pulmonale. *N. Engl. J. Med.,*
    291:1402–1408.
Friedman, H. S., Parikh, N. H., Chander, N., and Calderon, J. (1976).
    Sarcoidosis with incomplete bilateral bundle branch block pattern
    disappearing following steroid therapy: An electrophysiological study.
    Eur. J. Cardiol., **4**:141–150.
Harter, J. G., Reddy, W. J., and Thorn, G. W. (1963). Studies on inter-
    mittent corticosteroid dosage regimen. *N. Engl. J. Med.,* **269**:591– 596.
Hughes, J. T., Esiri, M., Oxbury, J. M., and Whitty, C. W. M. (1971).
    Chloroquine myopathy. *Q.J. Med.,* **40**:85–93.
Hoyle, C., Smyllie, H., and Leak, D. (1967). Prolonged treatment of
    pulmonary sarcoidosis with corticosteroids. *Thorax,* **22**:519–524.
Israel, H. L. (1970). The treatment of sarcoidosis. *Postgrad. Med. J.,*
    46:537–540.
Israel, H. L. (1974). Observations on the diagnosis and treatment of
    sarcoidosis. *J. Maine Med. Assoc.,* **65**:59–61.

Israel, H. L., Fouts, D. W., and Beggs, R. A. (1973). A controlled trial of prednisone treatment of sarcoidosis. *Am. Rev. Respir. Dis.,* **107**: 609–614.

Johns, C. J., Zachary, J. B., and Ball, W. C., Jr. (1974). A ten-year study of corticosteroid treatment of pulmonary sarcoidosis. *Johns Hopkins Med. J.,* **134**:271–283.

Johns, C. J., Macgregor, M. I., Zachary, J. B., and Ball, W. C. (1976). Extended experience in the long-term corticosteroid treatment of pulmonary sarcoidosis. *Ann. N.Y. Acad. Sci.,* **278**:722–731.

Lacher, M. (1968). Spontaneous remission or response of sarcoidosis with methotrexate. *Ann. Intern. Med.,* **69**:1247–1248.

MacGregor, R. R., Sheagren, J. N., Lipsett, M. B., and Wolff, S. M. (1969). Alternate day prednisone therapy. Evaluation of delayed hypersensitivity response, control of disease and steroid side effects. *N. Engl. J. Med.,* **280**:1427–1431.

Maddrey, W. C., Johns, C. J., Biotnott, J. K., and Iber, F. L. (1970). Sarcoidosis and chronic liver disease: A clinical and pathologic study of 20 patients. *Medicine,* **49**:375–395.

Mayock, R. L., Bertrand, P., Morrison, C. E., and Scott, H. (1963). Manifestations of sarcoidosis: Analysis of 145 patients with a review of nine series selected from the literature. *Am. J. Med.,* **35**:67–89.

Mitchell, D. N., and Scadding, J. G. (1974). Sarcoidosis. *Am. Rev. Respir. Dis.,* **110**:774–802.

Morse, S. I., Cohn, Z. A., Hirsch, J. G., and Schaedler, R. W. (1961). The treatment of sarcoidosis with chloroquine. *Am. J. Med.,* **30**:779–784.

Rosenthal, M., Trabert, U., Müller, W., Müller, S., and Wurm, K. (1976). Levamisole in sarcoidosis (letter). *N. Engl. J. Med.,* **294**:112–113.

Rosof, B. M. (1976). Allopurinol for sarcoidosis? (letter). *N. Engl. J. Med.,* **294**:447.

Sharma, O. P. (1972). Treatment of sarcoidosis. *Am. Rev. Respir. Dis.,* **105**:855.

Sheagren, J. N., Simon, H. B., and Rich, R. R. (1973). Therapy of sarcoidosis initiated with alternate-day prednisone. *J. Natl. Med. Assoc.,* **65**:391–398.

Siltzbach, L. E. (1967). Sarcoidosis: Clinical features and management. *Med. Clin. North Am.,* **51**:483–502.

Siltzbach, L. E., and Teirstein, A. S. (1964). Chloroquine therapy in 43 patients with intrathoracic and cutaneous sarcoidosis. *Acta Med. Scand. (Suppl. 425),* **176**:302.

Turiaf, J., Johns, C. J., Teirstein, A. S., Tsuji, S., and Wurm, K. (1976). The problem of the treatment of sarcoidosis: Report of the subcommittee on therapy. *Ann. N.Y. Acad. Sci.,* **278**:743–751.

Turner, M. C. (1977). Renal failure as a presenting sign of diffuse
     sarcoidosis in an adolescent girl. *Am. J. Dis. Child.*, **131**:997–1000.
Veirn, N. K. (1977). Cutaneous sarcoidosis treated with methotrexate.
     Br. J. Dermatol., **97**:213–216.
Winnacher, J. L., Becker, K. L., and Katz, S. (1968). Endocrine aspects of
     sarcoidosis. *N. Engl. J. Med.*, **278**:427–434.

Part Seven

POSSIBLE ETIOLOGIC AGENTS

17

Studies of Transmissible Agents in Sarcoidosis

DONALD N. MITCHELL

Brompton Hospital
London, England

R. J. W. REES*

National Institute for Medical Research
London, England

I. Isolation of Transmissible Agents in Culture Directly from Patients with Sarcoidosis

No specific infectious agent has yet been isolated in culture from patients with sarcoidosis. Löfgren and Lundbäck (1950) reported the isolation of a virus belonging to the influenza-mumps-Newcastle disease group from four patients with erythema nodosum and bilateral hilar lymphadenopathy (Löfgren's syndrome) and from two patients with long-standing sarcoidosis. Although these were well-controlled experiments in which gastric lavage fluids and sarcoid tissues were inoculated into embryonated eggs by the allontoic and amniotic routes, they later concluded (Lundbäck and Löfgren 1952) that this virus must have been a laboratory contaminant since the results could not be repeated in a laboratory in which the mumps virus was not handled.

Later, Lundbäck and co-workers (1959) cultivated granulomatous lymph node tissues from 27 patients with sarcoidosis, and granulomatous skin lesions from three additional patients with sarcoidosis using the plasma clot technique. In cultures from all patients except one, characteristic patch degeneration of outgrown fibroblasts was observed, and in the

---

Present Affiliation
    *Clinical Research Centre, Harrow, Middlesex, England.

majority of the changed fibroblasts large eosinophilic cytoplasmic inclusions could be demonstrated. No changes of the kind observed in the cells of the sarcoid tissue cultures were found in cultures of lymph nodes from 10 patients with diseases other than sarcoidosis: The latter showed changes closely similar to those described by Grand (1944, 1949).

Homma and associates (1971) reported the isolation of unidentified mycoplasmas from throat swabs of five (29%) of 17 patients with sarcoidosis, but were able to isolate mycoplasmas from scalene node tissue in only 1 of 17 patients. Culture of lung and hilar lymph node tissue from two patients and from tissues obtained by liver biopsy from a further 5 patients were all negative for mycoplasma. All tissues examined showed epithelioid and giant cell granulomas.

Yansson and co-workers (1972) isolated an organism related to *Mycoplasma orale* type 1 from four of seven skin biopsy specimens and from each of two lymph nodes from patients with sarcoidosis, but it is relevant that Taylor-Robinson et al. (1964) isolated *M. orale* type 1 from 25% of healthy subjects. However, as a group the patients with sarcoidosis showed higher indirect hemagglutination titers against an isolated mycoplasma (strain 215-M) than did controls. Similarly, Uesaka and associates (1974) isolated nocardia-like organisms from the granulomatous scalene and mediastinal lymph node tissues of three patients with sarcoidosis.

The significance, if any, of all these findings in relation to the pathogenesis of sarcoidosis is doubtful. It is possible that these organisms found in sarcoid tissues are able to survive there because of altered immunity in sarcoidosis, although a defect of cell-mediated immunity as detected by cutaneous tests of delayed hypersensitivity do not appear to be prerequisite to the development of sarcoidosis. Moreover, the ability of patients with sarcoidosis to show enhanced humoral antibody responses is well recognized (Sands, Palmer and Maycock 1955, Hirshaut et al. 1970).

Steplewski and Israel (1976) examined 28 sarcoid lymph nodes, four sarcoid lung biopsies, three Kveim papules, and three sarcoid spleen preparations using cell fusion techniques which have been used successfully for the culture of oncogenic viruses (Knowles et al. 1968). Specimens were cultured directly into fresh Eagle's minimum essential medium (MEM) containing 20% fetal calf serum (FCS). Fibroblasts growing out from the cultured tissues were used for co-cultivation with human foreskin fibroblasts (HFF) and monkey Vero cells. No sarcoid lymphocytes or fibroblasts, fused or co-cultivated with HFF or Vero cells, showed the presence of a cytopathic effect (CPE), and supernatants from cocultivated or fused cells also failed to induce CPE on indicator cells. Electron microscopy was also negative for the presence of viral agents.

II. Inoculation of Experimental Animals

There have been numerous reports (Ravaut et al. 1929, Leigheb 1933, Pautrier and Glasser 1936, Grillo 1938, 1939, Santoianni 1938, Amati 1947, 1948, Croxatto 1948, Rosenthal 1949, Santoianni and Ayala 1949, Muratore and Vulpis 1952) in which sporadic and inconclusive attempts were made to transmit sarcoidosis directly to guinea pigs or hamsters: All these experiments were uncontrolled and usually based on single patients.

Mitchell and Rees (1969, 1970) reported the results of initial controlled experiments modelled on normal and immunologically deficient mice, the latter prepared by adolescent thymectomy and 900 rad of whole body irradiation. The hind footpads of these 12-week-old female CBA strain mice were used as the site for inoculation of 0.03 ml of homogenates. These methods were chosen because they have provided a means of reproducing human leprosy experimentally (Shepard 1960, Rees and Weddell 1968). In these and in subsequent controlled experiments (Mitchell and Rees 1974a, 1974b, Mitchell and Rees 1976, Mitchell et al. 1976, Mitchell and Rees 1980), fresh sarcoid lymph nodes were obtained by mediastinoscopy performed for diagnosis (Mikhail and Mitchell 1971); a spleen removed for hypersplenism was the source of fresh sarcoid splenic tissue. Each tissue showed characteristic microscopic changes.

As controls, lymph nodes were obtained from the groin at operation for ligation of varicose veins or during the course of vascular surgery in otherwise healthy individuals. Microscopically, each showed an essentially normal structure, although simple inflammatory changes were sometimes present. Splenic tissue was obtained as a control from a Kveim-negative patient with recurrent illness in whom splenectomy was undertaken for gross splenomegaly, but who showed no evidence of sarcoidosis. Normal CBA mouse footpad tissue served as an additional control.

Homogenates were prepared in an identical manner from each fresh unfrozen tissue in 1% bovine albumin in saline solution, yielding approximately a 13.5% suspension. All homogenates were injected into guinea pigs and cultured on Löwenstein-Jensen medium. No mycobacteria were detected. Homogenates were inoculated into the hind footpads, intraperitoneally (0.5 ml) or intravenously (0.5 ml); for intravenous injection homogenates were filtered to remove coarse particles and diluted (1:3 or 1:4) to avoid toxicity. For passage, homogenates were prepared in an identical manner from mouse footpad tissues showing epithelioid cell granulomas 12–20 months after the injection of human sarcoid homogenate and, as controls, from the footpad tissues of mice after a similar interval following the inoculation of control tissue homogenates. Fresh supernatants were obtained by centrifugation of whole fresh homogenates

(120 X *g* for 5 min), and filtrates were obtained by passing the fresh supernatants additionally through an 0.2 μm-membrane filter.

Full thickness biopsy specimens, initially of the same, and later of the contralateral footpad, were obtained 9–24 months or more after inoculation. Kveim tests were made in the ears of mice with lots 0025, 004, and 005 of a type 1 suspension (Commonwealth Serum Laboratories, designated CSL), usually between 9 and 18 months after inoculation of homogenates. A punch biopsy of the Kveim test sites was obtained 35–46 days after inoculation. The histology of the footpads, viscera, and Kveim test site was assessed according to the criteria conventionally accepted in humans: In a "positive" response the essential feature was the presence of one or more granulomas composed principally of epithelioid cells with occasional Langhans' type giant cells.

Closely similar results were obtained in normal and immunologically deficient mice. Microscopically, positive changes were present in a substantial proportion of the footpads of mice given whole fresh supernatant or supernatant filtrate (0.2 μm) of human sarcoid or mouse "sarcoid" passage tissue (first, second, third, fourth, and fifth passages) 9–20 months after inoculation into footpads, intraperitoneally or intravenously. Granulomas were also found in the viscera of these mice at each passage, including mice given a second or third passage of supernatant filtrate (0.2 μm) or a fourth or fifth passage of whole fresh mouse "sarcoid" tissue homogenate, and were present in lung, liver, spleen, lymph nodes, and muscle 12–20 months after inoculation. Kveim tests of mice ears were positive or equivocal in some of these mice 9–20 months after initial inoculation and after these same intervals after each passage, but were elicited only in mice showing granulomatous changes in footpads and/or viscera. The development of epithelioid and giant cell granulomas 9–24 months or more after inoculation of human sarcoid or mouse "sarcoid" passage tissue homogenates and the persistence of relatively fresh or progressively hyaline granulomas were striking features of these studies. In contrast, mice given human control tissue homogenates or passaged homogenates originating from control autoclaved (10 lb for 25 min), ^{60}Co-irradiated (2.5 megarad) human sarcoid or mouse "sarcoid" passage tissues or from the footpad homogenate did not show these changes.

An inflammatory cellular response was sometimes present in the footpads of mice inoculated into footpads with these control tissue homogenates and examined during the first 3 months following inoculation. This inflammatory cellular response, which was an early feature in these footpads, was no longer apparent in specimens from the contralateral footpad or in the previously unbiopsied footpads of mice given control tissue homogenates into footpads intraperitoneally or intravenously when examined 12–20 months after inoculation when all these mice had negative

Kveim test histology and showed no granulomatous changes in footpads
or viscera.

Mice given fresh sarcoid homogenate or fresh sarcoid homogenate after
storage at +4°C or −70°C for 1 week yielded slowly developing epithelioid
and giant cell granulomas and showed Kveim reactivity; in contrast, mice
inoculated with sarcoid homogenates that had been stored for 1 week at
−20°C had microscopically negative tissues and negative Kveim tests the
same length of time after inoculation. In controlled studies Taub and
Siltzbach (1974) confirmed that homogenates prepared from the granulomatous lymph nodes or spleens of patients with sarcoidosis are capable
of inducing epithelioid cell granulomas in the footpads of mice, but
granulomas were not transmitted by frozen (−25°C) or phenolized sarcoid
tissue homogenates. These authors found slowly evolving epithelioid cell
granulomas in the hind footpads of a proportion of normal CBA mice
1–8 months after their inoculation with homogenates prepared from fresh
sarcoid lymph node tissues. In several mice the epithelioid cell granulomas
present in the footpad more than 8 months after inoculation showed bony
invasion.

Iwai and Takahashi (1976), using scalene lymph nodes from sarcoidosis patients and control lymph nodes obtained at the time of
thoracotomy from the lung hilum, the mediastinum, or the thoracic wall
of patients with tuberculosis, bronchiectasis, or giant bullae, were unable
to confirm these findings. Homogenate of 30 sarcoid lymph nodes was
injected into the footpads of mice and 42% of the mice showed granulomatous changes similar to those in human sarcoid granulomas in their
footpad tissues. These changes occurred 3 months after inoculation and
persisted for more than 1 year without regression. However, the control
lymph node homogenates also showed similar granulomatous changes in
the footpad sites, although the positive rate was somewhat lower and the
granulomas appeared to be somewhat immature. Granuloma-inciting
activity remained after the sarcoid homogenate had been sterilized in
several different ways and it was present in sediments of centrifugation of
less than 2200 X *g*, but not in the supernate. These experiments suggested
that the inoculated homogenate persisted in the footpads and may act as
an antigenic stimulant provoking a local immunologic reaction and leading
to the formation of epithelioid cell granulomas.

Mitchell and co-workers (1976) and Mitchell and Rees (1980)
showed that a transmissible agent from human sarcoid tissue can be
passaged repeatedly. Up to five successful and sequential passages were
achieved following the inoculation of whole fresh tissue or of supernatant
(0.2 μm) filtrates of granulomatous mouse "sarcoid" tissue. The dilution
of any transmissible factor originally present in the human sarcoid tissue
homogenates and required to incite granuloma formation must by then

approach infinity. The passageable transmissible agent demonstrated in these experiments must approximate the size of a virus or be capable of being deformed (L forms) so as to pass an 0.2-μm membrane filter. This agent is inactivated when human or mouse passage tissue homogenates are autoclaved or ^{60}Co-irradiated (2.5 megarad). It is thus a replicating agent and may be viable.

Samples of serum from 29 mice inoculated with passage homogenates originating from each of seven sarcoidosis patients were tested against two different populations of human lymphocytes for the presence of cytotoxic antibody using the modified method of Teresaki (1964, 1970). The sera of 7 of 10 mice given a second passage and the sera of 10 of 19 mice given a third passage of "sarcoid" mouse tissue homogenate showed the presence of cytotoxins against both human lymphocyte populations. These findings are in keeping with recent reports of the incidence of naturally occurring lymphocytotoxic antibody in the serum of patients with sarcoidosis (Daniele and Rowlands 1976).

Although it cannot be assumed that all cases of sarcoidosis are associated with the same infective agent (Mitchell and Scadding 1974) it is relevant that acid-fast rods were present in the lungs of mice 17 months after the inoculation of a first passage of which fresh mouse "sarcoid" homogenate originating from the inoculation of whole fresh sarcoid homogenate into the footpads of normal CBA mice, some 3 yr previously. Similarly, acid-fast rods were present in the lungs and spleens of mice given a third passage of whole fresh mouse "sarcoid" homogenate originating from the intravenous inoculation of human sarcoid tissue from a second patient more than 5 yr previously. From a pooled homogenate of the granulomatous pulmonary tissue from mice given a second passage of homogenate and likewise originating from a third patient with sarcoidosis some 5 yr previously, a mycobacterium with the cultural characteristics of human mycobacterium tuberculosis was isolated. Acid-fast rods were present in the lungs and spleens of mice given a third or a fourth passage of homogenate originating from this second passage of pooled pulmonary tissue and again yielded positive cultures on Löwenstein-Jensen medium, irrespective of whether mice were inoculated with whole fresh homogenate at third or fourth passage or with supernatant of these homogenates that had been passed additionally through an 0.2-μm membrane filter. No mycobacteria had been detected or isolated from the fresh sarcoid tissue or homogenates from which any of these passages originated 3–8 yr previously.

These findings are consistent with the hypothesis of Burnet (1959) who suggested the possibility that in an individual with abnormally efficient production of humoral antibody and poor development of delayed hypersensitivity, a protoplast form of tubercle bacillus might persist as an intracellular parasite of mesenchymal cells, multiplying only sifficiently to keep more or less in pace with the cells that contain it. He also pointed out that a low-grade virus might behave like the hypothetical protoplast of this hypothesis.

The hypothesis advanced by Hanngren and co-workers (1974) is also relevant. They discussed ways in which viral and mycobacterial infections might interact in the pathogenesis of sarcoidosis, suggesting that the disturbance of the balance between T and B lymphocytes of the immune system, which is often found in sarcoidosis, might be due to the effects of viral infection in depressing T-cell function and of mycobacterial infection in stimulating B-cell function. Both genetic predisposition and exposure to infective agents or other factors may be involved in the causation of this immunologic abnormality, but their relative importance is unknown.

References

Amati, G. (1947). Ricerche sperimentali nella malattia di Besnier-Boeck-Schaumann. (Experimental research in Besnier-Boeck-Schaumann disease). *Boll. Soc. Ital. Biol. Sper.*, **23**:377–379.

Amati, G. (1948). Esperienze bioloche sulla malattia di Besnier-Boeck-Schaumann. Risultati batteriologici ed istologici nella prova intra-ganglionare secondo Ninni. (Biological and histological results with Ninni's intraganglionic test). *Rev. Ist. Sieroter Hol.*, **23**:229–246.

Burnet, F. M. (1959). In *The Clonal Selection Theory of Acquired Immunity.* Cambridge University Press, p. 160.

Croxatto, O. C. (1948). Similtudes entre la sarcoidosis y la tuberculosis experimental en el 'Cricetus Auratus' (hamster). (Similarities between sarcoidosis and experimental tuberculoses in the hamster, *Cricetus auratus.*) *Arch. Soc. Argent. Anat.*, **10**:247–252.

Daniele, R. P., and Rowlands, D. T. (1976). Antibodies to T cells in sarcoidosis. *Ann. N.Y. Acad. Sci.*, **278**:88–100.

Grand, C. G. (1944). Tissue culture studies of cytoplasmic inclusion bodies in lymph nodes of Hodgkin's disease. *Proc. Soc. Exp. Biol.*, **56**:229–230.

Grand, C. G. (1949). Cytoplasmic inclusions and the characteristics of Hodgkin's diseased lymph nodes in tissue culture. *Cancer Res.*, **9**:183–192.

Grillo, V. (1938). Contributo alla malattia di Besnier-Boeck: Una fase sarcoidea della infezione tubercolare? (Contribution to Besnier-Boeck disease: Sarcoid phase of infectious tuberculosis?) *G. Ital. Dermatol. Sif.*, **79**:547–569.

Grillo, V. (1939). Riproduzione delle lesioni istologiche della malattia di Besnier-Boeck-Schaumann in gangli linfatici di cavie inoculate in peritoneo con spappolato di tessuto 'sarcoideo.' (Production of histologic lesions of Besnier-Boeck-Schaumann disease in lymph nodes of guinea pigs after intraperitoneal inoculation with broth from 'sarcoid' tissue.) *Arch. Ital. Med. Sper.,* **4**:515–522.

Hanngren, Å., Biberfeldt, G., Carlens, E., Hedfors, E., Nilsson, B. S., Ripe, E., and Wahren, B. (1974). Is sarcoidosis due to an infectious interaction between virus and mycobacterium? In *Proceedings of the VI International Conference on Sarcoidosis,* Tokyo, September 11–15, 1972. Edited by K. Iwai and Y. Hosoda. Tokyo, University of Tokyo Press, pp. 8–11.

Hirshaut, Y., Glade, P., Vieira, L. O. B. A., Ainbender, E., Dvorak, B., and Siltzbach, L. E. (1970). Sarcoidosis, another disease associated with serologic evidence for herpes-like virus infection. *N. Engl. J. Med.,* **283**:502–506.

Homma, H., Okano, H., and Motchuzuki, H. (1971). An attempt to isolate mycoplasmas from patients with sarcoidosis. In *Fifth International Conference on Sarcoidosis,* Prague, June 16–21, 1969. Edited by L. Levinsky and F. Macholda. Prague, Universita Karlova, p. 101.

Iwai, K., and Takahashi, S. (1976). Transmissibility of sarcoid-specific granulomas in the footpads of mice. *Ann. N.Y. Acad. Sci.,* **278**: 249–259.

Knowles, B. B., Jensen, F. C., Steplewski, Z., and Koprowski, H. (1968). Rescue of infectious SV40 after fusion between different SV40 transformed cells. *Proc. Latl. Acad. Sci. U.S.A.,* **61**:42–45.

Leigheb, V. (1933). Ricerche sperimentali sul problema istologico delle tuberculidi (nota prima). (Experimental research on histologic problem of tuberculid: First note.) *G. Ital. Dermatol. Sif.,* **74**: 633–667.

Löfgren, S., and Lundbäck, H. (1950). Isolation of a virus from six cases of sarcoidosis. *Acta Med. Scand.,* **138**:71–75.

Lundbäck, H., and Löfgren, S. (1952). Attempts at isolation of virus strains from cases of sarcoidosis and malignant lymphoma. *Acta Med. Scand.,* **143**:98–109.

Lundbäck, H., Löfgren, S., and Nordenstam, H. (1959). Cultivation of sarcoidotic tissue from lymph nodes and skin. *Br. J. Exp. Pathol.,* **40**:61–65.

Mikhail, J. R., and Mitchell, D. N. (1971). Mediastinoscopy: A diagnostic procedure in hilar and paratracheal lymphadenopathy. *Postgrad. Med. J.,* **47**:698–704.

Mitchell, D. N., and Rees, R. J. W. (1969). A transmissible agent from sarcoid tissue. *Lancet,* **2**:81–84.

Mitchell, D. N., and Rees, R. J. W. (1970). An attempt to demonstrate a transmissible agent from sarcoid material. *Postgrad. Med. J.,* **46**:510–514.

Mitchell, D. N., and Rees, R. J. W. (1974a). The production of granulomas in mice by sarcoid tissue suspensions. In *Proceedings of the VI International Conference on Sarcoidosis,* Tokyo, September 11–15, 1972. Edited by K. Iwai and Y. Hosoda. Tokyo, University of Tokyo Press, pp. 12–19.

Mitchell, D. N., and Rees, R. J. W. (1974b). On the aetiology. In *Proceedings of the VI International Conference on Sarcoidosis,* Tokyo, September 11–15, 1972. Edited by K. Iwai and Y. Hosoda. Tokyo, University of Tokyo Press, pp. 634–635.

Mitchell, D. N., and Rees, R. J. W. (1976). The nature and physical characteristics of a transmissible agent from human sarcoid tissue. *Ann. N.Y. Acad. Sci.,* **278**:88–100.

Mitchell, D. N., and Rees, R. J. W. (1980). Further observations on the nature and physical characteristics of transmissible agents from human sarcoid and Crohn's disease tissues. In *Eighth International Conference on Sarcoidosis and Other Granulomatous Diseases,* Cardiff, 1978. Edited by W. J. Williams and B. H. Davies. Cardiff, Alpha Omega, pp. 121–132.

Mitchell, D. N., and Scadding, J. G. (1974). Sarcoidosis. *Am. Rev. Respir. Dis.,* **110**:774–802.

Mitchell, D. N., Rees, R. J. W., and Goswami, K. K. A. (1976). Transmissible agents from human sarcoid and Crohn's disease tissues. *Lancet,* **2**:761–765.

Muratore, R., and Vulpis, N. (1952). Modificazioni prodotte neele cavie dalla iniezione di liquido preparato da materiale sarcoidosico secondo la technica di Lofgren e Lundback. I. Ricerche anatomoistologiche. (Modifications produced in guinea pigs by injection of fluids prepared from sarcoidosis materials, according to the technique of Löfgren and Lundbäck. I. Anatomical and histological research.) *Boll. Soc. Ital. Biol. Sper.,* **28**:169–172.

Pautrier, L. M., and Glasser, R. (1936). Inoculation positive probable au lapin au point d'inoculation, de lesions cutanées de maladie de Besnier-Boeck-Schaumann. (Probable positive inoculation in a rabbit, at inoculation site of skin lesions from Besnier-Boeck-Schaumann disease.) *Bull. Soc. Franc. Dermatol. Syph.,* **43**:505–506.

Ravaut, P., Valtis, J., and Nellis, P. (1929). Resultats de l'inoculation au cobaye d'un sarcoide et d'une tuberculide papulo-necrotique. (Results of inoculation of sarcoid and papulonecrotic tuberculid in the guinea pig.) *C. R. Soc. Biol. (Paris),* **101**:444–445.

Rees, R. J. W., and Weddell, A. G. M. (1968). Experimental models for studying leprosy. *Ann. N.Y. Acad. Sci.,* **154**:214–236.

Rosenthal, S. R. (1949). Pathological and experimental studies of Boeck's
    sarcoid. 1. Report of a case with panarteritis, periarteritis, terminal
    hypertension and uremia, and the reproduction of a sarcoid-like
    lesion in guinea pigs. *Am. Rev. Tuberc.*, **60**:236–248.
Sands, J. H., Palmer, P. P., Maycock, R. L., and Creger, W. P. (1955).
    Evidence for serologic hyperactivity in sarcoidosis. *Am. J. Med.*,
    19:401–409.
Santoianni, G. (1938). La malattia di Besnier-Boeck-Schaumann (trasmissione
    sperimentale negli animali). (Besnier-Boeck-Schaumann disease:
    Experimental transmission in animals.) *Arch. Ital. Dermatol. Sif.,***15**:78–90.
Santoianni, G., and Ayala, L. (1949). Ricerche sperimentali sulla etiologia
    della malattia di Besnier-Boeck-Schaumann. Risultati della prova
    biologica negli animali. (Experimental studies on the etiology of
    Besnier-Boeck-Schaumann disease. Results of the biologic test in
    animals.) *Ann. Ital. Dermatol. Sif.*, **4**:9–16.
Shepard, C. C. (1960). Acid-fast bacilli in nasal secretions in leprosy, and
    results of inoculation of mice. *Amer. J. Hyg.*, **71**:147–157.
Steplewski, Z., and Israel, H. L. (1976). The search for viruses in
    sarcoidosis. *Ann. N.Y. Acad. Sci.*, **278**:260–264.
Taub, R. N., and Siltzbach, L. E. (1974). Induction of granulomas in
    mice by injection of human sarcoid and ileitis homogenates. In
    Proceedings of the VI International Conference on Sarcoidosis.
    Tokyo, September 11–15, 1972. Edited by K. Iwai and Y. Hosoda.
    Tokyo, University of Tokyo Press, pp. 20–21.
Taylor-Robinson, D., Canchola, J., Fox, H., and R. M. Chanock (1964).
    A newly identified oral mycoplasma (*M. orale*) and its relationship
    to other human mycoplasmas. *Am. J. Hyg.*, **80**:135–148.
Teresaki, P. I. (1970). In *Histocompatibility Testing.* Edited by P. I.
    Terasaki. Munschgaard, p. 301.
Teresaki, P. I., and McClelland, J. D. (1964). Microdroplet assay of human
    serum cytotoxins. *Nature,* **204**:998–1000.
Uesaka, I., Izumi, T., and Tsuji, S. (1974). Nocardia-like organisms
    isolated from lesions of sarcoidosis. In *Proceedings of the VI
    International Conference on Sarcoidosis,* Tokyo, September 11–15,
    1972. Edited by K. Iwai and Y. Hosoda. Tokyo, University of
    Tokyo Press, p. 3.
Yansson, E., Hannuksela, M., Eklung, H., Halme, H., and Tuari, S. (1972).
    Isolation of a mycoplasma from sarcoid tissue. *J. Clin. Pathol.,* **25**:837–842.

Part Eight

EXPERIMENTAL MODELS

18

Experimental Granulomatous Disease

DOV L. BOROS

Wayne State University School of Medicine
Detroit, Michigan

I. Introduction

The granuloma is a chronic, complex inflammatory reaction which may be
formed in response to persistent irritants/agents that impinge on the tissues.
The agents are surrounded and, if possible, ingested by the inflammatory
cells, and their slow degradability is the major factor in the chronicity of
the inflammatory response (Epstein 1967, Spector 1969, Adams 1976,
James and Neville 1977, Boros 1978). The spectrum of irritants is large
and includes live, replicating intracellular invaders (bacteria, fungi, protozoa),
metazoans (larvae and ova of worms), inanimate chemical compounds,
metals (silica, beryllium) and autogenous cell (sperm cells).

Based on the nature of the inducer agent, granulomatous inflammations
are broadly classified into nonimmunologic, foreign body, and immunological,
hypersensitivity reactions. With some exceptions, granulomatous inflammations evoked by foreign bodies (metal salts, surgical sutures, sponges,
plastic beads, etc.) have a simple cellular composition, are less intense,

This research was supported by USPHS grants AI 12913, HL 19732,
and HL 20104.

have a shorter duration, and are accompanied by less tissue damage than their immunologic counterparts. The immune granulomas are induced by the prolonged antigenic stimulus of slowly degradable substances which results in the induction of the state of delayed hypersensitivity in the host. Such lesions have a complex histology, may last for a long time, show an intense inflammatory reaction with tissue damage, and resolve by fibrous repair which often contributes to the pathology of the disease.

Many major diseases of mankind such as tuberculosis, leprosy, syphilis, and schistosomiasis are characterized by granulomatous tissue inflammations. Whereas these diseases are caused by well-defined etiologic agents (bacilli, spirochetes, schistosome eggs), in other clinically important diseases, including sarcoidosis, Crohn's disease, Wegener's granulomatosis, and primary biliary cirrhosis, no causative agent(s) have been identified.

The foreign body type lesions are composed predominantly of macrophages and their derivatives, and of fibroblasts. In contrast, the hypersensitivity lesions are more complex and consist of lymphocytes, macrophages and their derivatives (the epithelioid and giant cells), and at times eosinophils, mast cells, and fibroblasts. Analysis of the cellular composition of the hypersensitivity lesions has shown the presence of T lymphocytes. Recently, B lymphocytes and plasma cells have been located within the sarcoid, hypersensitivity pneumonitis, schistosome egg-induced, and lepromatous leprosy type granulomas (Tannenbaum et al. 1976, Salvaggio et al. 1975, Chensue and Boros 1979a, Ridley et al. 1978). The presumed intralesional production of antibodies may have an important bearing on the pathology of the disease. Antibodies may neutralize excess antigen or create complexes which could exacerbate or modulate the inflammatory response.

Sequential analysis of the cellular components of these lesions also demonstrates the dynamic nature of the host response. The rate of influx, local multiplication, and death of the cells are most probably governed by the inflammatory signals that prevail within the lesions. In the hypersensitivity lesions such signals are likely to originate from the T lympho-cytes and are mediated by inflammatory lymphokines. In the nonimmune granulomas the low cellular turnover may be influenced by inflammatory signals derived from serum components (complement, kinin) and chemical mediators (vasoactive amines, prostaglandins).

Granuloma macrophages derive from blood monocytes which immigrate into the lesions and undergo local maturation and differentiation. Epithelioid cells are such mature cells which assume complex morphological and functional changes resulting in the loss of phagocytic ability (Spector 1974). Traditionally, pathologists have considered the presence of epithelioid cells as a diagnostic sign for the identity of the hypersensitivity type granulomas. However, recent observations indicate that epithelioid cells also appear in response to foreign bodies evoked by implanted plastic sheets (van der Rhee et al. 1979) and ingested muramyl dipeptide (Tanaka and Emori 1980). The role of such cells within the lesions is still unclear. Their unique ability of membrane interdigitation creates a solid sheet of cells around the core of the lesion and thus may help to wall off the irritant. The layers of cells could prevent the leakage of antigen or potentially noxious substances to the neighboring tissue. Being highly secretory, the cells may also participate in the extracellular, enzymatic degradation of the irritants. Under certain circumstances, usually young and more mature macrophages fuse and generate the giant cells (recently termed the macrophage polykaria) (Papadimitriou and Walters 1979). Fusion occurs in both the foreign body and hypersensitivity lesions. In the latter, lymphokines have been shown to mediate the reaction (Parks and Weiser 1975). The role of these poorly phagocytic cells within the lesions is unknown.

The protective role of the granulomatous response against a variety of injurious agents has been established without doubt. The cells of the granuloma sequester, wall off, kill, and degrade the offenders. The indispensable role of the granulomatous response is strongly emphasized in clinical situations where feeble or inefficient granuloma formation allows the rapid multiplication and dissemination of intracellular invaders. This is seen in cases of miliary tuberculosis, disseminated histoplasmosis, leishmaniasis, and lepromatous leprosy.

Efficient mobilization and activation of the macrophages within the hypersensitivity lesions is carried out by antigen-stimulated T lymphocytes which secrete various soluble mediators, the lymphokines. Lymphokine activity has been defined mostly in vitro using peritoneal or alveolar macrophages. The various effects include chemotaxis, inhibition of migration, cellular aggregation, cellular multiplication, and activation. The available evidence allows us to believe that similar effects take place also in vivo, the end result being the recruitment, activation, efficient killing, and removal of the replicating invaders and the resolution of the infection (Boros 1981).

The protective role of the granulomas in silicosis or berylliosis is less evident because these inanimate materials do not disseminate or pose life-threatening infections. Their containment, often with detrimental consequences, may be the result of the stereotyped responses of the host to chronic irritation.

Regardless of the nature of the irritant, once the macrophages undergo activation, they have an elevated content of various hydrolytic enzymes needed for the degradation of the ingested material. Such enzymes, released from the cells along with oxygen breakdown products, can cause considerable tissue destruction. Tissue damage, in turn, triggers the activity of fibroblasts which participate in reparative fibrosis, the final phase of the granulomatous response. The mechanisms that activate fibroblasts, regulate collagen synthesis, and influence remodeling of the fibrous tissue are the least understood facets of the granulomatous inflammatory response. Conceivably, these various activities proceed in stages that comprise fibroblast chemotaxis, proliferation, collagen production and resorption, and, finally, fibrosis. In vitro observations indicate that fibroblasts react to signals originating from both macrophages and lymphocytes. The cells once triggered undergo chemotaxis, cellular proliferation, and, in the minority of cases, enhanced collagen synthesis. The first steps toward the understanding of the fibrous process in the granulomas have been taken. A full understanding of fibrogenesis and irreversible fibrosis, which often aggravate the pathology of the disease, will greatly improve the handling of chronic inflammatory reactions.

Since there is no currently recognized animal model of spontaneous sarcoidosis, studies of granulomatous disease in the experimental animal require the establishment of granulomas produced by several agents known to cause such lesions. These experimental granulomas will be discussed in this chapter. Whether any of these truly represent the lesions of sarcoidosis remains to be established.

II. Mycobacterium-Induced Granulomas

Over the past decades, numerous animal species were used for the study of experimental tuberculosis. As expected, considerable variations were observed in susceptibility to tubercle bacilli, as well as in the histopathology that develop in the various species. Whereas rabbits and guinea pigs, which are sensitive to the bacilli, develop histopathology similar to humans, rats and mice are fairly resistant to infection and do not develop caseating tubercles (Dannenberg 1980). Important factors, sometimes overlooked, are the virulence of the strain and its viable or killed form used in the experiments. Curiously, research in the past focused more on the histopathology of the tubercle than on the antibacterial function of the granuloma.

The two major questions that researchers asked were the cellular origin of the granuloma macrophage and the complex maturation/differentiation that the cells undergo within the lesions. By radiolabeling and autoradiography, most of the macrophages of the tubercle bacilli-induced granulomas were shown to originate from circulating blood monocytes (Spector 1969, 1974). However, at the incipient stage, a small undetermined number of resident tissue macrophages (Kupffer cells, alveolar macrophages) may also contribute to the lesions (Adams 1976). During an acute or chronic inflammatory reaction, macrophages recapitulate in an accelerated manner the events of the normal steady state (van Furth 1976). Thus, precursor monoblasts and promonocytes are produced in the bone marrow and, as monocytes, leave the marrow and enter the circulation. Subsequently, some monocytes leave the circulation and mature into macrophages in the tissues.

Sequential histological studies of the BCG-induced dermal granulomas show infiltration of blood monocytes, some neutrophils, and lymphocytes within the first few days of the injection of the bacilli. By day 5 aggregates of immature macrophages are seen. In the ensuing 2 weeks macrophages mature further, develop large oval eccentric nuclei, and arrange themselves into sheets. By the third week, the organization of the granuloma is evident, and immature epithelioid and numerous giant cells appear. The classic arrangement of the granuloma with a halo of lymphocytes surrounding nests of interdigitating mature epithelioid cells is developed only 4 weeks after the initiation of the lesion (Adams 1974).

If killed, virulent *Mycobacterium tuberculosis* bacilli are injected into guinea pigs, instead of viable attenuated BCG (bacille Calmette-Guérin), the sequence of macrophage maturation/differentiation is greatly accelerated. As early as 3 days after the initial injection, macrophages are arranged into granulomas, and by day 9 a fully matured granulomatous reaction develops. The lesions begin to resolve between days 11–15, at which time the number of detectable bacilli within the granulomas drops significantly. An intriguing feature of these lesions is the reversion of the differentiation of epithelioid cells. They revert first to the morphology of the mature macrophage and finally into immature macrophages. These observations indicate that at least some of the macrophages within such lesions can dedifferentiate and perhaps leave the lesions, thereby accelerating the resolution of the response (Adams 1975).

The origin and turnover of the component cells has been examined in BCG-induced dermal granulomas. Cell traffic is traced by labeling bone marrow cells with tritiated thymidine, and radiolabeled cells in tissue sections are identified by autoradiography. By this method, mononuclear cells are identified without resolving them into macrophages and lymphocytes. In the subcutaneous granulomas of rats induced by emulsified complete adjuvant, the inflammatory cells originate from the blood (Spector 1969). The daily influx of fresh blood monocytes into the granulomas is about 1% of the total population of the lesion (Spector et al. 1967). When the supply of bone marrow precursor cells is cut off by x-irradiation, no significant granulomatous inflammation develops (Ryan and Spector 1970). The rapid decline in the number of labeled mononuclear cells within the lesions is mainly due to local proliferation and cell death. Thus, the adjuvant-induced granuloma is maintained by recruitment of fresh blood monocytes and local cellular multiplication. A similar kinetic pattern was observed also in intradermal granulomas induced by dead pertussis organisms and, thus, seems to be characteristic of the so-called high turnover granulomata (Spector and Ryan 1970).

It has been demonstrated in rabbits injected with live BCG organisms that the rapid cellular turnover is maintained by the cell-mediated immune response of the infected animals. In this model the radiolabeling of precursor cells is complemented by histochemical staining (specific for the lysosomal enzyme β galactosidase) which identifies macrophages among the labeled mononuclear cells. Sequential biopsies of dermal lesions show that blood-borne mononuclear cells, with low enzyme content, enter the lesion in an immature form. Within the granulomas the monocytes divide once or twice, enlarge, and eventually assume the morphology of the epithelioid cells. Such cells are rich in intracellular organelles and lysosomal enzyme content.

The rapid rate of entry, local multiplication, and death (or disappearance) of radiolabeled macrophages correlates well with the development of delayed tuberculin skin sensitivity in the animals, and peaks when the lesions attain maximum size (14 days). Concurrently, the macrophages acquire a high β galactosidase content, indicative of their state of activation. The demonstration of an acceleration of these events in lesions of previously sensitized animals further confirms the cellular immune nature of these lesions (Ando et al. 1972, Dannenberg et al. 1972).

The protective function of the granulomas has been elegantly proven by the correlation between the high rate of cellular turnover and the bactericidal effect of the activated macrophages. Dermal lesions, initiated by the injection of radiolabeled BCG organisms, show the disappearance of bacilli in concert with the development of cellular immunity. In the 3–7-day-old lesions, the percentage of macrophages that contain bacilli is high. With the onset of tuberculin hypersensitivity both the number of bacilli-laden activated macrophages and the bacillary load per cell diminish considerably (Ando et al. 1977). Apparently, the immature, less activated macrophages possess a lower bactericidal potency than those that undergo a presumed lymphokine-mediated activation process.

This point has been illustrated also in BCG-infected adult mice that were rendered immunodeficient by thymectomy and irradiation. Whereas control mice showed normal tuberculin hypersensitivity, but no mortality from the intravenously injected bacilli, the deficient, bone-marrow-reconstituted animals failed to develop tuberculin hypersensitivity, had persistent lung granulomas containing a diffuse collection of many foamy macrophages and plasma cells, and eventually succumbed to a progressive fatal infection (Collins et al. 1975). Essentially similar results have been observed using BCG-infected congenitally athymic nude mice. These mice did not develop tuberculin hypersensitivity and did not mount an effective granulomatous response, though their macrophages are packed with acid-fast bacilli (Ueda et al. 1976).

It is emphasized throughout this review that granulomas exist due to the persistence of the inciting agents. In the case of the mycobacterium-induced granulomas, successful killing/degradation of the bacilli apparently diminishes the antigenic stimulus. This causes the turnover of cells to change from a high to a low level. In the aging (4–9-week-old) BCG granulomas, cell division, activation, and death are considerably diminished, apparently due to the cessation of antigenic stimulus and the waning hypersensitivity response (Ando et al. 1972). The rapid cellular turnover of the mycobacterium-induced granulomas is usually accompanied by cellular death and is manifested by the appearance of a necrotic caseous center within the lesions.

Caseation may occur in the lung lesions as early as 6 days after the injection of the bacilli (Shima et al. 1972). Caseation may proceed to liquefaction, destruction of whole lung segments, as well as promotion of the systemic dissemination of tubercle bacilli (Myrvik et al. 1975, Dannenberg 1980). Some researchers consider cavity formation to result from a particularly intense hypersensitivity response. Experimentally, cavity formation was prevented by immunosuppressive drugs and desensitization with tuberculopeptides (Yamamura et al. 1968, 1974). The exact cause of caseation is still uncertain; it may be due to released hydrolytic and degradative enzymes and/or oxygen breakdown products which attack the cells and cause their autolytic degradation. The source of these enzymes is the activated macrophage which possesses a battery of proteases, esterases, lipases, nucleases, etc., needed for the breakdown of endocytosed material (Tsuda et al. 1974). Macrophages may increase their intracellular enzyme content as a consequence of T-cell-mediated activation or ingestion of tissue debris.

Certain macrophages with specialized tasks situated within various locations in the lesion have been shown to contain different enzymes. Whereas the β-galactosidase-positive macrophages and epithelioid cells are associated with destruction of tubercle bacilli, macrophages that surround the border of the necrotic center contain cathepsin D, a proteolytic enzyme presumed to participate in the digestion or liquefaction of the caseous debris (Rojas-Espinosa et al. 1974). Double staining techniques that identify two separate enzymes within the same macrophage reveal the highest enzyme content at the peak of the granulomatous response.

The pattern of intracellular enzyme content differs from cell to cell. While certain macrophages have esterase–β galactosidase enzyme pairs, others contain acid phosphatase–cathepsin D enzymes. Hence the enzyme content and the secretory-digestive capacity of macrophages may be under a dual control, and certain specialized functions may be carried out by various subpopulations of macrophages within the lesions (Suga et al. 1980). The actual release of enzymes from dermal granulomas of rabbits has also been demonstrated with plastic collection chambers. The secretion of collagenase, DNase, RNase, lysozyme, and lactic dehydrogenase (released only after cell death) was maximal when the lesions reached peak size and the animals displayed strong tuberculin hypersensitivity. These results confirm the role of T-cell-mediated immunity in the activation of the granuloma cells and indicate that during strong reactions released enzymes may cause liquefaction/destruction of the underlying tissue and cavity formation (Sugimoto et al. 1978a). Vigorous cortisone treatment of BCG-injected rabbits reduced granuloma sizes, caseous necrosis, and ulceration of dermal lesions (McCue et al. 1978).

BCG organisms, both killed and alive, have also been used to induce granulomatous pulmonary alveolitis. In this model rabbits are injected intravenously with 100–200 μg of killed BCG organisms in mineral oil. In 2–4 weeks animals develop chronic alveolitis composed of macrophages and loosely organized granulomas in the interstitium. In the absence of further challenge, the lesions regress without developing necrosis (Myrvik et al. 1962, Leake and Myrvik 1968). This inflammatory reaction is the result of locally induced, specific cell-mediated response. Rabbits sensitized by this route do not develop dermal tuberculin reactivity, but their antigen-stimulated bronchoalveolar lymphocytes produce migration inhibition factor (MIF) (Galindo and Myrvik 1970). These lymphocytes also produce a macrophage fusion factor, that may mediate giant cell formation (Galindo et al. 1974) and a factor that causes macrophage aggregation (Galindo et al. 1975). The alveolitis reaction is specific for BCG, because a challenge injection of Corynebacteria failed to elicit an accelerated exudative response (Moore et al. 1973). Though the response lacks the compact palisaded histology of granulomas, the alveolar macrophages obtained by bronchial lavage are activated as shown by enhanced hexose monophosphate shunt activity and strong, nonspecific bacteriostatic action against ingested Listeria organisms (Myrvik 1972).

The inflammatory response peaks at 3 weeks after the injection of the bacilli. Homogenates of the heavily inflammed lungs obtained at that time have enhanced acid and neutral protease activity, and alveolar macrophages also contain elevated protease content (McGee and Myrvik 1976). The exudative alveolitis is not suppressible by antiserum prepared against alveolar macrophages (Moore and Myrvik 1970). However, cortisone treatment of rabbits suppresses both the pulmonary inflammation and MIF production by lymphocytes (Moore and Myrvik 1973).

Although it has been emphasized that macrophages die at an accelerated rate, at the height of the cell-mediated granulomatous response, the exact cause of cell death is still unknown. Apparently, activated alveolar macrophages in BCG-injected lungs are more susceptible to phagocytosis-induced cell death than are their normal counterparts. Alveolar macrophages show an enhanced rate of cell death, having ingested in vitro BCG organisms, insolubilized tuberculoprotein, or zymosan. Cellular mortality may be partially prevented by catalase and ascorbic acid. These agents neutralize peroxides and free radicals liberated by lymphokine-activated macrophages during the bactericidal activity of the cell (Johnston et al. 1978). Thus, in addition to degradative enzymes, peroxides and other oxygen breakdown products may also contribute to cell death and tissue necrosis (McGee and Myrvik 1979).

Recent experiments strongly indicate that the granulomatous inflammatory response in the mouse is under genetic control. Strains of mice injected with killed BCG in oil may be classified as high or low responders by measuring total lung inflammation (increase in lung weight) rather than lesion size. In high responders the lung interstitium is thick and contains infiltrated macrophages and lymphocytes, and the consolidated lung contains numerous granulomas. Low responders have moderate lung infiltration without granuloma formation. An analysis of the response in congenic strains does not show that genes within the major histocompatibility complex are involved in the control of the inflammation (Allen et al. 1977). Another study, using emulsified BCG cell wall preparations rather than whole organisms, confirmed these data. Backcross studies between hybrid and parental strains of mice indicate that, although responsiveness to cell wall components is under genetic control, multiple loci rather than a single locus are involved, and the role of the major histocompatibility complex in this regulation may be only marginal (Yamamoto and Kakinuma 1978).

Though the experimental, mycobacterium-induced granulomas do not closely approximate the course of human infections, they provide valuable information on the cell-mediated nature, dynamics, and protective/destructive functions of these complex tissue reactions.

III. The Schistosome Egg Granuloma

Schistosomiasis mansoni is a chronic granulomatous disease of the tropics caused by trematode worms. The male and female worms live in copula in the mesenteric venous plexus of infected individuals. The mature female deposits daily several hundred eggs which contain a live, antigen-secreting embryo. Some of the eggs laid in the blood vessels penetrate the vessel wall and, aided by proteolytic enzymes (Asch and Dresden 1979), move through the tissues and finally drop into the lumen of the intestines. Whereas these eggs are evacuated with the fecal material, many eggs are trapped in the liver and intestinal wall where they evoke a circumscribed granulomatous tissue reaction. The eggs are large, measuring approximately 150 X 60 μm, and thus are surrounded rather than ingested by the inflammatory cells. Due to the influx of freshly deposited eggs, there is an ongoing asynchronous granulomatous process in the liver, intestines, and other organs. Since the life span of an egg is about 3–4 weeks, the inflammatory response slowly wanes with the elimination of the irritant. This constant cycle of egg deposition, granuloma formation, involution of the lesion, and fibrous healing are the major factors in the pathogenesis of the disease. Heavily infected individuals develop the hepatosplenic form of the disease characterized by hepatosplenomegaly, obstruction of portal blood flow, portal hypertension, collateral circulation, esophageal varices, and occasionally fatal bleeding.

The mouse is an excellent host for *Schistosoma mansoni* worms. The animals are not only susceptible to the infection but also duplicate most of the pathologic symptoms that occur in humans (Warren 1973, 1978). The granulomatous response can be studied in either the infected or the normal mouse. The former model presents the full spectrum of the disease syndrome with remarkable similarities to the human condition. In normal mice synchronously evolving granulomas are induced by the intravenous injection of viable eggs isolated from the livers of infected mice. Eggs injected into the tail or mesenteric veins evoke pulmonary (Warren et al. 1967) or hepatic lesions (Edungbola and Schiller 1979) in 4–16 days. These are well circumscribed and can be quantitated with great precision in stained histological sections. With this model, the time course of development, etiology, cellular composition, susceptibility to immunosuppressive measures, and fibrous repair of the granulomas have been studied.

In general, the schistosome egg granuloma is composed of macrophages, epithelioid and giant cells, many eosinophils, some neutrophils and mast cells, lymphocytes, and fibroblasts (Stenger et al. 1967). Recent observations indicate that the granulomas are subject to local organ influences. Lung granulomas are consistently smaller than liver lesions (Colley 1975, Chensue and Boros 1979a), and a recently finished study shows that considerable segmental differences exist in the size of ileal vs. colonic lesions (Weinstock et al. 1981). The accumulated evidence has clearly established that the *S. mansoni* egg-induced granuloma is a T-lymphocyte-mediated immune response. Following the intravenous injection of eggs, an inflammatory reaction appears (Hang et al. 1974) in 4 days, peaks between 16 and 20 days, and then slowly subsides. This granulomatous response is accelerated and enhanced in mice previously primed intraperitoneally with schistosome, but not Ascaris, eggs and can be adoptively transferred by sensitized lymphocytes but not by antiserum (Warren et al. 1967).

Homogenization of viable eggs yields a crude water-soluble egg antigen (SEA) preparation which, in microgram amounts, has been shown to induce and elicit delayed hypersensitivity in mice and guinea pigs (Boros and Warren 1970, Boros et al. 1973a) without the use of adjuvant. Subsequent fractionations of SEA yield various antigens that are reactive with immune sera and also retain their inductive properties (Pelley et al. 1976, Boros et al. 1977). Because the isolated antigens are soluble proteins and glycoproteins, no special granulomagenic properties can be attributed to these substances. Rather, the granuloma-inducing properties of the schistosome eggs derive from the combination of a large insoluble, noningestible nidus (surface of the egg) and the slowly released soluble antigens. Substitution of bentonite particles for the nidus and adsorption of SEA onto the particles elicits granulomatous reactions in the lungs of mice, thereby proving the validity of the assumption (Boros and Warren 1973). The T-cell-mediated immune nature of the schistosome granulomas is further confirmed by the correlation of the evolution of the granulomatous response with delayed skin responses, specific blastogenesis (Colley 1971), and MIF production (Boros et al. 1973a). Moreover, isolated liver granulomas cultured in vitro have been shown to secrete MIF-active and eosinophilotactic lymphokines (Boros et al. 1973b, James and Colley 1975).

Infected immunosuppressed mice or congenitally athymic nude mice without immunocompetent T cells do not develop normal granulomatous responses (Phillips et al. 1977, Amsden et al. 1980). The loose mononuclear aggregates that appear around the eggs are apparently unable to sequester the egg antigens. The result is focal liver damage or necrosis with excessive mortality (Buchanan et al. 1973, Byram and von Lichtenberg 1977). These observations emphasize the protective nature of the granulomatous response. The cells that aggregate around the eggs wall off the offender and sequester its antigens (von Lichtenberg 1964), enzymes, and other potentially toxic excretory products, thereby preventing tissue damage. The eosinophils that surround the eggs also invade them (Bogitsh 1971) and thus help to eliminate the focus of antigenic irritation. Several reports indicate that the cells of the egg granuloma are activated. Liver granulomas of infected mice cultured in vitro release both lysozyme and β glucuronidase enzymes. The level of these two enzymes is maximal in the circulation when mice have maximal granulomatous lesions. The presumed source of the enzymes is the mononuclear cell of the granuloma (Perrotto et al. 1976). Macrophages isolated from young, egg-induced lung granulomas show high esterase content, display a high density/avidity of Fc receptors on their membranes, and are phagocytic. As the inflammation subsides, receptors become greatly diminished (Amsden and Boros 1979).

Preliminary observations also show that T lymphocytes isolated from liver granulomas produce MIF-active substance in vitro and adoptively transfer the enhanced granulomatous response in vivo (Wellhausen and Boros 1981). Unlike the granulomas of tubercle bacilli, the lesions in murine schistosomiasis mansoni rarely if ever undergo caseation and central necrosis. It is highly unlikely that this is due to the less activated state of the granuloma macrophage present in the egg-induced lesions. However, it is possible that no enhancement of cell death takes place in these lesions because the cells do not harbor a replicating intracellular invader.

The granulomatous inflammatory response and its fibrous sequel are the major pathogenetic factors in the disease. Studies of the microcirculation demonstrate that the large liver granulomas cause a presinusoidal block to portal blood flow in the liver. This blockage eventually leads to portal hypertension (Cheever 1965), portalsystemic collateral circulation, and congestive splenomegaly (Bloch et al. 1972).

As the granulomatous condition proceeds to chronicity, fibrosis in the liver and gut of the infected animals becomes pronounced. Though fibrosis is a stereotyped sequel to inflammation it may be compounded by exaggerated fibroblast activity induced by the parasite's eggs. In the present stage of research, the signals for fibroblast activation, collagen synthesis and breakdown, and the degree of reversibility of tissue fibrosis are important topics for investigations. Chemotherapy given to schistosome-infected mice before the onset of the chronic stage of the disease eliminates the worms and results in the resorbtion of the granulomas without any residual fibrotic damage (Warren 1962, Cameron and Ganguly 1964).

Livers of schistosome-infected mice at the peak of granulomatous response have elevated hydroxyproline content, and granulomatous liver slices incorporate maximal amounts of labeled hydroxyproline into collagen (Dunn et al. 1977). Moreover, isolated liver granulomas secrete substances in vitro that induce thymidine incorporation and proliferation in monolayers of xenogeneic fibroblasts (Wyler et al. 1978). Recently collagen synthesis was examined in egg-induced pulmonary granulomas. Peak synthesis was observed in the 1–3-week-old explanted lesions. This coincided with the fully developed state of delayed hypersensitivity (Boros et al. 1981).

Taken together, these data strongly indicate a role for the cell-mediated immune response in the activation and regulation of fibroblast activity and the process of fibrosis. It has been pointed out that fibrosis is the result of an imbalance between collagen formation, deposition, and degradation (Takahashi et al. 1980). Whether overt fibrosis in murine schistosomiasis is due to the lack of available protease-active enzymes in the tissues still needs to be confirmed.

Considerable effort has been invested in the suppression of the inflammatory response in schistosomiasis. The various treatments have included use of immunosuppressive drugs, irradiation, thymectomy, the in vivo administration of antilymphocyte, antimacrophage, and antieosinophil antisera, and the induction of tolerance. The relative efficacy of these treatments has been recently reviewed in detail (Boros 1978). In summary, data from these experiments show that measures that suppress the cell-mediated immune response of the mouse also suppress the granuloma formation. As a rule, suppression of the primary lung granuloma is achieved, whereas only partial suppression is obtained in the size of secondary lesions growing in sensitized mice. These observations confirm the cell-mediated nature of the schistosome egg granuloma and indicate that greatly diminished granulomatous responses ameliorate the morbid manifestations of the disease.

As the protective function of the schistosome granuloma has been recognized, interest has shifted from attempts to suppress the inflammation severely to mechanisms that maintain a toned-down inflammation of low intensity. Such a mechanism seems to be operative in the chronically infected mice in which the size of liver and lung granulomas progressively decreases as the disease proceeds into the chronic stage (20–32 weeks of infection) (Andrade and Warren 1964, Domingo and Warren 1968). Analysis has shown that such animals do not mount a specific delayed skin response, and their splenic lymphocytes are not producing MIF and eosinophilotactic lymphokines. In the face of diminished T-lymphocyte mediated responses, an exponential rise in specific antibody production is observed (Boros et al. 1975, Colley 1975). This phenomenon, termed spontaneous modulation (Boros et al. 1975), is also accompanied by a changed ratio of T to B lymphocytes (favoring the latter) in the blood, lymphoid organs, and granulomas of the chronically infected mice (Chensue and Boros 1979a). Adoptive transfer studies using splenic T lymphocytes of donors undergoing modulation show significant suppression of the vigorous granulomatous response of acutely infected recipients (Colley 1976, Chensue and Boros 1979b). Apparently the modulated granulomatous response is the result of a dynamic equilibrium between inflammatory and regulatory T lymphocytes. When the equilibrium is disturbed in the infected mice by cyclophosphamide treatment (Colley et al. 1979, Chensue et al. 1981) or by splenectomy (Hood and Boros 1980) (measures that eliminate T suppressor cells), an enhanced granulomatous response is obtained.

This dynamic interaction has been further analyzed in vitro and in vivo. Using the assay of macrophage migration inhibition, two separate subpopulations of splenic T lymphocytes have been defined. One subset, designated by alloantiserum as Lyt 1^+ Ia$^-$ T cells, was shown to be the effector population that produces MIF-active lymphokine. Another subset, belonging to the Lyt 2, 3^+ Ia$^+$ group, does not produce lymphokine, but in mixed cultures abrogates MIF production by the effector T-cell population (Chensue et al. 1980). Similar results have also been obtained in adoptive transfer experiments. Elimination of the Lyt 1^+ subset of T cells from spleen lymphocytes significantly diminishes their ability to transfer enhanced granulomatous responses in normal recipients. Cotransfer of a mixture of equal numbers of T lymphocytes, containing a mixture of effector and suppressor cells, results in a significantly diminished granulomatous response in the recipient mice (Wellhausen et al. 1980).

A full understanding of the immunoregulatory mechanisms active in the modulation of the granulomatous inflammatory response in murine schistosomiasis may lead to a universal concept on the spontaneous control of chronic tissue inflammation. Recently, an elegant method has been developed which allows the examination of in vitro granuloma formation. Worm pairs cultured with added erythrocytes and sensitized spleen cells produce eggs which are slowly enveloped by several layers of cells. Apparently the initial interaction is between a macrophage and the egg shell. Subsequently, lymphocytes appear which bind to the macrophage surface. Within days a sphere of cells is created around each egg which contains epithelioid cells, giant cells, eosinophils, and fibroblasts. The cellular reaction is specific for schistosome eggs and appears to be mediated by T lymphocytes. This in vitro model appears to reenact the steps in the in vivo formation of the schistosome granuloma. The mechanisms active during the formation and modulation of the granulomatous response are presently analyzed by this model, which may help to shed light on both the inflammatory and reparatory aspects of granuloma formation (Phillips et al. 1980).

The schistosome egg-induced inflammation has proved to be one of the most useful models for the study of the granulomatous tissue response. It provides insight not only into the immunopathology of human schistosomiasis, but also into the granulomatous process in general. The model confirms the concept that practically all hypersensitivity type granulomatous inflammations are T-lymphocyte-mediated reactions. It emphasizes the dynamic nature of the tissue response, delineates mechanisms active in the generation, and possibly the regulation, of the inflammation, and contributes to our understanding of the process of fibrous healing.

IV. Experimental Hypersensitivity Pneumonitis

Hypersensitivity pneumonitis, also called allergic alveolitis, is a disease syndrome caused by the intermittent chronic inhalation of organic dust. The disease may be associated with high levels of circulating precipitins to the offending antigen, and the pulmonary pathology consists of inflammation of the interstitium, alveolitis, granuloma formation, and often irreversible fibrosis (Lopez and Salvaggio 1976, Fink 1978, Johnson et al. 1979, Salvaggio 1979). Whereas the immunologic background of the disease has been recognized, the actual mechanism(s) responsible for the pathology are still unclear. Virtually the whole range of hypersensitivity immune reactions has been implicated in the disease syndrome (Pepys 1977).

Numerous animal models have been used to assess the mechanism of the reaction and these experiments have been summarized in recent reviews (Roberts and Moore 1977, Olenchok 1977). Though the models provide insight into the possible mechanisms in the disease, they approximate rather than reproduce the actual clinical syndrome. Comparison of the models shows great variations in the choice of antigen and its presentation, the animal species used, the mode of chronic exposure to the offending agent, the histopathologic picture obtained, and the immune parameters examined. This obviously makes interpretations more difficult and the relevance of the models to the disease more tenuous.

Some investigators have employed the actual offending agents, such as antigens found in pigeon droppings and fungal spores, in their models. Dust inhaled from pigeon droppings causes pigeon breeder's disease manifested by the pneumonitis syndrome. The offending antigen is apparently the avian serum protein which is modified in the intestinal tract of birds (Fink 1978). Extracts from this antigen have been used for immunization of rats, rabbits, or monkeys.

Daily exposure of rats to aerosolized extracts of pigeon droppings induces a marked septal infiltration of macrophages, lymphocytes, and plasma cells, as well as epithelioid and giant-cell-containing granulomas. The animals concurrently also developed circulating specific antibodies (Fink et al 1970). In contrast, rabbits exposed chronically to the same antigen develop circulating antibodies without bronchial or alveolar pathology. Challenge of the chronically exposed animals by intravenous injection of killed BCG in oil and further exposure to the extract causes severe acute exudative pneumonitis composed of neutrophils. The local presence of mycobacteria not only promotes the inflammatory response but also helps to induce delayed hypersensitivity to the pigeon antigen as measured by a positive macrophage migration inhibition test with lavaged bronchoalveolar cells (Moore et al. 1975).

The nonspecific enhancing effect of adjuvant-active agents in the induction of pneumonitis has been further underscored by the injection of carrageenan (a sulfated polysaccharide) along with the sensitizing pigeon antigen. The complex nature of the pneumonitis syndrome is well illustrated in these experiments. Although rabbits exposed to aerosolized extracts develop delayed hypersensitivity to the antigen, lung histology shows acute inflammation and no granulomatous pathology (Peterson et al. 1977). A stronger sensitizing regimen using a combination of aerosol exposures and subcutaneous injections of adjuvant-antigen mixtures induces specific delayed hypersensitivity and granulomatous inflammations in rabbits. Similar results are obtained when animals are sensitized and challenged with human gamma globulin. Because the reaction is not transferrable by immune serum, the evidence favors the assumption that the granulomatous response is associated with T-lymphocyte-mediated cellular hypersensitivity (Peterson et al. 1979).

Experiments in the monkey, however, point to a role for circulating antibodies and immune complexes in the induction of pneumonitis. This has been demonstrated by alveolar hemorrhage and a neutrophil-dominated exudate in the lungs of animals that were sensitized with a mixture of pigeon serum in complete adjuvant and exposed to inhalation challenge. Since normal monkeys receiving immune serum also develop pneumonitis after challenge, an Arthus type, immune complex-mediated local inflammation is postulated to be the active mechanism (Hensley et al. 1974).

Bagassosis, a lung disease of workers who inhale fiber dust from sugar canes infected with thermophilic actinomycetes, has been investigated in rats and rabbits. Rats exposed to aerosolized particulate bagasse develop increased cellularity of the pulmonary interstitium, perivascular lymphocytic infiltration, and thickening of alveolar septa. Rabbits exposed repeatedly to *Micropolyspora faeni* antigen (the offending agent) develop extensive pneumonitis consisting of macrophages, lymphocytes, and numerous giant cells. However, no compact granuloma formation is observed in this model. Intratracheal sensitization with high antigen doses induces the production of circulating precipitins, a delayed skin response and specific blastogenesis in lymph node lymphocytes (Kawai et al. 1972).

Rabbits repeatedly challenged by intratracheal injections develop multifocal pneumonitis which progresses from mononuclear infiltration to granuloma formation and fibrosis. The cell-mediated nature of these reactions has been confirmed by the development of delayed dermal responses and a positive macrophage migration inhibition test (Salvaggio et al. 1975). Sensitization by the intratracheal route also causes enhanced recruitment of pulmonary macrophages. The accumulated macrophages are activated as judged by morphological and metabolic criteria. The influx of activated cells precedes florid granuloma formation in the lung (Harris et al. 1976). Macrophage activation has also been demonstrated by the enhanced non-specific phagocytic and bactericidal activity of cultured bronchoalveolar macrophages obtained between 2 and 4 weeks of immunization. Animals with a waning inflammatory response when boosted with antigen showed renewed macrophage activity. These observations support a correlation between the presence of activated macrophages and the histopathology of pneumonitis (Stankus et al. 1978). Hypersensitivity pneumonitis has also been induced in the guinea pig by aerosolized thermophilic actinomycetes.

Although the reaction may have a cell-mediated immune basis, the pathology of the disease can be transferred to normal recipients either by immune lymphocytes or antisera, indicating a dual immune etiology of the reaction (Wilkie et al. 1973, Burrell and Hill 1975).

Induction of experimental hypersensitivity pneumonitis has also been attempted in various animal species with well-defined soluble antigens. Both the mode of sensitization and the type of immunity induced proved to be crucial.

Aerosol exposure to the antigens was insufficient for the induction of sensitization (Fink et al. 1970); therefore animals were sensitized by subcutaneous injections of antigens emulsified in adjuvant. In several experiments a correlation was found between the type (humoral, cellular) of immunity induced and the pulmonary pathology seen after antigenic challenge. Guinea pigs that develop complement-fixing antibodies to ovalbumin react with a severe Arthus type hemorrhagic pneumonia and polymorphonuclear infiltration within 4–6 hr of aerosolized challenge (Richerson 1972). In similar experiments the severity of the reaction is moderately suppressed by cobra venom factor, indicating a role for complement in the inflammatory response. Successful transfer of hemorrhagic pneumonitis by immune serum confirms the immune complex-mediated basis of this reaction (Roska et al. 1977). In contrast, animals rendered hypersensitive to mycobacteria, PPD, or a soluble hapten-carrier complex 24 hr after challenge develop alveolitis composed of mononuclear cells, thickening of alveolar walls, and early granuloma formation (Richerson 1972, Miyamoto et al. 1971).

A recent study that employed chemically crosslinked, particulate ovalbumin in intratracheal challenge emphasized that pulmonary pathology develops in a continuous process. Whereas 4 hr after challenge focal hemorrhagic pneumonitis develops with neutrophil accumulation in the alveoli and interstitium, the cellular composition in the alveoli becomes increasingly mononuclear, and by 96 hr only mononuclear cells are visible. As early as 24 hr postchallenge, elevated numbers of antigen-reactive T lymphocytes are recovered from the lung parenchyma. The changing histology of the inflamed lungs is probably due to the effect of coexisting humoral and cell-mediated immune reactivities; the former eliciting the acute, the latter the chronic phase of the response (Bernardo et al. 1979).

The role of cell-mediated immunity in the development of mononuclear cell pneumonitis has also been demonstrated in rabbits. Only those animals that develop delayed hypersensitivity to ovalbumin generate mononuclear infiltration in the alveoli. Bronchoalveolar lymphocytes recovered from the lungs produce macrophage migration inhibitory factor and undergo blastogenesis in the presence of specific antigen (Richerson 1974, Thomas et al. 1974, Bice et al. 1976).

One of the more significant observations to have emerged from these experiments is the minimal, rather than aggravated, histopathology produced by continued chronic inhalation exposure of sensitized rabbits to soluble or insolubilized antigen. The acute alveolitis observed within 6–48 hr after challenge disappears and on continued exposure cannot be recalled. The phenomenon has been explained to be due either to the increased clearance of antigen or to the development of a desensitization or tolerance state in the chronically exposed animals (Richerson 1974, Richerson et al. 1978).

A critical evaluation of the numerous animal models used in the experimental induction of hypersensitivity pneumonitis shows a great deal of progress in understanding this disease syndrome. The models approximate the acute and, to some extent, the chronic granulomatous manifestations of the disease. The success in inducing granulomatous pulmonary reactions by aerosolized particulate antigens of fungi, but not with soluble antigens, underscores the important role of the physical nature of the antigens in the induction of chronic inflammatory reactions. Whereas alveolitis is often produced after challenge, the actual granulomatous responses obtained are composed of immature macrophages. This may be due to the short duration of the experiments. A limitation of the experiments is the need to rely on strong adjuvants for the induction of granulomatous responses. This is dissimilar to the natural condition. Aided by these models we more closely understand the complexity of the chronic alveolar inflammatory reactions. Whereas an immune complex-mediated Arthus type hemorrhagic alveolitis is produced in the acute models (Johnson and Ward 1974), the production of lymphokines by bronchoalveolar lymphocytes, granuloma formation, and the occasional transferrability of pneumonitis by sensitized lymphocytes indicates a prominent role for delayed hypersensitivity in the chronicity of the disease.

A more complex situation in which continuous immune complex formation (in antibody excess) in the lower respiratory tract would eventually result in granulomatous inflammations rather than proliferative pneumonitis has not yet been achieved in any experimental condition (Brentjens et al. 1974). Additional amplifier mechanisms, active in inflammation, may be found among the complement components, especially split products of C3. Complement can be triggered through the alternate pathway by thermoactinomyces (Schorlemmer et al. 1977, Marx and Flaherty 1976) and can induce release of lysosomal enzymes from macrophages. In turn, lysosomal enzymes can further split complement. Thus, a complex amplification of the pulmonary inflammatory reaction, due in part to activated complement products, may be possible (Henson et al. 1979).

A fascinating feature of some of the reviewed experiments is the spontaneous "desensitization" of animals exposed to a chronic regiment of inhalation challenge. This phenomenon is worthy of further exploration and may be akin to the T suppressor cell-mediated modulation of the granulomatous response seen in murine schistosomiasis. In experimental pneumonitis both immune complex and cell-mediated immune responses participate. The two may occur sequentially, with cell-mediated granulomatous alveolitis predominating in the chronic stage. It also appears that, in addition to the antigenic insult, other factors, such as adjuvant action, rate of pulmonary clearance, toxicity of the antigen, action on complement, and the genetic background of the host, may all play a role in the final outcome of pathologic manifestations.

V. The Artificial Hypersensitivity Granulomas

Although soluble, degradable antigens are incapable of inducing granulomatous reactions, the role of soluble antigens in the granulomatous process can be explored by adsorbing or chemically coupling them onto insoluble carriers which serve as nidi for the cellular response. The model is advantageous since it examines both the foreign body and the hypersensitivity inflammatory aspects of the granulomatous response. The particles (bentonite, latex, synthetic beads) are insoluble and measure 40–60 μm. Following the intravenous injection into rodents, the particles embolize the microcapillaries and induce an inflammatory response, in which the cells surround but do not ingest the irritant. Bare particles invariably induce a mild, usually transient foreign body granulomatous response, whereas particles coupled with an antigen and injected into previously sensitized animals evoke florid granulomas similar to the "infectious" or hypersensitivity inflammatory response. Using this model, questions regarding the role of T lymphocytes, lymphokines, and fibroblasts in the inflammatory response have been explored.

Intravenous injection of bentonite particles, with adsorbed soluble antigens of *S. mansoni* eggs, into specifically sensitized mice rapidly evokes large hypersensitivity pulmonary granulomas composed of lymphocytes, macrophages, occasional giant cells and eosinophils (Boros and Warren 1971, von Lichtenberg et al. 1971). On the other hand, bare or antigen-coated particles given to normal mice evoke very small reactions consisting of young macrophages. Similar results were obtained using tuberculin and histoplasmin. In each instance the specific accelerated, enhanced nature of the hypersensitivity granulomas has been confirmed. The occurrence of the granuloma correlates with the onset of delayed footpad swelling, the standard skin response measured in mice. Moreover, sensitized lymphoid cells, but not antiserum, transfers enhanced granuloma formation around the antigen-coated beads (Boros and Warren 1973).

The foreign body nature of the granuloma induced by intradermally injected bentonite has been confirmed recently by ultrastructural studies showing the presence of large macrophages and giant cells but no epithelioid cells or lymphocytes in the lesions (Browett et al. 1980). The T-cell-mediated nature of the artificial hypersensitivity granuloma induced by schistosomal egg antigens has been confirmed with latex carrier particles. These studies emphasize one of the major characteristics of these models, that is, that the intensity of the granulomatous response is strongly correlated with the local retention and slow release of the antigens from the insoluble nidus (Dunsford et al. 1974). Synthetic beads with the covalently coupled antigens have been used as additional models. Whereas antigens are known to be released from bentonite particles over a period of days, no data are available about the release of the chemically bound antigens. The results of these studies confirm that proteins (hemocyanin, human serum albumin) or hapten-protein antigens coupled onto particles evoke hypersensitivity type granulomatous inflammations.

The pulmonary reactions in sensitized guinea pigs are large, peak early, and seem to assume the palisading arrangement of mononuclear cells, some of which resemble epithelioid cells (Unanue and Benacerraf 1973, Kasdon and Schlossman 1973. The granulomatous response is transferrable by sensitized lymphocytes, not by antiserum, and is dependent on the recognition by T cells of the carrier determinant (protein) on the hapten-carrier antigen complex (Unanue and Benacerraf 1973). Essentially, similar hypersensitivity type granulomas are obtained by the intradermal injection of particles coupled with hapten-protein complexes (Kasdon et al. 1974). In all these experiments bare beads or particles evoke only mild, transient inflammations in the unprimed animals. One report also shows the feasibility of intrapulmonary sensitization by antigen-coated beads. Normal rats receiving latex particles coated with human gamma globulin develop specific delayed hypersensitivity, as demonstrated by accelerated granuloma formation around a challenge dose of antigen-coated particles, pronounced eosinophilia, and specific blastogenesis of blood lymphocytes (Schriber and Zucker-Franklin 1975).

Artificial granuloma models were also used to confirm the participation of lymphokines in granulomatous inflammation. These artificial granulomas are generated by a hapten-protein complex bound covalently onto agarose beads in antigen-adjuvant sensitized guinea pigs. The lesions are composed of mononuclear cells with occasional giant cells and epithelioid cells. Control lesions, induced by bare beads, contain a collection of young macrophages. Extracts of lung homogenates obtained 2 days after the generation of the granuloma yield MIF activity, while extracts of control lungs are inactive. Gel filtration of the extract shows recoverable MIF activity at the region (30,000–60,000 mol wt) where MIF activity usually resides (Masih et al. 1979). Homogenates obtained from lungs with older lesions do not yield lymphokine-active materials.

Lymphokine-active substances are also obtained from granulomas explanted from the lungs of sensitized, antigen-bead-injected mice. These lesions are isolated from the lungs by gentle homogenization and sedimentation. The 7-day-old hypersensitivity type granulomas contain esterase-positive mature macrophages and occasional giant cells. No epithelioid cells are evident. Overnight cultures of the explanted, antigen-stimulated lesions yield MIF-active and chemotactic substances. Column chromatography yields active fractions that correspond in molecular weight and enzyme sensitivity to murine lymphokines obtained from splenic lymphocytes. Significantly, cultures obtained from the small foreign body granulomas are devoid of lymphokine activity (Carrick and Boros 1980).

Production of lymphokine-active substances by hypersensitivity type lesions strongly indicates that these substances play an important role in the local generation and maintenance of the granulomatous response. This premise has been proven by injecting normal mice with bead-bound fractionated granuloma supernates with MIF and chemotactic activity. Granulomatous reactions composed of several layers of young macrophages are evoked in 4 days. The complex (in vivo) role of lymphokine-active substances in immune inflammatory reactions was further emphasized by the demonstration that granuloma formation also occurs around naked beads if mice receive an intratracheal, or slowly released intraperitoneal injection of the lymphokines concurrently with beads. The data strongly indicate both a systemic and local role for lymphokines in cellular recruitment and granuloma formation (Boros and Carrick 1980).

Additional experiments indicate that macrophage activation, as measured by the display of Fc receptors on the cell membrane, is correlated with the etiology and intensity of the granulomatous responses. Receptor display is maximal 7 days after the generation of the granulomas and declines in the waning lesions. More macrophages display a higher density of receptors for a longer duration in the artificial hypersensitivity lesions than in the foreign body lesions. This enhanced membrane activity is attributed to the activated state of the macrophage mediated by locally produced lymphokines (Amsden and Boros 1979).

The etiology of the lesion seems also to influence the collagen synthetic ability of the granulomas. When foreign body and hypersensitivity type bead granulomas were isolated from lungs of mice at various intervals after initiation of the lesions, protein and collagen were found to be synthesized at the highest rate in the 7-day-old explants. However, explants of the hypersensitivity lesions showed markedly higher synthetic capacity compared with those of the foreign body lesions. Also, intravenous antigen challenge given to hypersensitive mice significantly elevated collagen synthesis in the explanted lesions. Since lymphokine-active substances injected into mice bearing foreign body type granulomas similarly enhanced the collagen synthetic ability of the explants, the results strongly indicate that the state of delayed hypersensitivity not only initiates and maintains the granulomatous inflammatory response but may also influence fibroblast activity and the process of fibrous repair (Boros et al. 1981).

The types of collagen deposited in artificial granulomas induced by beads coupled with soluble schistosomal egg antigens have been examined recently. Indirect immunofluorescence studies reveal the presence of types I and III collagen deposited in the waning hypersensitivity granulomas. No fibrosis is observed in the foreign body type lesions by this method (van Marck et al. 1980).

The model of artificial hypersensitivity granulomas demonstrated that soluble antigens are granulomagenic if bound to insoluble nidi. A similar mechanism may be active in hypersensitivity pneumonitis with spores of thermoactinomycetes (Salvaggio 1979). The artificially induced granulomas have a limited life span, the duration of the inflammation being dependent on the availability of the bound antigens. The model allows the parallel examination of foreign body and hypersensitivity lesions, and demonstrates that the latter is a "pure" T-cell mediated reaction, which is generated by lymphokine-active substances. Though the lesions do not show an intense inflammatory response, they nevertheless undergo dynamic changes during the evolution and involution of the reaction and terminate in fibrotic healing. This model serves as the blueprint for the prototypic granuloma.

VI. Foreign Body Granulomas Induced by Bacterial Cell Wall Components

A. Streptococcal Peptidoglycan

Although mycobacterium-induced tuberculosis has become the prototype of granulomatous diseases, "infectious" granulomas are evoked also by several gram-negative (Brucella, Salmonella) and gram-positive (Corynebacterium, Streptococcus) microorganisms. Streptococci play an important role in the pathogenesis of endocarditis, myocarditis, arthritis, and periodontal gingivitis in humans. A major factor in these diseases is the chronic granulomatous inflammatory response mounted against streptococcal cell wall components (Ginsburg 1972). Due to the great clinical importance of group A streptococci-induced chronic diseases, interest has been focused on experimental animal models that duplicate the clinical manifestations of chronic inflammation. Rabbits, mice, and rats injected intradermally, intravenously, or intraarticularly with intact group A streptococci develop chronic granulomatous inflammations at the site of the injection or in the heart and livers of animals (Ohanian and Schwab 1967, Sellin et al. 1968, Haferkamp et al. 1970, Ginsburg 1979). Histological studies show initially a purulent inflammatory response in which polymorphonuclear leukocytes predominate. Degradation of phagocytized streptococci takes place within polymorphonuclear cells.

Several days later macrophages become numerous and subsequently comprise the major cellular component of the lesions. The macrophages are enlarged and have a foamy cytoplasm. Whereas occasional giant cells are present, epithelioid cells are not detectable within the lesions. It is noteworthy that granulomatous lesions appear only after the breakdown of the intact organisms. Degradation of the microorganisms is accomplished within 2-3 weeks. This has been demonstrated by the localization of cell wall fragments within macrophages by labeled antibodies directed to the group-specific C polysaccharide and the peptidoglycans of the organisms (Ohanian and Schwab 1967, Schwab and Ohanian 1968, Sellin et al. 1970, Ginsburg et al. 1977). The persistence of cell wall components has been confirmed also in monolayer of rat macrophages using differentially labeled peptidoglycan and polysaccharide moieties. The persistence of undegraded cell wall fragments could be demonstrated for up to 40 days of culture. Supplementation of the monolayers with antiserum or sensitized lympho-cytes from vaccinated animals do not induce any degradation (Schwab and Smialowicz 1975, Smialowicz and Schwab 1977).

The cell wall component responsible for the granulomatous reaction has been identified as a complex of peptidoglycan and group C polysaccharide (Krause and McCarty 1961, Abdulla and Schwab 1966). Protoplasts of L-forms devoid of cell wall components are unable to evoke similar lesions (Schwab et al. 1962). It is possible that the polysaccharide protects the peptidoglycan from degradation in the tissues and blocks its granulo-magenicity (Schwab and Ohanian 1968). Removal of the terminal N-acetyl-glucosamine molecule from group C polysaccharide does not enhance the elimination of streptococci from muscle granulomas (Rickles et al. 1969). Though the role of purified peptidoglycans in the induction of granu-lomatous inflammations in streptococcal infections still awaits final elucidation, the adjuvant arthritis model indicates that this moiety has potent biologic effects. Substitution of the mycobacterial component in the adjuvant mixture with streptococcal peptidoglycans duplicates the effects of adjuvant arthritis (Koga et al. 1976). The arthritogenic effect is located in a chain length of 2 or more disaccharide units that are coupled with the peptidoglycan (Kohashi et al. 1976).

Peptidoglycans derived from streptococci are potent biologic agents that can induce chronic and often destructive inflammatory reactions. The etiology of the granulomatous response has been extensively investigated. Because animals and humans are exposed continuously to streptococci as well as to potentially cross-reactive peptidoglycans from other bacilli and plants, it is conceivable that the granulomatous response has a specific, immune etiology. However, the failure of repeated attempts to sensitize animals with the peptidoglycans refuted this assumption. Spleen cells of peptidoglycan or cell-wall-injected animals neither transfer an enhanced granulomatous response to recipients nor can be stimulated to produce MIF or lymphotoxin (Heymer et al. 1971, Jones and Schwab 1970). Peptidoglycans also fail to elicit MIF production in lymphocyte cultures of rats preimmunized with streptococci (Heymer et al. 1973). Thus, currently the most plausible explanation is that the granulomagenic activity of the peptidoglycans is due to their ability to activate inflammatory macrophages.

Indeed, peptidoglycans have been shown to exert an adjuvant effect (Holton and Schwab 1966) and to inhibit nonspecifically the in vitro migration of normal peritoneal macrophages (Heymer et al. 1973, Bültmann et al. 1970). Monolayers of macrophages exposed to the polysaccharide-peptidoglycan complex of group A streptococci increase their lysosomal and nonlysosomal enzyme content and also secrete some of the lysosomal hydrolases (Davies et al. 1974, Page et al. 1978). The exact mode of cellular recruitment, activation, and multiplication that takes place in the peptidoglycan-induced granulomas is unknown. The recent observations that showed activation of the alternate pathway of complement by peptidoglycans (Greenblatt et al. 1978) may indicate one pathway for cell recruitment. Once the lesion is generated, the inflammation would perpetuate itself by secreted macrophage products. The end result is a chronic, foreign body type granulomatous lesion with pronounced tissue-destructive side effects.

B. Muramyl Dipeptide (MDP)

Until recently, mycobacteria emulsified in water-in-oil (Freund's complete adjuvant) served as the most effective aid in the amplification of humoral and cell-mediated immune responses. The mode of action of this adjuvant remains largely unelucidated. Some believe that the various mycobacterial lipids serve as adjuvant-active substances, while others implicate the granulomatous response and the concurrent induction of tuberculin hyper-sensitivity as necessary modes for the nonspecific enhancement of an immune response. Recent developments, however, indicate that water-soluble cell wall components fractionated from mycobacteria have potent in vivo adjuvant activity (Adam et al. 1972). The water-soluble adjuvant (WSA) is composed of arabinogalactan linked to peptidoglycan. Further analysis reveals that a portion of the cell wall subunit composed of N-acetyl-muramyl-L-alanyl-D-isoglutamine (muramyl dipeptide) is the minimal adjuvant-active unit (Ellouz et al. 1974). This has led to the synthesis of MDP and to the demonstration that the dipeptide substituted for whole mycobacteria in the complete adjuvant mixture (Merser et al. 1975).

In routine immunization of animals, MDP has proven to be adjuvant-active when incorporated into water-in-oil emulsion, but more importantly it is equally effective when injected together with the antigen in an aqueous medium (Chedid et al. 1978, 1979). In recent years the range of adjuvant activity, potential mode of action, and granulomagenicity of MDP and its analogs have been thoroughly tested. Two recent publications from the same laboratory indicate that MDP injected into guinea pigs induces granulomatous inflammations. Significantly, in both studies MDP was incorporated into the classic water-in-oil emulsion used for the incomplete adjuvant. Injection of emulsified MDP into the footpad of animals evokes, both at the site of the injection and in the draining lymph node, an intense inflammation which by 2 weeks assumes the form of large compact granulomas. This is especially clear-cut in the nodes, where the presence of closely packed epithelioid cells with a few giant cells is noted. The epithelioid cells seem to conform to the classic description of such cells found in the mycobacterial tubercle.

Four weeks after the injection, the granulomatous inflammation starts to resolve and fibroblasts appear in the lesion. Rats injected with the same dose of MDP show the development of similar, though less mature looking lesions, with a somewhat more accelerated appearance. Extensive skin tests done in rats or guinea pigs indicate that MDP is nonantigenic in these animals. Preliminary observations also indicated that the diastereomer of MDP, N-acetyl-muramyl-L-alanyl-L-isoglutamine, which lacks adjuvant activity, is incapable of granuloma induction (Emori and Tanaka 1978). In further experiments, 3 weeks after the injection of MDP, enlargement of the draining lymph nodes coincided with the histological picture of the mature granuloma. Interestingly, no difference is seen if MDP is injected alone or in conjunction with ovalbumin in the emulsion. During the first days a polymorphonuclear infiltration is seen, which by 7 days gives way to infiltrated macrophages that phagocytize oil droplets. By the third week mature epithelioid cells are visible and are organized into tubercles, along with some giant cells. In electron microscopy, epithelioid cells have a large oval nucleus, prominent nucleolus, and intracytoplasmic organelles which include lysosomes, mitochondria, rough endoplasmic reticulum, free ribosomes, and Golgi apparatus. The closely packed cells also show the interdigitation of membrane pseudopodia.

It is emphasized that MDP dissolved in water does not evoke granulomas. The molecule in its aqueous form is rapidly excreted from the organism. Thus, mineral oil may be necessary to provide a depot and ensure the prolonged presence of the molecule in the tissues. The possibility that MDP requires some lipids for its granulomagenic effect has also been suggested. Quantitative comparisons showed that emulsified MDP is a stronger inducer of granulomas than heat-killed virulent tubercle bacilli (Tanaka and Emori 1980). In any case, MDP has a direct activating effect on macrophages which, in turn, leads to the massive granulomatous response. MDP has been shown to inhibit in a nonspecific manner (which seems to exclude the action of lymphokine) the in vitro migration of normal peritoneal macrophages of rats and guinea pigs (Adam et al. 1978, Yamamoto et al. 1978, Nagao et al. 1979). Moreover, MDP enhances the nonspecific resistance of mice to encapsulated Klebsiella organisms even when given by the oral route (Chedid et al. 1977) and activates the murine RES (reticuloendothelial system) as demonstrated by enhanced carbon clearance (Tanaka et al. 1979). Very significantly, macrophage activation is dependent on the stereochemical specificity of MDP. Neither the D-D nor the L-L configuration of MDP is active in the inhibition of macrophage migration, RES activation, or adjuvant activity. A further demonstration of MDP-mediated macrophage activation shows the induction of collagenase activity, prostaglandin E_2 production, and the secretion of a factor that causes fibroblast proliferation (Wahl et al. 1978). These observations, coupled with previous ones that show that MDP acts as an adjuvant in the induction of immune reactions via the macrophage (Modolell et al. 1974), underscore the concept that granulomagenic substances possess the intrinsic potential of macrophage activation and adjuvant activity.

C. Cord Factor

Mycobacteria possess unique lipid and waxy envelopes that may provide protection during intracellular residence against the degradative mechanisms of the macrophage. These lipids and waxes are also considered to contribute to the adjuvant action of the dead organisms. Various myco-bacterial lipids have been shown to elicit granulomatous reactions which histologically do not seem to differ from the classic mycobacterium-induced tubercle (Boros 1978). With the advent of more precise biochemical preparative procedures, attempts have been made to extract and isolate homogeneous substances from the lipid envelopes of mycobacteria and to examine their granulomagenic as well as adjuvant-active properties. One of these substances which has gained prominence in recent years is a toxic glycolipid named cord factor (trehalose-6, 6'-dimycolate). Cord factor emulsified in oil, water, and detergent and injected intravenously in microgram amounts evokes isolated or confluent pulmonary lesions in mice. The bulk of the lesions is composed of mononuclears and it has been claimed that occasional epithelioid cells can also be detected within the lesions (Bekierkunst 1968, Bekierkunst et al. 1969). Injection of cord factor into the footpads of normal mice evoked local granuloma formation with hyperplasia of the paracortical zones in the draining lymph nodes (Bekierkunst et al. 1971).

Whereas early descriptions claim that repeated injections of cord factor induce a state of sensitivity, further experiments failed to substantiate this. Nor can cord factor sensitize mice to an accelerated granulomatous response (Bekierkunst and Yarkoni 1973). The discrepancy in the early results may be due to the presence of minute amounts of contaminating substances such as the highly antigenic wax D. Cord factor preparations are known to be heterogeneous, containing a mixture of several dimycolates. Indeed, a preparation of cord factor, designated P3 and considered to be freed from impurities, elicits only small foreign body granulomas in mouse lung and guinea pig skin and is devoid of antigenicity in the guinea pig (Meyer et al. 1975). Cord factor emulsified in oil and water and injected intravenously into rabbits fails to elicit granulomas similar to those evoked by killed BCG. Neither can such an emulsion induce sensitization to BCG organisms (Moore et al. 1972).

It is to be pointed out that cord factor employed in the various experiments for the induction of granulomas needs to be emulsified in oil and water. The size distribution of oil droplets within the emulsion apparently plays an important role. When cord factor is emulsified with droplets 1 μm or larger, an intense granulomatous pulmonary response is obtained (Granger et al. 1976, Yarkoni and Rapp 1977). Apparently, the complete molecule is needed for the granulomagenic action because trehalose alone, or separated mycolic acids and their esters, do not induce granulomas (McLaughlin et al. 1978).

Cord factor is a highly potent biologic agent. Injected into mice, it causes swelling and disruption of liver mitochondria. In vitro, it damages mitochondrial respiration and phosphorylation (Kato and Fukushi 1969, Kato 1969). Specific antibodies obtained after immunization with cord factor complexed with a basic protein carrier neutralizes these toxic manifestations and provides some protection to mice against *M. tuberculosis* infection (Kato 1972, 1973).

More recent observations deal with the adjuvanticity of this glycolipid. Several laboratories have demonstrated that the immune response to soluble or particulate antigens is enhanced if the antigens are emulsified with cord factor. Thus, the glycolipid enhances the humoral response to sheep red blood cells and hapten carrier complexes (Löwy et al. 1977, Sugimoto et al. 1978b) and promotes the induction of delayed hypersensitivity to bovine serum albumin and ABA-N-acetyl tyrosine (Granger et al. 1976, Azuma et al. 1976). The potent biologic role of the glycolipid has been extended also to antitumor activity. Cord factor alone or in admixture with endotoxin causes either the suppression of tumor cell growth or the regression of hepatoma or fibrosarcoma tumors (Ribi et al. 1975, Rapp et al. 1978, Yarkoni et al. 1979). The antitumor effect is likely to be mediated through the activated macrophages. Cord factor is chemotactic for mouse peritoneal macrophages and human blood monocytes (Ofek and Bekierkunst 1976), stimulates peritoneal macrophages to enhanced phagocytosis of Listeria organisms (Yarkoni et al. 1977), and induces nonspecific resistance against *S. typhi* and *S. typhimurium* organisms as well as *M. tuberculosis* (McLaughlin et al. 1978, Yarkoni and Bekierkunst 1976).

Thus, cell wall fragments as well as whole bacteria can be granulomagenic. However, whereas the microorganisms are highly immunogenic, their cell wall fragments lack the capacity to induce cell-mediated immunity. Thus, we encounter a paradoxical situation in which one organism can induce both a hypersensitivity and a foreign body type granulomatous inflammatory response. The two effects are practically inseparable from each other when assessing tissue pathology. The common characteristics of cell wall fragments are their small size, relative nondegradability, and the capacity to strongly activate macrophages. Though the exact mode of macrophage activation is unknown, the degree of activation is often comparable to that achieved by lymphokines. The chronicity of the inflammatory response is maintained by the activated state of the macrophage. Secretory products of these cells (hydrolases, proteases) probably interact with the clotting, kinin, complement, and fibrinolytic pathways and can trigger reactions which generate inflammatory substances (Page et al. 1978). Continued, enhanced secretions by macrophages are the major factor in tissue damage which does not differ in severity from that caused by the immunologically activated cells.

These models again illustrate that the magnitude of macrophage activation is the decisive factor in the intensity of the granulomatous inflammation, and in tissue damage.

VII. Overview and Conclusions

Experimentally induced granulomatous diseases or inflammations have been reviewed in this chapter. At the present time there is no animal species that spontaneously develops sarcoid type granulomas. Thus, the experimental models serve as blueprints for a better understanding of the chronic granulomatous tissue responses that characterize sarcoidosis. The following comments attempt to correlate the relevant features of the models to sarcoidosis.

1. The various experimental models support the view that the granulomatous response is induced by nondegradable or only slowly degradable tissue irritants. These agents provide a sustained stimulus for macrophage mobilization and activation. The range of inducer agents is wide and includes fungal spores, bacilli, parasite ova, and soluble peptides. The common feature of these agents is their capacity to persist in tissues and, in most cases, to induce a specific immune reaction of the cell-mediated type. What is the causative agent of sarcoidosis? This question is not currently answerable. The efforts invested so far into the isolation, identification, and propagation of putative transmissible or infectious agents of sarcoidosis remain largely unsuccessful. However, according to observations of the experimental models, the inciting agent of sarcoidosis should be of a persisting nondegradable nature. The experimental models demonstrate that numerous noninfectious agents, including degraded microbial cell wall components, antigen-antibody complexes, and modified or resorbed cells of self, can serve as granulomagenic agents. Any of these may be the etiologic agent of sarcoidosis. Thus, while the search for the elusive agent(s) of sarcoidosis is continued, it is possible that sarcoidosis may not be caused by a classic replicating, transmissible agent.

2. Pathologists still emphasize the diagnostic importance of the organized epithelioid cells within the hypersensitivity type human granulomatous lesion. The demonstration that epithelioid type cells can be artificially induced by foreign bodies makes these claims tenuous. The immune, most probably T-cell-mediated character of a clinical granulomatous condition should be verified by tests that detect specifically reactive lymphocytes in the patient. Naturally, for such tests one needs an eliciting antigen with a high degree of specificity. However, in the absence of such a reagent, positive parameters indicative of T-lymphocyte activation may also suggest an immune etiology. Though the Kveim antigen used for diagnosis of sarcoidosis has often proved to be less than satisfactory, reports showing the presence of circulating lymphokines (Yoshida et al. 1979) and the secretion of lymphokine-active substances by bronchoalveolar lymphocytes of sarcoid patients (Hunninghake et al. 1980) strongly indicate a cell-mediated etiology of the disease. Further efforts aimed at better purification of the crude antigen should help provide a more specific and standardized diagnostic tool.

3. Most, if not all granulomatous reactions are accompanied by some tissue injury. The models show that, irrespective of the etiology, if the inflammatory response is strong enough, cell death and tissue injury will ensue. Although most of the models emphasize the role of the macrophage in this process, additional granuloma cells (lymphocytes, eosinophils, fibroblasts) should also be considered as potential contributors to injury. Tissue damage is caused by the released hydrolytic and degradative enzymes as

well as by oxygen breakdown products released by the activated macrophages. Yet the degree of tissue injury seen in the various models is
variable. Whereas the Mycobacterium-induced lesions invariably caseate at
the core, central necrosis does not occur in the sarcoid, beryllium, or
schistosome granulomas. Whether this is due to the absence of certain
degradative enzymes or toxic macrophage products, or to the innate
toxicity of the inciting agents as seen in the cord factor or silica-induced
lesions, is still to be investigated.

Sequential determinations of enzyme contents of granulomas or
granuloma cells show the dynamic nature of the lesions but often provide
contradictory results regarding the role of proteolytic enzymes in caseation.
Though enzyme determinations have been done in the free alveolar macrophages of sarcoid patients (Gee et al. 1978), these cells may play only an
ancillary role in the compact granulomatous inflammatory process. Except
for the dermal lesions, granulomas of various human diseases are not easily
accessible to analysis. In the experimental models, isolation of the lesions
from organs make their sequential analysis possible. In organ cultures the
secretory and synthetic activity of the lesions can be examined, whereas
dispersal of the granulomas into cellular components opens the possibilities
of characterization and functional analysis.

In the clinical situation, a modest amount of tissue can be obtained
by biopsy. Though there are obvious ethical and practical limitations to
the collection of such material, the difficulty is not insurmountable and the
feasibility of this approach should be pursued by clinicians. Analysis of the
isolated granuloma would yield effector lymphocytes and macrophages that
bear more relevance to the inflammatory process than blood monocytes or
free alveolar macrophages obtained by lavage. Moreover, if nondegradable
antigenic substances are involved in sarcoidosis, they would be more likely
located within, rather than outside of, the lesion.

4. Studies aimed at the suppression of the granulomatous response
have shown that the hypersensitivity type lesions are suppressible by various
measures directed against the T-effector lymphocyte. Good results have been
obtained also by the administration of corticosteroids which have a broad
action, affecting cellular traffic and proliferation and activation of lymphocytes, macrophages, and other cells. In this respect, the experimental
models reconfirm the experience gained in clinical practice. Whereas the
intensity of the inflammatory response and the extent of tissue injury is
diminished by cortisone treatment, fibrosis remains unaffected. Development
of drugs with more specified action may improve the treatment of chronic
granulomatous diseases. Special attention should be directed to fibroblast
activity and the process of fibrosis which often contributes considerably to
the pathology of the disease. Very recent observations indicate that

lymphocytes may also be involved in the activation/regulation of fibroblasts. These aspects, as yet unaddressed in sarcoidosis, deserve a great deal of research effort.

5. One of the most fascinating features of the experimental granuloma models is the appearance of regulatory mechanism(s) which spontaneously diminish the intensity of the granulomatous inflammations. The mechanism seems to be based on a complex interaction between effector, inflammatory, and suppressor cells and factors. Because, in many instances, a total suppression of the granulomatous response is ill-advised if not outright dangerous, this naturally occurring modulated response is of great importance. Anti-inflammatory regulator mechanisms detected in some experimental models may represent universal phenomena. It is tempting to speculate that the anergic condition often described in patients with sarcoidosis may also be a manifestation of the anti-inflammatory, suppressor mechanisms of the body. Diminished skin responses to a battery of antigens, diminished in vitro lymphocyte responses, and elevated immunoglublin levels which occur during an ongoing granulomatous process in sarcoidosis show great similarities to the spontaneous modulation described in murine schistosomiasis. It is possible that granuloma formation in chronic sarcoidosis is modulated and diminished, but so far has escaped detection due to the unavailability of the lesions for sequential quantitative measurements. The recent description of adherent suppressor cells in the circulation of patients with sarcoidosis indicates the existence of some active regulator mechanism (Goodwin et al. 1979). Whether these regulator mechanisms are beneficial and whether they play some role in the complex immunopathology of the disease should constitute a major portion of future investigations.

6. There is good reason to believe that the capacity to mount an inflammatory response as well as the intensity and rapidity of resolution of the granulomatous reaction are under genetic control. Both the experimental models and some clinical observations (James and Neville 1977) confirm this contention. Future studies should elucidate whether the unresolved chronic, granulomatous response in a low percentage of humans with sarcoidosis and other granulomatous diseases may signify a genetic inability to generate an adequate, effective inflammatory reaction.

The experimental animal models provide invaluable information on the various facets of the granulomatous inflammatory response. Granuloma formation to tissue irritants is a stereotyped reaction of mammals. Thus, results from animal experiments should be applicable (with some caution) to granulomatous diseases of humans. The insight into the complex processes of granulomatous inflammation acquired during the past decade should help the improved management, if not the prevention, of human sarcoidosis.

References

Abdulla, E. M., and Schwab, J. H. (1966). Biological properties of
streptococcal cell wall particles. III. Dermonecrotic reaction to cell
wall mucopeptides. *J. Bacteriol.*, **91**:374–383.

Adam, A., Ciorbaru, R., Petit, J. F., and Lederer, E. (1972). Isolation and
properties of a macromolecular, water-soluble, immunoadjuvant
fraction from the cell wall of *Mycobacterium smegmatis. Proc. Natl.
Acad. Sci. U.S.A.*, **69**:851–854.

Adam, A., Souvannavong, V., and Lederer, E. (1978). Non-specific MIF-
like activity induced by the synthetic immunoadjuvant: n-acetyl
muramyl-L-alanyl-D-isoglutamine (MDP). *Biochem. Biophys. Res.
Commun.*, **85**:684–690.

Adams, D. O. (1974). The structure of mononuclear phagocytes differentiating in vivo. I. Sequential fine and histologic studies of the effect
of Bacillus Calmette-Guerin (BCG). *Am. J. Pathol.*, **76**:17–48.

Adams, D. O. (1975). The structure of mononuclear phagocytes differentiating in vivo. II. The effect of *Mycobacterium tuberculosis. Am.
J. Pathol.*, **80**:101–116.

Adams, D. O. (1976). The granulomatous inflammatory response. A
review. *Am. J. Pathol.*, **84**:164–192.

Allen, E. M., Moore, V. L., and Stevens, J. O. (1977). Strain variation in
BCG-induced chronic pulmonary inflammation in mice. I. Basic
model and possible genetic control by non H-2 genes. *J. Immunol.*,
119:343–347.

Amsden, A. F., and Boros, D. L. (1979). Fc-receptor-bearing macrophages
isolated from hypersensitivity and foreign-body granulomas. Delineation of macrophage dynamics, Fc receptor density/avidity and
specificity. *Am. J. Pathol.*, **96**:457–474.

Amsden, A. F., Boros, D. L., and Hood, A. T. (1980). Etiology of the
liver granulomatous response in *Schistosoma mansoni*-infected athymic
nude mice. *Infect. Immun.*, **27**:75–80.

Ando, M., Dannenberg, A. M., Jr., and Shima, K. (1972). Macrophage
accumulation, division, maturation and digestive and microbicidal
capacities in tuberculous lesions. II. Rate at which mononuclear
cells enter and divide in primary BCG lesions and those of reinfection.
J. Immunol., **109**:8–19.

Ando, M., Dannenberg, A. M., Jr., Sugimoto, M., and Tepper, B. S. (1977).
Histochemical studies relating the activation of macrophages to the
intracellular destruction of tubercle bacilli. *Am. J. Pathol.*, **86**:
623–634.

Andrade, Z. A., and Warren, K. S. (1964). Mild prolonged schistosomiasis
in mice: Alterations in host response with time and the development
of portal fibrosis. *Trans. R. Soc. Trop. Med. Hyg.*, **58**:53–57.

Asch, H. L., and Dresden, M. H. (1979). Acidic thiol proteinase activity of *Schistosoma mansoni* egg extracts. *J. Parasitol.*, **65**:543–549.

Azuma, I., Sugimura, K., Taniyama, T., Yamawaki, M., Yamamura, Y., Kusumoto, S., Okada, S., and Shiba, T. (1976). Adjuvant activity of mycobacterial fractions: Adjuvant activity of synthetic n-acetylmuramyl dipeptide and the related compounds. *Infect. Immun.*, **14**:18–27.

Bekierkunst, A. (1968). Acute granulomatous response produced in mice by trehalose-6, 6′-dimycolate. *J. Bacteriol.*, **96**:958–961.

Bekierkunst, A., and Yarkoni, E. (1973). Granulomatous hypersensitivity to trehalose-6, 6′-dimycolate (cord factor) in mice infected with BCG. *Infect. Immun.*, **7**:631–638.

Bekierkunst, A., Levy, I. S., Yarkoni, E., Vilkas, E., Adams, A., and Lederer, E. (1969). Granuloma formation induction in mice by chemically defined mycobacterial fractions. *J. Bacteriol.*, **100**: 95–102.

Bekierkunst, A., Levy, I. S., Yarkoni, E., Vilkas, E., and Lederer, E. (1971). Cellular reaction in the footpad and draining lymph node of mice induced by mycobacterial fractions and BCG bacilli. *Infect. Immun.*, **4**:245–255.

Bernardo, J., Hunninghake, G. W., Gadek, J. E., Ferrans, V. J., and Crystal, R. G. (1979). Acute hypersensitivity pneumonitis: Serial changes in lung lymphocyte subpopulations after exposure to antigen. *Am. Rev. Respir. Dis.*, **120**:985–994.

Bice, D. E., Salvaggio, J. E., and Hoffman, E. (1976). Passive transfer of experimental hypersensitivity pneumonitis with lymphoid cells in the rabbit. *J. Allergy Clin. Immunol.*, **58**:250–262.

Bloch, E. H., Abdel Wahab, M. F., and Warren, K. S. (1972). In vivo microscopic observations of the pathogenesis and pathophysiology of hepatosplenic schistosomiasis in the mouse liver. *Am. J. Trop. Med. Hyg.*, **21**:546–557.

Bogitsh, B. J. (1971). *Schistosoma mansoni*: Cytochemistry of eosinophils in egg-caused early hepatic granulomas of mice. *Exp. Parasitol.*, **29**: 493–500.

Boros, D. L. (1978). Granulomatous inflammations. *Prog. Allergy*, **24**: 183–267.

Boros, D. L. (1981). The role of lymphokines in granulomatous inflammations. In *Lymphokines: A Forum for Immunoregulatory Cell Products,* vol. 3. Edited by E. Pick. New York, Academic, pp. 257–281.

Boros, D. L., and Carrick, L., Jr. (1980). The artificial granuloma. II. Induction of pulmonary granuloma formation by exogenous, circulating and localized granuloma-derived lymphokines. In *Biochemical Characterization of Lymphokines.* Edited by A. De Weck. New York, Academic, pp. 599–604.

Boros, D. L., and Warren, K. S. (1970). Delayed hypersensitivity type granuloma formation and dermal reaction induced and elicited by a soluble factor isolated from *Schistosoma mansoni* eggs. *J. Exp. Med.,* **132**:488–507.

Boros, D. L., and Warren, K. S. (1971). Specific granulomatous hypersensitivity elicited by bentonite particles coated with soluble antigens from schistosome eggs and tubercle bacilli. *Nature,* **229**:200–201.

Boros, D. L., and Warren, K. S. (1973). The bentonite granuloma: Characterization of a model system for infectious and foreign body granulomatous inflammation using soluble Mycobacterial, Histoplasma, and Schistosoma antigens. *Immunology,* **24**:519–529.

Boros, D. L., Schwartz, H. J., Powell, A. E., and Warren, K. S. (1973a). Delayed hypersensitivity as manifested by granuloma formation, dermal reactivity, macrophage migration inhibition, and lymphocyte transformation, induced and elicited in guinea pigs with soluble antigens of *Schistosoma mansoni* eggs. *J. Immunol.,* **110**:1118–1125.

Boros, D. L., Warren, K. S., and Pelley, R. P. (1973b). The secretion of migration inhibition factor by intact schistosome egg granulomas maintained in vitro. *Nature,* **246**:224–226.

Boros, D. L., Pelley, R. P., and Warren, K. S. (1975). Spontaneous modulation of granulomatous hypersensitivity in schistosomiasis mansoni. *J. Immunol.,* **114**:1437–1441.

Boros, D. L., Tomford, R., and Warren, K. S. (1977). Induction of granulomatous and elicitation of cutaneous sensitivity by partially purified SEA of *Schistosoma mansoni.* *J. Immunol.,* **118**:373–376.

Boros, D. L., Lande, M. A., and Carrick, L., Jr. (1981). The artificial granuloma. III. Collagen synthesis during the cell-mediated granulomatous response as determined in explanted granulomas. *Clin. Immunol. Immunopathol.,* **18**:276–286.

Brentjens, J. R., O'Connell, D. W., Pawlowski, I. B., Hsu, K. C., and Andres, G. (1974). Experimental immune complex disease of the lung. The pathogenesis of a laboratory model resembling certain human interstitial lung diseases. *J. Exp. Med.,* **140**:105–125.

Browett, P. J., Simpson, L. O., and Blennerhassett, J. B. (1980). Experimental granulomatous inflammation: The ultrastructure of the reaction of guinea pigs to bentonite injection. *J. Pathol.,* **130**: 57–64.

Buchanan, R. D., Fine, D. P., and Colley, D. G. (1973). *Schistosoma mansoni* infection in mice depleted of thymus-dependent lymphocytes. II. Pathology and altered pathogenesis. *Am. J. Pathol.,* **71**:207–214.

Bültmann, B., Heymer, B., Haferkamp, O., and Schmidt, W. C. (1970). Untersuchungen zur zellgebundenen überempfindlichkeit gegen Streptokokkenzellwandantigene. *Verh. Dtsch. Ges. Pathol.,* **54**: 329–332.

Burrell, R., and Hill, J. O. (1975). The effect of respiratory immunization on cell-mediated immune effector cells of the lung. *Clin. Exp. Immunol.*, **24**:116–124.

Byram, J. E., and von Lichtenberg, F. (1977). Altered schistosome granuloma formation in nude mice. *Am. J. Trop. Med. Hyg.*, **26**: 944–956.

Cameron, G. R., and Ganguly, N. C. (1964). An experimental study of the pathogenesis and reversibility of schistosomal hepatic fibrosis. *J. Pathol. Bacteriol.*, **87**:217–237.

Carrick, L., Jr., and Boros, D. L. (1980). The artificial granuloma. I. In vitro lymphokine production by pulmonary artificial hypersensitivity granulomas. *Clin. Immunol. Immunopathol.*, **17**:415–426.

Chedid, L., Parant, M., Parant, F., Lefrancier, P., Choay, J., and Lederer, E. (1977). Enhancement of nonspecific immunity to *Klebsiella pneumoniae* infection by a synthetic immunoadjuvant (n-acetyl-muramyl-L-alanyl-D-isoglutamine) and several analogs. *Proc. Natl. Acad. Sci. U.S.A.*, **74**:2089–2093.

Chedid, L., Audibert, F., and Johnson, A. G. (1978). Biological activities of muramyl dipeptide, a synthetic glycopeptide to bacterial immuno-regulating agents. *Prog. Allergy*, **25**:63–105.

Chedid, L., Carelli, C., and Audibert, F. (1979). Recent developments concerning muramyl dipeptide, a synthetic immunoregulating molecule. *J. Reticuloendothel. Soc.*, **26**:631–641.

Cheever, A. W. (1965). A comparative study of *Schistosoma mansoni* infections in mice, gerbils, multimammate rats and hamsters. I. The relation of portal hypertension to size of hepatic granulomas. *Am. J. Trop. Med. Hyg.*, **14**:211–226.

Chensue, S. W., and Boros, D. L. (1979a). Population dynamics of T and B lymphocytes in the lymphoid organs, circulation, and granulomas of mice infected with *Schistosoma mansoni*. *Am. J. Trop. Med. Hyg.*, **28**:291–299.

Chensue, S. W., and Boros, D. L. (1979b). Modulation of granulomatous hypersensitivity. I. Characterization of T lymphocytes involved in the adoptive suppression of granuloma formation in *Schistosoma mansoni* infected mice. *J. Immunol.*, **123**:1409–1414.

Chensue, S. W., Boros, D. L., and David, C. S. (1980). Regulation of granulomatous inflammation in murine schistosomiasis: In vitro characterization of T lymphocyte subsets involved in the production and suppression of migration inhibition factor (MIF). *J. Exp. Med.*, **151**:1398–1412.

Chensue, S. W., Wellhausen, S. R., and Boros, D. L. (1981). Modulation of granulomatous hypersensitivity. II. Participation of $Ly1^+$ and $Ly2^+$, T lymphocytes in the suppression of granuloma formation and lymphokine production in *Schistosoma mansoni* infected mice. *J. Immunol.*, **127**:363–367.

Colley, D. G. (1971). Schistosomal egg antigen-induced lymphocyte blastogenesis in experimental murine *Schistosoma mansoni* infection. *J. Immunol.,* **107**:1477–1480.

Colley, D. G. (1975). Immune responses to a soluble schistosomal egg antigen preparation during chronic primary infection with *Schistosoma mansoni. J. Immunol.,* **115**:150–156.

Colley, D. G. (1976). Adoptive suppression of granuloma formation. *J. Exp. Med.,* **143**:696–700.

Colley, D. G., Lewis, F. A., and Todd, C. W. (1979). Adoptive suppression of granuloma formation by T lymphocytes and lymphoid cells sensitive to cyclophosphamide. *Cell. Immunol.,* **46**:192–200.

Collins, F. M., Congdon, C. C., and Morrison, N. E. (1975). Growth of *Mycobacterium bovis* (BCG) in T lymphocyte-deprived mice. *Infect. Immun.,* **11**:57–64.

Dannenberg, A. M., Jr. (1980). Pathogenesis of tuberculosis. In *Pulmonary Diseases and Disorders.* Edited by A. P. Fishman. New York, McGraw-Hill, pp. 1264–1281.

Dannenberg, A. M., Jr., Ando, M., and Shima, K. (1972). Macrophage accumulation, division, maturation, and digestive and microbicidal capacities in tuberculous lesions. III. The turnover of macrophages and its relation to their activation and antimicrobial immunity in primary BCG lesions and those of reinfection. *J. Immunol.,* **109**: 1109–1121.

Davies, P., Page, R. C., and Allison, A. C. (1974). Changes in cellular enzyme levels and extracellular release of lysosomal acid hydrolases in macrophages exposed to group A streptococcal cell wall substances. *J. Exp. Med.,* **139**:1262–1282.

Domingo, E. O., and Warren, K. S. (1968). Endogenous desensitization: Changing host granulomatous response to schistosome eggs at different stages of infection with *Schistosoma mansoni. Am. J. Pathol.,* **52**:369–380.

Dunn, M. A., Rojkind, M., Warren, K. S., Hait, P. K., Rifas, L., and Seifter, S. (1977). Liver collagen synthesis in murine schistosomiasis. *J. Clin. Invest.,* **59**:666–674.

Dunsford, H. A., Lucia, H. L., Doughty, B. L., and von Lichtenberg, F. (1974). Artificial granulomas from bentonite and latex carrier particles. *Am. J. Trop. Med. Hyg.,* **23**:203–217.

Edungbola, L. D., and Schiller, E. L. (1979). Histopathology of hepatic and pulmonary granulomata experimentally induced with eggs of *Schistosoma mansoni. J. Parasitol.,* **65**:253–261.

Ellouz, F., Adam, A., Ciorbaru, R., and Lederer, E. (1974). Minimal structural requirements for adjuvant activity of bacterial peptidoglycan derivatives. *Biochem. Biophys. Res. Commun.,* **59**:1317–1325.

Emori, K., and Tanaka, A. (1978). Granuloma formation by synthetic
bacterial cell wall fragment: Muramyl dipeptide. *Infect. Immun.*,
19:613–620.

Epstein, W. L. (1967). Granulomatous hypersensitivity. *Prog. Allergy*,
11:36–88.

Fink, J. N. (1978). Hypersensitivity pneumonitis. In *Allergy: Principles
and Practice.* Edited by E. Middleton, C. E. Reed, and E. F. Ellis.
St. Louis, Mosby, pp. 855–967.

Fink, J. N., Hensley, G., and Barboriak, J. (1970). An animal model of
hypersensitivity pneumonitis. *J. Allergy,* **46**:156–161.

Galindo, B., and Myrvik, Q. N. (1970). Migratory response of
granulomatous alveolar cells from BCG-sensitized rabbits. *J.
Immunol.,* **105**:227–237.

Galindo, B., Lazdins, J., and Castillo, R. (1974). Fusion of normal rabbit
alveolar macrophages induced by supernatant fluids from BCG-
sensitized lymph node cells after elicitation by antigen. *Infect.
Immun.,* **9**:212–216.

Galindo, B., Myrvik, Q. N., and Love, S. H. (1975). A macrophage
agglutinating factor produced during a pulmonary delayed hypersensitivity reaction. *J. Reticuloendothel. Soc.,* **18**:295–304.

Gee, J. B. L., Bodel, P. T., Zorn, S. K., Hinman, L. M., Stevens, C. A.,
and Matthay, R. A. (1978). Sarcoidosis and mononuclear phagocytes.
Lung, **155**:243–253.

Ginsburg, I. (1972). Mechanisms of cell and tissue injury induced by
group A streptococci. Relation to poststreptococcal sequelae. *J.
Infect. Dis.,* **126**:294–340.

Ginsburg, I. (1979). The role of lysosomal factors of leukocytes in the
biodegradation and storage of microbial constitutents in infectious
granulomas. In *Lysosomes in Applied Biology and Therapeutics.*
Edited by J. T. Dingle, P. J. Jacques, and I. H. Shaw. New York,
North Holland Publishing, pp. 327–398.

Ginsburg, I., Zor, U., and Floman, Y. (1977). Experimental models of
streptococcal arthritis: Pathogenetic role of streptococcal products
and prostaglandins and their modification by antiinflammatory agents.
In *Experimental Models of Chronic Inflammatory Diseases.* Edited
by L. E. Glynn and H. D. Schlumberger. Berlin, Springer Verlag,
pp. 256–299.

Goodwin, J. S., DeHoratius, R., Israel, H., Peake, G. T., and Messner, R. P.
(1979). Suppressor cell function in sarcoidosis. *Ann. Intern. Med.,*
90:169–173.

Granger, D. L., Yamamoto, K.-I., and Ribi, E. (1976). Delayed hypersensitivity and granulomatous response after immunization with
protein antigens associated with a mycobacterial glycolipid and oil
droplets. *J. Immunol.,* **116**:482–488.

Greenblatt, J., Boackle, R. J., and Schwab, J. H. (1978). Activation of the alternate complement pathway by peptidoglycan from streptococcal cell wall. *Infect. Immun.*, **19**:296–303.

Haferkamp, O., Heymer, B., Schäfer, H., Hsu, K., and Schmidt, W. C. (1970). Ein Beitrag zur Immunopathologie der granulomatösen Entzündung. *Verh. Dtsch. Ges. Pathol.*, **54**:325–329.

Hang, L. M., Warren, K. S., and Boros, D. L. (1974). *Schistosoma mansoni*: Antigenic secretions and the etiology of egg granulomas in mice. *Exp. Parasitol.*, **35**:288–298.

Harris, J. O., Bice, D., and Salvaggio, J. E. (1976). Cellular and humoral bronchopulmonary immune response of rabbits immunized with thermophilic actinomyces antigen. *Am. Rev. Respir. Dis.*, **114**: 29–43.

Hensley, G. T., Fink, J. N., and Barboriak, J. J. (1974). Hypersensitivity pneumonitis in the monkey. *Arch. Pathol.*, **97**:33–38.

Henson, P. M., McCarthy, K., Larsen, G. L., Webster, R. O., Giclas, P. C., Dreisin, R. B., King, T. E., and Shaw, J. O. (1979). Complement fragments, alveolar macrophages and alveolitis. *Am. J. Pathol.*, **97**: 93–110.

Heymer, B., Bültmann, B., and Haferkamp, O. (1971). Toxicity of streptococcal mucopeptides in vivo and in vitro. *J. Immunol.*, **106**: 858–861.

Heymer, B., Bültmann, B., Schachenmayr, W., Spanel, R., Haferkamp, O., and Schmidt, W. C. (1973). Migration inhibition of rat peritoneal cells induced by streptococcal mucopeptides. Characteristics of the reaction and properties of the mucopeptide preparations. *J. Immunol.*, **111**:1743–1754.

Holton, J. B., and Schwab, J. H. (1966). Adjuvant properties of bacterial cell wall mucopeptides. *J. Immunol.*, **96**:134–138.

Hood, A. T., and Boros, D. L. (1980). The effect of splenectomy on the pathophysiology and egg-specific immune response of *Schistosoma mansoni*-infected mice. *Am. J. Trop. Med. Hyg.*, **29**:586–591.

Hunninghake, G. W., Gadek, J. E., Young, R. C., Kawanami, O., Ferrans, V. J., and Crystal, R. G. (1980). Maintenance of granuloma formation in pulmonary sarcoidosis by T lymphocytes within the lung. *N. Engl. J. Med.*, **302**:594–598.

James, S. L., and Colley, D. G. (1975). Eosinophils and immune mechanisms: Production of the lymphokine eosinophil stimulation promotor (ESP) in vitro by isolated intact granulomas. *J. Reticuloendothel. Soc.*, **18**:283–293.

James, D. G., and Neville, E. (1977). Pathobiology of sarcoidosis. *Pathobiol. Annu.*, **7**:31–61.

Johnson, K. J., and Ward, P. (1974). Acute immunologic pulmonary
  alveolitis. *J. Clin. Invest.,* **54**:349–357.
Johnson, K. J., Chapman, W. E., and Ward, P. A. (1979). Immunopathology
  of the lung: A review. *Am. J. Pathol.,* **95**:793–844.
Johnston, R. B., Jr., Godzik, C. A., and Cohn, Z. A. (1978). Increased
  superoxide anion production by immunologically activated and
  chemically elicited macrophages. *J. Exp. Med.,* **148**:115–127.
Jones, J. M., and Schwab, J. H. (1970). Immune response to cell wall
  and tissue antigens in rabbits injured with streptococcal cell wall
  fragments. *Int. Arch. Allergy Appl. Immunol.,* **39**:445–448.
Kasdon, E. J., and Schlossman, S. F. (1973). An experimental model of
  pulmonary arterial granulomatous inflammation. *Am. J. Pathol.,*
  71:365–374.
Kasdon, E. J., Jones, G., and Schlossman, S. F. (1974). Experimental
  intradermal granuloma formation. *J. Invest. Dermatol.,* **63**:411–414.
Kato, M. (1969). Studies of a biochemical lesion in experimental
  tuberculosis in mice. XI. Motochondrial swelling induced by cord
  factor in vitro. *Am. Rev. Respir. Dis.,* **100**:47–53.
Kato, M. (1972). Antibody formation to trehalose-6, 6′-dimycolate (cord
  factor) of *Mycobacterium tuberculosis. Infect. Immun.,* **5**:203–212.
Kato, M. (1973). Effect of anti-cord factor antibody on experimental
  tuberculosis in mice. *Infect. Immun.,* **7**:14–21.
Kato, M., and Fukushi, K. (1969). Studies of a biochemical lesion in
  experimental tuberculosis in mice. X. Mitochondrial swelling induced
  by cord factor in vivo and accompanying biochemical change. *Am.
  Rev. Respir. Dis.,* **100**:42–46.
Kawai, T., Salvaggio, J., Lake, W., and Harris, J. O. (1972). Experimental
  production of hypersensitivity pneumonitis with bagasse and
  thermophilic actinomycete antigen. *J. Allergy Clin. Immunol.,* **50**:
  276–288.
Koga, T., Kotani, S., Narita, T., and Pearson, C. P. (1976). Induction of
  adjuvant arthritis in the rat by various bacterial cell walls and their
  water-soluble components. *Int. Arch. Allergy Appl. Immunol.,* **51**:
  206–213.
Kohashi, O., Pearson, C. M., Watanabe, Y., Kotani, S., and Koga, T. (1976).
  Structural requirements for arthritogenicity of peptidoglycans from
  Staphylococcus aureus and *Lactobacillus plantarum* and analogous
  synthetic compounds. *J. Immunol.,* **116**:1635–1639.
Krause, R. M., and McCarty, M. (1961). Studies on the chemical structure
  of the streptococcal cell wall. I. The identification of a mucopeptide
  in the cell walls of groups A and A-variant streptococci. *J. Exp.
  Med.,* **114**:127–140.

Leake, E. S., and Myrvik, Q. N. (1968). Changes in morphology and in lysozyme content of free alveolar cells after the intravenous injection of killed BCG in oil. *J. Reticuloendothel. Soc.,* **5**:33–53.

Lopez, M., and Salvaggio, J. (1976). Hypersensitivity pneumonitis: Current concepts of etiology and pathogenesis. *Ann. Rev. Med.,* **27**:453–463.

Löwy, I., Constantin, B., and Chedid, L. (1977). Target cells for the activity of a synthetic adjuvant: Muramyl dipeptide. *Cell. Immunol.,* **29**:195–199.

Marx, J. J., Jr., and Flaherty, D. K. (1976). Activation of the complement sequence by extracts of bacteria and fungi associated with hypersensitivity pneumonitis. *J. Allergy Clin. Immunol.,* **57**:328–334.

Masih, N., Majeska, J., and Yoshida, T. (1979). Studies on experimental pulmonary granulomas. I. Detection of lymphokines in granulomatous lesions. *Am. J. Pathol.,* **95**:391–406.

McCue, R. E., Dannenberg, A. M., Jr., Higuchi, S., and Sugimoto, M. (1978). The effect of cortisone on the accumulation and necrosis of macrophages in tuberculous lesions. *Inflammation,* **3**:159–176.

McGee, M. P., and Myrvik, Q. N. (1976). Hydrolase levels in necrotizing and non-necrotizing BCG-induced pulmonary granulomas. *J. Reticuloendothel. Soc.,* **20**:187–195.

McGee, M. P., and Myrvik, Q. N. (1979). Phagocytosis-induced injury of normal and activated alveolar macrophages. *Infect. Immun.,* **26**: 910–915.

McLaughlin, C. A., Parker, R., Hadlow, W. J., Toubiana, R., and Ribi, E. (1978). Moieties of mycobacterial mycolates required for inducing granulomatous reactions. *Cell Immunol.,* **38**:14–24.

Merser, C., Sinäy, P., and Adam, A. (1975). Total synthesis and adjuvant activity of bacterial peptidoglycan derivatives. *Biochem. Biophys. Res. Commun.,* **66**:1316–1322.

Meyer, T. J., Ribi, E., and Azuma, I. (1975). Biologically active components from mycobacterial cell walls. V. Granuloma formation in mouse lungs and guinea pig skin. *Cell. Immunol.,* **16**:11–24.

Miyamoto, T., Kabe, J., Noda, M., Kobayashi, N., and Miura, K. (1971). Physiologic and pathologic respiratory changes in delayed hypersensitivity reaction in guinea pigs. *Am. Rev. Respir. Dis.,* **103**:509–515.

Modolell, M., Luckenbach, G. A., Parant, M., and Munder, P. G. (1974). The adjuvant activity of a mycobacterial water soluble adjuvant (WSA) in vitro. I. The requirement of macrophages. *J. Immunol.,* **113**:395–403.

Moore, V. L., and Myrvik, Q. N. (1970). Effect of antimacrophage serum on dermal tuberculin sensitivity and allergic pulmonary granuloma formation in rabbits. *Infect. Immun.,* **2**:810–814.

Moore, V. L., and Myrvik, Q. N. (1973). Relationship of BCG induced pulmonary delayed hypersensitivity to accelerated granuloma formation in rabbits' lungs: Effect of cortisone acetate. *Infect. Immun.,* 7:764–770.

Moore, V. L., Myrvik, Q. N., and Kato, M. (1972). Role of cord factor (trehalose-6, 6'-dimycolate) in allergic granuloma formation in rabbits. *Infect. Immun.,* 6:5–8.

Moore, V. L., Myrvik, Q. N., and Leake, E. S. (1973). Specificity of a BCG induced pulmonary granulomatous response in rabbits. *Infect. Immun.,* 7:743–746.

Moore, V. L., Hensley, G. T., and Fink, J. N. (1975). An animal model of hypersensitivity pneumonitis in the rabbit. *J. Clin. Invest.,* 56:937–944.

Myrvik, Q. N. (1972). Function of the alveolar macrophage in immunity. *J. Reticuloendothel. Soc.,* 11:459–468.

Myrvik, Q. N., Leake, E. S., and Oshima, S. A. (1962). A study of macrophages and epithelioid-like cells from granulomatous (BCG-induced) lungs of rabbits. *J. Immunol.,* 89:745–751.

Myrvik, Q. N., Kohlweiss, L. A., and Harpold, D. (1975). Pathological potential of exaggerated immunological reactions. In *Microbiology–1975.* Edited by D. Schlessinger. Washington, D. C., American Society for Microbiology, pp. 227–235.

Nagao, S., Tanaka, A., Yamamoto, Y., Koga, T., Onoue, K., Shiba, T., Kusumoto, K., and Kotani, S. (1979). Inhibition of macrophage migration by muramyl peptides. *Infect. Immun.,* 24:308–312.

Ofek, I., and Bekierkunst, A. (1976). Chemotactic response of leukocytes to cord factor (trehalose-6, 6'-dimycolate). *J. Natl. Cancer Inst.,* 57:1379–1381.

Ohanian, S. H., and Schwab, J. H. (1967). Persistence of group A streptococcal cell walls related to chronic inflammation of rabbit dermal connective tissue. *J. Exp. Med.,* 125:1137–1148.

Olenchok, S. A. (1977). Animal models of hypersensitivity pneumonitis: A review. *Ann. Allergy,* 38:119–126.

Page, R. C., Davies, P., and Allison, A. C. (1978). The macrophage as a secretory cell. *Int. Rev. Cytol.,* 52:119–157.

Papadimitriou, J. M., and Walters, M. N.-I. (1979). Macrophage polykarya. *CRC Crit. Rev. Toxicol.,* 6:211–255.

Parks, D. E., and Weiser, R. S. (1975). The role of phagocytes and natural lymphokines in the fusion of alveolar macrophages to form Langhans giant cells. *J. Reticuloendothel. Soc.,* 17:219–228.

Pelley, R. P., Pelley, R. J., Hamburger, J., Peters, P. A., and Warren, K. S. (1976). *Schistosoma mansoni* soluble egg antigens. I. Identification and purification of three major antigens, and the employment of radioimmunoassay for their further characterization. *J. Immunol.,* 117:1553–1560.

Pepys, J. (1977). Clinical and therapeutic significance of patterns of allergic reactions of the lungs to extrinsic agents. *Am. Rev. Respir. Dis.*, **116**:573–588.

Perrotto, J. L., Falchuk, K. R., Pelley, R. P., and Warren, K. S. (1976). Serum lysozyme and beta-glucuronidase in experimentally induced granulomatous inflammation. *Ann. N.Y. Acad. Sci.*, **278**:592–598.

Peterson, L. B., Thrall, R. S., Moore, V. L., Stevens, J. O., and Abramoff, P. (1977). An animal model of hypersensitivity pneumonitis in the rabbit. Induction of cellular hypersensitivity to inhaled antigens using carrageenan and BCG. *Am. Rev. Respir. Dis.*, **116**:1007–1012.

Peterson, L. B., Braley, J. F., Calvanico, N. J., and Moore, V. L. (1979). An animal model of hypersensitivity pneumonitis in rabbits. Development of chronic pulmonary inflammation and cell-mediated hypersensitivity after repeated aerosol challenge. *Am. Rev. Respir. Dis.*, **119**:991–999.

Phillips, S. M., Diconza, J. J., Gold, J. A., and Reid, W. A. (1977). Schistosomiasis in the congenitally athymic (nude) mouse. I. Thymic dependency of eosinophilia, granuloma formation, and host morbidity. *J. Immunol.*, **118**:594–599.

Phillips, S. M., Reid, W. A., Doughty, B. L., and Bentley, A. G. (1980). The immunologic modulation of morbidity in schistosomiasis. *Am. J. Trop. Med. Hyg.*, **29**:820–831.

Rapp, H. J., Yarkoni, E., Ruco, L., and Hunter, J. T. (1978). Immunotherapy of a guinea pig hepatoma with vaccines containing mycobacterial fractions: Comparison of cell walls and trehalose-6, 6'-dimycolate. *Cancer Immunol. Immunother.*, **3**:179–181.

Ribi, E. E., Granger, D. L., Milner, K. C., and Strain, S. M. (1975). Tumor regression caused by endotoxins and mycobacterial fractions. *J. Natl. Cancer Inst.*, **55**:1253–1257.

Richerson, H. B. (1972). Acute experimental hypersensitivity pneumonitis in the guinea pig. *J. Lab. Clin. Med.*, **79**:745–757.

Richerson, H. B. (1974). Varieties of acute immunologic damage to the rabbit lung. *Ann. N.Y. Acad. Sci.*, **221**:340–360.

Richerson, H. B., Seidenfeld, J. J., Ratajczak, H. V., and Richards, D. W. (1978). Chronic experimental interstitial pneumonitis in the rabbit. *Am. Rev. Respir. Dis.*, **117**:5–13.

Rickles, N., Zilberstein, Z., Krause, S., Arad, G., Kaufstein, M., and Ginsburg, I. (1969). Persistence of group A streptococci labeled with fluorescein isothiocyanate in inflammatory sites in the heart and muscle of mice and rabbits. *Proc. Soc. Exp. Biol. Med.*, **131**:525–530.

Ridley, M. J., Ridley, D. S., and Turk, J. L. (1978). Surface markers on lymphocytes and cells of the mononuclear phagocyte series in skin sections in leprosy. *J. Pathol.*, **125**:91–98.

Roberts, R. C., and Moore, V. L. (1977). Immunopathogenesis of hypersensitivity pneumonitis. *Am. Rev. Respir. Dis.,* **116**:1075–1090.

Rojas-Espinosa, O., Dannenberg, A. M., Sternburger, L. A., and Tsuda, T. (1974). The role of cathespin D in the pathogenesis of tuberculosis. A histochemical study employing unlabeled antibodies and the peroxidase-antiperoxidase complex. *Am. J. Pathol.,* **74**:1–18.

Roska, A. K. B., Garancis, J. C., Moore, V. L., and Abramoff, P. (1977). Immune-complex disease in guinea pig lungs. I. Elicitation by aerosol challenge, suppression with cobra venom factor, and passive transfer with serum. *Clin. Immunol. Immunopathol.,* **8**:213–224.

Ryan, G. B., and Spector, W. G. (1970). Macrophage turnover in inflamed connective tissue. *Proc. R. Soc. Lond. Ser. B.,* **175**:269–292.

Salvaggio, J. E. (1979). Immunological mechanisms in pulmonary diseases. *Clin. Allergy,* **9**:659–668.

Salvaggio, J., Phanuphak, P., Stanford, R., Bice, D., and Claman, H. (1975). Experimental production of granulomatous pneumonitis. *J. Allergy Clin. Immunol.,* **56**:364–380.

Schorlemmer, H. U., Edwards, J. H., Davies, P., and Allison, A. C. (1977). Macrophage responses to mouldy hay dust, *Micropolyspora faeni* and zymosan, activators of complement by the alternative pathway. *Clin. Exp. Immunol.,* **27**:198–207.

Schriber, R. A., and Zucker-Franklin, D. (1975). Induction of blood eosinophilia by pulmonary embolization of antigen-coated particles: The relationship to cell-mediated immunity. *J. Immunol.,* **114**: 1348–1353.

Schwab, J. H., and Ohanian, S. H. (1968). Biological properties related to chemical structures of the streptococcal cell. In *Current Research on Group A Streptococcus.* Edited by R. Caravano. Amsterdam, Excerpta Medica, pp. 80–88.

Schwab, J. H., and Smialowicz, R. (1975). Interaction of bacterial cell wall polymers and rat macrophages. *Z. Immunol. Forsch.,* **1495**: 283–288.

Schwab, J. H., Gooder, H., and Maxted, W. R. (1962). Further studies on toxic C polysaccharide complexes of the haemolytic streptococci. *Br. J. Exp. Pathol.,* **43**:181–188.

Sellin, D., Smith, T. B., and Schmidt, W. C. (1968). Immunhistologische Untersuchungen an Lebergranulomen der Maus nach Streptokokken-Injektion. *Verh. Dtsch. Ges. Pathol.,* **52**:547–549.

Sellin, D., Heymer, B., Smith, T. B., Bültmann, B., Haferkamp, O., and Schmidt, W. C. (1970). Streptococcal A-carbohydrate antigen in granulomata of mouse liver after intravenous injection of heat-killed group A streptococci. *Arch. Pathol.,* **90**:17–21.

Shima, K., Dannenberg, A. M., Jr., Ando, M., Chandrasekhar, S., Seluzicki, J. A., and Fabrikant, J. I. (1972). Macrophage accumulation, division, maturation and digestive and microbicidal capacities in tuberculous lesion. I. Studies involving their incorporation of tritiated thymidine and their content of lysosomal enzymes and bacilli. *Am. J. Pathol.*, **67**:159–180.

Smialowicz, R. J., and Schwab, J. H. (1977). Processing of streptococcal cell walls by rat macrophages and human monocytes in vitro. *Infect. Immun.*, **17**:591–598.

Spector, W. G. (1969). The granulomatous inflammatory exudate. *Int. Rev. Exp. Pathol.*, **8**:1–55.

Spector, W. G. (1974). The macrophage: Its origins and role in pathology. *Pathobiol. Annu.*, **4**:33–64.

Spector, W. G., and Ryan, G. B. (1970). The mononuclear phagocyte in inflammation. In *Mononuclear Phagocytes.* Edited by R. van Furth. Philadelphia, Davis, pp. 219–232.

Spector, W. G., Lykke, A. W. J., and Willoughby, D. A. (1967). A quantitative study of leukocyte emigration in chronic inflammatory granulomata. *J. Pathol. Bacteriol.*, **93**:101–107.

Stankus, R. P., Cashner, F. M., and Salvaggio, J. E. (1978). Bronchopulmonary macrophage activation in the pathogenesis of hypersensitivity pneumonitis. *J. Immunol.*, **120**:685–688.

Stenger, R. J., Warren, K. S., and Johnson, E. A. (1967). An ultrastructural study of hepatic granulomas and schistosome egg shells in murine hepatosplenic *Schistosomiasis mansoni. Exp. Mol. Pathol.*, **7**:116–132.

Suga, M., Dannenberg, A. M., Jr., and Higuchi, S. (1980). Macrophage functional heterogeneity in vivo: Macrolocal and microlocal macrophage activation, identified by double-staining tissue sections of BCG granulomas for pairs of enzymes. *Am. J. Pathol.*, **99**:305–324.

Sugimoto, M., Dannenberg, A. M., Jr., Wahl, L. M., Ettinger, W. H., Jr., Hastie, A. T., Daniels, D. C., Thomas, C. R., and Demoulin-Brahy, L. (1978a). Extracellular hydrolytic enzymes of rabbit dermal tuberculous lesions and tuberculin reactions collected in skin chambers. *Am. J. Pathol.*, **90**:583–606.

Sugimoto, M., Germain, R. N., Chedid, L., and Benacerraf, B. (1978b). Enhancement of carrier-specific helper T cell function by the synthetic adjuvant, n-acetyl muramyl-L-alanyl-D-isoglutamine (MDP). *J. Immunol.*, **120**:980–982.

Takahashi, S., Dunn, M. A., and Seifter, S. (1980). Liver collagenase in murine schistosomiasis. *Gastroenterology,* **78**:1425–1431.

Tanaka, A., and Emori, K. (1980). Epithelioid granuloma formation by a synthetic bacterial cell wall component, muramyl dipeptide (MDP). *Am. J. Pathol.*, **98**:773–748.

Tanaka, A., Nagao, S., Nagao, R., Kotani, S., Shiba, T., and Kusumoto, S. (1979). Stimulation of the reticuloendothelial system of mice by muramyl dipeptide. *Infect. Immun.,* **24**:302–307.

Tannenbaum, H., Rocklin, R. E., Schur, P. H., and Sheffer, A. L. (1976). Immunological identification of subpopulations of mononuclear cells in sarcoid granulomas. *Ann. N.Y. Acad. Sci.,* **278**:136–146.

Thomas, A. R., Rhodes, M. L., and Richerson, H. B. (1974). Ultrastructural studies of acute hypersensitivity pneumonitis in rabbits. *J. Allergy Clin. Immunol.,* **54**:147–156.

Tsuda, T., Dannenberg, A. M., Ando, M., Rojas-Espinosa, O., and Shima, K. (1974). Enzymes in tuberculous lesions hydrolyzing protein, hyaluronic acid and chondroitin sulfate. A study of isolated macrophages and developing and healing rabbit BCG lesions with substrate film techniques: The shift of enzyme pH optima towards neutrality in 'intact' cells and tissue. *J. Reticuloendothel. Soc.,* **16**:220–231.

Ueda, K., Yamazaki, S., and Someya, S. (1976). Experimental mycobacterial infection in congenitally athymic "nude" mice. *J. Reticuloendothel. Soc.,* **19**:77–90.

Unanue, E. R., and Benacerraf, B. (1973). Immunological events in experimental hypersensitivity granulomas. *Am. J. Pathol.,* **71**:349–364.

van der Rhee, H. J., van der Burgh-de Winter, C. P. M., and Daems, W. T. (1979). The differentiation of monocytes into macrophages, epithelioid cells and multinucleated giant cells in subcutaneous granulomas. *Cell Tissue Res.,* **197**:355–378.

van Furth, R. (1976). Origin and kinetics of mononuclear phagocytes. *Ann. N.Y. Acad. Sci.,* **278**:161–175.

von Lichtenberg, F. (1964). Studies on granuloma formation. III. Antigen sequestration and destruction in the schistosome pseudotubercle. *Am. J. Pathol.,* **45**:75–94.

von Lichtenberg, F., Smith, T. M., Lucia, H. L., and Doughty, B. L. (1971). New model for schistosome granuloma formation using a soluble egg antigen and bentonite particles. *Nature,* **229**:199–200.

van Marck, E. A. E., Stoker, S., Grimaud, J. A., Kestens, L., Gigase, P. L. J., and Deelder, A. M. (1980). The implantation of sepharose beads in mouse livers as an aid in the study of hepatic schistosomal fibrosis. *Experientia,* **36**:1116–1118.

Wahl, S. M., Wahl, L. M., McCarthy, J. B., Chedid, L., and Mergenhagen, S. E. (1978). Macrophage activation by mycobacterial water soluble compounds and synthetic muramyl dipeptide. *J. Immunol.,* **122**: 2226–2231.

Warren, K. S. (1962). The influence of treatment on the development and course of murine hepato-splenic *Schistosomiasis mansoni. Trans. R. Soc. Trop. Med. Hyg.,* **56**:510–519.

Warren, K. S. (1973). The pathology of schistosome infections. *Helm. Abstr.,* **42**:592–633.

Warren, K. S. (1978). Hepatosplenic schistosomiasis: A great neglected disease of the liver. *Gut,* **19**:572–577.

Warren, K. S., Domingo, E. O., and Cowan, R. B. T. (1967). Granuloma formation around schistosome eggs as a manifestation of delayed hypersensitivity. *Am. J. Pathol.,* **51**:735–756.

Weinstock, J. V., Boros, D. L., and Gee, J. B. (1981). Enhanced angiotensin I converting enzyme activity associated with modulation in murine schistosomiasis. *Gastroenterology,* **81**:48–53.

Wellhausen, S. R., and Boros, D. L. (1981). Characterization and functional analysis of inflammatory lymphocytes isolated from liver granulomas of *Schistosoma mansoni* infected mice. *Fed. Proc.,* **40**:1002.

Wellhausen, S. R., Chensue, S. W., and Boros, D. L. (1980). Modulation of granulomatous hypersensitivity: Analysis by adoptive transfer of effector and suppressor T lymphocytes involved in granulomatous inflammation in murine schistosomiasis. In *Basic and Clinical Aspects of Granulomatous Diseases.* Edited by D. L. Boros and T. Yoshida. Amsterdam, Elsevier North Holland, pp. 219–234.

Wilkie, B., Pauli, B., and Gygax, M. (1973). Hypersensitivity pneumonitis: Experimental production in guinea pigs with antigens of *Micropolyspora faeni. Pathol. Microbiol.,* **39**:393–411.

Wyler, D. J., Wahl, S. M., and Wahl, L. M. (1978). Hepatic fibrosis in schistosomiasis: Egg granulomas secrete fibroblast stimulating factor in vitro. *Science,* **202**:438–440.

Yamamoto, K., and Kakinuma, M. (1978). Genetic control of granuloma response to oil-associated BCG cell wall vaccine in mice. *Microbiol. Immunol.,* **22**:335–348.

Yamamoto, Y., Nagao, S., Tanaka, A., Koga, T., and Onoue, K. (1978). Inhibition of macrophage migration by synthetic muramyl dipeptide. *Biochem. Biophys. Res. Commun.,* **80**:923–928.

Yamamura, T., Ogawa, Y., Maeda, H., and Yamamura, Y. (1974). Prevention of tuberculous cavity formation by desensitization with tuberculin-active peptide. *Am. Rev. Respir. Dis.,* **109**:594–601.

Yamamura, Y., Ogawa, Y., Yamagata, H., and Yamamura, Y. (1968). Prevention of tuberculous cavity formation by immunosuppressive drugs. *Am. Rev. Respir. Dis.,* **98**:720–723.

Yarkoni, E., and Bekierkunst, A. (1976). Nonspecific resistance against infection with *Salmonella typhi* and *Salmonella typhimurium* induced in mice by cord factor (trehalose-6, 6'-dimycolate) and its analogues. *Infect. Immun.,* **14**:1125–1129.

Yarkoni, E., and Rapp, H. J. (1977). Granuloma formation in lungs of mice after intravenous administration of emulsified trehalose-6, 6'-dimycolate (cord factor): Reaction intensity depends on size distribution of the oil droplets. *Infect. Immun.,* **18**:552–554.

Yarkoni, E., Wang, L., and Bekierkunst, A. (1977). Stimulation of macrophages by cord factor and by heat-killed and living BCG. *Infect. Immun.,* **16**:1–8.

Yarkoni, E., Ruco, L. P., Rapp, H. J., and Meltzer, M. S. (1979). Histopathology of tumor regression by cord factor, turpentine, or endotoxin, dissociation of therapy and granuloma formation. *Eur. J. Cancer,* **15**:1401–1407.

Yoshida, T., Siltzbach, L. E., Masih, N., and Cohen, S. (1979). Serum-migration inhibitory activity in patients with sarcoidosis. *Clin. Immunol. Immunopathol.,* **13**:39–46.

Part Nine

OTHER GRANULOMATOUS LUNG DISEASE

19

Beryllium Disease

NANCY L. SPRINCE

Massachusetts General Hospital
Boston, Massachusetts

HOMAYOUN KAZEMI

Harvard Medical School
and Massachusetts General Hospital
Boston, Massachusetts

I. History of Beryllium Disease

Beryllium was first implicated as a cause of occupational pulmonary disease
in reports from Germany and Russia in the 1930s. In the German
literature, Weber and Englehardt (1933) described conjunctivitis, eczema,
bronchitis, and bronchiolitis associated with diffuse densities on chest
radiographs in beryllium extraction workers. Gelman (1936) described
dermatitis, conjunctivitis, and respiratory disease characterized by dyspnea,
cough, cyanosis, rales, and diffuse nodules found on radiographic examination in Russian beryllium workers. Berkovitz and Israel (1940) reported
physical findings and radiographic abnormalities in 46 patients with
"fluorine beryllium poisoning." Meyer (1942) described acute respiratory
disease, followed by either recovery or death in the acute phase, or chronic
respiratory illness in German beryllium extraction workers. Pathology in
the fatal cases was reported by Wurm and Ruger (1942) and showed
organizing pneumonia, or cellular exudate filling alveoli and alveolar ducts.

The first report of clinical disease among beryllium workers in the
United States was published by Van Ordstrand and co-workers (1943):
They described acute bronchiolitis and chemical pneumonitis in three

beryllium workers engaged in manufacturing beryllium oxide from beryl ore in Ohio. Shilen and associates (1944) described acute respiratory disease in beryllium extraction workers in Pennsylvania, but erroneously attributed the etiology to fluorine compounds. Kress and Crispell (1944) reported acute chemical pneumonitis in men working with beryllium phosphors in fluorescent powder. Van Ordstrand and co-workers (1945) reported dermatitis and chemical pneumonitis in 170 additional Ohio extraction workers.

Hardy and Tabershaw (1946) reported the first cases of chronic beryllium disease in the United States in 17 fluorescent lamp workers in Salem, Massachusetts. Hardy later specifically linked these patients' beryllium exposure with their pulmonary and systemic granulomatous disease which resembled sarcoidosis. Throughout the 1940s large numbers of patients, whose exposures occurred mainly in beryllium extraction from beryl ore, fluorescent lamp manufacturing, and atomic bomb production, were reported with acute and chronic beryllium disease. Hardy established the Beryllium Case Registry at the Massachusetts General Hospital in 1952 to collect information from the cases in the United States and to follow the course and complications of patients with this disease.

By 1950 awareness of the relationship between beryllium exposure and disease led to changes in industrial practice and resulted in a reduction in exposures to beryllium and a subsequent decline in reported cases of beryllium disease. Use of beryllium in fluorescent lamp manufacturing was discontinued, and initial engineering controls were instituted in beryllium-using industries in an attempt to reduce exposure. However, new cases of beryllium disease resulting from recent exposures have continued to be reported to the Beryllium Case Registry.

II. Beryllium: Its Properties, Production, and Uses

A. Properties of Beryllium

Beryllium is the fourth element in the periodic table with an atomic weight of 9. It is a lightweight metal, with high tensile strength and heat resistance. Hence, beryllium oxide is a good electrical insulator and heat conductor. Copper is frequently alloyed with beryllium, since the resultant beryllium-copper has high tensile strength, electrical and heat conductivity, and corrosion and fatigue resistance. Because of these unique properties, many industrial applications have been found for beryllium.

B. Production

Beryl ore, the major natural source for beryllium, is mined in Brazil, Germany, India, the USSR, and, to a limited extent, in the United States in Utah. Beryllium, which is extracted from the ore, is used mainly in three forms: beryllium metal, beryllium oxide, and beryllium alloys.

Table 1 Major Industrial Uses for Beryllium

Production and use of beryllium alloys (especially beryllium-copper)

Computer manufacturing

Beryllium ceramics production

X-ray tube window manufacturing

Electronic equipment manufacturing

Nuclear reactor manufacturing

Atomic energy research and development

Rocket parts, heat shields, guidance and navigation systems manufacturing

Gas mantle manufacturing

Rocket fuel development research

Salvage of fluorescent and neon lamps

C. Uses

Before 1950, major exposures to beryllium occurred in the extraction of
beryllium from ore, the manufacturing of fluorescent lamps, and the
production of atomic bombs. After 1950, modern uses for beryllium were
found in nuclear, electronics, and aerospace industries. The major
industrial uses for beryllium are listed in Table 1. Beryllium metal and all
beryllium compounds except beryl ore have been associated with respiratory
disease. Potentially harmful exposures occur where fine particles of
beryllium are generated from the welding, grinding, casting, or machining
of beryllium and its compounds. The total number of exposed workers
in the United States is unknown, although estimates vary widely from
30,000 (NIOSH, 1972) to 870,000 (National Occupational Hazard Survey,
1972).

III. Acute Disease

Acute disease secondary to beryllium exposure may affect skin, mucous
membranes, or the respiratory tract. Initial exposure of the dermis to
high concentrations of beryllium is associated with dermatitis of the
primary irritant type. Beryllium also sensitizes skin, causing dermatitis
1-2 weeks after the initial exposure. Dermatitis usually improves after
dermal exposure is discontinued. Skin ulceration may be a complication
and removal of any beryllium implanted in the skin is required to promote
healing.

    As a direct irritant, beryllium may cause inflammation and edema of
any contacted surface or mucous membrane and has been associated with

conjunctivitis, periorbital edema, nasopharyngitis, tracheobronchitis, and pneumonitis. The dose of beryllium exposure determines the prevalence and severity of the clinical manifestations of acute chemical pneumonitis. Early observations of beryllium workers exposed to high concentrations of inhaled beryllium indicated that acute chemical pneumonitis occurred in almost all workers exposed to air concentrations above 1000 $\mu g/m^3$ and in none exposed to less than 100 $\mu g/m^3$. Brief, high-dose exposures may cause severe acute chemical pneumonitis, while prolonged, lower-dose exposure may cause beryllium disease that is subacute in onset and course.

Symptoms, signs, lung function abnormalities, and radiographic and histopathologic changes are identical to those found in acute chemical pneumonitis after exposure to other pulmonary irritants. Common symptoms and signs are dyspnea, cough and sputum, which may be blood-tinged, chest pain, tachycardia, tachypnea, rales, and cyanosis. Diffuse or localized infiltrates are seen radiographically. Lung function tests reveal hypoxemia and reduced lung volumes. In fatal cases, histopathologic examination has revealed interstitial and intraalveolar edema, alveolar cell proliferation and desquamation, lymphocyte and plasma cell infiltrates, organizing pneumonia, and hyaline membranes. As seen in chronic beryllium disease, lung tissue of patients who have died from the acute pneumonitis may also contain beryllium.

Therapy for acute pneumonitis, beginning with complete removal from further exposure to beryllium, includes bedrest, oxygen therapy if needed, and corticosteroids for severe disease. Beryllium Case Registry data indicate that 17% of patients with acute disease develop chronic beryllium disease. Although approximately 24% of all cases of beryllium disease in the Beryllium Case Registry are acute disease, only one case of acute disease has been reported since 1973.

IV. Chronic Disease

Chronic beryllium disease, caused by beryllium inhalation, is a pulmonary and systemic granulomatous disease. Although exposure in most cases has taken place over several months to years, the latent period between initial exposure and clinical evidence of disease varies. Some patients become symptomatic during ongoing exposure at work, while in others a delay of 25 years is noted. An average latent period is 10–15 years.

Dyspnea is the most common symptom of chronic beryllium disease. Weight loss, chest pain, cough, arthralgias, fatigue, and skin rash may also occur. Physical findings include bibasilar rales, skin lesions, hepatosplenomegaly, clubbing of the nail beds, and lymphadenopathy. In severe cases, signs of pulmonary hypertension may appear late in the course.

Although respiratory disease, in the form of interstitial granulomatous pneumonitis, is the most frequent finding, noncaseating granulomas plus elevated tissue content of beryllium have also occurred in skin, liver, spleen, thoracic and extrathoracic lymph nodes, myocardium, skeletal muscle, kidney, bone, and salivary glands.

Other associated abnormalities have been reported. Hyperuricemia may occur secondary to impaired renal clearance of uric acid. Hypercalcemia and hypercalciuria have also occurred in chronic beryllium disease, probably on the basis of mechanisms similar to those in sarcoidosis. Renal calculi, which may contain beryllium, are associated with hypercalciuria in some cases. Elevated erythrocyte sedimentation rate, erythrocytosis and increases in serum gamma globulin concentrations, especially IgA and IgG, also occur.

V. Laboratory Diagnosis—Pulmonary Function Tests

The pattern of impairment of lung function emphasized in early descriptions of patients with chronic beryllium disease was that of restrictive disease. This was noted to be associated with reduced diffusing capacity for carbon monoxide and hypoxemia at rest which worsened on exercise. Later reports noted an obstructive defect in some patients, with reduced air flow rates and elevated residual volume.

Andrews and co-workers (1969) reported three patterns of impairment of lung function in 41 Beryllium Case Registry patients with the chronic disease. An obstructive pattern, occurring in smokers and nonsmokers and associated with peribronchial granulomas, was found in 39% of these patients. A restrictive defect was seen in 20% of the cases. Patients in both the restrictive and obstructive groups showed worsening of lung function on follow-up testing done an average of 5 years later. The third pattern, an interstitial defect, was characterized by normal lung volumes and air flow rates and reduced diffusing capacity for carbon monoxide. Patients in this category (36% of the total) had the least deterioration in lung function at a 5-year follow-up. Kanarek and co-workers (1973), reporting early manifestations of beryllium disease in asymptomatic extraction and production workers undergoing medical surveillance, noted mild hypoxemia and mildly elevated alveolar-arterial oxygen tension difference with well-preserved lung volumes and air flow rates.

VI. Radiographic Manifestations

Characteristic chest radiographic findings are diffuse infiltrates and hilar lymphadenopathy (Fig. 1). Densities have been described as granular, nodular, linear, and mixed patterns. Approximately 40% of patients have

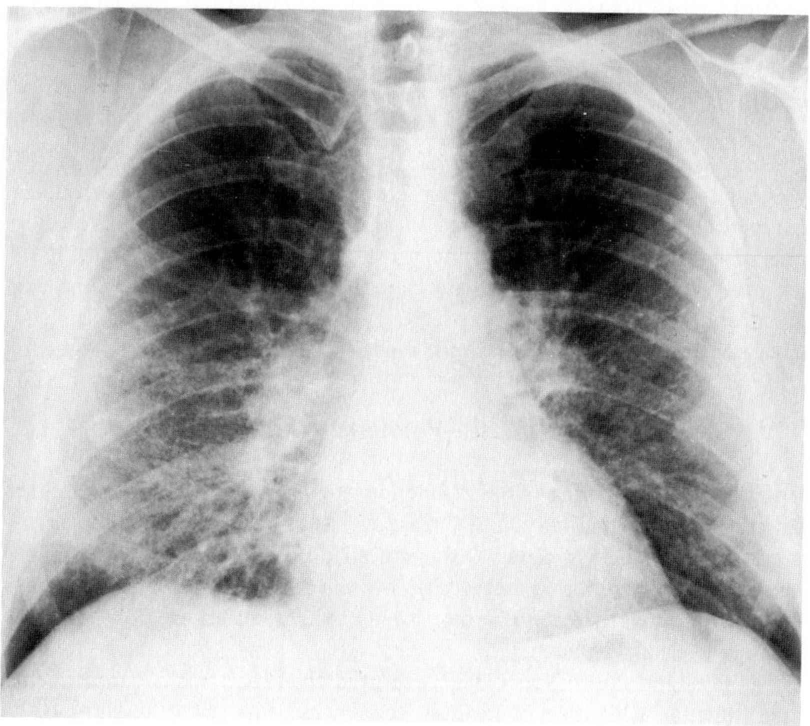

Figure 1 Chest radiograph of a 56-year-old man with chronic beryllium disease, showing bilateral hilar lymphadenopathy and bilateral linear infiltrates.

hilar lymphadenopathy, which is usually mild, bilateral, and associated with parenchymal infiltration. Hilar lymphadenopathy as the sole radiographic manifestation occurs rarely. Other abnormalities include contraction of lobes, most frequently in the upper lung fields with adjacent hyperinflation, pneumothorax, lung cysts, pleural thickening, and calcified lung densities. The initial infiltrates may remain stable, improve, or progress.

Complete radiographic resolution has been reported by Stoeckle et al. (1969) in one patient after treatment with ACTH. Spontaneous improvements have been noted in patients receiving no therapy. Institution of corticosteroid therapy has been associated with radiographic improvement in some patients. A recent report by Sprince and co-workers (1978) suggests that mild interstitial disease on radiographs may be seen in workers exposed to elevated beryllium air concentrations, and that improvements in radiographic findings may be seen after air concentrations of beryllium are decreased.

VII. Pathology

Freiman and Hardy (1970) described histopathologic changes in lung tissue from 124 patients with chronic beryllium disease. The most frequent findings were chronic interstitial pneumonitis and noncaseating granulomas (Fig. 2). Infiltrates were made up of histiocytes, lymphocytes, and plasma cells. Giant cells, some containing asteroid bodies, and intra- and extra-cellular calcific inclusions were common. Moderate to severe fibrosis was noted in approximately 50% of their cases. They divided the cases into group I (prominent interstitial cellular infiltration) and group II (slight or absent interstitial cellular infiltration). Subgroup IA was further categorized by poorly formed or absent granulomas, while subgroup IB had well-formed granulomas. The cases in Group II, comprising 20% of their series and indistinguishable from sarcoidosis, had well-formed granulomas and slight or absent interstitial cellular infiltration. Patients with group II histopathology seemed to respond better to corticosteroid therapy and to live longer than group I patients.

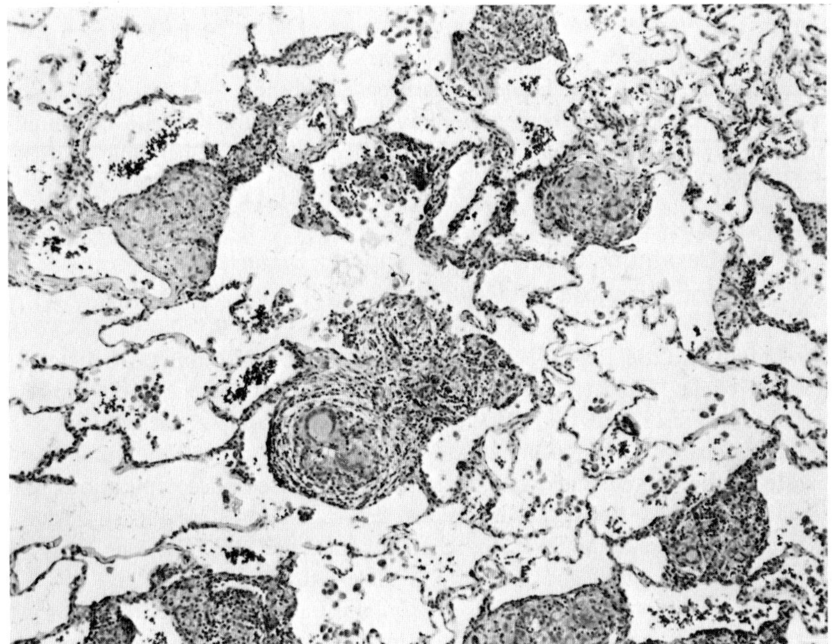

Figure 2 Lung biopsy from a patient with chronic beryllium disease. There are numerous well-formed granulomas containing giant cells.

Although the lung is the most frequently involved organ in chronic beryllium disease, granulomas may also be seen in extrapulmonary tissues, including lymph nodes, skin, liver, spleen, and muscle.

VIII. Neighborhood Cases

The current permissible standard for community air beryllium levels is 0.01 $\mu g/m^3$. Such an exposure limit was required because of reports of chronic beryllium disease occurring in individuals with no occupational exposure to beryllium who lived near a plant using beryllium. The exposure in non-occupational cases may be secondary to plant discharges into the air or to beryllium brought home on workclothes of family members or to a combination of these exposures. Beryllium Case Registry data show that the prevalence of neighborhood cases has decreased since 1949, most likely because of stricter controls reducing beryllium air concentrations of plant discharges.

IX. Extent of the Problem

The precise prevalence of beryllium disease is unknown. The current (January 1981) 898 cases in the Beryllium Case Registry most likely represent an underestimate of the true number of affected patients because of difficulties in recognition of the disease and of under-reporting of patients in whom the diagnosis has been established. Medical surveillance of currently exposed workers engaged in beryllium extraction and beryllium-copper alloy production has revealed incidences of chronic beryllium disease of 5% and 2.5% found on initial screening.

X. Beryllium Case Registry and Its Criteria for Diagnosis of Disease

The Beryllium Case Registry was established at the Massachusetts General Hospital by Dr. Harriet Hardy in 1952. Begun shortly after the epidemics of beryllium disease of the 1940s, the Registry's major purpose was to collect clinical information about cases of acute and chronic beryllium disease in the United States and to follow the course and complications of beryllium disease. Investigators working with Beryllium Case Registry data have been able to characterize the clinical course and complications, lung function abnormalities, and radiographic and histopathologic findings of beryllium disease. The work of the Beryllium Case Registry at the Massachusetts General Hospital has continued to the present and currently there are 898 collected cases, of which 212 are acute, 642 are chronic, and

44 are patients who presented initially with acute disease but later developed chronic disease.

Investigators working in the Beryllium Case Registry have developed criteria for the diagnosis of chronic beryllium disease. Of the six criteria listed in Table 2, four must be met to make the diagnosis, including criterion 1 or 6 in every case to establish beryllium exposure.

Fulfilling criterion 1, or establishing significant beryllium exposure, is frequently difficult. Although results of air concentrations of beryllium taken from the workers' breathing zone provide optimal information, these measurements are usually unavailable. Occupational history, which in some cases is reviewed by an industrial hygienist familiar with beryllium-using industries, has provided the basis for establishing criterion 1 for many Beryllium Case Registry cases. Problems impairing occupational history-taking include long latent periods between exposure and clinical disease, inadequate labeling and trade secrecy in industry, and lack of information for workers concerning exposure hazards.

Criteria 2–5 are self-explanatory. Objective evidence of beryllium exposure is provided by criterion 6. Beryllium remains in lung and thoracic lymph nodes for many years and is excreted slowly in the urine. Hence, lung tissue, thoracic lymph node, and urinary beryllium levels are useful to confirm exposure. Sprince and co-workers (1976) found that 82% of 66 cases of chronic beryllium disease had elevated beryllium levels in lung tissue, while normal controls and patients with sarcoidosis had no elevations. Elevated urinary beryllium levels have been detected up to 20 years after the last exposure. Since the presence of beryllium in tissues or in urine indicates exposure only, this finding must be correlated with

Table 2 Diagnostic Criteria for Beryllium Disease (Beryllium Case Registry)

1. Significant exposure to beryllium based on occupational history, results of air samples, or other evidence

2. Objective evidence of lower respiratory tract disease and a consistent clinical course

3. Chest radiographs showing interstitial fibronodular disease

4. Lung function findings of restrictive, obstructive, or interstitial defect

5. Histopathologic changes consistent with beryllium disease in lung tissue and/or thoracic lymph nodes

6. Presence of beryllium in a urine specimen, lung tissue, or thoracic lymph nodes

available clinical, radiographic, physiologic, and pathologic data before establishing a diagnosis of chronic beryllium disease.

XI. Regulation of Exposure Levels

The present Occupational Safety and Health Administration (OSHA) standards for permissible exposure limits for beryllium in the workplace are 2 $\mu g/m^3$ as an 8-hr time-weighted average and 25 $\mu g/m^3$ as the peak allowable concentration for a maximum of 30 min during any 8-hr shift. These limit values, proposed initially in 1948 by an advisory committee of the U.S. Atomic Energy Commission, were adopted by the American Conference of Government Industrial Hygienists in 1959. Although the 2 $\mu g/m^3$ level was an arbitrary standard based on no scientific evidence, experience over subsequent years has indicated that chronic beryllium disease does not occur in workers exposed at or below this level. The peak exposure limit of 25 $\mu g/m^3$, designed to prevent acute beryllium disease, was based on the observation of acute beryllium disease occurring only in workers exposed to air concentrations exceeding 100 $\mu g/m^3$. It is generally accepted that acute disease has been prevented among workers exposed to levels no greater than 25 $\mu g/m^3$. Although engineering controls capable of reducing air concentrations to the prescribed limits are available, industrial exposures exceeding current permissible standards continue to occur.

In 1975, after reviewing the beryllium standard, OSHA proposed a reduction in the 8-hr time-weighted average value to 1 $\mu g/m^3$. The rationale for the proposal was that since animal and human evidence suggested that beryllium was a carcinogen, the lowest feasible limit value should be required. Currently (January 1981) OSHA has not promulgated this new standard and a final version of the standard is pending.

XII. Pathogenesis

The mechanism of action of beryllium in causing acute disease is that of a direct irritant causing inflammation, edema, and necrosis of the mucosal surfaces of the respiratory tract. The current proposed mechanism for the development of chronic beryllium disease is that inhaled beryllium combines with immunoglobulins and causes release of cytotoxic cellular enzymes. The beryllium-protein complex is then transported from the lung to extra-pulmonary tissues. This mechanism helps explain the clinical observation that pulmonary disease is the most frequent manifestation of beryllium disease and that extrapulmonary involvement is variable. This proposed mechanism also accounts for the observation that, in patients with chronic beryllium disease, beryllium has been detected in many tissues including lung, lymph nodes, muscle, spleen, liver, and skin.

Although a dose-response relationship has been accepted for acute beryllium disease, the mode of disease production for the chronic disease is uncertain, and both dose-response and immunologic or hypersensitivity mechanisms have been suggested.

Several observations support a dose-response mechanism. An epidemiologic observation is that total numbers of cases of acute and chronic beryllium disease decreased dramatically after 1950, the year after which ventilation and engineering measures reduced beryllium air concentrations in industry and after which beryllium was no longer used in fluorescent lamp manufacturing. In addition, a Beryllium Case Registry study of 332 cases of chronic beryllium disease reported by Williams (1959) evaluated their proximity to the source of beryllium at the workplace and found that directly exposed workers accounted for 80.5% of 332 cases, and that indirectly exposed workers in the same building as a beryllium source accounted for 13.0%. Indirectly exposed individuals in a building separate from the source accounted for 4.5% and neighborhood cases for 2.0%. These data suggested a dose-response relationship.

Another explanation may be required for the historical observation that only 1–5% of a total workforce exposed to beryllium developed chronic beryllium disease. Several investigators have presented data suggesting that immunologic or hypersensitivity factors are important in beryllium disease pathogenesis. Increased blast transformation of lymphocytes from patients with chronic beryllium disease challenged in vitro with beryllium salts was reported by Hanifin and co-workers (1970). Deodhar et al. (1973) reported strongly positive blast transformation reactions of lymphocytes exposed to beryllium sulfate in 60% of patients with chronic beryllium disease, but in only one (4.5%) healthy, unexposed control. A good correlation between amount of blast transformation and severity of disease was noted. Preuss and associates (1980) reported that 57% of 47 patients with chronic beryllium disease had strongly positive reactions of blast transformation, compared with no strongly positive reactions among 553 healthy beryllium workers. Price and co-workers (1976) demonstrated that lymphocytes from two patients with chronic beryllium disease who were not receiving steroid therapy produced macrophage migration inhibition factor (MIF), while 14% of 50 healthy beryllium workers and no healthy, unexposed controls demonstrated production of MIF. They postulate that healthy workers with positive tests have been sensitized to beryllium.

The best explanation to encompass all these observations may be a combination of dose-response and hypersensitivity or immunologic mechanisms. Whether the same immunologic abnormalities present in sarcoidosis occur in beryllium disease is unknown.

XIII. Beryllium and Cancer

Groth (1980) reviewed the evidence for beryllium as a carcinogen and cited animal experiments showing induction of bone sarcomas after inhalation or intravenous injection of beryllium in rabbits, and lung carcinomas after inhalation or intratracheal exposure in monkeys and rats. Mancuso (1970) showed a higher than expected rate of lung cancer in beryllium extraction workers who had a history of acute respiratory disease secondary to beryllium. Infante and co-workers (1980) found an excessive rate of lung cancer deaths among white male Beryllium Case Registry patients with a history of acute chemical pneumonitis or bronchitis secondary to beryllium. Wagoner and associates (1980) found excess lung cancer mortality among beryllium extraction and production workers. These observations suggest an association between beryllium exposure and lung cancer in humans, especially in those with a history of prior acute respiratory tract disease secondary to beryllium.

XIV. Differential Diagnosis

In many cases, differentiating beryllium disease from sarcoidosis is difficult because of overlap in signs, symptoms, and radiographic, lung function, and histopathologic changes. Uveitis, uveoparotid fever, cystic bone lesions, and cranial and peripheral nerve involvement have been reported in sarcoidosis but not in chronic beryllium disease. The Kveim test and tissue levels for beryllium have been used to differentiate these diseases. The Kveim test has been negative in all patients with beryllium disease, although it is positive in a large percentage of patients with sarcoidosis. Limited availability restricts the clinical usefulness of the Kveim test. Lung tissue beryllium levels are normal in sarcoidosis and elevated in chronic beryllium disease.

Serum angiotension 1-converting enzyme (ACE) levels are elevated in approximately 50% of patients with sarcoidosis, whereas Sprince and co-workers (1980) found only one elevation of serum ACE among 22 patients with chronic beryllium disease. However, Lieberman and co-workers (1979) reported elevated ACE levels in three of four beryllium patients. Until results are obtained from larger numbers of patients, the usefulness of serum ACE in differentiating these diseases will remain uncertain. Carrington and co-workers (1976) reported that both necrosis in granulomas and angiitis were more frequently seen in sarcoidosis than in chronic beryllium disease.

Because of the marked similarities of these two diseases, a useful practical approach is to seek a history of beryllium exposure and to analyze available biopsy specimens and urine for beryllium in all patients whose clinical diagnosis is sarcoidosis.

XV. Prognosis

Beryllium Case Registry data indicate that the course of chronic beryllium disease is variable. Some patients maintain a stable course initially and show subsequent deterioration. Other patients have multiple exacerbations and remissions. Early reports from the Beryllium Case Registry emphasized worsening of disease during pregnancy, surgery, or other intercurrent illness. Symptomatic patients with only radiographic abnormalities may remain stable or may develop symptoms and impairment in lung function. Progression of disease is characterized by increased dyspnea, worsening of impairment in lung function, and progression of radiographic abnormalities. End-stage disease is marked by respiratory failure, pulmonary hypertension, and cor pulmonale.

Improvements in symptoms and radiographic abnormalities have been reported after treatment with corticosteroids. In some cases, symptoms and radiographic findings worsen after corticosteroids are withdrawn. In contrast to sarcoidosis, spontaneous improvement without therapy is rare in chronic beryllium disease.

In some patients with chronic beryllium disease, deterioration has been observed in association with further beryllium exposure. One study by Sprince and co-workers (1978) suggested improvements in early interstitial disease secondary to beryllium after reduction in inhaled beryllium concentrations. These observations suggest that patients with chronic beryllium disease should avoid further exposure to beryllium to prevent worsening of disease.

XVI. Therapy

To prevent worsening of the disease, removal from further beryllium exposure is recommended for all patients with chronic beryllium disease. Corticosteroids are the major available medical therapy. Although not associated with long-standing reversal of disease, corticosteroids improve the clinical course in some patients. Chronic daily or alternate day oral corticosteroid therapy is usually needed for symptomatic patients with abnormalities in lung function. General recommendations for patients with chronic beryllium disease include prompt antibiotic therapy for bacterial infections of the respiratory tract and immunization against influenza and pneumococcus. Other therapy varies with the specific clinical situation or complication. Supplemental oxygen therapy is useful if hypoxemia is significant. Oxygen, diuretics, and digitalis have been used to treat complicating right ventricular failure.

References

Andrews, J. L., Kazemi, H., and Hardy, H. L. (1969). Patterns of lung dysfunction in chronic beryllium disease. *Am. Rev. Respir. Dis.,* **100**:791–800.

Berkovitz, M., and Israel, B. (1940). Changes in the lungs in fluorine beryllium poisoning. *Klin. Med. (USSR),* **18**:117–122.

Carrington, C. B., Gaensler, E. A., Mikus, J. P., Schachter, A. W., Burke, G. W., and Goff, A. M. (1976). Structure and function in sarcoidosis. *Ann. N.Y. Acad. Sci.,* **278**:265–283.

Deodhar, S. D., Barna, B., and Van Ordstrand, H. S. (1973). A study of the immunologic aspects of chronic berylliosis. *Chest,* **63**:309–313.

Freiman, D. G., and Hardy, H. L. (1970). Beryllium disease. *Hum. Pathol.,* **1**:25–44.

Gelman, I. (1936). Poisoning by vapors of beryllium oxyfluoride. *J. Ind. Hyg. Toxicol.,* **18**:371–379.

Groth, D. H. (1980). Carcinogenicity of beryllium: Review of the literature. *Environ. Res.,* **21**:56–62.

Hanifin, J. M., Epstein, W. L., and Cline, M. J. (1970). In vitro studies of granulomatous hypersensitivity to beryllium. *J. Invest. Dermatol.,* **55**:284.

Hardy, H. L., and Tabershaw, I. R. (1946). Delayed chemical pneumonitis occurring in workers exposed to beryllium compounds. *J. Ind. Hyg. Toxicol.,* **28**:197–211.

Infante, P. F., Wagoner, J. K., and Sprince, N. L. (1980). Mortality patterns from lung cancer and non-neoplastic respiratory disease among white males in the Beryllium Case Registry. *Environ. Res.,* **21**:35–43.

Kanarek, D. J., Wainer, R. A., Chamberlin, R. I., Weber, A. L., and Kazemi, H. (1973). Respiratory illness in a population exposed to beryllium. *Am. Rev. Respir. Dis.,* **108**:1295–1302.

Kress, J. E., and Crispell, K. R. (1944). Chemical pneumonitis in men working with fluorescent powders containing beryllium. *Guthrie Clin. Bull.,* **13**:91.

Lieberman, J. A., Nosal, J. A., Schleissner, L. A., and Sastre-Foken, A. (1979). Serum angiotensin-converting enzyme for diagnosis and therapeutic evaluation of sarcoidosis. *Am. Rev. Respir. Dis.,* **120**:329.

Mancuso, T. F. (1970). Relation of duration of employment and prior respiratory illness to respiratory cancer among beryllium workers. *Environ. Res.,* **3**:251–275.

Meyer, H. E. (1942). On beryllium disease of the lungs. *Beitr. Klin. Tuberk.,* **98**:388–395.

National Institute for Occupational Safety and Health (1972). Occupational exposure to beryllium. U.S. Dept. of Health, Education and Welfare. PHS, HSM 72-10268.

National Occupational Hazard Survey (1972). DHEW (NIOSH). Publication #78-114, volume 3. U.S. Dept. of Health, Education and Welfare. PHS, CDC, NIOSH.

Preuss, O., Deodhar, S. D., and Van Ordstrand, H. S. (1980). Lymphoblast transformation in beryllium workers. In *Proceedings of the Eighth International Conference on Sarcoidosis and Other Granulomatous Disease.* Cardiff, Wales, Alpha Omega, pp. 711–714.

Price, C. D., Pugh, A., Piolo, E. M., and Williams, W. J. (1976). Beryllium macrophage migration inhibition test. *Ann. N.Y. Acad. Sci.,* **278**: 204–210.

Shilen, J., Galloway, A. E., and Mellor, G. (1944). Beryllium oxide from beryl: Health hazards incident to extraction. *Ind. Med.,* **13**:464–469.

Sprince, N. L., Kazemi, H., and Hardy, H. L. (1976). Current (1975) problem of differentiating between beryllium disease and sarcoidosis. *Ann. N.Y. Acad. Sci.,* **278**:654–664.

Sprince, N. L., Kanarek, D. J., Weber, A. L., Chamberlin, R. I., and Kazemi, H. (1978). Reversible respiratory disease in beryllium workers. *Am. Rev. Respir. Dis.,* **117**:1011–1017.

Sprince, N. L., Kazemi, H., and Fanburg, B. L. (1980). Serum angiotensin 1 converting enzyme in chronic beryllium disease. In *Proceedings of the Eighth International Conference on Sarcoidosis and Other Granulomatous Disease.* Cardiff, Wales, Alpha Omega, pp. 287–290.

Stoeckle, J. D., Hardy, H. L., and Weber, A. L. (1969). Chronic beryllium disease. *Am. J. Med.,* **46**:545–561.

Van Ordstrand, H. S., Hughes, R., DeNardi, J. M., and Carmody, M. G. (1943). Chemical pneumonia in workers extracting beryllium oxide. *Cleveland Clin. Q.,* **10**:10.

Van Ordstrand, H. S., Hughes, R., DeNardi, J. M., and Carmody, M. G. (1945). Beryllium poisoning. *JAMA,* **129**:1084–1090.

Wagoner, J. K., Infante, P. F., and Bayliss, D. L. (1980). Beryllium: An etiologic agent in the induction of lung cancer, non-neoplastic respiratory disease and heart disease among industrially exposed workers. *Environ. Res.,* **21**:15–34.

Weber, H. H., and Englehardt, W. E. (1933).   Investigation of dusts arising
    out of beryllium extraction. *Zentr. Gewerbehyg. Unfallverhüt.*, **10**:
    41–47.
Williams, C. R. (1959).   Evaluation of exposure data in Beryllium Registry:
    Their relation to present maximum allowable concentrations. *Arch.
    Ind. Hyg.*, **19**:263–267.
Wurm, H., and Ruger, H. (1942).   Investigations on the question of
    beryllium dust pneumonia. *Beitr. Klin. Tuberk.*, **98**:396–404.

20

Drug-Induced Pulmonary Granulomas

EDWARD C. ROSENOW III
and K. KRISHNAN UNNI

Mayo Graduate School of Medicine
Mayo Clinic
Rochester, Minnesota

I. Introduction

Five drugs are currently recognized to be associated with the production or
induction of pulmonary granulomas. They are (a) mineral oil, (b) cromolyn
sodium, (c) BCG (bacille Calmette-Guérin), (d) talc (magnesium trisilicate),
and (e) methotrexate. There appear to be no similarities between the
structural, chemical, or pharmacological actions of any of these drugs.
For this reason they will be discussed separately.

II. Mineral Oil

Aspirated oil may be one of the most common causes of drug-induced
pulmonary disease; but because it is rarely fatal and usually does not
produce symptoms of respiratory insufficiency unless the aspiration is
extensive, its incidence and significance are underestimated. It can produce
abnormalities ranging from an asymptomatic solitary pulmonary nodule
(Fig. 1) to diffuse disease, and it does not always produce a granulomatous
reaction (Wagner et al. 1955, Buechner and Strug 1956, Weill et al. 1964,
Elston 1966, Schwindt et al. 1967, Ayvazian et al. 1967, Salm and Hughes
1970, CPC, 1977).

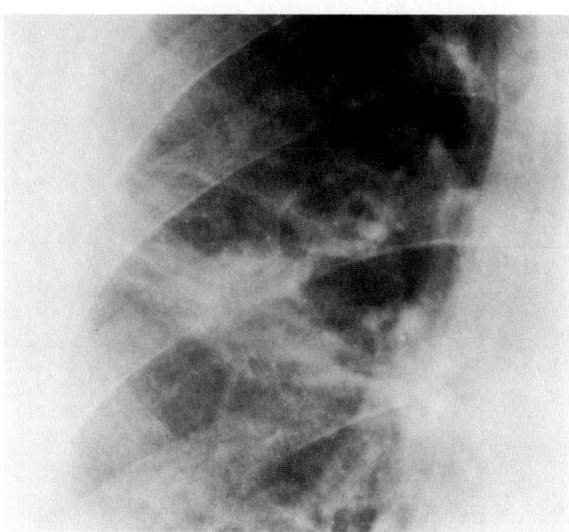

Figure 1 Tomogram of a 12-mm mineral oil granuloma presenting as a discrete, well-localized process mimicking bronchogenic carcinoma.

Most patients with a chest radiographic abnormality due to oil aspiration are asymptomatic; the finding is usually incidental and may be confused with a more serious process such as bronchogenic carcinoma. The patient almost never considers mineral oil or oily nose drops as medication. Thus, the physician must learn to ask specific questions concerning these agents when an abnormality appears on the chest roentgenogram that even remotely could be aspirated oil.

There are three different types of oils: neutral oils, animal fats, and mineral oils (Salm and Hughes 1970). Neutral or vegetable oils, such as castor oil or olive oil, do not elicit a local reaction and are removed by expectoration. Animal fats, such as butter or milk, are rapidly hydrolyzed by lipase in the lung; the liberated fatty acids, in turn, produce necrosis followed by fibrosis. These substances are not commonly aspirated, probably because, unlike mineral oils, they do not suppress the cough reflex. Nor do they appear to be a source of pulmonary granuloma formation.

Mineral oils are the most commonly aspirated oils. Necrosis is not produced; instead, the oils are emulsified and taken up by macrophages. As the macrophages disintegrate the oil is released, but since it inhibits ciliary activity, it is not expectorated and thus is again ingested by macrophages. Eventually, a fibrosis or granulomatous reaction, or both, occur (Fig. 2). It is not known why a granulomatous reaction occurs in some cases and not in others. In this respect, the intensity of the insult of the dose per unit area of the lung involved may be important.

A granulomatous reaction in the lungs is almost always a localized lesion rather than a diffuse one. There appear to be no case reports of a diffuse granulomatous reaction occurring as a result of mineral oil aspiration, nor has there been a case report describing a localized lipoid granuloma occurring in an area of diffuse pneumonitis. If a "critical" amount of oil

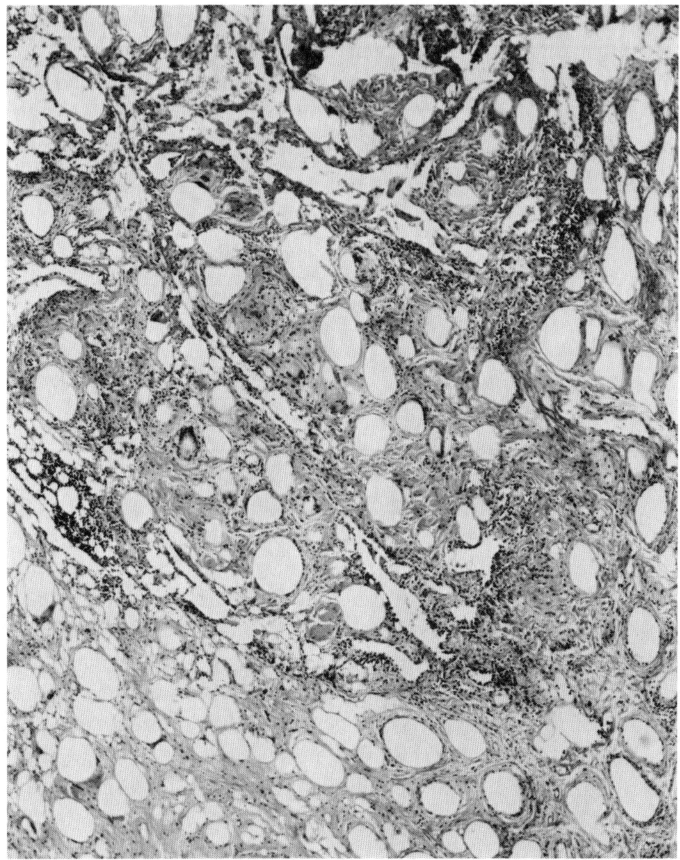

Figure 2 Mineral oil "granuloma." The "holes" in the tissue represent the mineral oil that has been removed during tissue processing. There is diffuse fibrosis and foreign body type giant cells present around the oil (H & E X 664).

significantly impairs the clearance mechanism, then it is likely that this oil is "allowed" to remain sequestered to the point of irritation and granuloma formation. An additional factor might be that the repeated disintegration of the macrophage releases a substance or substances that promote a granulomatous reaction.

Most patients who have aspirated oil are asymptomatic; the rest, who almost always have diffuse pulmonary infiltration, complain of cough, dyspnea, and occasionally fever. Clinically and radiologically, one of three patterns emerges: acute pneumonitis, chronic pneumonitis, or localized reaction, which is frequently granulomatous. The acute and chronic pneumonitis may be either localized or diffuse, and is usually in the dependent portions of the lungs. The diagnosis is established with the demonstration of oil in the lung tissue.

Salm and Hughes (1970) mention that mineral oil can get into the lymphatics and hilar nodes, so it is not surprising that a lipoid granulomatous reaction in a scalene node draining a localized granulomatous pneumonitis can occur (Varkey and Kutty 1976).

Computerized tomography has been found to be of benefit in diagnosing a mineral oil granuloma by virtue of a negative attenuation coefficient compared to the density of water (Wheeler et al. 1981). More experience will be needed before we can be absolutely comfortable with this procedure for diagnosing oil-induced lesions.

III. Cromolyn Sodium

Cromolyn sodium, inhaled as a powder, inhibits mast cell degranulation and, in turn, prevents the release of mediators of bronchospasm. The overall side effects of this drug are small. In one study it was found that only 8 of 375 patients taking cromolyn sodium developed an adverse reaction; none involved the lung or caused a granulomatous reaction (Settipaine et al. 1979). There is only one case report of a postulated tissue proven cromolyn sodium-induced diffuse pulmonary granulomatous reaction (Burgher et al. 1974). This patient had peripheral eosinophilia and a granulomatous involvement of the lung interstitium, bronchial walls, and pulmonary vessels (Figs. 3 and 4). There are three other single case reports of cromolyn sodium-related pulmonary infiltrate/eosinophilia without lung biopsy (Löbel et al. 1972, Sheffer et al. 1975, Repo and Nieminen 1976). The first and third of these three cases had a radiologic description of "scattered, ill-defined foci of soft infiltrations in both lungs." Repo and Nieminen (1976) thought the roentgenographic findings were consistent

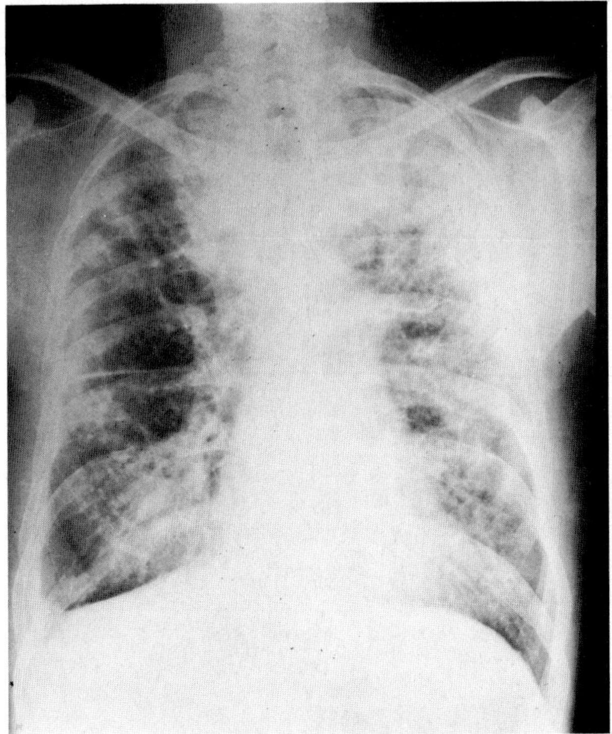

Figure 3 A cromolyn sodium-induced diffuse interstitial process that histologically showed granulomas. (From Burgher et al. 1974.)

with the same granulomatous reaction as in Burgher's case, even though there was no lung biopsy.

Cromolyn sodium is widely used for the treatment of asthma. Thus, with only one case reported of drug-induced granulomatous reaction, its role in causing such reactions must be viewed with some suspicion. However, the authors (Burgher et al. 1974) have as thoroughly as possible removed other possible causes of granulomatous reaction. The involvement of the pulmonary vessels as well as bronchial and lung tissue by granulomatous reaction, along with a peripheral eosinophilia, would lead one to suspect some kind of vasculitis such as Wegener's. This patient responded to corticosteroids.

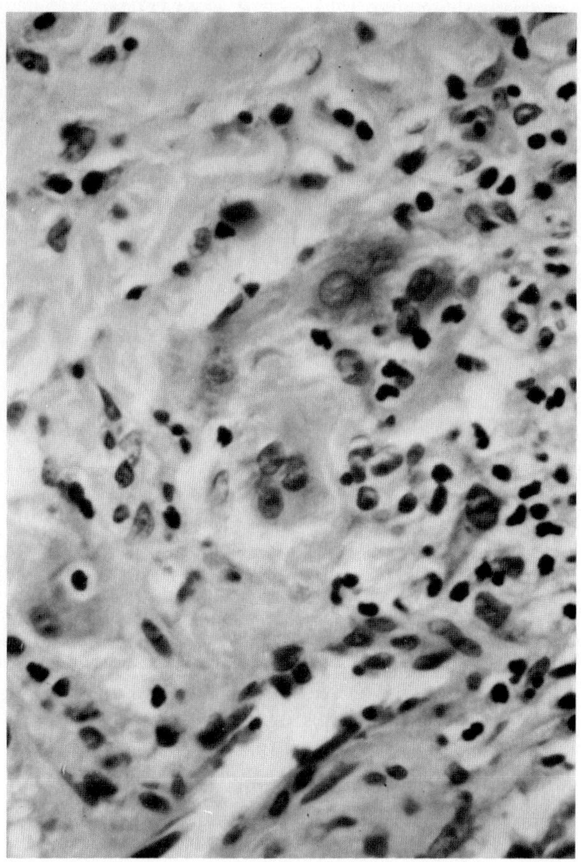

Figure 4 Pulmonary granuloma associated with cromolyn sodium. The granuloma is poorly formed and consists of giant cells, lymphocytes, and slight fibrosis (H & E X 450 approximate). (From Burgher et al. 1974.)

IV. BCG

BCG, which contains an attenuated form of tubercle bacillus, has been used for many years as a preventative vaccination against *Mycobacterium tuberculosis* infection. More recently, it has been widely used experimentally to treat or prevent metastatic disease through its stimulation of the body's own immune mechanism. The results so far have been limited and somewhat disappointing. However, in some patients pulmonary abnormalities develop that have been shown histologically to be granulomas, both caseating and noncaseating. On chest roentgenograms the abnormalities can mimick metastasis.

The incidence of this occurrence is unknown. Gormsen (1955) examined the lungs of 20 individuals who had received BCG and died incidentally and found that 13 of the 20 had evidence of granulomas in the lungs, liver, and hilar nodes. In another study pulmonary granulomas were found in four of five patients who had undergone a thoracotomy for indeterminate pulmonary nodules after receiving BCG within the previous 3 weeks (Au et al. 1978). No mention was made about stains or cultures for acid-fast organisms or the ultimate outcome of these granulomas. The explanation was that "BCG causes granulomatous inflammatory reactions."

Schapira and McPherson (1977) reported a case of presumed BCG-induced pulmonary granulomas in which the cultures were negative. It has been stated that BCG-induced granulomas rarely yield a positive culture, but it would appear that these attenuated mycobacteria are the source of the granulomas and that the granulomas are not a result of a "hypersensitivity" reaction (Mansell and Krementz 1973, Grant et al. 1974).

Aungst and co-workers (1975) reviewed the records of more than 300 patients who received BCG for neoplasm to better define the potential complications. They described one patient (patient 6) who developed "miliary tuberculosis" involving the liver, lungs, spleen, and bone marrow. Cultures of liver and lung tissue grew BCG organisms. They recommend prophylactic isoniazide to immunosuppressed patients receiving BCG and to any patient receiving BCG who develops any clinical findings consistent with acid-fast infection.

V. Talc

Talc, magnesium trisilicate, acts as a bonding agent in the manufacture of pills intended for oral use, but when given intravenously repeatedly over a period of time can incite a granulomatous reaction in the pulmonary interstitium, arteries, and arterioles. This subject has been reviewed by several authors (Douglas et al. 1971, Marschke et al. 1975, Arnett et al. 1976, Paré et al. 1979, Overland et al. 1980, Waller et al. 1980). Other inert fillers, such as corn starch, rarely produce a similar reaction (Johnston and Waisman 1971); but there is a report of a pulmonary granulomatous reaction occurring as a result of cellulose, the major filler of pentazocine (Houck et al. 1980). The drugs most commonly known to contain talc and, in turn, to cause pulmonary granulomas are methadone, methylphenidate (Ritalin), hydromorphone (Dilaudid), tripelennamine (Pyribenzamine), propoxyphene (Darvon), phenmetrazine (Preludin), and amphetamines. Tripelennamine combined with paragoric is "blue velvet" and is used by some addicts to get a "high."

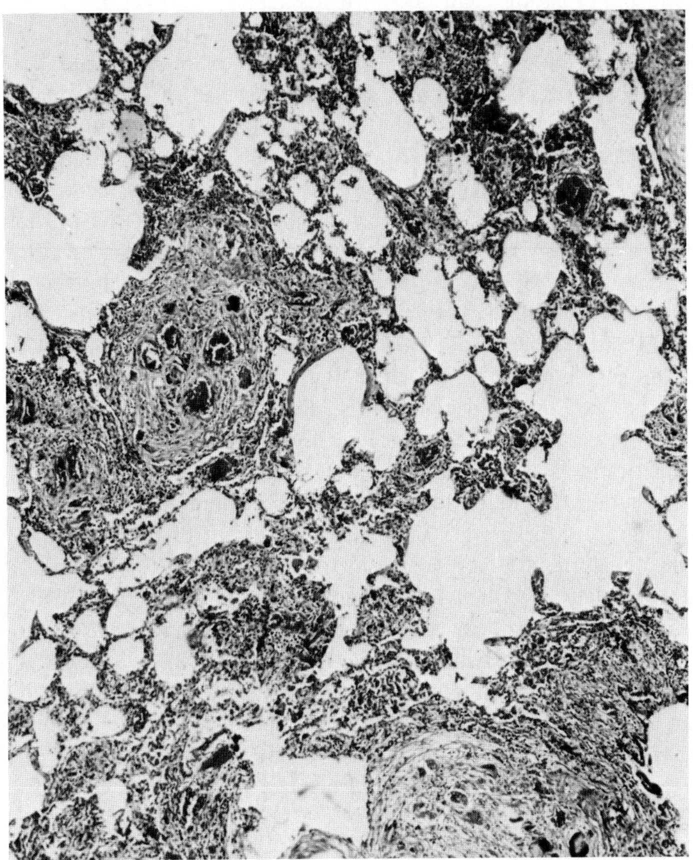

Figure 5 Talc granuloma in lung. There is interstitial fibrosis, and two well-formed granulomas contain giant cells. (From Waller et al. 1980.)

The mechanism for the induction of granulomas by talc is unknown (Hildick-Smith 1976). There is some evidence that granulomas are immune-mediated (Unanue and Benacerraf 1973), and possibly this is the mechanism of the formation of talc granulomas. The extent of granuloma formation as measured by degree of dyspnea, chest x-ray change, pulmonary function abnormalities, or severity of pulmonary hypertension cannot always be directly correlated with the amount of estimated talc injected over a period of years. Paré et al. (1979) studied 17 individuals who each had a long history of intravenously injecting substances that contained talc. Only two had granuloma confirmed by tissue examination. Ten complained of

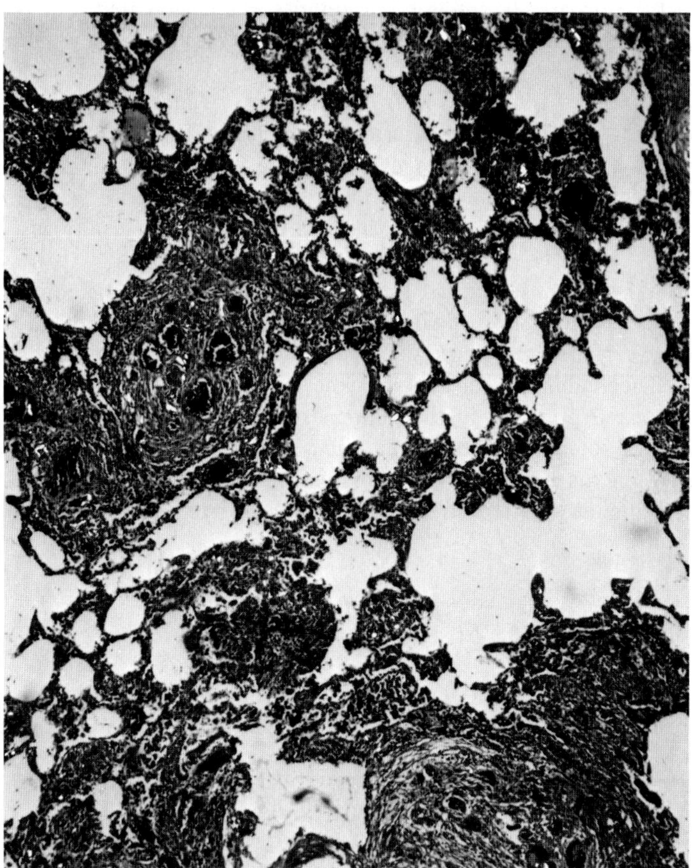

Figure 6 With polarized light crystalline material is visible within granulomas and in the pulmonary interstitium without granulomatous reaction (H & E X 64). (From Waller et al. 1980.)

dyspnea. Nine showed funduscopic evidence of talc emboli. The chest roentgenogram was distinctly abnormal in seven and showed two different patterns: a micronodularity similar to that seen in alveolar microlithiasis, and larger nodularity associated with loss of lung volume, sometimes in a contracted form, similar to that seen in progressive massive fibrosis of coal worker's pneumoconiosis. Pulmonary function studies were done in all 17 patients. In 10 there was a significant decrease in the steady state diffusing capacity. Nine of these and two others had evidence of airway obstruction (all smoked). A significant reduction in the vital capacity was found in only two patients. It was the authors' impression that pulmonary talcosis is an irreversible disease whose severity increases despite discontinuing drug abuse.

Overland and co-workers (1980) did pulmonary function studies on 512 drug addicts who used illicit drugs intravenously. However, they did not attempt to identify the studies that might be associated with patients with talc granulomatosis. They found low carbon monoxide diffusing capacities in 42% of the addicts, and this was the only abnormality in 38% of them.

Waller et al. (1980) reviewed the literature regarding the necropsy findings in 16 reported cases of talc granulomas and added another case (Figs. 5 and 6). It is their impression that patients who have been mainlining talc-containing medication for the longest time tend to have talc granulomas located primarily in the pulmonary interstitium; and those who have been doing so for the shortest duration tend to have the granulomas predominantly in the lumina of the pulmonary arteries. Morphological evidence of pulmonary arterial hypertension was present in 13 of 16 patients.

VI. Methotrexate

Methotrexate (MTX) is an antimetabolite used primarily in the treatment of acute lymphatic leukemia, but more recently it has been incorporated into a number of polypharmacy protocols for the treatment of different neoplasms. It has also been used in the treatment of nonneoplastic conditions such as psoriasis and connective tissue diseases. Of all the adverse pulmonary drug reactions by chemotherapeutic agents (Rosenow 1980), MTX has the most variable types of reactions (Clarysse et al. 1969, Schwartz and Kajani 1969, Robertson 1970, Filip et al. 1971, Rawbone et al. 1971, Goldman and Moschella 1971, Whitcomb et al. 1972, Robbins et al. 1973, Everts et al. 1973, Lisbona et al. 1973, Bhat et al. 1974, Sostman et al. 1976, Gutin et al. 1976, Nesbit et al. 1976, Lascari et al. 1977, Bedrossian et al. 1979).

Usually, symptoms of cough, dyspnea, and fever begin 10 days to 6 months after initiating therapy. In all cases reported, the leukemia has always been in remission. An eosinophilia occurs in about one-half of the cases. The chest roentgenogram shows a diffuse interstitial pattern, or frequently, a combined alveolar and interstitial pattern (Fig. 7). Hilar adenopathy and pleural effusion can occur. Generally, the pulmonary problem spontaneously resolves when the drug is stopped, or almost certainly when corticosteroids are added. Occasionally, the patient gets better in spite of staying on the drug. However, there have been deaths

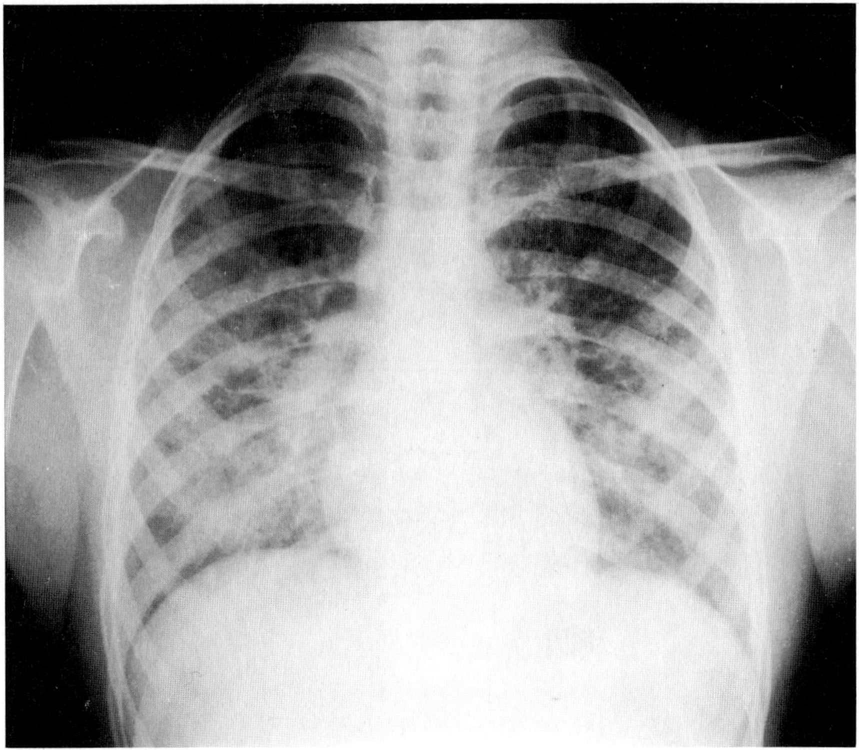

Figure 7 Chest x-ray of methotrexate pneumonitis showing a diffuse interstitial alveolar pattern. Hilar and paratracheal lymphadenopathy are present as well.

due to respiratory failure, attributed to methotrexate pneumonitis. Another interesting feature of methotrexate pneumonitis is that after recovery, the drug can be resumed without precipitating a reaction, a negative rechallenge. This has been shown in many instances and has led to the theory that a concomitant, unidentified infection (presumed viral) precipitates the methotrexate pneumonitis.

The histology is quite variable, ranging from an interstitial pneumonitis to a predominantly desquamative pneumonitis to a granulomatous reaction (Fig. 8). In a few of the fatal cases the histology takes on the appearance of the cytotoxic reactions seen with cyclophosphamide, busulfan, bleomycin, and others.

There appears to be no way to predict whether the tissue reaction will be granulomatous or nongranulomatous; there is no correlation with the

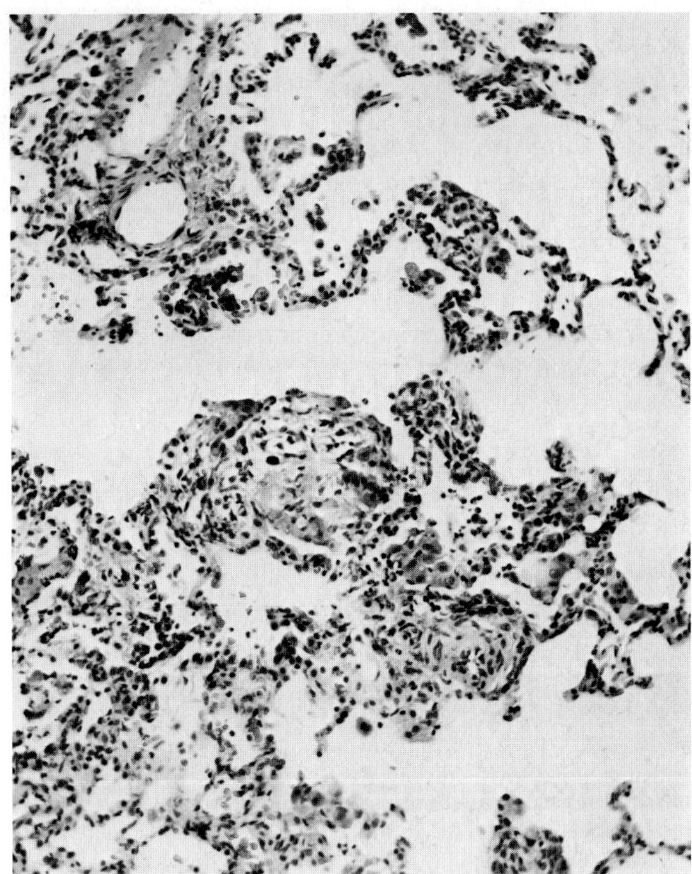

Figure 8 Focal interstitial pneumonitis associated with methotrexate lung disease. In the center of the figure there is a noncaseating epithelioid granuloma situated within the interstitium (H & E X 160).

presence or absence of eosinophilia, fever, or the interval from initiating therapy to the onset of pulmonary disease. Granulomas in the lungs have even been seen in the fatal cases related to intrathecal methotrexate (Gutin et al. 1976, Lascari et al. 1977).

To add to the confusion, Sybert and Butler (1978) reported a patient who developed pulmonary "sarcoidosis" after 1 yr of high-dose methotrexate for osteogenic sarcoma. The asymptomatic pulmonary nodule and hilar adenopathy began after the last dose of methotrexate. They theorize that the immunosuppressive therapy may have inhibited the development of sarcoidosis.

References

Arnett, E. N., Battle, W. E., Russo, J. V., and Roberts, W. C. (1976). Intravenous injection of talc-containing drugs intended for oral use. A cause of pulmonary granulomatosis and pulmonary hypertension. *Am. J. Med.*, **60**:711–718.

Au, F. C., Webber, B., and Rosenberg, S. A. (1978). Pulmonary granulomas induced by BCG. *Cancer,* **41**:2209–2214.

Aungst, C. W., Sokal, J. E., and Jager, B. V. (1975). Complications of BCG vaccination in neoplastic disease. *Ann. Intern. Med.*, **82**:666–669.

Ayvazian, L. F., Steward, D. S., Merkel, C. G., and Frederick, W. W. (1967). Diffuse lipoid pneumonitis successfully treated with prednisone. *Am. J. Med.*, **43**:930–934.

Bedrossian, C. W. M., Miller, W. C., and Luna, M. A. (1979). Methotrexate-induced diffuse interstitial pulmonary fibrosis. *Southern Med. J.*, **72**:313–318.

Bhat, K. S. S., Anderson, K. R., and Stewart, R. D. H. (1974). Lung disease associated with methotrexate therapy. *Aust. N. Z. J. Med.*, **4**:277–280.

Buechner, H. A., and Strug, L. H. (1956). Lipoid granuloma of the lung of exogenous origin. *Dis. Chest.*, **29**:402–415.

Burgher, L. W., Kass, I., and Schenken, J. R. (1974). Pulmonary allergic granulomatosis: A possible drug reaction in a patient receiving cromolyn sodium. *Chest,* **66**:84–86.

Clarysse, A. M., Cathey, W. J., Cartwright, G. E., and Wintrobe, M. M. (1969). Pulmonary disease complicating intermittent therapy with methotrexate. *JAMA,* **209**:1861–1864.

CPC (1977). Lipoid pneumonia due to aspiration of mineral oil. *N. Engl. J. Med.*, **296**:1105–1111.

Douglas, F. G., Kafilmout, K. J., and Patt, N. L. (1971). Foreign particle embolism in drug addicts: Respiratory pathophysiology. *Ann. Intern. Med.*, **75**:865–872.

Elston, C. W. (1966). Pneumonia due to liquid paraffin with chemical analysis. *Arch. Dis. Child.*, **41**:428–434.

Everts, C. S., Westcott, J. L., Bragg, D. G. (1973). Methotrexate therapy and pulmonary disease. *Radiology,* **107**:539–543.

Filip, D. J., Logue, G. L., Harle, T. S., and Farrar, W. H. (1971). Pulmonary and hepatic complications of methotrexate therapy of psoriasis. *JAMA,* **216**:881–882.

Goldman, G. C., and Moschella, S. L. (1971). Severe pneumonitis occurring during methotrexate therapy. *Arch. Dermatol.*, **103**:194–197.

Gormsen, H. (1955). On the occurrence of epitheloid cell granulomas in the organs of BCG-vaccinated human beings. *Acta. Pathol. Microbiol. Scand. (Suppl.),* **111**:117–120.

Grant, R. M., Mackie, R., Cochran, A. J., Murray, E. L., Hoyle, D., and Ross, C. (1974). Results of administering BCG to patients with melanoma. *Lancet,* **2**:1096–1100.

Gutin, P. H., Green, M. R., Bleyer, W. A., Bauer, V. L., Wiernik, P. H., and Walker, M. D. (1976). *Cancer,* **38**:1529–1534.

Hildick-Smith, G. Y. (1976). The biology of talc. *Br. J. Industr. Med.,* **33**:217–229.

Houck, R. J., Bailey, G. L., Daroca, P. J., Jr., Brazda, F., Johnson, F. B., and Klein, R. C. (1980). Pentazocine abuse. Report of a case with pulmonary arterial cellulose granulomas and pulmonary hypertension. *Chest,* **77**:227–230.

Johnston, W. H., and Waisman, J. (1971). Pulmonary corn starch granulomas in drug user. *Arch. Pathol.,* **92**:196–202.

Lascari, A. D., Strano, A. J., Johnson, W. W., and Collins, J. G. P. (1977). Methotrexate-induced sudden fatal pulmonary reaction. *Cancer,* **40**:1393–1397.

Lisbona, A., Schwartz, J., Lachance, C., Frank, H., and Palayew, M. J. (1973). Methotrexate-induced pulmonary disease. *J. Can. Assoc. Radiol.,* **24**:215–220.

Löbel, H., Machtey, I., and Eldror, M. Y. (1972). Pulmonary infiltrates with eosinophilia in an asthmatic patient treated with disodium cromoglycate. *Lancet,* **2**:1032.

Mansell, P. W. A., and Krementz, E. T. (1973). Reactions to BCG. *JAMA,* **226**:1570–1571.

Marschke, G., Haber, L., and Feinberg, M. (1975). Pulmonary talc embolization. *Chest,* **68**:824–826.

Nesbit, M., Krivit, W., Heyn, R., and Sharp, M. (1976). Acute and chronic effects of methotrexate on hepatic, pulmonary skeletal systems. *Cancer (Suppl.),* **37**:1048–1057.

Overland, E. S., Nolan, A. J., and Hopewell, P. C. (1980). Alteration of pulmonary function in intravenous drug abusers. Prevalence, severity, and characterization of gas exchanged abnormalities. *Am. J. Med.,* **68**:231–237.

Paré, J. A. P., Fraser, R. G., Hogg, J. C., Howlett, J. G., and Murphy, S. B. (1979). Pulmonary "mainline" granulomatosis: Talcosis of intravenous methadone abuse. *Medicine,* **58**:229–239.

Rawbone, R. G., Shaw, M. T., Jackson, J. G., and Bagshawe, K. D. (1971). Complication of methotrexate-maintained remission in lymphoblastic leukaemia. *Br. Med. J.,* **4**:467–468.

Repo, U. K., and Nieminen, P. (1976). Pulmonary infiltrates with eosinophilia and urinary symptoms during disodium cromoglycate treatment. A case report. *Scand. J. Respir. Dis.,* **57**:1–4.

Robbins, K. M., Gribetz, I., Strauss, L., Leonidas, J. C., and Sanders, M. (1973). Pneumonitis in acute lymphatic leukemia during methotrexate therapy. *J. Pediatr.,* **82**:84–88.

Robertson, J. H. (1970). Pneumonia and methotrexate. *Br. Med. J.,* **2**:156.

Rosenow, E. C., III. (1980). Chemotherapeutic drug-induced pulmonary disease. *Semin. Respir. Med.,* **2**:89–96.

Salm, R., and Hughes, E. W. (1970). A case of chronic paraffin pneumonitis. *Thorax,* **25**:762–768.

Schapira, D. V., and McPherson, T. A. (1977). Pneumonitis with oral BCG. *N. Engl. J. Med.,* **296**:397 (letter).

Schwartz, I. R., and Kajani, M. D. (1969). Methotrexate therapy and pulmonary disease. *JAMA,* **210**:1924 (letter).

Schwindt, W. D., Barbee, R. A., and Jones, R. J. (1967). Lipoid pneumonia. Its protean nature and clinical resemblance to carcinoma of the lung. *Arch. Surg.,* **95**:652–657.

Settipane, G. A., Klein, D. E., Boyd, G. K., Sturam, J. H., Freye, H. B., and Weltman, J. K. (1979). *JAMA,* **241**:811–813.

Sheffer, A. L., Rocklin, R. E., and Goetzl, E. J. (1975). Immunologic components of hypersensitivity reactions to cromolyn sodium. *N. Engl. J. Med.,* **293**:1220–1224.

Sostman, H. D., Matthay, R. A., Putman, C. E., and Walker Smith, G. J. (1976). Methotrexate-induced pneumonitis. *Medicine,* **55**:371–388.

Sybert, A., and Butler, T. P. (1978). Sarcoidosis following adjuvant high-dose methotrexate therapy for osteosarcoma. *Arch. Intern. Med.,* **138**:488–489.

Unanue, E. R., and Benacerraf, B. (1973). Immunologic events in experimental hypersensitivity granulomas. *Am. J. Pathol.,* **71**:349–359.

Varkey, B., and Kutty, A. V. P. (1976). Lipoid pneumonia with lipoid granulomata in scalene node. *Ann. Intern. Med.,* **84**:176–177.

Wagner, J. C., Adler, D. I., and Fuller, D. N. (1955). Foreign body granulomata of the lungs due to liquid paraffin. *Thorax,* **10**:157–170.

Waller, B. F., Brownlee, W. J., and Roberts, W. C. (1980). Self-induced pulmonary granulomatosis. A consequence of intravenous injection of drugs intended for oral use. *Chest,* **78**:90–94.

Weill, H., Ferrans, V. J., Gay, R. M., and Ziskind, M. M. (1964). Early lipoid pneumonia. Roentgenologic, anatomic, and physiologic characteristics. *Am. J. Med.,* **36**:370–376.

Wheeler, P. S., Stitik, F. P., Hutchins, G. M., Klinefelter, H. F., and
    Siegelman, S. S. (1981). Diagnosis of lipoid pneumonia by
    computerized tomography. *JAMA,* **245**:65–66.
Whitcomb, M. E., Schwartz, M. I., and Tormey, D. C. (1972). Metho-
    trexate pneumonitis: Case report and review of the literature.
    Thorax, **27**:636–639.

C

Calderon, J., 384, *386*
Caldwell, P. R. B., 266, *269*
Calvanico, N. J., 418, *444*
Cameron, G. R., 414, *437*
Campbell, P. B., 159, *196*
Canchola, J., 392, *400*
Cantor, H., 204, *221*, 226, 227, *239*
Carasso, B., 67, *73*
Cardillo, M. E., *262*
Carelli, C., 427, *437*
Carlens, E., 397, *398*
Carliner, N. H., 69, *75*
Carmody, M. G., 453, 454, *467*
Carney, J. F., 221, *221*
Carpenter, R. J., III, 167, *200*
Carr, C., *97*
Carr, D. T., 117, *127*
Carrick, L., Jr., 414, 423, *435, 436, 437*
Carrington, C. B., 81, 85, *94*, 151, 160, 162, 179, 181, 182, 186, *196, 197, 199*, 287, 302, *316*, 464, *466*
Carstairs, L. S., 4, 19, *34, 35*
Carter, J. R., 264, *270*
Cartwright, G. E., 478, *481*
Casalone, G., 105, 110, *128*
Cashner, F. M., 418, *446*
Cassan, S. M., 81, *95*
Castelman, B., 324, *331*
Castillo, R., 410, *439*
Cathey, W. J., 478, *481*
Celikoglu, S. I., 105, 106, 107, 108, 109, 110, 111, 219, *224, 130*, 353, *379*
Centea, A., 105, 106, 107, 108, 109, 110, 111, *127, 130*, 353, *379*
Cerottini, J. C., 214, *221*
Ceuppens, J., 158, 159, *196*
Chakravarty, S. C., *128*
Chalsner, B. A., 297, *319*
Chamberlin, R. I., 457, 458, 465, 466, *467*

Chander, N., 384, *386*
Chandor, S., 160, *200*
Chandrasekhar, S., 409, *446*
Chanock, R. M., 392, *400*
Chapman, J. S., 228, *239*
Chapman, W. E., 193, *199*, 417, *441*
Chaudhary, B. A., 330, *331*
Chaves, A. D., 118, 119, *132*
Chedid, L., 427, 428, 429, *437, 442, 446, 447*
Cheever, A. W., 414, *437*
Chensue, S. W., 404, 412, 415, 416, *437, 448*
Cherniack, N. S., 82, *95*
Chess, L., 214, *221*
Cheung, H. S., 263, 266, *269*
Chiba, Y., 113, *128*, 137, *144*
Childress, W. G., 88, *97*
Choay, J., 428, *437*
Choy, A. R., 330, *333*
Chretien, J., 155, *201*, 249, *259*, 301, 302, *317, 321*
Chuang, M., 82, 83, 90, *96*, 277, 280, *285*, 324, 330, *333*
Chumbley, L. C., 167, 170, *196*
Chun, B. K., 9, 10, *34*, 62, *73*
Chung, A., 266, *271*
Churg, J., 160, 161, 162, 167, 168, 178, *196, 197, 202*
Chusid, E. L., 10, *34*, 151, *197*
Ciorbaru, R., 426, 427, *434, 438*
Claman, H., 404, 418, *445*
Clark, J., 273, 274, 276, *282*
Clark, M., 115, 116, 117, *132*
Clark, T. J. H., 83, 91, *94*
Clarysse, A. M., 478, *481*
Cline, M. J., 463, *466*
Clretien, J., 304, *322*
Coates, E. O., 82, *94*
Cochran, A. J., 475, *482*
Cochrane, C. G., 178, *197*
Cockburn, C., 123, *131*, 141, *145*
Cohen, J., 306, *321*, 328, *332*
Cohen, M. L., 182, *197*
Cohen, S., 158, *202*, 431, *449*

H

Heart involvement in sarcoidosis
(*see* Organ involvement in
sarcoidosis)
Heerfordt's syndrome (*see* Organ
involvement in sarcoidosis)
Hemoptysis, 83
HLA antigens in sarcoidosis, 123,
140–143
Humoral immune responses,
225–227

I

Immune complexes, 159, 230–234,
238
Incidence of sarcoidosis, 102

K

Kidney in sarcoidosis (*see* Organ
involvement in sarcoidosis)
Kveim reaction, 337 (*see also*
Diagnosis of sarcoidosis)
clinical studies, 103, 274, 278
comparison with delayed hypersensitivity, 218
false positive reactions, 275
histological interpretation, 277
test materials, 276
tests in animals, 394–395

L

Laryngeal sarcoidosis (*see* Organ
involvement in sarcoidosis)
Liver involvement in sarcoidosis
(*see* Organ involvement in
sarcoidosis)
Loefgren's syndrome (*see* Acute
sarcoidosis)
Lung volumes, 78
Lupus pernio, 13
Lymphadenopathy, 7, 39, 42 (*see also*
Organ involvement in
sarcoidosis)

Lymphokines, 158–159, 210
Lymphomatoid granulomatosis
clinical presentation, 181
comparisons with other granulomatous diseases, 193–196
extrapulmonary disease, 186
pathology, 182

M

Macrophages, 203
Miliary sarcoidosis (*see* Radiologic
patterns of sarcoidosis)
Mycetoma, 66

N

Necrotizing sarcoidal granulomatosis
clinical presentation, 160
comparison with other granulomatous diseases, 193–196
etiology and immunopathology,
162
pathology, 161
Nervous system in sarcoidosis (*see*
Organ involvement in
sarcoidosis)

O

Organ involvement in sarcoidosis,
33, 139
bone, 18
endobronchial, 9
endocrine
hypothalamus, 30
pituitary, 30
eyes, 21, 341
choroidoretinitis, 22
conjunctivitis, 22
iridocyclitis, 22–23
uveoparotid fever, 22
gastrointestinal tract, 31
genitourinary tract, 31
heart, 69, 343
angina pectoris, 27
arrhythmias, 27